AF791056

WILL MACLEAN
JANE LYTTLETON

CLINICAL HANDBOOK of INTERNAL MEDICINE

The Treatment of Disease with Traditional Chinese Medicine

Volume 2
Spleen and Stomach

UNIVERSITY OF WESTERN SYDNEY

Copyright ©2002 University of Western Sydney

This work is copyright. All rights reserved. Apart from any permitted use under the *Copyright Act 1968*, no part of this publication may be reproduced, stored in a retrieval system, or transmitted in any form or by any means without the prior written permission of the publisher. Requests and inquiries concerning reproduction and rights should be addressed to the Chinese Medicine Unit of the University of Western Sydney.

National Library of Australia Cataloguing-in-Publication data:
Maclean, Will and Lyttleton, Jane
Clinical Handbook of Internal Medicine, Volume 2

Bibliography
Includes Index
ISBN 0-9579720-0-8

1. Internal diseases 2. Medicine, Chinese

Published by
Chinese Medicine Unit
College of Social and Health Sciences
University of Western Sydney
Locked Bag 1797
Penrith South DC
NSW, Australia 1797

Distributed worldwide by Impulse Books (www.impulsebooks.com)

Distributed in Australia by Pangolin Press (pangolinpress@bigpond.com)
P.O. Box 667
Glebe, NSW
Australia 2037

Cover Design: Yolande Gray Design
Photography: Louise Lister
Illustrations: Karen Vance

Contents

ACKNOWLEDGEMENTS

A book of this size and scope is impossible without the help, input and patience of many people. My sincere thanks to all those who were integral to, or involved in some way with, this project. Particular thanks and gratitude are due to my co-author and editor Jane Lyttleton. Without her dedication, incisive criticism and encouragement, this work would have been impossible. Thanks also to David Legge, Dr. Nyrie Dodd, Dr. Trevor Morris, Kathryn Taylor, Margaret Bruce, Karen Vance, Yolande Gray, Ben Maclean, and especially Bill Maclean.

All care has been taken to ensure accuracy and efficacy of the material presented. Any omissions or errors are wholly my own.

W.M

I would like to make grateful acknowledgement to all the above mentioned people, each of whom contributed in a unique and essential way.

Also to Will Maclean who has, with heroic perseverance, translated, sorted and compiled the material that over the last 2-3 years have been analysed, sorted, edited and expounded upon to produce the volume you now hold.

My personal thanks must go to my patient and supportive family, David, Lara and Charlie, who's dinners often got sacrificed in the name of this work, but who never complained. And to my colleagues at Paddington Medical Centre who continue to foster a nurturing and vibrant clinical space where all the theory and practice in these volumes comes to life.

J.L

INTRODUCTION TO THE CLINICAL HANDBOOK SERIES

Traditional Chinese medicine (TCM) is growing in popularity and importance throughout the world, and is now being taught at university level in several countries outside China. The English language literature that has supported this development has, until the last decade or so, been scant and has tended to be Sinocentric, which is natural enough for a medical system that has grown out of and is rooted in the perceptions and culture of the Chinese. However, as TCM has expanded into the Western world, it has had to confront cultural and lifestyle differences that give rise to a different clinical reality, a non Chinese presentation of disharmony. These differences can cause pattern variations that don't appear in the Chinese model, and which require a different type of response. The process that we are now faced with, of taking the essence of the TCM analytical model and making it our own, has occurred in other countries over the centuries. Japan, Korea and Vietnam have developed their own unique styles of acupuncture and herbal medicine, firmly rooted in the ancient Chinese classics, but adapted to suit the cultural and sociological features of their own people.

Similarly, in the West, with our different perceptions of the world and our relationships, diets, environmental and genetic influences, TCM cannot be successfully applied in exactly the same way as it is in China. The lengthy process of accumulation of clinical experience (in the rich light of China's millennia of experience) has only just begun, and our learning curve is steep. This is quite an exciting time to be practising TCM in the Western world, as new ideas and understanding enrich the classical model, and we discover just how far we can go with what is a very powerful and effective medical system.

Aim of the Clinical Handbook series

For the reasons noted above, the way Chinese medicine is practised in the clinics of the Western world is somewhat different to the way it is in China. As practitioners, we are all too aware of the gaps in the English language TCM literature, and the Chinese cultural bias that flavours much of the material available. For this reason, we felt that a clinical reference that at least began to take our cultural and social differences into account was required. Our clinical experience is shaped by the climatic and social environment in which we practise. The collaborators of this handbook series live and work in Sydney, Australia, with a temperate climate, mild winters and hot humid summers, and a predominantly European culture. Australia is an affluent country with a high consumption of fat, sugar, protein and alcohol, and an excess of sedentary behaviour relative to physical exercise. The types of illnesses patients present with in our clinics, and the way these illnesses present, are sometimes quite different to those we observe in China. Practitioners in other parts of the world with different cultural backgrounds and environments will have different experiences and expertise in different types of pathology.

We believe that TCM could take its next developmental step in the West, and the gathering and recording of our accumulated experience is an important part of that process. Because TCM is relatively new to the West, and from a cultural point of view we are still quite inexperienced, we can only get better and more mature in our profession. We have much to learn, so we consider this series to be very much a *work in progress*, and one which will grow as we gather experience as a profession. In future editions of the Clinical Handbook series, we would like to include other pieces of clinical information, such as detailed prognosis, other therapies, patterns that may be more prevalent in some parts of the world and case histories, and to this end contributions from readers are encouraged.

Using this book

The purpose of the Clinical Handbook series is to provide easy access to the clinical information needed to treat a patient. These books are not a substitute for a solid background in the theory of TCM, indeed a good understanding of TCM theory is essential for their efficient clinical use. The main body of the text is the description of 'patterns' of disharmony. In this context, a pattern is defined as a group of signs and symptoms that point to a particular imbalance in the function and/or structure of the body. The patterns described here are not in reality discrete entities (or 'diseases'). Rather, patterns are the framework for modelling the reality of disharmony and organising the information gathered in a clinically useful way.

Furthermore and importantly, the treatment strategies described in this book represent the accumulated experience of generations of physicians who recorded their knowledge in so many classical texts. Those texts have in turn been modernised and modified by contemporary physicians and the treatments adapted for use in the West. The majority of treatments outlined in this book are not the fruits of contemporary research in the form of randomised controlled trials, animal studies or laboratory experiments, but rather the oral and written legacy of Chinese medical masters and the experienced gained from centuries of application and practice.

STRUCTURE OF THE TEXT

Chapters in this volume are named after TCM defined disease symptoms and are presented in alphabetical order. If the patient's clinical picture is uncomplicated then choosing the appropriate chapter for reference and finding the correct treatment is straightforward. In chronic problems however, there are often several pathologies coexisting. For example, there will often be some overlap with the TCM defined disease symptoms of abdominal distension, abdominal pain, Intestinal abscess, constipation and diarrhoea. The determining factor for selection of the appropriate TCM disease is the dominance of the symptom. The patient may list abdominal pain as the primary complaint. If not, the interrogation skills of the practitioner and a degree of clinical experience and clear judgement are required to decide the best starting point for analysis.

Aetiology

At the beginning of each chapter a brief account is given of the aetiological factors pertaining to the patterns therein. These accounts serve as quick summaries of the relevant TCM theory and highlight the most common causes. The same aetiological factors (e.g. diet, emotion, Spleen deficiency, etc.) crop up in many or most of the chapters which necessarily brings with it some repetition. Most practitioners will use this volume as a reference manual, dipping into different chapters as clinical enquiries arise. However we ask the understanding and patience of the student or teacher who decides to study the book from beginning to end and inevitably encounters the same descriptions of aetiological theory in many chapters.

Pathophysiology

The pathophysiology section describes the mechanism producing the principal disease symptom. It also contains some information about the variability of certain patterns and interesting or unique aetiological features.

Clinical features

The clinical features are collections of signs and symptoms that define a particular pattern of disharmony. Much of the material in this book has been derived from original sources, although we have attempted where possible to introduce aspects of our experience. Some patterns described in the text are not found in Chinese texts, but have been observed and treated with sufficient frequency in clinics here to warrant inclusion. Some of the patterns described are uncommon or only dealt with in hospital, so we have little or no experience with them.

Treatment principles

Defining the pattern of disharmony is the final step before selection of a principle of treatment and a prescription to treat the disorder. Treatment principles follow directly from the diagnosis and describe a set of treatment priorities depending on the nature of a disorder and its complications, and serve to focus the treatment strategy. Thus, for example, the principle that follows the diagnosis of Spleen *qi* deficiency with a degree of Dampness is to 'Supplement Spleen *qi* and transform Dampness. The main principle is to supplement the Spleen, with transforming Dampness the second priority. The clarity of this statement leads directly to the appropriate solution in the Spleen supplementing category of prescriptions. The selection process (or any modification to the primary prescription) is focused further by the secondary priorities.

A clearly stated hierarchy of treatment principles is an essential prerequisite to accurate prescribing, modification of prescription, point selection, dietary modification and good therapeutic results.

Herbal Prescriptions

The majority of prescriptions given in the text have been modified to focus on the particular disease symptom and pattern variation being treated. As always in Chinese medicine, the application of prescriptions and their modifications should be flexible and varied to meet the precise needs of each individual.

In some cases several prescriptions are offered as possible solutions. These prescriptions will usually have similar therapeutic actions, but take into account variations in the clinical presentation.

The English names of the prescriptions are drawn from two main sources. First, when a widely available powdered form of a prescription is available we have taken the name from Hong Yen-hsu's *Commonly Used Chinese Herbal Formulas*. We have selected these names because many practitioners nowadays use powdered herbal extracts because they are convenient, patient compliance is good and in general powders are manufactured to GMP standards ensuring consistency and quality.

Second, where a prescriptions is not listed by Hsu we have drawn the name from Dan Bensky and Andrew Gamble's *Formulas and Strategies*. Where a formula is not found in either Hsu or Bensky, the translation spirit of *Formulas and Strategies* is retained.

The prescriptions described in the text are derived from numerous Chinese and non-Chinese sources (*see* bibliography), their selection being determined by a combination of consistency between the sources and clinical experience.

See Appendix 3 for details on the practical aspects of decoction preparation, granulated herbs and dosage.

Endangered animals

The prescriptions in this volume do not contain any materials derived from endangered animals. Where endangered animal derivatives were present in the original script, we have substituted or deleted them and noted the variation in the methods section below the prescription. We have taken the liberty of altering the names of a prescription to reflect the change, thus **XI JIAO DI HUANG TANG** (*Rhinoceros Horn and Rehmannia Decoction* 犀角地黄汤) becomes **SHUI NIU JIAO DI HUANG TANG** (*Water Buffalo Horn and Rehmannia Decoction* 水牛角地黄汤). For a list of endangered animals and potential substitutes, see the appendices to Volume 1 of this series.

Modifications

The modifications section gives information about the addition or deletion of herbs to or from the primary prescription so as to tailor the prescription as closely as possible to the individual patient's needs.

Variations and additional prescriptions

This section provides information about variations to the main pattern and its presentation, and lists additional prescriptions appropriate for these variations.

Patent medicines

Information on patent medicines is drawn from the *Clinical Manual of Chinese Herbal Patent Medicines* (Maclean 2001). The English name of any patent medicine may vary from country to country depending on differences between factories and regional licencing regulations. Be aware that patent formulae of the same name may have quite different compositions depending on the company of origin, so it is advisable to check the list of ingredients before use.

We recommend using only those patent medicines produced by factories complying with the principles of Good Manufacturing Practice (GMP). The basic concept of GMP is that quality must be built into each batch of product during all stages of the manufacturing process. It involves quality control and checking at all stages of production, from selection of the herbs and testing for active ingredients, to extraction and binding methods, to packaging and labelling. GMP has become the standard against which all pharmaceutical practices are judged. Patent medicines produced in accord with GMP contain only the ingredients listed on the label, and thus have no contaminants. They are also free of endangered animal parts. The main quality producers are the Lanzhou Foci Pharmaceutical Factory, Beijing Tong Ren Tang Pharmaceutical Factory and Tianjin Drug Manufactory. These factories are registered with the Australian TGA and are judged to be of pharmaceutical grade. For more information see the *Clinical Manual of Chinese Herbal Patent Medicines*.

Acupuncture

The acupuncture points suggested for each pattern are derived from standard works on acupuncture, such as Deadman's *A Manual of Acupuncture* and

Bensky's *Acupuncture: A Comprehensive Text* and are by no means exhaustive. A selection of points is given as a list rather than as a prescription. More points are usually suggested than should actually be used in a single session. It is up to the practitioner to select points according to the normal rules of point selection and the requirements of each individual.

Key to the Symbols following Acupuncture Points

- + denotes a supplementing method (*bu fa* 补法)
- - denotes a reducing method (*xie fa* 泻法)
- absence of a symbol denotes an even method (*ping bu ping xie fa* 平补平泻法)
- ▲ denotes moxa, either stick, warm needle, rice grain or moxa box
- Ω denotes cupping
- ↓ indicates a point should be bled

Clinical notes

Clinical notes are an attempt to relate TCM patterns to possible biomedical diseases, and to give some general indication about management, required treatment length and prognosis.

In attempting to associate a certain pattern with a group of biomedically defined diseases, we are mindful of the traps involved, principally the temptation to equate a pattern and a disease directly. For example, the oral ulcerations associated with Beçhets disease are frequently equated with Heart Fire. This is only partly correct, as patients with ulceration associated with Beçhets disease may present with a number of patterns, including *yin* deficiency, Phlegm, stagnant Heat, *yang* deficiency or a combination, depending on factors like constitution and the patient's *zheng qi* and environment. All of these factors influence the ultimate manifestation and pattern and, therefore, the diagnosis and treatment. There is an increasing trend in the current TCM literature towards differentiating biomedically defined diseases (for example using Beçhets disease rather than mouth ulcers as the 'disease' symptom starting point). This approach can be useful as far as it goes, but ultimately it lacks the flexibility of application of the traditional approach.

Nevertheless, the reality of TCM practice in the West is that patients often arrive at the clinic with a biomedically defined disease name, and although correct TCM diagnosis proceeds in its own fashion, the biomedical diagnosis is often useful in terms of prognosis.

Terminology

In the Clinical Handbook series, we have attempted to make the text as easy to read and accessible as possible, while maintaining accuracy. Terms in common usage are left untranslated–*qi*, *shen*, *yin*, *yang*, *jing*, *jiao*, *san jiao*, *tai yang*, *shao yang* and so on.

Translated technical terms with precise meaning specific to Chinese medicine, such as Blood, Liver, Wind and Damp, are capitalised.

In instances where an English translation captures the meaning accurately, and has been widely adopted elsewhere in the English TCM literature, we have retained that rendering. Examples of this include painful obstruction syndrome for *bi zheng* (痹症), atrophy syndrome for *wei zheng* (痿证), and indeterminate gnawing hunger for *cao za* (嘈杂).

LIMITATIONS OF THE TEXT

Traditional Chinese medicine is a fluid analytical model used to describe the interaction between pathogenic influence and the strength of the patient, and the influence of lifestyle, diet and emotional life on the actual manifestations of any particular disease. Its strengths are to take into account the responses of an individual to the various conditions that produce ill health, and to prescribe a treatment strategy that reflects a closely as possible the individual's needs.

The identification of a pattern or patterns, which is the final step in the diagnostic process, is the weaving together of numerous strands of observation and information. Since these strands include not only information about pathogenic influences but also constitution, emotions, diet and life circumstance, in short, a summary of all the influences to which an individual is subject, a comprehensive and unique picture can be constructed.

In the real world of course, things are often complicated. Patients frequently exhibit signs of multiple patterns, or contradictory signs and symptoms. The art and skill of the practitioner is reflected in his or her ability to weave the information into a meaningful diagnosis. The fact that real life and the pathologies derived from it are usually more complicated than that described in standard text books, creates a problem when presenting a work like this. In order to analyse common patterns, they need to be described discretely, whereas in reality they are not so discrete, and overlap more than the text would suggest. In fact, we find that in gastro-intestinal disorders certain pathologies combine with such frequency as to warrant a special discussion. This is found in Appendix 2, p.912.

INTRODUCTION TO VOLUME 2

Volume 1 of the Clinical Handbook series examined pathologies of the Lung, Kidney, Liver and Heart organ systems. The discussion included disorders of the Gallbladder and Urinary Bladder. Volume 2 completes the analysis of *zang fu* pathologies with the addition of the Spleen and Stomach organ systems. Disorders of the Large and Small Intestines are also found in this volume.

The Spleen and Stomach (*pi wei* 脾胃) are central to the maintenance and continuance of health and life. The Spleen and Stomach are the harvesters of the *qi* that is used on a daily basis for the everyday processes of growth and repair, defence, locomotion, temperature regulation, respiration and reproduction. Every other organ system relies on a steady stream of *qi* derived from the digestion to function correctly, so any disruption to the function of the Spleen and Stomach affects all other organ systems, and thus the whole body.

Within the framework of Traditional Chinese medicine, the Spleen and Stomach (sometimes referred to collectively as the 'middle *jiao*'), incorporates all functional aspects of the gastro-intestinal system. Thus, the Spleen and Stomach includes various functional aspects of the biomedical stomach, small and large intestines, pancreas, liver and gall bladder, and extends as far as transport of nutrients by the circulatory system.

PHYSIOLOGY OF DIGESTION

This aim of this text is practical rather than theoretical and assumes a working knowledge of TCM theory, so the following overview of Spleen and Stomach physiology is brief. For a more detailed discussion of digestive physiology, see Maciocia (1989) or Ellis and Wiseman (1994).

Spleen and Stomach

The Spleen and Stomach are the key organ systems of the digestive process. Digestion begins in the mouth, where food is ground and broken up to prepare it for further transformation in the Stomach. The Stomach receives food and further processes it, preparing it for separation into physiological *qi* (the 'pure' portion) and waste material (the 'turbid' portion). The pure extract is then sent upwards to the Lungs where the final fusion with *da qi* (the *qi* of air) occurs. The result is further refined into the various physiological subtypes of *qi* (*wei qi*, *ying qi*, *zang fu qi* etc.), which are then distributed to the relevant tissues and parts of the body by the Spleen. This process is described in Chinese as *yun hua* 运化, usually translated as 'transformation and transportation', or 'digestion and distribution'.

Liver and Gallbladder

The Liver has a significant influence over the function of digestion and harmonious activity of the Spleen and Stomach. The relationship between the Liver, and the Spleen and Stomach is one of the fundamental axes regulating the supply and movement of *qi*. According to the relationships described by the five phases (*wu xing* 五行), impediment to the movement of Liver *qi* quickly and inevitably affects the Spleen and Stomach. This can occur in three ways, through the generating cycle (*sheng* 生), the controlling cycle (*ke* 克) or a combination of both. When Liver *qi* is sufficiently constrained, it will not flow on through the generating cycle to the organ systems downstream, thus depriving them of *qi*. Similarly, the pent up *qi* will seek alternative pathways, the most common being the controlling cycle. The release of the pent up (and thus pathological) *qi* through the controlling cycle leads to an uneven distribution of *qi* in the Spleen and Stomach, and injury to their normal functioning.

The Gallbladder's role is to store and release the 'pure fluid' bile to assist in digestion. It plays a secondary role in the digestive process, subsidiary to the Liver. Gallbladder pathology in a TCM sense appears more often in the Liver section of Volume 1.

Intestines

The Small and Large Intestines are energetically aligned with the Heart and Lungs. In terms of gastro-intestinal function however, the Intestines are more closely aligned with the Stomach, and the natural downward flow of Stomach *qi*. In TCM there is little distinction made between the Small and Large Intestines in terms of gastro-intestinal function and pathology. As *fu* organs, their major function is to drain and eliminate the waste by-products of digestion (the 'turbid'). The Intestines also play an important role in assisting the Spleen in regulating fluid metabolism and distribution.

The close relationship of the Intestines and the Spleen and Stomach as a functional unit can be seen in descriptions of the pathology of the Intestines. Intestinal pathology is often implicit within the context of Spleen and or Stomach pathology (for example, Spleen *yang* deficiency usually involves a functional weakness or laxity of the Intestines as well; Stomach *yin* deficiency will often involve dryness in the Intestines). Intestinal pathology may also be discrete however, and not necessarily involve the Spleen and Stomach. This usually occurs when a pathogen has invaded directly, or accumulated in the Intestines.

THE FUNDAMENTAL RELATIONSHIPS

Normal functioning of the digestive process and gastro-intestinal system is especially dependent on two dynamic relationships, the *qi* mechanism and the Liver and Spleen/Stomach relationship. Many of the treatments in this text are aimed at restoring one or both of these relationships to harmony.

1. The Qi mechanism

The *qi* mechanism (*qi ji* 气机) is one of the fundamental axes of normal physiological function in the body. Essentially, it is the dynamic created by the natural tendency of Spleen *qi* to rise ('the raising of the pure'), and Stomach *qi* to descend ('descent of the turbid'). The correct movement of Spleen and Stomach *qi* thus acts as the dynamo, or pivot, of ascending and descending throughout the body, and the *qi* mechanism facilitates the general movement and distribution of *qi* throughout the body.

Pathology of the *qi* mechanism

Disruption to the *qi* mechanism features prominently in many gastro-intestinal problems. Nausea and vomiting are associated with blockage to, and consequent rising of, Stomach *qi*; abdominal distension occurs when *qi* fails to descend and accumulates in the middle *jiao*. Constipation often reflects a failure of the descent of Stomach *qi*.

Obstruction of the *qi* mechanism (or *qi* blockage) is an obstruction to the correct movement of *qi* through the middle *jiao* and can be associated with either an excess pattern, a deficient pattern, or both.

Excess type

The excess type of *qi* blockage is usually related to Liver *qi* stagnation and its obstructing action on the movement of Spleen and Stomach *qi*. Pathogenic accumulations, such as Dampness, Phlegm or stagnant food can also obstruct *qi* and disrupt the *qi* mechanism.

A less common type of *qi* blockage is that associated with obstruction of Lung *qi*. Lung *qi* is spread to the surface and should descend. When this process is blocked by a pathogen, the subsequent accumulation of *qi* in the Lungs has a disruptive effect on the ascent of Spleen *qi*. The result is disruption of the *qi* mechanism, the natural movement of *qi*, and consequent accumulation of *qi* in the middle *jiao*. This situation may occur in patients with acute Wind invasions, residual or incompletely cleared pathogens, or patients with chronic respiratory disorders.

Deficiency type

The deficient type of *qi* mechanism dysfunction is due to a weakness of middle *jiao qi*, that is, there is insufficient motive force behind the rising of Spleen *qi*, or the descent of Stomach *qi*. Deficient type *qi* blockage will often be further complicated by excess accumulation. The obstruction in this case occurs because the *qi* is too feeble to move adequately, or the weakened

Spleen/Stomach invite the attention and overcontrol of Liver *qi*, or because they are too weak to process food adequately so that food or Dampness and Phlegm accumulate.

2. The Liver and Spleen/Stomach

The relationship between the Liver and Spleen/Stomach system is important in the maintenance of healthy digestion and correct functioning of the *qi* mechanism. The Liver restrains the Spleen/Stomach through the controlling (*ke* 克) cycle, and governs smooth distribution of *qi* to the Spleen/Stomach when demand increases during digestion. The relationship is easily disturbed however, as the Liver is prone to be overbearing, especially when there is any weakness in the Spleen. When Liver *qi* is constrained or obstructed it will seek alternate pathways, most commonly horizontal rebellion through the *ke* cycle, described as overcontrolling. This has the effect of injuring the Spleen and Stomach and disrupting the *qi* mechanism.

TREATMENT OF SPLEEN AND STOMACH DISORDERS

Treatment strategies for gastro-intestinal problems usually need to be multifaceted, incorporating diet, lifestyle management and active relaxation methods in addition to the basis therapies of acupuncture and herbal medicine.

Diet

Modification and manipulation of the diet plays a major role in rectification of many disorders. This is especially so in the case of gastro-intestinal disorders. Analysis and modification of the diet, when appropriate, is always the first line of therapy. See chapter 26 for more detail.

Herbal medicines

This text describes the use of many herbal prescriptions and patent formulae for gastro-intestinal disorders. Traditionally herbal medicine has been the primary modality for internal or organ system disorders. The addition of herbs to any treatment programme is secondary to appropriate modification of the diet.

Acupuncture

Acupuncture is of excellent value in many gastro-intestinal disorders, especially those featuring pain or obstruction of the *qi*. Where there is damage to tissues or organs, acupuncture should be combined with herbal therapy. Long courses of acupuncture therapy are able to alter the habitual response patterns of some patients, promoting a type of 'physiological retraining'.

Exercise

Exercise is fundamental to the health of the Spleen and Stomach, indeed one of the main factors contributing to weakness of the Spleen is 'excessive sitting'. Walking for 30 minutes a day is sufficient to keep the *qi* circulating for many people. Keep in mind that although some exercise is beneficial, it does not always follow that a large amount is better. Over work or excessive training places undue strain on the Spleen and has the potential to weaken function as surely as no exercise. Vigorous exercise in small regular doses can be useful in helping to disperse pent up or stagnant Liver *qi* and release an obstructed *qi* mechanism. Similarly, some forms of yoga and *qi gong* can be effective in facilitating *qi* movement in the Liver and through the *san jiao*.

Relaxation, meditation

Some type of relaxation technique or meditation practice is a useful adjunct to the treatment of gastro-intestinal complaints, especially those with a component of Liver *qi* stagnation. A practical method that can be used to short circuit the usual responses to stressful or emotional triggers, that is to calm and regulate the Liver and stimulate the *qi* mechanism, is useful. This may be something as simple as focused breathing or *qi gong* exercises, or guided relaxation. Persistent practice of a relaxation or meditation technique will, over time, begin to alter the way an individual responds to their environment, and alleviate many *qi* stagnation related complaints.

Abdominal massage

Abdominal massage encourages movement of Intestinal *qi* and stimulates peristalsis. It is especially effective in releasing the *qi* mechanism and facilitating the descent of Stomach and Intestinal *qi* for the alleviation of constipation and abdominal distension.

Retention enema

Retention enemas are useful for pathology of the Large Intestine, and in cases where a patient is unable or unwilling to ingest medicine orally. Although a seemingly unpleasant task, enemas are in fact easy and convenient to perform. Herbs are boiled in the usual fashion (or powdered herbs dissolved) and a suitable amount (usually 100-200mls) inserted into the rectum using a commercial enema device. The patient lies on the back or left side, with the liquid in place for 30-60 minutes. The urge to defecate may occur but subsides quite quickly. The advantages are direct contact with the intestinal wall, no destruction of sensitive ingredients by gastric acids and a large surface area for absorption.

COURSE OF TREATMENT

In our experience, the length of treatment is critical and often underestimated. New graduates often seem to expect resolution of complex and chronic conditions in unrealistically short times. The difference between success and failure is sometimes simply a question of perseverance. Most of the patients we see in Western clinics have chronic problems. They are frequently medicated with pharmaceuticals which may alter their responses to TCM treatment. There is a tendency for inexperienced practitioners to chop and change prescriptions if results are not forthcoming in one or two weeks. This is wrong. When there is a reasonable degree of confidence in the diagnosis and guiding prescription, the basic strategy should be maintained for at least six weeks before making large changes. This is especially true when there are structural changes like Blood stagnation or Phlegm masses. The rule of thumb for the length of treatment in general is that for every year a symptom has been present, one month of treatment is required.

1. Abdominal Distension

Excess patterns

Food stagnation
Phlegm Damp
Liver *qi* stagnation
Accumulation of Lung *qi*
Damp Heat

Deficient patterns

Spleen and Stomach *qi* deficiency
Spleen and Stomach *yang* deficiency
Stomach (Spleen) *yin* deficiency

1 ABDOMINAL DISTENSION

fu zhang 腹胀, (*pi man* 痞满)

Fu zhang refers to a sense of fullness, discomfort, blockage or obstruction across the either the upper or lower abdomen, or across the abdomen as a whole. *Pi man* is distension specifically in the epigastric area. For practical purposes, however, *fu zhang* and *pi man* can be dealt with as a single TCM defined disease symptom, hencefore abdominal distension, because the pathology and treatment strategies are generally the same.

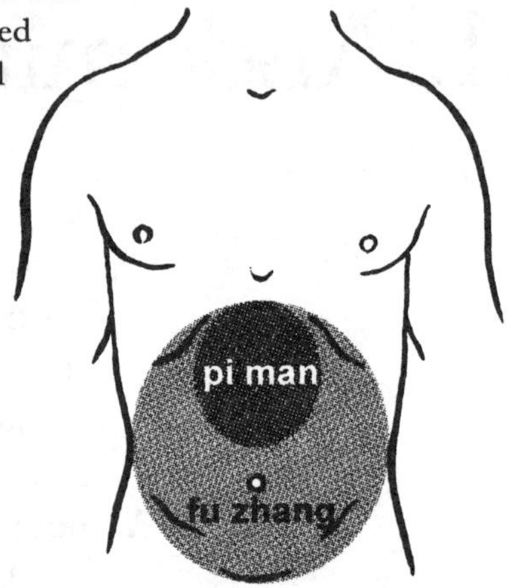

Figure 1.1 *Fu Zhang and Pi Man*

The complaint of distension, often described as 'bloating', 'fullness' or 'discomfort', usually refers to a subjective feeling of fullness or pressure within the abdomen. It may or may not be associated with visible swelling of the abdomen. In practice, abdominal distension can be difficult to localise to a specific area, and will frequently be felt in different places at different times. When the disease diagnosis is abdominal distension, the distension is generally not associated with pain.

Distension may be acute or chronic. When acute it is usually due to dietary indiscretion, or is part of an external invasion. Patients with chronic patterns are the ones most likely to present in clinic, and this chapter focuses on these, often difficult, prolonged patterns.

As a general rule, abdominal distension is due to an obstruction to the correct movement of Spleen and Stomach *qi*. The obstruction itself may be due to the presence of some pathogen, internal or external, or due to weakness or stagnation of *qi*.

In TCM terms, there are four main mechanisms that can produce abdominal distension, each of which can occur separately or in combination. These are–

- obstruction of the *qi* mechanism (*see* Introduction, p.xix)
- fluid retention
- constipation
- pathogenic accumulation (usually Phlegm and/or Dampness)

In practice, these mechanisms are often intermingled, and become mutually engendering. For example, if the *qi* mechanism is obstructed by a pathogen (say Damp or stagnant food from the diet), this can eventually weaken the Spleen, which then fails to regulate and distribute fluids adequately. These now pathogenic fluids accumulate in the tissues of the abdominal wall and Intestines, aggravating the distension. Similarly, obstruction of the *qi* mechanism is often complicated by constipation, as Stomach *qi* fails to descend and aid the passage of stool. With a constipated stool, *qi* backs up through the digestive tract, further obstructing *qi* movement and disabling the *qi* mechanism.

BOX 1.1 SOME BIOMEDICAL CAUSES OF ABDOMINAL DISTENSION

- chronic gastritis
- functional and motility disorders
  - gastroparesis
  - intestinal pseudo-obstruction
  - visceral neuropathies and myopathies
- irritable bowel syndrome
- chronic peptic ulcer disease
- chronic colitis
- hiatus hernia
- eating disorders
- premenstrual syndrome
- hormone replacement therapy, oral contraceptive pill
- hepatitis
- hepatic cirrhosis
- chronic pancreatitis
- gall stones
- mesenteric artery insufficiency
- carcinoma - gastric, pancreatic, colonic
- anxiety, depression

AETIOLOGY

Diet, Food stagnation

Food stagnation is a common component of abdominal distension. Eating more food than the Spleen and Stomach can cope with, either because too much is consumed, or because the Spleen is already weak, will obstruct the *qi* mechanism and thus the descent and ascent of middle *jiao qi*. Once the *qi* mechanism is obstructed by unprocessed food, various complications can arise to further aggravate the distension. One of the most common complications is constipation. Thus disruption of the *qi* mechanism, food stagnation and constipation form a common clinical picture.

Overeating, eating irregularly or at odd hours, especially late at night, weakens Spleen and Stomach *qi* and leads to food stagnation. Too much cold natured or raw food weakens Spleen *qi* and *yang*. Overconsumption in general and excessive consumption of rich, heating and supplementing foods in particular, can lead to the accumulation of food and Damp Heat in the Intestines.

Food stagnation is a common precursor to a large number of other pathologies and is a common aetiological factor in the development of many of the diseases that occur in modern life. In traditional TCM texts food stagnation as a cause of disease has been underrated because overeating or a rich diet was not common among the Chinese people. However, in developed countries in modern times, food stagnation is more common and more insidious. Patients can become conditioned to ignoring, or may not even be conscious of, the typical symptoms of bloating, belching, bad breath, and flatulence. The eating patterns that give rise to such symptoms may be so ingrained that individuals cease to be aware of them, or the symptoms experienced are considered to be normal.

By habitually overloading the Spleen and Stomach and exceeding their capacities to process the food ingested, a cycle is begun that can have profound ramifications. Firstly, instead of being sent through the Intestines, the food lingers longer than it should, fermenting and rotting. The stagnation in the digestive tract may produce Heat which can intensify this process of putrefaction. The Spleen and Stomach are weakened, further inhibiting their abilities to perform their digestive tasks efficiently. The weakened Spleen produces Damp which in turn may be congealed into Phlegm by the Heat. The Phlegm or Phlegm Heat so produced can then affect other systems, for example the cardiovascular system (Phlegm stagnation in the chest causing chest pain), neurological system (some types of tremors, anxiety states, insomnia, vertigo, paralysis) and skin (cysts, various ulcerations, chronic sores and swellings). In addition, chronic Heat or Damp Heat can injure Intestinal *yin* and the Intestinal lining, compromising the circulation of *qi* and Blood. Phlegm accumulation may eventually evolve into Blood stagnation, causing polyps, nodules and tumours.

Emotion

Liver *qi* stagnation is a common component of recurrent abdominal distension. It impacts on the abdomen in numerous ways. Liver *qi* can invade the Spleen and Stomach and disrupt the *qi* mechanism. It can impair the Spleen's ability to process fluids, resulting in fluid accumulation in the abdominal wall and Intestines, or in development of Dampness and Phlegm from the retardation of fluid movement. *Qi* stagnation can slow the passage of food through the Intestine, causing constipation and distension.

Prolonged or severe Liver *qi* stagnation can also generate stagnant Heat, which can then combine with any Dampness present to form Damp Heat, or can injure fluids and *yin*.

Liver *qi* stagnation is caused by repressed emotion, frustration, anger and resentment. These emotions, especially when chronically unexpressed, cause a low grade spasm and tension in the smooth muscle of the gut. Patients with chronic *qi* stagnation type digestive problems will often note that their stress and tension is stored in the gut and be aware of the consequences of stress–the knot in the stomach, stomach cramps, loss of appetite and bowel disturbances. Liver *qi* stagnation type distension tends to be intermittent and is clearly related to the emotional state and stress levels of the patient.

BOX 1.2 KEY DIAGNOSTIC POINTS

- with constipation or sluggish bowels - excess, blockage to the *qi* mechanism
- abdominal distension or discomfort worse for pressure - excess
- worse for eating - excess
- worse when tired or at the end of the day and evening - deficiency
- alleviated by belching, passing gas or defecation - food stagnation, blockage to the *qi* mechanism
- distension with an emotional component - Liver *qi* stagnation
- associated with an upper respiratory tract disorder - accumulation of Lung *qi*
- worse in the afternoon - Damp Heat
- associated with belching, flatulence or constipation - blockage to the *qi* mechanism
- associated with quick fluctuations in weight, puffy eyes and fingers, scanty urination - pathogenic fluid accumulation, Spleen deficiency

In addition to the emotional factors that upset the Liver, worry, obsessive thinking and prolonged concentration, in combination with a sedentary lifestyle and poor diet, will weaken Spleen *qi*, predisposing it to (or inviting) invasion by Liver *qi*. This may result in further damage as well as disruption to the *qi* mechanism. Spleen *qi* naturally ascends creating the appropriate equilibrium for the descent of turbid waste materials, so it is said the Spleen governs 'the raising of the clear and descent of the turbid'. If this activity fails, the *qi* and 'clear and turbid' (turbid here implying Dampness as well as waste materials) intermingle and accumulate, causing a feeling of fullness and distension.

Dysfunction of the Lungs can also contribute to abdominal distension. Bereavement, social isolation, unresolved issues of loss or abandonment and sudden changes of familiar routine are all factors which can cause Lung *qi* to knot up and accumulate. Because the Lung system incorporates the Large Intestine, *qi* accumulation and constipation can result.

If Lung *qi* has been weakened through illness or lack of exercies, a similar situation may arise. Weak Lung *qi* may not descend because it is too feeble to do so. When the Lungs are involved in the genesis of distension, there is often a postural component as well. Lung disorders frequently cause patients to hunch forward, slouching over and rolling their shoulders internally. This further restricts the free movement of Lung *qi* and compounds the accumulation.

Spleen and Stomach deficiency

Spleen and Stomach weakness is at the root of many cases of abdominal distension, and can contribute to all patterns. In simple cases, the Spleen is weak and unable to process food adequately; *gu qi* is not sent to the Lungs and accumulates in the middle *jiao* causing distension. Similarly Stomach *qi* may fail to descend, compounding the distension and contributing to constipation. This is a deficiency type of *qi* mechanism blockage.

Other aspects of Spleen and Stomach weakness may complicate the basic pattern. When the Spleen fails to move and metabolise fluids, the fluids may accumulate in and around the tissues of the abdominal wall or Intestines. Fluid accumulation is a common cause of generalised abdominal distension. In contrast to the *qi* blockage type of distension, fluid retention is more widespread and not focused in a specific region (such as the epigastrium). On it own, fluid accumulation tends to lack the typical gastro-intestinal clues that characterise *qi* blockage, such as frequent belching, flatulence or constipation. Fluid accumulation type distension also tends to be more prolonged and harder to shift than *qi* blockage. It seems to affect females more frequently than males.

A weakened Spleen may generate Dampness and Phlegm. Dampness and Phlegm are especially good at creating obstruction, and, once present, easily block the *qi* mechanism, aggravating the condition.

A weak Spleen can also 'invite' the unwanted attentions of a normal Liver, causing *qi* stagnation and further disrupting the *qi* mechanism.

Spleen *qi* and *yang* are weakened by excessive consumption of cold raw food and irregular eating habits, or by too many cold natured herbs or antibiotics in the treatment of a febrile or other hot disease. Additional factors are lack of physical activity, prolonged or serious illness, and prolonged starvation or digestive insult, as occurs in patients with a history of anorexia nervosa or bulimia.

Pathogens

Various pathogens, both internal and external, can contribute to patterns which include abdominal distension. External invasion of Wind (plus Cold, or less commonly, Heat) can obstruct the natural descent of Lung *qi* causing disruption to the *qi* mechanism. What this means is that when Lung *qi* is obstructed and prevented from descending naturally, this influences the natural ascent of Spleen *qi*. *Qi* begins to accumulate in the middle *jiao* and this is experienced as distension.

External Damp Heat can invade the Spleen and Stomach, indeed Damp has a preference forlodging the gastro-intestinal system. Once in the body it often accumulates in the middle *jiao* blocking the *qi* mechanism.

Internally generated Dampness, Phlegm or Damp Heat may be the product of *qi* blockage applied to physiological fluids, congealing them over time. Dampness caused by ingestion of an excess of dietary Damp inducing agents, or Spleen weakness that creates Damp, may block the normal movement of middle *jiao qi*.

Constipation

Constipation is a common contributing factor in abdominal distension, both generally over the abdomen as a whole, and specifically, over the site of the constipated stool. Constipation itself can be related to *qi* obstruction–if *qi* is not descending there is no impetus behind the stool to move it forward and out; similarly if the stool isn't moving, *qi* will back up behind the obstruction.

TCM DIFFERENTIAL DIAGNOSIS

- ***Gu Zhang*** (臌张, ascites, or drum like abdominal distension, *see* Volume 1): *Gu zhang* or ascites, is characterised by fluid accumulation in the abdominal cavity, with a decrease in urinary output. The abdomen may be quite distended, however the presence of fluid distinguishes ascites from simple abdominal distension. *Gu zhang* is a sign of serious disease, and occurs in such conditions as hepatic cirrhosis, congestive cardiac failure, abdominal and liver cancer, schistosomiasis, chronic malaria and tuberculous peritonitis. The name *gu zhang* (literally drum distension) derives from the resemblance of the abdomen to a drum–firm and taut on the outside and empty within–the emptiness here referring to deficiency of the various *zang fu* involved.
- ***Jie Xiong*** (结胸): *Jie xiong* describes a syndrome of the lower thorax and epigastrium characterised by focal pain, fullness and rigidity. The pain is usually the major feature. *Jie Xiong* may be associated with biomedical disorders such as pleurisy, intercostal neuralgia and peptic ulcer disease.
- ***Xiong Bi*** (胸痹): *Xiong* or chest *bi* syndrome is a feeling of fullness, stuffiness and pain in the chest, often associated with diseases of the Heart and/or Lungs.

TREATMENT

Treatment involves determining precisely which mechanism (or combination of mechanisms) is at play. When the *qi* mechanism is disrupted, the correct ascent and descent of *qi* must be promoted, in addition to dealing with the underlying pathology. When fluid retention is contributing to the distension, a diuretic method is employed. When constipation is an issue, a laxative, purgative or *qi* regulating method is used depending on the type and pathology.

Regulation of diet, the types of food ingested and the way food is eaten, is essential, as all other treatments will be less than completely successful if this fundamental component of gastro-intestinal health is neglected.

Exercise is important in the excess patterns, especially when Liver *qi* stagnation or *qi* accumulation is involved. Exercise moves *qi* and strengthens Spleen and Lung function. Sustained walking and deep breathing is often sufficient, at least temporarily, to move *qi*.

1.1 FOOD STAGNATION

饮食积滞

Pathophysiology

- Food stagnation is a common cause of both acute and chronic abdominal distension, and an important aetiological feature of a variety of chronic disorders (see aetiology). It is caused by an excess of food or indigestible food that overwhelms the digestive and distribution capacity of the Spleen and Stomach. Food sits in the gut for too long and, like compost, rots. The site of the stagnation, and thus distension, is usually the upper gastrointestinal tract. The accumulated food blocks the descent of Stomach *qi,* so distension and constipation are the main features. Food stagnation can be the result of simple overeating in robust patients, or can occur in those with Spleen deficiency even when they eat normal or small amounts of food, as the capacity of the Spleen to process what is ingested is quickly overwhelmed.
- Chronic food stagnation can be complicated by Spleen deficiency, Damp Heat, Phlegm or Phlegm Heat.

Clinical features

- Upper abdominal and epigastric distension and/or discomfort, which are relieved following belching or passing gas and are worse for overeating (or eating certain poorly tolerated foods). Distension and discomfort are worse for pressure.
- constipation, difficult or irregular stools, or occasional diarrhoea
- foul belching, halitosis
- acid reflux, heartburn
- nausea or vomiting
- foul flatulence

T thick white or yellow greasy coat
P wiry and slippery or slippery and rapid

Treatment principle

Relieve food stagnation and harmonise the Stomach

Prescription

BAO HE WAN 保和丸
(*Citrus and Crategus Formula*)

This prescription is best for relatively mild food stagnation, with mild levels of deficiency, Damp or Heat accumulation.

chao shan zha (dry fried Fructus Crataegi) 炒山楂 18-24g
chao shen qu (dry fried Massa Fermentata) 炒神曲 12-15g

chao lai fu zi (dry fried Semen Raphani Sativi)
炒莱服子 9-12g
ban xia (Rhizoma Pinelliae Ternatae) 半夏 9-12g
fu ling (Sclerotium Poriae Cocos) 茯苓 12-15g
chen pi (Pericarpium Citri Reticulatae) 陈皮 6-9g
lian qiao (Fructus Forsythia Suspensae) 连翘 6-9g

Method: Grind herbs to a powder and form into 9-gram pills with water. The dose is one pill 2-3 times daily. May also be decocted with the quantities as shown. **Shan zha, shen qu** and **lai fu zi** improve digestion and alleviate food stagnation; **ban xia** and **chen pi** eliminate Phlegm; **lian qiao** disperses accumulation and clears Heat; **fu ling** strengthens the Spleen. (Source: *Shi Yong Zhong Yi Nei Ke Xue*)

Modifications

- With severe distension and discomfort, add **zhi shi** (Fructus Immaturus Citri Aurantii) 枳实 9-12g and **hou po** (Cortex Magnoliae Officinalis) 厚朴 9-12g.
- With some Heat (irritability, red tongue tip and sides, rapid pulse), add **shan zhi zi** (Fructus Gardeniae Jasminoides) 山栀子 9-12g and **huang lian** (Rhizoma Coptidis) 黄连 3-6g.
- With mild Spleen deficiency, add **bai zhu** (Rhizoma Atractylodes Macrocephalae) 白术 9-12g.
- With constipation or difficult stools, add **da huang** (Radix et Rhizoma Rhei) 大黄 6-9g and **bing lang** (Semen Arecae Catechu) 槟榔 9-12g.
- If the food stagnation is associated with ingestion of excessive meat, double the dose of **shan zha**.
- If the food stagnation is associated with ingestion of starchy foods, such as noodles and grains, double the dose of **lai fu zi**.
- With severe vomiting and nausea, increase the dose of **ban xia** to 15g, and add **sheng jiang** (Rhizoma Zingiberis Officinalis Recens) 生姜 9-12g.

Variations and additional prescriptions

With Damp Heat or Phlegm Heat

- In more severe or chronic cases, Damp Heat or Phlegm Heat may be generated (in much the same way as rotting compost generates Heat). The features are fairly severe epigastric and abdominal distension, abdominal pain that is worse for pressure, constipation or difficult stools, scanty concentrated urine, a red tongue with a greasy yellow coat and a deep strong pulse. The aim of treatment is to guide stagnation downward, clear Heat and dispel Damp with **ZHI SHI DAO ZHI WAN** (*Immature Bitter Orange Pill to Guide out Stagnation* 枳实导滞丸).

da huang (Radix et Rhizoma Rhei) 大黄 30g
zhi shi (Fructus Immaturus Citri Aurantii) 枳实 15g

shen qu (Massa Fermentata) 神曲 15g
huang qin (Radix Scutellariae Baicalensis) 黄芩 9g
huang lian (Rhizoma Coptidis) 黄连 9g
fu ling (Sclerotium Poriae Cocos) 茯苓 9g
bai zhu (Rhizoma Atractylodes Macrocephalae) 白术 9g
ze xie (Rhizoma Alismatis Orientalis) 泽泻 6g

Method: Grind the herbs to powder and form into 9-gram pills with water. The dose is one pill 2-3 times daily. May also be decocted with the **da huang**, reduced to 6-9 grams, added towards the end (*hou xia* 后下). Use this prescription for a few weeks only, then when the Heat is clearing, switch to something less bitter and cold (such as **BAO HE WAN**). **Da huang** purges accumulations and Heat from the Stomach and Intestines; it is assisted in this by **zhi shi** which also regulates *qi* and alleviates epigastric distension; **shen qu** alleviates food stagnation; **huang qin** and **huang lian** clear accumulated Damp Heat; **fu ling** and **ze xie** promote urination to clear Damp Heat; **bai zhu** and **fu ling** strengthen the Spleen, and dry and leach Damp respectively. (Source: *Formulas and Strategies*)

With Spleen deficiency

- When there is significant Spleen and Stomach deficiency, either as a result of chronic food stagnation or preceding it, the treatment is to strengthen the Spleen and Stomach while resolving food stagnation with a prescription such as **JIAN PI WAN** (*Strengthen the Spleen Pill* 健脾丸).

zhi shi (Fructus Immaturus Citri Aurantii) 枳实 90g
dang shen (Radix Codonopsis Pilosulae) 党参 60g
chao bai zhu (dry fried Rhizoma Atractylodes Macrocephalae) 炒白术 60g
chao mai ya (dry fried Fructus Hordei Vulgaris Germinantus) 炒麦芽 30g
chen pi (Pericarpium Citri Reticulatae) 陈皮 30g
shan zha (Fructus Crataegi) 山楂 30g
shen qu (Massa Fermentata) 神曲 30g

Method: Grind the herbs to a fine powder and form into 6-gram pills with water or ginger juice. The dose is 2-3 pills daily. May also be decocted with a 60-90% reduction in quantities. **Dang shen** and **bai zhu** strengthen the Spleen; **bai zhu** dries Damp; **mai ya, shan zha** and **shen qu** improve digestion; **chen pi** and **zhi shi** regulate *qi*; **zhi shi** regulates and directs *qi* downwards. (Source: *Shi Yong Fang Ji Xue*)

Patent medicines

Bao He Wan 保和丸 (Bao He Wan)
Mu Xiang Shun Qi Wan 木香顺气丸 (Mu Xiang Shun Qi Wan)
Zi Sheng Wan 资生丸 (Zi Sheng Wan, Zi Sheng Stomachic Pills)
Jian Pi Wan 健脾丸 (Jian Pi Wan)
- with Spleen deficiency
Shen Qu Cha 神曲茶 (Shen Qu Cha)

Liu He Bao He Wan 六合保和丸 (Bo Wo Yuen Medical Pills)
Xiang Sha Yang Wei Wan 香砂养胃丸 (Xiang Sha Yang Wei Wan, Hsiang Sha Yang Wei Wan)

Acupuncture (select from)

Ren.12 (*zhong wan* -) .... *mu* point of the Stomach, clears Heat and alleviates stagnation
St.25 (*tian shu* -) .... *mu* point of the Large Intestine, regulates Intestinal function
Ren.6 (*qi hai* -) .... regulates *qi* and alleviates distension
St.36 (*zu san li* -) .... *he* sea point of the Stomach, regulates and strengthens the Stomach, directs Stomach *qi* downwards
LI.10 (*shou san li* -) .... benefits digestion and regulates gastro-intestinal function
St.44 (*nei ting* -) .... *rong* spring and Water point of the Stomach, clears Heat from the Stomach and alleviates food stagnation

- with nausea, add PC.6 (*nei guan* -)
- with Spleen deficiency, add Sp.6 (*san yin jiao*)
- with abdominal pain, add Sp.8 (*di ji* -), St.34 (*liang qiu* -) and Sp.4 (*gong sun* -)
- with borborygmus, add Sp.5 (*shang qiu* -)
- with constipation, add St.37 (*shang ju xu* -) and SJ.6 (*zhi gou* -)
- *Ear points*: spleen, stomach, large intestine, small intestine, liver, abdomen

Clinical notes

- This is a disorder of gluttony and dietary irregularity. In isolation it needs no treatment other than a sensible approach to diet and eating habits, however if bad habits persist it can become a more entrenched condition requiring treatment.
- The Chinese and other Asian cultures have long known the benefits of sipping small amounts of certain teas while eating. The action of such teas helps assist digestion, especially of fats, and reduces the risk of food stagnation. European cultures use table wine in much the same way, hence 'a little wine for thy stomach's sake'. Similarly, 'bitters', combinations of bitter herbs and alcohol, are a common accompaniment to food, either as a digestive aid following a meal, or as an aperitive. The bitterness of the herbs assists the descent of Stomach *qi* and dries Damp.

痰湿内阻

1.2 PHLEGM DAMP

Pathophysiology

- Phlegm Damp can be the result of consumption of an excess of Phlegm producing foods, such as dairy products, sweets, rich or greasy foods and alcohol. It can also be the result of poor Spleen function. Phlegm Damp and Spleen deficiency are a common mixed pathology. The difference between this pattern and the Spleen deficiency with Phlegm pattern (Variations and additional prescriptions, p.31) is the relative dominance of the Phlegm Damp here. Once the Phlegm has been cleared, the focus of treatment will often shift to strengthening the Spleen and especially it's function of moving fluids.
- The Phlegm Damp blocks the ascent of Spleen *qi* and the descent of Stomach *qi* ('the raising of the pure and descent of the turbid')–the *qi* mechanism is disrupted. *Qi* and Phlegm accumulate in the middle *jiao* causing distension. When Phlegm Damp is dominant, symptoms are often worse first thing in the morning or after periods of inactivity as the Phlegm tends to settle and congeal when there is no movement.

Clinical features

- relatively severe distension, fullness and discomfort in the epigastrium and abdomen that may be apparent upon waking
- fatigue, lethargy, tiredness (may be worse in the morning), increased desire to sleep, heaviness in the body, heavy tired limbs, foggy-headedness
- poor appetite, loss of taste
- nausea, vomiting, often worse first thing in the morning
- belching, acid reflux
- loose stools
- dizziness, headaches that can be triggered by strong smells
- stifling sensation in the chest
- maybe chronic mucus production from the sinuses and lungs
- greasy skin, musty body odour
- tendency to obesity, pear shape

T thick, greasy, white coat, possible swollen or flabby tongue body
P slippery or wiry or moderate

Treatment principle

Dry Dampness and transform Phlegm
Promote the correct movement of *qi*, harmonise the Stomach

Prescription

PING WEI SAN 平胃散
(*Magnolia and Ginger Formula*) modified

cang zhu (Rhizoma Atractylodis) 苍术 12-15g
hou po (Cortex Magnoliae Officinalis) 厚朴 9-12g
chen pi (Pericarpium Citri Reticulatae) 陈皮 9-12g
zhi gan cao (honey fried Radix Glycyrrhizae Uralensis)
炙甘草 3-6g
ban xia (Rhizoma Pinelliae Ternatae) 半夏 9-12g
fu ling (Sclerotium Poria Cocos) 茯苓 12-15g

Method: Grind the herbs into powder and take 9-grams as a draft in boiled water on an empty stomach. May also be decocted. **Cang zhu** powerfully parches and dries Dampness, thereby freeing the Spleen to function properly; **hou po** regulates *qi*, transforms Dampness and alleviates distension; **ban xia** and **chen pi** transform Phlegm and dry Dampness, regulate middle *jiao qi* and correct the *qi* mechanism; **zhi gan cao** strengthens the Spleen and harmonises the Stomach; **fu ling** strengthens the Spleen and leaches out Dampness. (Source: *Shi Yong Zhong Yi Nei Ke Xue*)

Modifications

- With severe distension, add **zhi shi** (Fructus Immaturus Citri Aurantii) 枳实 9-12g.
- With Cold, add **rou gui** (Cortex Cinnamomi Cassiae) 肉桂 3g and **gan jiang** (Rhizoma Zingiberis Officinalis) 干姜 6-9g.
- With food stagnation and constipation, add **lai fu zi** (Semen Raphani Sativi) 莱服子 9-12g, **da fu pi** (Pericarpium Arecae Catechu) 大腹皮 9-12g and **zhi shi** (Fructus Immaturus Citri Aurantii) 枳实 9-12g.
- With foggy-headedness, add **shi chang pu** (Rhizoma Acori Graminei) 石菖蒲 6-9g and **yuan zhi** (Radix Polygalae Tenuifoliae) 远志 6-9g.
- If the distension is initially unresponsive to treatment, correct the flow of *qi* by stimulating the normal ascent and descent of *qi* by adding herbs that direct the *qi* in a specific direction. Typical combinations include **jie geng** (Radix Platycodi Grandiflori) 桔梗 6-9g (to direct *qi* up) and **xuan fu hua** (Flos Inulae) 旋复花 12-15g (to direct *qi* down), or **jie geng** (Radix Platycodi Grandiflori) 桔梗 6-9g and **zhi shi** (Fructus Immaturus Citri Aurantii) 枳实 9-12g (to direct *qi* down).

Variations and additional prescriptions

Resistant distension with Stomach qi deficiency

- With Stomach *qi* deficiency and Phlegm Damp causing epigastric distension, relentless belching, vomiting and a wiry thready pulse, the aim of treatment is to transform Phlegm and harmonise the Stomach, benefit and redirect *qi* downward with **XUAN FU DAI ZHE TANG** (*Inula and Haematite Decoction* 旋复代赭汤).

xuan fu hua (Flos Inulae) 旋复花 12-15g
dai zhe shi (Haematitum) 代赭石 12-15g
ban xia (Rhizoma Pinelliae Ternatae) 半夏 9-12g
sheng jiang (Rhizoma Zingiberis Officinalis Recens)
生姜 9-12g
dang shen (Radix Codonopsis Pilosulae) 党参 12g
zhi gan cao (honey fried Radix Glycyrrhizae Uralensis)
炙甘草 6g
da zao (Fructus Zizyphi Jujubae) 大枣 4pce

Method: Decoction. **Xuan fu hua** is decocted in a cloth bag (*bao jian* 包煎). **Xuan fu hua** and **dai zhe shi** are the main herbs and are a synergistic pair that forcefully drive down rising Stomach *qi*; **xuan fu hua** also transforms Phlegm; **ban xia** transforms Phlegm, dries Dampness, directs rising Stomach *qi* downwards and stops nausea and vomiting; **sheng jiang** harmonises the Stomach and stops vomiting; **dang shen**, **da zao** and **zhi gan cao** supplement *qi* and strengthen the Spleen. (Source: *Shi Yong Zhong Yi Nei Ke Xue*)

With exterior Wind Cold

- If a patient with a pre-existing tendency to Phlegm and *qi* accumulation is invaded by Wind Cold, the resulting obstruction to the movement of Lung *qi* can in turn constrain the *qi* mechanism of the Spleen and Stomach. This can lead to a mixed pattern with exterior signs (fever and chills with no sweating, floating pulse, occipital headache) and digestive disruption (epigastric distension, belching, loss of appetite). This is usually an acute pattern, but may present as an exacerbation of a pre-existing chronic condition. The aim of treatment is to regulate *qi* and clear the exterior with **XIANG SU SAN** (*Cyperus and Perilla Formula* 香苏散) modified.

zi su ye (Folium Perillae Frutescentis) 紫苏叶 9-12g
xiang fu (Rhizoma Cyperi Rotundi) 香附 9-12g
chen pi (Pericarpium Citri Reticulatae) 陈皮 6-9g
zhi gan cao (honey fried Radix Glycyrrhizae Uralensis)
炙甘草 3-6g
cong bai (Bulbus Allii Fistulosi) 葱白 3pce
dan dou chi (Semen Sojae Preparatum) 淡豆豉 9-12g
zhi shi (Fructus Immaturus Citri Aurantii) 枳实 9-12g
jie geng (Radix Platycodi Grandiflori) 桔梗 6-9g

Method: Decoction. **Zi su ye** dispels Wind Cold and regulates middle *jiao qi*; **xiang fu** regulates *qi* and alleviates *qi* stagnation; **chen pi** transforms Phlegm and dries Dampness, regulates middle *jiao qi* and corrects the *qi* mechanism; **zhi gan cao** strengthens the Spleen and harmonises the Stomach; **cong bai** and **dan dou chi** unblock *yang qi* and gently promote diaphoresis; **zhi shi** and **jie geng** work synergistically to alleviate distension; **zhi shi** regulates and directs *qi* downward, **jie geng** elevates and guides the action of other herbs to the upper body and together they promote the correct movement of *qi* in the middle *jiao* to correct the *qi* mechanism. (Source: *Shi Yong Zhong Yi Nei Ke Xue*)

Shao yang syndrome

- If a pathogen invades the Stomach and lodges at the *shao yang* level this can give rise to distension and a stifling sensation in the epigastrium and hypochondrium, alternating fever and chills, nausea or vomiting, loss of appetite, dizziness, fatigue, temporal headaches and a wiry or slippery pulse. The correct treatment is to harmonise *shao yang* and restore the *qi* mechanism with **CHAI HU ZHI JIE TANG** (*Bupleurum, Bitter Orange, and Platycodon Decoction* 柴胡枳桔汤).

chai hu (Radix Bupleuri) 柴胡 9g
ban xia (Rhizoma Pinelliae Ternatae) 半夏 9g
huang qin (Radix Scutellariae Baicalensis) 黄芩 9g
zhi ke (Fructus Citri Aurantii) 枳壳 9g
chen pi (Pericarpium Citri Reticulatae) 陈皮 9g
lu cha (Folium Camellia Sinensis) 绿茶 9g
sheng jiang (Rhizoma Zingiberis Officinalis Recens) 生姜 6g
jie geng (Radix Platycodi Grandiflori) 桔梗 6g

Method: Decoction. **Chai hu** harmonises and closes off the *shao yang* level to retained pathogens, as well as regulating *qi*; **huang qin** clears Heat from the Liver and Gallbladder and *shao yang*. Together these two herbs are the main synergistic pair for dispersing pathogens from *shao yang*. **Ban xia** and **sheng jiang** harmonise the Stomach; **zhi ke** regulates and directs *qi* downward; **jie geng** elevates and guides the action of other herbs to the upper body. Together they promote the correct movement of *qi* in the middle *jiao* and correct the *qi* mechanism. **Chen pi** and **ban xia** transform Phlegm and dry Dampness, regulate middle *jiao qi* and correct the *qi* mechanism; **lu cha** clears Heat and alleviates headache. (Source: *Shi Yong Zhong Yi Nei Ke Xue*)

Patent medicines

Ping Wei San 平胃散 (Ping Wei San, Tabellae Pingwei)
Er Chen Wan 二陈丸 (Er Chen Wan, Pinellia-Pachyma Compound Pills)
Xiang Sha Yang Wei Wan 香砂养胃丸 (Xiang Sha Yang Wei Wan, Hsiang Sha Yang Wei Wan)
- with *qi* stagnation

Xiao Chai Hu Wan 小柴胡丸 (Xiao Chai Hu Wan)
- combine with one of the above patent formulae for *shao yang* syndrome

Acupuncture (select from)

Ren.12 (*zhong wan* -) .... *mu* point of the Stomach, clears pathogens, directs Stomach *qi* downwards and harmonises the Stomach
St.25 (*tian shu* -) .... *mu* point of the Large Intestine, regulates Intestinal function

Sp.15 (*da heng*) .... strengthens the Spleen and resolves Dampness
Liv.13 (*zhang men*) .... *mu* point of the Spleen, regulates the Liver and Spleen
St.40 (*feng long* -) .... *luo* point of the Stomach, transforms Phlegm and clears Heat and Phlegm from the Stomach
Sp.3 (*tai bai*) .... *yuan*, *shu* stream and Earth point of the Spleen, supplements the Spleen and transforms Dampness
Sp.5 (*shang qiu* -) .... *jing* river point of the Spleen, transforms Dampness

- with Spleen deficiency, add St.36 (*zu san li* -)
- with fluid retention and oedema, add St.28 (*shui dao* -), Sp.9 (*yin ling quan* -) and Sp.6 (*san yin jiao*)
- with sluggish stools or constipation, add SJ.6 (*zhi gou* -), St.37 (*shang ju xu* -) and St.41 (*jie xi* -)
- with Liver *qi* stagnation, add Liv.3 (*tai chong*) and PC.6 (*nei guan*)
- with plum stone throat, add PC.5 (*jian shi* -)
- with foggy-headedness, add GB.20 (*feng chi*) and Bl.62 (*shen mai*)
- with Wind Phlegm, add GB.40 (*qiu xu* -), St.8 (*tou wei*) and St.41 (*jie xi* -)
- with Cold Phlegm, apply moxa cones to Bl.20 (*pi shu* ▲) and Bl.21 (*wei shu* ▲)
- with muscle aches and heaviness, add Sp.21 (*da bao*)
- with somnolence, add Kid.6 (*zhao hai*) and Bl.62 (*shen mai*)
- *Ear points*: spleen, stomach, large intestine, small intestine, liver, abdomen

Clinical notes

- Distension of a Phlegm Damp type may be diagnosed biomedically as acute or chronic gastroenteritis, chronic colitis, food poisoning, functional dyspepsia, irritable bowel syndrome, gastric neurosis or peptic ulcer disease.
- Phlegm disorders generally respond well to correct treatment. Treatment usually needs to be prolonged and accompanied by dietary modification to be successful in the long term.
- For dietary recommendations, see p.880.

肝郁气滞

1.3 LIVER QI STAGNATION

Pathophysiology

- Liver *qi* stagnation causes distension primarily of the *qi* blockage variety. The Liver fails to regulate *qi* and the lack of *qi* movement leads to a disruption of the *qi* mechanism and accumulation of *qi* in the upper abdomen. Because movement of *qi* through the gastro-intestinal system is retarded, *qi* stagnation patterns are often complicated by constipation, as well as fluid retention or Phlegm Damp, through damage to Spleen function.
- This pattern is also described as Liver and Spleen/Stomach disharmony.

Clinical features

- chronic epigastric and abdominal distension, fullness and discomfort, all of which have a clear relationship to the emotional state and stress levels of the patient
- hypochondriac discomfort, ache or tightness, generally worse on the right side
- irritability, moodiness, depression
- belching, frequent sighing, flatulence
- borborygmus, loss of appetite, indigestion
- acid reflux, heartburn
- alternating constipation and diarrhoea

T thin white coat

P wiry

Treatment principle

Soothe the Liver and regulate *qi*

Disperse accumulation and ease distension

Prescription

YUE JU WAN 越鞠丸

(*Escape Restraint Pill*)

This prescription is excellent for mild cases of *qi* stagnation, especially when there is accompanying emotional depression. It is often used unmodified, however it can be easily tailored to focus on specific or dominant features (see modifications).

xiang fu (Rhizoma Cyperi Rotundi) 香附 100g
cang zhu (Rhizoma Atractylodis) 苍术 100g
chuan xiong (Radix Ligustici Chuanxiong) 川芎 100g
shan zhi zi (Fructus Gardeniae Jasminoides) 山栀子 100g
shen qu (Massa Fermentata) 神曲 100g

Method: Grind the herbs to powder and form into 6-gram pills with water. The dose is one pill 2-3 times daily. May also be decocted with a 80-90% reduction in quantities. **Xiang fu** is the main herb and disperses stagnant Liver *qi*; **cang zhu** dries Dampness and Phlegm, and works with **xiang fu** to improve Spleen and Stomach function; **chuan xiong** invigorates *qi* and Blood and reinforces the *qi* moving function of **xiang fu**; **shan zhi zi** clears Heat from all three *jiao*; **shen qu** alleviates food stagnation, aids digestion and harmonises the Stomach. (Source: *Shi Yong Zhong Yi Nei Ke Xue*)

Modifications (applicable to YUE JU WAN).

All quantities 100g unless otherwise stated

- With severe bloating, distension, sluggish bowels and flatulence, add **hou po** (Cortex Magnoliae Officinalis) 厚朴, **bing lang** (Semen Arecae Catechu) 槟榔, **zhi shi** (Fructus Immaturus Citri Aurantii) 枳实 and **qing pi** (Pericarpium Citri Reticulatae Viride) 青皮.
- With fluid retention, add **ze xie** (Rhizoma Alismatis Orientalis) 泽泻, **che qian zi** (Semen Plantaginis) 车前子 and **fu ling** (Sclerotium Poria Cocos) 茯苓.
- With acid reflux, add **huang lian** (Rhizoma Coptidis) 黄连 60g, **wu zhu yu** (Fructus Evodiae Rutaecarpae) 吴茱萸 15g and **chuan lian zi** (Fructus Meliae Toosendan) 川楝子.
- With Liver *qi* stagnation, distending abdominal pain and depression, add **chai hu** (Radix Bupleuri) 柴胡 and **bai shao** (Radix Paeoniae Lactiflora) 白芍.
- With Blood stagnation, add **tao ren** (Semen Persicae) 桃仁 and **hong hua** (Flos Carthami Tinctorii) 红花.
- With Damp accumulation, add **hou po** (Cortex Magnoliae Officinalis) 厚朴 and **fu ling** (Sclerotium Poria Cocos) 茯苓.
- With stagnant Heat or Liver Fire, add **huang lian** (Rhizoma Coptidis) 黄连 60g and **qing dai** (Pulverata Indigo) 青黛 20g.
- With food stagnation, add **shan zha** (Fructus Crataegi) 山楂 and **mai ya** (Fructus Hordei Vulgaris Germinantus) 麦芽 150g.
- With Phlegm, add **ban xia** (Rhizoma Pinelliae Ternatae) 半夏, **dan nan xing** (Pulvis Arisaemae cum Felle Bovis) 胆南星 60g and **gua lou** (Fructus Trichosanthis) 瓜楼.
- With Cold, add **wu zhu yu** (Fructus Evodiae Rutaecarpae) 吴茱萸 60g and **gan jiang** (Rhizoma Zingiberis Officinalis) 干姜 60g.
- To further correct the *qi* mechanism, add **zhi shi** (Fructus Immaturus Citri Aurantii) 枳实 and **jie geng** (Radix Platycodi Grandiflori) 桔梗.

Variations and additional prescriptions

Liver invading the Spleen

- The distension caused by Liver *qi* invading the Spleen will have a clear emotional component. The patient will be uptight and irritable with muscular tension and stiffness in the neck and upper back, cold fingers and toes, tension headaches and hypochondriac aching. The correct treatment is to soften the Liver, move Liver *qi*, and harmonise the Liver and Spleen/Stomach with **CHAI HU SHU GAN SAN** (*Bupleurum and Cyperus Formula* 柴胡疏肝散).

chai hu (Radix Bupleuri) 柴胡 9-12g
cu bai shao (vinegar fried Radix Paeoniae Lactiflora)
醋白芍 12-18g
xiang fu (Rhizoma Cyperi Rotundi) 香附 9-12g
zhi shi (Fructus Immaturus Citri Aurantii) 枳实 9-12g
chuan xiong (Radix Ligustici Chuanxiong) 川芎 6-9g
gan cao (Radix Glycyrrhizae Uralensis) 甘草 3-6g

Method: Decoction, or ground to a fine powder and taken in 9-gram doses as a draft with hot water. **Chai hu** regulates and invigorates Liver *qi* and clears Heat; **cu bai shao** softens the Liver and nourishes *yin* and Blood, thus preventing excessive dispersal of, and damage to, *qi* and Liver *yin* by **chai hu**; **xiang fu** regulates *qi* and disperses stagnant Liver *qi*; **zhi shi** breaks up stagnant *qi*, directs *qi* downwards and alleviates distension, it's descending action neatly balances the ascending nature of **chai hu** thus facilitating the correct functioning of the *qi* mechanism; **chuan xiong** invigorates *qi* and Blood and reinforces the *qi* moving function of **xiang fu**; **gan cao** harmonises the Stomach and strengthens the Spleen, and with **bai shao** eases spasms thereby alleviating cramping pain. (Source: *Shi Yong Zhong Yi Nei Ke Xue*)

With chronic sluggish bowels or constipation

- If *qi* stagnation causes chronic constipation and the constipation is difficult to consistently shift, consider **LIU MO TANG** (*Six Milled-Herb Decoction* 六磨汤). This prescription is useful for sedentary individuals who sit a lot, working in stressful occupations.

chen xiang (Lignum Aquilariae) 沉香 6g
bing lang (Semen Arecae Catechu) 槟榔 9-12g
wu yao (Radix Linderae Strychnifoliae) 乌药 9g
zhi shi (Fructus Immaturus Citri Aurantii) 枳实 6-9g
mu xiang (Radix Aucklandiae Lappae) 木香 9g
da huang (Radix et Rhizoma Rhei) 大黄 6g

Method: Grind the herbs to a fine powder and steep in hot water before use. The dosage varies depending on the individual. Generally a larger dose should be given at first (1-2 teaspoons, 3 times daily, or more) until the bowels move, then the dose is reduced to the minimum required for a smooth evacuation. **Chen xiang** directs *qi* downward and eases *qi* flow; **bing lang** breaks up stagnant *qi* and directs Intestinal *qi* downwards; **wu yao**, **zhi shi** and **mu xiang** regulate *qi* and alleviate distension; **da huang** purges accumulation from the Intestines and opens the bowels. The **da huang** can be gradually withdrawn as the condition improves. (Source: *Shi Yong Zhong Yi Nei Ke Xue*)

With food stagnation and sluggish bowels

- With *qi* and food stagnation (general abdominal distension and discomfort, sour belching, foul flatulence, foul, sluggish or incomplete bowel movements, thick tongue coat), the approach is to regulate *qi* and disperse *qi* accumulation downwards (rather than purging) with **MU XIANG SHUN QI WAN** (*Saussurea Pill to Order the Qi* 木香顺气丸).

xiang fu (Rhizoma Cyperi Rotundi) 香附 12g
wu yao (Radix Linderae Strychnifoliae) 乌药 6g
mu xiang (Radix Aucklandiae Lappae) 木香 6g
zhi ke (Fructus Citri Aurantii) 枳壳 6g
chen pi (Pericarpium Citri Reticulatae) 陈皮 6g
chao shen qu (dry fried Massa Fermentata) 炒神曲 6g
chao shan zha (dry fried Fructus Crataegi) 炒山楂 6g
chao mai ya (dry fried Fructus Hordei Vulgaris Germinatus) 炒麦芽 6g
chao lai fu zi (dry fried Semen Raphani Sativi) 炒莱服子 6g
fu ling (Sclerotium Poria Cocos) 茯苓 6g
bing lang (Semen Arecae Catechu) 槟榔 4.5g
qing pi (Pericarpium Citri Reticulatae Viride) 青皮 4.5g
gan cao (Radix Glycyrrhizae Uralensis) 甘草 4.5g

Method: Grind the herbs to a fine powder and form into 6-gram pills with water. The dose is one pill 2-3 times daily. May also be decocted. **Mu xiang, xiang fu** and **wu yao** regulate *qi* and alleviate distension and pain; **zhi ke, qing pi** and **bing lang** break up stagnant *qi* and direct *qi* downwards; **chen pi** transforms Phlegm, dries Dampness and regulates middle *jiao qi*; **shen qu, shan zha, mai ya** and **lai fu zi** improve digestion and alleviate food stagnation; **fu ling** strengthens the Spleen and leaches out Dampness; **gan cao** harmonises the Stomach. (Source: *Shi Yong Fang Ji Xue*)

Patent medicines

Chai Hu Shu Gan Wan 柴胡疏肝丸 (Chai Hu Shu Gan Wan)
- Liver invading the Spleen/Stomach

Mu Xiang Shun Qi Wan 木香顺气丸 (Mu Xiang Shun Qi Wan)
- with sluggish or incomplete bowel movements

Chen Xiang Hua Qi Wan 沉香化气丸 (Chen Xiang Hua Qi Wan)
- with constipation

Xiao Yao Wan 逍遥丸 (Xiao Yao Wan, Hsiao Yao Wan, Bupleurum Sedative Pills)
- especially good for women

Xiang Sha Yang Wei Wan 香砂养胃丸 (Xiang Sha Yang Wei Wan, Hsiang Sha Yang Wei Wan)
- with Spleen deficiency and Damp

Acupuncture (select from)

Ren.12 (*zhong wan* -) .... *mu* point of the Stomach, clears pathogens, directs Stomach *qi* downwards and and harmonises the Stomach

Liv.13 (*zhang men*) .... *mu* point of the Spleen, regulates the Liver and Spleen

St.25 (*tian shu* -) .... *mu* point of the Large Intestine, regulates Intestinal function

Ren.6 (*qi hai* -) .... regulates *qi* and alleviates distension

PC.6 (*nei guan* -) .... *luo* point of the Pericardium, master point of *yin wei mai*, regulates the middle *jiao*, spreads Liver *qi*

Liv.3 (*tai chong* -) .... together these points regulate Liver *qi*, pacify
GB.34 (*yang ling quan*) the Liver and harmonise the Liver and
Liv.5 (*li gou* -) Stomach

- In most cases, points to calm the *shen* should be added: select one or two points from *yin tang* (M-HN-3), Du.19 (*hou ding*), Du. 24 (*shen ting*)
- with Blood or *yin* deficiency, add Sp.6 (*san yin jiao* +), St.36 (*zu san li* -), Bl.18 (*gan shu* +) and Bl.23 (*shen shu* +)
- with Phlegm or plum stone throat, add PC.5 (*jian shi* -), St.40 (*feng long* -) and Sp.3 (*tai bai*)
- with fat intolerance, pale or pasty stools and right side hypochondriac pain or distension, add GB.24 (*ri yue*), GB.40 (*qiu xu* -) and *dan nang xue* (M-LE-23)
- *Ear points*: liver, spleen, stomach, large intestine, small intestine, abdomen

Clinical notes

- Distension of a *qi* stagnation type may be diagnosed biomedically as chronic gastritis, irritable bowel syndrome, peptic ulcer disease, functional disorder of the stomach, motility disorder, gastro-oesophageal reflux, premenstrual distension, cholecystitis, gall stones or chronic hepatitis.
- Exercise is important in moving *qi*, and regular exercise greatly enhances clinical results. The key feature is not the type or duration of the physical activity, but its regularity. It needs to be built into the daily routine and maintained every day or second day.
- For dietary recommendations, see p.878.

肺气不降

1.4 ACCUMULATION OF LUNG QI, (LUNG AND SPLEEN DEFICIENCY)

Pathophysiology

- Accumulation of Lung *qi* gives rise to abdominal distension by inhibiting the natural function of the *qi* mechanism. Just as blockage or weakness of Spleen or Stomach *qi* can cause *qi* to accumulate in the middle *jiao*, so too can weakness or blockage of Lung *qi*. As Spleen *qi* attempts to rise to the Lungs, it is impeded by the failure of downward and outward movement of Lung *qi*. Similarly, lack of descent by Lung *qi* contributes to poor downward movement of Large Intestine *qi* and consequent backing up of *qi* through the gastro-intestinal system. The result is accumulation of *qi* in the middle *jiao*.
- There are a couple of ways this pattern may present, although the mechanism outlined above is the same in each case. The pattern can be relatively acute, with the distension appearing as a main symptom in an external Wind invasion. Patients usually present with a cold or flu. More common in the clinic is residual abdominal distension following an incompletely cleared Wind invasion, an emotional episode that knots Lung *qi*, or is associated with a chronic respiratory disorder. The patient may present some time after the initial Wind invasion or emotional trauma, when the initiating episode is forgotten or trivialised. The patient may experience abdominal distension with asthma or coughing. The pattern presented below is the more common chronic presentation.

Clinical features

- chronic abdominal distension, maybe focused in the upper abdomen, worse with eating; the distension may be associated with mild or dull abdominal pain
- nausea, belching
- spontaneous sweating, or lack of sweating
- shortness of breath
- weak voice, reluctance to speak, general air of sadness or melancholy
- waxy pale complexion, dry skin
- tendency to loose stools, or dry sluggish stools
- history of respiratory disorders–wheezing, cough, shortness of breath
- rounded or hunched over shoulders

T pale with a thin or thick greasy white coat

P elevated in the right middle position, deep and weak in the right distal position

Treatment principle

Promote the descent and dispersal of Lung *qi* and the ascent of Spleen *qi*

Harmonise the *qi* mechanism, disperse accumulation
Strengthen Spleen and Lung *qi*

Prescription

WU JI SAN 五积散
(*Five Accumulation Powder*) modified

zhi ma huang (honey fried Herba Ephedra) 炙麻黄 6-9g
gui zhi (Ramulus Cinnamomi Cassiae) 桂枝 9-12g
bai shao (Radix Paeoniae Lactiflora) 白芍 12-15g
jie geng (Radix Platycodi Grandiflori) 桔梗 9g
zhi ke (Fructus Citri Aurantii) 枳壳 9g
chen pi (Pericarpium Citri Reticulatae) 陈皮 9g
gan jiang (Rhizoma Zingiberis Officinalis) 干姜 9g
fu ling (Sclerotium Poriae Cocos) 茯苓 15g
cang zhu (Rhizoma Atractylodis) 苍术 9g
hou po (Cortex Magnoliae Officinalis) 厚朴 12g
huang qi (Radix Astragali Membranacei) 生黄芪 18-30g
xing ren (Semen Pruni Armeniacae) 杏仁 9-12g

Method: Decoction. This prescription is quite dispersing, and if the diagnosis is correct, positive results should be fairly swift. It is not suitable for prolonged use in patients with significant underlying deficiency. **Huang qi** strengthens and promotes the distribution and descent of Lung *qi* as well as promoting urination; **zhi ma huang** and **gui zhi** dispel Wind Cold and promote dispersing function of the Lungs; **gui zhi** and **bai shao** harmonise *ying* and *wei qi*, enabling dispersal of pathogens without damage to *yin* fluids; **xing ren** aids descent of Lung *qi* and stops cough; **jie geng** and **zhi ke** work synergistically to alleviate distension–**jie geng** elevates and guides the action of other herbs to the upper body, **zhi ke** regulates and directs *qi* downward; together they promote the correct movement of *qi* in the middle *jiao* and correct the *qi* mechanism; **gan jiang** warms the Spleen and Stomach; **chen pi** transforms Phlegm and dries Dampness, regulates middle *jiao qi* and corrects the *qi* mechanism; **fu ling** strengthens the Spleen and leaches out Damp; **cang zhu** powerfully parches and dries Dampness; **hou po** regulates *qi*, transforms Dampness and alleviates distension. (Source: *Zhong Yi Nei Ke Shou Ce*)

Modifications

- If the patient presents with acute distension and clear signs of a Wind Cold exterior pattern (chills, mild fever, myalgia, cough) substitute **zhi ma huang** with unprocessed **ma huang**, and add **xi xin** (Herba cum Radice Asari) 细辛 3g. *See also* **XIANG SU SAN** (*Cyperus and Perilla Formula* 香苏散, p.14).
- With severe distension, add **bai jie zi** (Semen Sinapsis Albae) 白芥子 6-9g, **su zi** (Fructus Perillae Fructescentis) 苏子 6-9g and **lai fu zi** (Semen Raphani Sativi) 莱服子 6-9g.
- With copious sputum, add **ban xia** (Rhizoma Pinelliae Ternatae) 半夏

9-12g and **su zi** (Fructus Perillae Fructescentis) 苏子 9g.

- With fullness in the chest and nausea, add **ban xia** (Rhizoma Pinelliae Ternatae) 半夏 9-12g and **zi su ye** (Folium Perillae Frutescentis) 紫苏叶 9-12g.
- With severe Lung *qi* deficiency, add **dang shen** (Radix Codonopsis Pilosulae) 党参 15-24g.
- With sluggish stools, add **bing lang** (Semen Arecae Catechu) 槟榔 9-12g.

Patent medicines

Su Zi Jiang Qi Wan 苏子降气丸 (Su Zi Jiang Qi Wan)
Zhui Feng Su He Wan 追风苏合丸 (So Hup Yuen Medical Pills)

Acupuncture (select from)

Lu.7 (*lie que*) .... *luo* point of the Lungs, master point of *ren mai*, promotes the dispersing function of the Lungs, directs Lung *qi* downwards and dispels Wind Cold
Lu.5 (*chi ze*) .... *he* sea and Water point of the Lungs, clears Lung Heat, directs Lung *qi* downwards, stops cough
Du.14 (*da zhui* -) .... meeting point of the *yang* channels, dispels exterior pathogens, promotes distribution of Lung *qi*
Du.12 (*shen zhu* -) .... promotes distribution of Lung *qi*
Ren.12 (*zhong wan* -) .... *mu* point of the Stomach, clears pathogens, directs Stomach *qi* downwards and harmonises the Stomach
St.25 (*tian shu* -) .... *mu* point of the Large Intestine, regulates Intestinal function
Ren.6 (*qi hai* -) .... regulates *qi* and alleviates distension
PC.6 (*nei guan* -) .... *luo* point of the Pericardium, master point of *yin wei mai*, regulates the middle *jiao*, spreads Liver *qi*

- with Spleen and Lung *qi* deficiency, add St.36 (*zu san li* +), Bl.13 (*fei shu* +), Bl.20 (*pi shu* +), Lu.9 (*tai yuan* +)
- *Ear points*: lung, spleen, stomach, intestines, abdomen

Clinical notes

- Distension due to blockage of Lung *qi* is a diagnosis which is often overlooked. If treatment of the Spleen produces no improvement in symptoms then a closer look at Lung involvement may be useful.

- The emotional element in this pattern should not be underestimated and may only become apparent after a period of time, as the patient begins to 'let go and open up', as their Lung *qi* begins to flow. In cases where some significant trauma is suspected, it is wise to exercise caution on the strong distal Lung points (especially Lu.7 *lie que*) during the early stages of treatment as, in some patients, these points can be too dispersing. Long buried, unresolved or unrecognised emotions that are released too quickly may be overwhelming. If in doubt begin with proximal and trunk points.
- Breathing exercises, aerobic exercises, *tai ji chuan* or *qi gong* are an important way of strengthening Lung and Spleen *qi* and facilitating the correct movement of *qi*.
- For dietary recommendations, see p.870.

湿热蕴结

1.5 DAMP HEAT

Pathophysiology

- Damp Heat type abdominal distension can be acute or chronic and is associated with Damp Heat lodged in the Spleen, Stomach or Intestines. When acute, it is typically associated with invasion by a seasonal Damp Heat pathogen, or by sudden excessive ingestion of Damp Heat inducing substances. When chronic, it may be associated with a lingering Damp Heat pathogen, or with internally generated Damp Heat. This pattern is relatively common in humid climates towards the end of Summer ('Indian Summer'), and in patients who travel to tropical climates and pick up a persisting intestinal infection.
- Damp Heat has a tendency to become chronic, and can linger in the system for prolonged periods, surfacing periodically when the patient is exposed to a climactic or dietary influence, or is run down.
- Regardless of the source, the presence of the lingering Damp Heat disrupts the functioning of the *qi* mechanism, compounding the accumulation in the middle *jiao*, leading to quite severe distension.
- The pattern and prescriptions presented here are for chronic Damp Heat patterns. For acute Damp Heat treatments, *see* Acute Exterior Disorders (Vol. 1), Diarrhoea or Nausea and Vomiting (Vol. 2).

Clinical features

- Intermittent or continuous abdominal distension and fullness (mostly upper abdomen); the distension is generally worse in the afternoon and after eating; the abdomen feels firm and may or may not appear swollen.
- loss of appetite, nausea
- dry mouth or thirst with no desire to drink, bitter taste
- fullness and stuffiness in the chest
- restlessness, irritability
- red complexion, greasy skin, possibly strong body odour
- possibly fever or afternoon fever
- heavy sensation in the body, lethargy
- loose stools or a tendency to sluggish stools or constipation; stools are not dry
- concentrated urine

T thick, greasy yellow coat
P slippery or soggy, rapid

Treatment principle

Clear Damp Heat from the Spleen and Stomach, disperse accumulation
Strengthen the Spleen and regulate *qi*

Prescription

LIAN PO YIN 连朴饮
(Coptis and Magnolia Bark Decoction)

This relatively gentle, yet effective prescription, is selected for a lingering Damp Heat pathogen which continues to smoulder at a low level, often for quite lengthy periods. The main features are persistent sensation of abdominal distension that is worse in the afternoon, fatigue and heaviness, nausea or vomiting, loose stools or diarrhoea, possible low grade or afternoon fever unrelieved by sweating, irritability and restlessness, greasy yellow tongue coat and dark urine.

huang lian (Rhizoma Coptidis) 黄连 3-6g
hou po (Cortex Magnoliae Officinalis) 厚朴 9-12g
shan zhi zi (Fructus Gardeniae Jasminoidis) 山栀子 9-12g
dan dou chi (Semen Sojae Preparatum) 淡豆豉 9-12g
shi chang pu (Rhizoma Acori Graminei) 石菖蒲 6-9g
ban xia (Rhizoma Pinelliae Ternatae) 半夏 9-12g
lu gen (Rhizoma Phragmitis Communis) 芦根 30-60g

Method: Decoction. **Huang lian** clears Damp Heat; **hou po** transforms Dampness, promotes movement of *qi* and alleviates distension; **shan zhi zi** and **dan dou chi** clear lingering Heat from the *qi* level and alleviate irritability; **shi chang pu** transforms Dampness, harmonises the middle *jiao* and revives the Spleen; **ban xia** transforms Phlegm, dries Dampness and directs rising Stomach *qi* downwards; the large dose of **lu gen** clears Heat from the *qi* level and stops vomiting. (Source: *Shi Yong Fang Ji Xue*)

Modifications

- With quite severe distension, add **mu xiang** (Radix Aucklandiae Lappae) 木香 9g and **cang zhu** (Rhizoma Atractylodis) 苍术 9-12g.
- With Heat predominant (concentrated urine, feverishness, thirst, rapid pulse), add **huang qin** (Radix Scutellariae Baicalensis) 黄芩 9-12g.
- With Damp predominant (severe distension, thick tongue coat, loose stools, soggy pulse), add **yi ren** (Semen Coicis Lachryma-jobi) 苡仁 30g and **cang zhu** (Rhizoma Atractylodis) 苍术 9-12g.
- With Spleen deficiency, add **bai zhu** (Rhizoma Atractylodes Macrocephalae) 白术 9g.
- With scanty urination, add **hua shi** (Talcum) 滑石 12g and **fu ling** (Sclerotium Poriae Cocos) 茯苓 12g.

ZHONG MAN FEN XIAO WAN 中满分消丸
(Separate and Reduce Fullness in the Middle Pill)

This prescription is somewhat stronger than that above, and is used for relatively severe Damp Heat accumulation. The distension in this pattern may be more marked and clearly related to diet and digestion. The distension may be constant, the abdomen firm and visibly swollen and the patient may need to let out clothing. The tongue coat is thick and yellow or brown.

hou po (Cortex Magnoliae Officinalis) 厚朴 .... 30(12)g
chao zhi shi (dry fried Fructus Immaturus Citri Aurantii) 炒枳实 .... 15(9)g
chao huang qin (dry fried Radix Scutellariae Baicalensis) 炒黄芩 .... 36(12)g
chao huang lian (dry fried Rhizoma Coptidis) 炒黄连 .... 15(6)g
chao zhi mu (dry fried Rhizoma Anemarrhenae Asphodeloidis) 炒知母 12g
ban xia (Rhizoma Pinelliae Ternatae) 半夏 .... 15(9)g
dang shen (Radix Codonopsis Pilosulae) 党参 9g
ze xie (Rhizoma Alismatis Orientalis) 泽泻 9g
chen pi (Pericarpium Citri Reticulatae) 陈皮 9g
gan jiang (Rhizoma Zingiberis Officinalis) 干姜 6g
fu ling (Sclerotium Poriae Cocos) 茯苓 6g
sha ren (Fructus Amomi) 砂仁 6g
jiang huang (Rhizoma Curcumae Longae) 姜黄 3g
bai zhu (Rhizoma Atractylodes Macrocephalae) 白术 3g
gan cao (Radix Glycyrrhizae Uralensis) 甘草 3g
zhu ling (Sclerotium Polypori Umbellati) 猪苓 3g

Method: Grind the herbs (except **zhu ling**) to a fine powder. Boil **zhu ling** in a small amount of water and combine the powder and the decoction to make 9-gram pills. May also be decocted with quantities as shown and those in brackets. **Hou po** and **chao zhi shi** promote movement of *qi* and alleviate distension; **hou po** transforms Dampness; **huang qin, huang lian, ban xia, jiang huang** and **gan jiang** combine bitter cold descending properties with pungent warm dispersal to separate Damp and Heat; **chao zhi mu** clears *qi* level Heat and protects *yin*; **dang shen, bai zhu, fu ling** and **gan cao** make up **SI JUN ZI TANG**, the fundamental *qi* supplementing prescription, and act here to regulate and strengthen Spleen function to resolve Dampness; **ze xie, zhu ling** and **fu ling** promote urination to drain Dampness; **chen pi** and **sha ren** assist the Spleen strengthening elements in regulating the *qi*. (Source: *Zhong Yi Nei Ke Shou Ce*)

Modifications

- With painful or difficult urination, add **che qian zi** (Semen Plantaginis) 车前子 9-12g and **liu yi san** (Six to One Powder) 六一散 9g.
- With constipation, add **da huang** (Radix et Rhizoma Rhei) 大黄 6-9g.
- With a degree of jaundice, delete **dang shen, bai zhu, gan jiang** and **gan cao**, and add **yin chen** (Herba Artemisiae Yinchenhao) 茵陈 18g, **shan zhi zi** (Fructus Gardeniae Jasminoidis) 山栀子 9-12g and **da huang** (Radix et Rhizoma Rhei) 大黄 6-9g.

Patent medicines

Bi Xie Sheng Shi Wan 萆解胜湿丸 (Bi Xie Sheng Shi Wan)
Long Dan Xie Gan Wan 龙胆泻肝丸 (Long Dan Xie Gan Wan, Lung Tan Xie Gan Wan) - with Liver involvement
Huang Lian Jie Du Wan 黄连解毒丸 (Huang Lian Jie Du Wan) plus *Ping Wei San* 平胃散 (Ping Wei San, Tabellae Pingwei)
Mu Xiang Shun Qi Wan 木香顺气丸 (Mu Xiang Shun Qi Wan)
Li Dan Pian 利胆片 (Li Dan Tablets)

Acupuncture (select from)

Ren.12 (*zhong wan* -) .... *mu* point of the Stomach, clears Damp Heat, alleviates distension, directs Stomach *qi* downwards and harmonises the Stomach
Ren.10 (*xia wan* -) .... regulates *qi* and alleviates distension
St.25 (*tian shu* -) .... *mu* point of the Large Intestine, clears Damp Heat, regulates Intestinal function
Ren.6 (*qi hai* -) .... regulates *qi* and alleviates distension
St.37 (*shan ju xu* -) .... lower *he* point of the Large Intestine, regulates and eliminates stagnation and accumulation from the Stomach and Intestines, clears Damp Heat
LI.11 (*qu chi* -) .... *he* sea point of the Large Intestine, clears Damp Heat from *yang ming*
St.36 (*zu san li* -) .... *he* sea point of the Stomach, regulates and strengthens the Spleen and Stomach

- with prominent Heat, add St.44 (*nei ting* -) and LI.4 (*he gu* -)
- with prominent Damp, add Sp.9 (*yin ling quan* -) and Sp.6 (*san yin jiao*)
- with nausea, add PC.6 (*nei guan*)
- with constipation, add SJ.6 (*zhi gou* -)
- with scanty urination, add Kid.7 (*fu liu* -) and Ren.9 (*shui fen* ▲)
- with tenesmus, add Bl.30 (*bai huan shu* -) and Ren.4 (*guan yuan*)
- with *shao yang* symptoms, add GB.39 (*xuan zhong* -), SJ.5 (*wai guan* -) and GB.34 (*yang ling quan* -)
- with lingering fever, add Du.13 (*tao dao* -)
- *Ear points*: spleen, stomach, large intestine, small intestine, liver, abdomen

Clinical notes

- Distension of a Damp Heat type may be diagnosed biomedically as inflammatory bowel disease, chronic colitis, chronic hepatitis (especially C), acute or chronic dysentery, intestinal infection or intestinal parasitosis.
- For dietary recommendations, see p.884.

脾胃气虚

1.6 SPLEEN AND STOMACH QI DEFICIENCY

Pathophysiology

- There are three potential mechanisms by which Spleen and Stomach *qi* deficiency can give rise to abdominal bloating. The first occurs simply because Spleen and Stomach *qi* are weak and therefore unable to move in their correct directions, instead accumulating in the middle *jiao*. The second mechanism is associated with a failure of the Spleen's role in fluid metabolism and distribution. The third and less common, is lack of *qi* movement in the Intestines which can, paradoxically for Spleen deficiency, cause sluggish bowel movements, compounding the distension.

Clinical features

- intermittent or continuous abdominal distension, fullness and discomfort which is improved with warmth and pressure; the distension is worse with eating raw or uncooked foods.
- poor appetite, early satiety
- fatigue, tiredness; weak, tired limbs
- loose stools or a tendency to sluggish bowel movements
- puffiness around the eyes or in the fingers; quick weight fluctuations
- pale, sallow complexion and lips
- shortness of breath, reluctance to speak, weak, low voice

T pale with a white coat; or pale and swollen with tooth marks
P weak, thready or deficient, or big and weak (especially right middle position)

Treatment principle

Supplement *qi* and strengthen the Spleen
Correct the *qi* mechanism (facilitate the 'raising of the clear and the descent of the turbid')

Prescription

BU ZHONG YI QI TANG 补中益气汤
(*Ginseng and Astragalus Combination*) modified

zhi huang qi (honey fried Radix Astragali Membranacei) 炙黄芪 18-30g
dang shen (Radix Codonopsis Pilosulae) 党参 12-15g
chao bai zhu (dry fried Rhizoma Atractylodes Macrocephalae) 炒白术 12-15g
dang gui (Radix Angelicae Sinensis) 当归 6-9g
chen pi (Pericarpium Citri Reticulatae) 陈皮 6-9g
sheng ma (Rhizoma Cimicifugae) 升麻 3-6g
chai hu (Radix Bupleuri) 柴胡 3-6g

zhi gan cao (honey fried Radix Glycyrrhizae Uralensis) 炙甘草 3-6g
zhi shi (Fructus Immaturus Citri Aurantii) 枳实 9-12g
hou po (Cortex Magnoliae Officinalis) 厚朴 9-12g

Method: Decoction or powdered and taken in doses of 9-grams as a draft. **Zhi huang qi**, **dang shen**, **chao bai zhu** and **zhi gan cao** strengthen the Spleen, supplement *qi* and assist the ascent of Spleen *qi*; **chai hu** and **sheng ma** support these principal herbs in elevating *qi*; **zhi shi** and **hou po** regulate *qi* and encourage *qi* to descend creating the balance for the ascending herbs–the ascent and descent of *qi* assists in getting *qi* moving and correcting the *qi* mechanism; **dang gui** supplements Blood; **chen pi** regulates *qi*. (Source: *Shi Yong Zhong Yi Nei Ke Xue*)

Modifications

- With severe distension, add **mu xiang** (Radix Aucklandiae Lappae) 木香 6-9g and **sha ren** (Fructus Amomi) 砂仁 6-9g.
- With fluid retention, add **fu ling** (Sclerotium Poriae Cocos) 茯苓 12-15g, **ze xie** (Rhizoma Alismatis Orientalis) 泽泻 9-12g and **che qian zi** (Semen Plantaginis) 车前子 9-12g, or combine with **WU LING SAN** (*Hoelen Five Formula* 五苓散, p.910).
- With Damp accumulation in the middle *jiao*, add **huo xiang** (Herba Agastaches seu Pogostemi) 藿香 9-12g and **cang zhu** (Rhizoma Atractylodis) 苍术 12-15g.
- With Liver *qi* stagnation, combine with **XIAO YAO SAN** (*Bupleurum and Dang Gui Formula* 逍遥散, p.159) or consider **SI MO TANG** (*Four Milled-Herb Decoction* 四磨汤, p.639).
- With loss of appetite, add **sha ren** (Fructus Amomi) 砂仁 6-9g and **chao shen qu** (dry fried Massa Fermentata) 炒神曲 15g.
- With suspected parasites, add a small dose of **da huang** (Radix et Rhizoma Rhei) 大黄 1-3g, **bai zhi** (Radix Angelicae Dahuricae) 白芷 6-9g, **zi su ye** (Folium Perillae Frutescentis) 紫苏叶 9-12g and **bo he** (Herba Mentha Haplocalycis) 薄荷 6-9g.
- With sluggish bowel movements, add **rou cong rong** (Herba Cistanches Deserticolae) 肉苁蓉 15-24g.

Variations and additional prescriptions

With Phlegm Damp and qi stagnation

- In patients with Spleen deficiency, Phlegm Damp and *qi* stagnation in the middle *jiao*, the features are focal distension and discomfort in the epigastrium and upper abdomen worse after eating, loss of appetite, decreased sense of taste, inability to eat more than a little food at a time, generalised weakness and a pale tongue with a thick white coat. The treatment is to strengthen the Spleen, harmonise the Stomach, dry Dampness, transform Phlegm and relieve distension with **XIANG SHA LIU JUN ZI TANG** (*Saussurea and Cardamon Combination* 香砂六君子汤)

modified.

dang shen (Radix Codonopsis Pilosulae) 党参 15-18g
bai zhu (Rhizoma Atractylodis Macrocephalae) 白术 12-15g
fu ling (Sclerotium Poriae Cocos) 茯苓 12-15g
ban xia (Rhizoma Pinelliae Ternatae) 半夏 9-12g
chen pi (Pericarpium Citri Reticulatae) 陈皮 6-9g
sha ren (Fructus Amomi) 砂仁 6-9g
mu xiang (Radix Aucklandiae Lappae) 木香 6-9g
zhi gan cao (honey fried Radix Glycyrrhizae Uralensis)
炙甘草 3-6g
cang zhu (Rhizoma Atractylodis) 苍术 9-12g
hou po (Cortex Magnoliae Officinalis) 厚朴 9-12g

Method: Decoction. **Sha ren** is added towards the end of cooking time (*hou xia* 后下). **Dang shen** supplements *qi* and strengthens the Spleen; **bai zhu** strengthens the Spleen and dries Dampness; **fu ling** strengthens the Spleen and leaches out Dampness through the urine; **ban xia** transforms Phlegm, dries Dampness, directs rising Stomach *qi* downwards and stops nausea and vomiting; **chen pi** transforms Phlegm and dries Dampness, regulates middle *jiao qi* and corrects the *qi* mechanism; **zhi gan cao** strengthens the Spleen and harmonises the Stomach; **sha ren** and **mu xiang** regulate *qi* and correct the *qi* mechanism; **cang zhu** parches and dries Dampness, liberates the Spleen and assists the *qi* mechanism; **hou po** regulates *qi*, transforms Dampness and alleviates distension. (Source: *Shi Yong Zhong Yi Nei Ke Xue*)

Complex of Heat, Cold and deficiency

- A common, yet somewhat more complex situation, is one in which Heat and Cold clump in the middle *jiao* against a background of Spleen and Stomach *qi* deficiency. This pattern is associated with poor dietary habits and the effect of stress on the gastro-intestinal system, and typically involves the primary pathological triad (p.912). The key feature is a sensation of blockage, distension, fullness and discomfort in the epigastrium, which, when palpated, feels soft and without pain. In addition, there may be nausea, vomiting or dry retching, borborygmus with diarrhoea, poor appetite, a thin greasy yellow tongue coat and a soft, slippery, slightly wiry and possibly rapid pulse. The treatment is to harmonise the Stomach, redirect *qi* downwards and disperse accumulation with **BAN XIA XIE XIN TANG** (*Pinellia Combination* 半夏泻心汤).

ban xia (Rhizoma Pinelliae Ternatae) 半夏 9-12g
huang qin (Radix Scutellariae Baicalensis) 黄芩 9-12g
huang lian (Rhizoma Coptidis) 黄连 3-6g
gan jiang (Rhizoma Zingiberis Officinalis) 干姜 6-9g
zhi gan cao (honey fried Radix Glycyrrhizae Uralensis)
炙甘草 3-6g
dang shen (Radix Codonopsis Pilosulae) 党参 15-24g

da zao (Fructus Zizyphi Jujubae) 大枣 4pce

Method: Decoction. **Ban xia** transforms Phlegm, dries Dampness, directs rising Stomach *qi* downwards; **gan jiang**, pungent and hot, warms Spleen and Stomach *yang* and dispels Cold; **huang qin** and **huang lian**, bitter and cold, clear Heat–together the pungent warm dispersing herbs and the bitter cold descending herbs stimulate the ascent and descent of *qi* and correct the *qi* mechanism; **dang shen** and **da zao** strengthen the Spleen, supplement *qi* and prevent the dispersing action of the principal herbs from injuring the Spleen and Stomach *qi* and *yin*; **zhi gan cao** strengthens the Spleen and harmonises the Stomach.

With severe Phlegm Damp and relentless distension

- With accompanying Phlegm Damp and rising Stomach *qi*, causing constant epigastric and upper abdominal distension distension with relentless belching, hiccough, reflux, nausea or vomiting, the main aim of treatment is to redirect *qi* downward and transform Phlegm, while supporting *qi* and harmonising the Stomach with **XUAN FU DAI ZHE TANG** (*Inula and Haematite Decoction* 旋复代赭汤, p.13).

Patent medicines

Bu Zhong Yi Qi Wan 补中益气丸 (Bu Zhong Yi Qi Wan, Central Qi Pills)

Xiang Sha Liu Jun Zi Wan 香砂六君子丸 (Xiang Sha Liu Jun Wan, Aplotaxis-Ammomum Pills, Six Gentlemen Tea Pills)

Jian Pi Wan 健脾丸 (Jian Pi Wan)
- Spleen *qi* deficiency with food stagnation

Xiang Sha Yang Wei Wan 香砂养胃丸 (Xiang Sha Yang Wei Wan, Hsiang Sha Yang Wei Wan) - with *qi* and Damp stagnation

Acupuncture (select from)

Ren.12 (*zhong wan* +▲) .. *mu* point of the Stomach, strengthens the Spleen and Stomach, directs Stomach *qi* downwards and harmonises the Stomach

Liv.13 (*zhang men* -) .... *mu* point of the Spleen and *hui* point of the *zang*, strengthens the Spleen and improves digestion, promotes Liver function

St.25 (*tian shu*) .... *mu* point of the Large Intestine, regulates Intestinal function

Sp.15 (*da heng*) .... strengthens the Spleen and resolves Dampness

Ren.6 (*qi hai*) .... regulates *qi* and alleviates distension

St.36 (*zu san li* +▲) .... *he* sea point of the Stomach, powerfully strengthens the Spleen and Stomach, supplements *qi* and corrects the *qi* mechanism

Sp.3 (*tai bai*) .... *yuan*, *shu* stream and Earth point of the Spleen, supplements the Spleen and transforms

Dampness

Sp.6 (*san yin jiao*) .... strengthens the Spleen, regulates Liver *qi*, benefits the Kidneys

Bl.20 (*pi shu* +) .... *shu* point of the Spleen, strengthens Spleen *qi*

Bl.21 (*wei shu* +) .... *shu* point of the Stomach, regulates the *qi* mechanism

- with severe distension, add Sp.1 (*yin bai*)
- with fluid retention and oedema, add St.28 (*shui dao* -) and Sp.9 (*yin ling quan* -)
- with Liver *qi* stagnation, add Liv.3 (*tai chong*) and PC.6 (*nei guan*)
- *Ear points*: spleen, stomach, large intestine, small intestine, abdomen

Clinical notes

- Spleen and Stomach *qi* deficiency type distension may be diagnosed biomedically as chronic gastroenteritis, food intolerance, coeliac disease, peptic ulcer disease, functional weakness of the stomach, hiatus hernia, an eating disorder or chronic colitis.
- For dietary recommendations, see p.870.

Table 1.1 *Comparison of Spleen supplementing prescriptions*

Prescription	Characteristics
Bu Zhong Yi Qi Tang	The main prescription for Spleen qi deficiency abdominal distension acts by strengthening the Spleen and correcting the qi mechanism, that is, by encouraging the ascent of the accumulating Spleen qi. Bu Zhong Yi Qi Tang is contraindicated when Stomach qi is already rising, with belching, nausea, headaches and reflux, as it can aggravate these symptoms.
Xiang Sha Liu Jun Zi Tang	For Spleen qi deficiency with Phlegm Damp. Particularly good when the Damp is very obvious, causing a thick tongue coat, inability to eat much without feeling more bloated, drowsiness after eating, nausea and heaviness.
Ban Xia Xie Xin Tang	For a complex mixture of Spleen and Stomach deficiency componded by both Heat and Cold signs and symptoms. The defining symptom for the use of this prescription is a sense of blockage or fullness in the epigastrium which is soft and painless when palpated.
Xuan Fu Dai Zhe Tang	For Stomach deficiency with rising Stomach qi causing epigastric distension with belching, hiccough, acid reflux, nausea or vomiting. The main aim of this prescription is to heavily weigh down Stomach qi to force its descent, rather than strengthening the Spleen and Stomach.

脾胃虚寒

1.7 SPLEEN AND STOMACH YANG DEFICIENCY

Pathophysiology

- Spleen and Stomach *yang* deficiency causes relatively severe abdominal distension. The mechanism is similar to that of Spleen *qi* deficiency, with the added complication of Cold. The Cold further constrains the movement of *qi* and leads to a more profound disruption to the *qi* mechanism.

Clinical features

- Severe, intermittent or unrelenting abdominal distension that is progressively worse as the day goes on until it may be difficult to bear in the evening. The abdomen may appear swollen or the patient may feel clothing is tight. The distension is worse with eating, exposure to cold and when fatigued.
- abdominal and/or epigastric discomfort or pain which is improved with warmth and pressure
- cold intolerance and cold extremities
- diarrhoea with undigested food in the stools; or conversely sluggish bowel movements with no urge to defecate; the stools are not dry
- loss of appetite, early satiety
- fatigue, tiredness, exhaustion
- puffiness around the eyes or in the fingers; quick weight fluctuations
- possible scanty urination, oedema

T pale and swollen with tooth marks

P deep, weak, slow

Treatment principle

Warm and supplement Spleen *yang*

Stimulate and correct the *qi* mechanism

Prescription

ZHI SHI LI ZHONG WAN 枳实理中丸
(*Immature Bitter Orange Pill to Regulate the Middle*)

dang shen (Radix Codonopsis Pilosulae) 党参 15-24g
chao bai zhu (dry fried Rhizoma Atractylodis Macrocephalae) 炒白术 12-15g
gan jiang (Rhizoma Zingiberis Officinalis) 干姜 9-12g
zhi gan cao (honey fried Radix Glycyrrhizae Uralensis) 炙甘草 6-9g
zhi shi (Fructus Immaturus Citri Aurantii) 枳实 9-12g
fu ling (Sclerotium Poriae Cocos) 茯苓 12-15g

Method: Decoction. **Dang shen, chao bai zhu, fu ling** and **zhi gan cao** strengthen the Spleen and supplement *qi*; **gan jiang** warms Spleen *yang*; **zhi shi** regulates *qi* and alleviates distension. (Source: *Shi Yong Fang Ji Xue*)

Modifications

- With severe Cold and cold intolerance, add **zhi fu zi** (Radix Aconiti Carmichaeli Praeparata) 制附子 6-12g (decocted for 30 minutes before the other herbs) and **rou gui** (Cortex Cinnamomi Cassiae) 肉桂 3g.
- With Dampness, add **cang zhu** (Rhizoma Atractylodis) 苍术 9g.
- For severe abdominal distension, add **mu xiang** (Radix Aucklandiae Lappae) 木香 6-9g and **sha ren** (Fructus Amomi) 砂仁 6-9g.
- With foggy-headedness or sleepiness, add **shi chang pu** (Rhizoma Acori Graminei) 石菖蒲 6-9g and **yuan zhi** (Radix Polygalae Tenuifoliae) 远志 6-9g.

Patent medicines

Fu Zi Li Zhong Wan 附子理中丸 (Carmichaeli Tea Pills, Fu Tzu Li Chung Wan, Li Chung Yuen Medical Pills)
Li Zhong Wan 理中丸 (Li Zhong Wan)

Acupuncture (select from)

Ren.12 (*zhong wan* +▲) .. *mu* point of the Stomach, warms and strengthens the Spleen and Stomach, directs Stomach *qi* downwards and harmonises the Stomach
St.25 (*tian shu* +▲) .... *mu* point of the Large Intestine, regulates Intestinal function and directs *qi* downwards
Sp.15 (*da heng* +▲) .... strengthens the Spleen and resolves Damp
Ren.6 (*qi hai* +▲) .... regulates *qi* and alleviates distension
Ren.4 (*guan yuan* +▲) ..... *mu* point of the Small Intestine, supplements *yuan qi*, warms *yang* and regulates *qi*
St.36 (*zu san li* +▲) .... *he* sea point of the Stomach, powerfully warms and strengthens the Spleen and Stomach, supplements *qi* and corrects the *qi* mechanism
Sp.6 (*san yin jiao* +▲) ...... strengthens the Spleen, regulates Liver *qi*, benefits the Kidneys
Bl.20 (*pi shu* +▲) .... *shu* point of the Spleen, strengthens the Spleen and supplements *qi*
Bl.21 (*wei shu* +▲) .... *shu* point of the Stomach, regulates the *qi* mechanism
Bl.23 (*shen shu* +▲) .... *shu* point of the Kidneys, warms and supports *yang*
Du.4 (*ming men* +▲) .... warms and supports Kidney *yang*

- a moxa box over the abdomen is useful

- with severe distension, add Sp.1 (*yin bai*)
- with fluid retention and oedema, add Ren.9 (*shui fen* ▲) and Sp.9 (*yin ling quan* -)
- with Liver *qi* stagnation, add Liv.3 (*tai chong*) and PC.6 (*nei guan*)
- *Ear points*: spleen, stomach, large intestine, small intestine, abdomen, adrenal

Clinical notes

- Spleen *yang* deficiency type abdominal distension may be diagnosed biomedically as chronic gastroenteritis, food intolerance, coeliac disease, post surgical intestinal dysfunction, chronic peptic ulcer disease, dumping syndrome, functional weakness of the stomach, an eating disorder, hiatus hernia or chronic colitis.
- Spleen *yang* deficiency type distension responds well to correct treatment, and the patient will often feel better quite quickly. For lasting results however, treatment usually needs to continue for at least a few months. Depending on the duration and severity of the initial condition, 6-12 months of treatment may be required to rebuild Spleen *yang*.
- For dietary recommendations, see p.873.

胃脾阴虚

1.8 STOMACH (SPLEEN) YIN DEFICIENCY

Pathophysiology

- The distension associated with Stomach *yin* deficiency is due to the Stomach being adversely affected by lack of physiological *yin* fluids. The digestive function of the Stomach is affected, food and fluids are poorly processed and can stagnate.
- Stomach *yin* deficiency is usually a complication of some other long standing pathology, most commonly Liver *qi* invading the Stomach or long term Stomach Heat, Damp Heat or Phlegm Heat. It can, however, be more acute, and follow sudden damage to Stomach *yin* following a febrile illness, typically *yang ming* syndrome.
- Stomach *yin* is a superficial form of *yin* (relative to the deeper Kidney *yin*) and may not produce *yin* deficiency Heat symptoms when deficient. The main feature will often be dryness rather than Heat, although in severe cases there may be significant Heat. Depending on the degree of deficiency and the length of the problem, Kidney *yin* may be drained with the onset of deeper Heat symptoms (like nightsweats or 'bone steaming'). Stomach *yin* deficiency is often complicated by *qi* deficiency and/or *qi* and Blood stagnation.

Clinical features

- chronic epigastric and/or abdominal distension; the distension may be worse with eating, worse at the end of the day, at night and when tired or hungry
- general dryness of mucous membranes and skin, thirst, dry mouth, lips and throat
- tendency to constipation or difficult stools, with dry pellet like stools
- poor appetite, or indeterminate gnawing hunger with no real desire to eat, or desire for cold and bland foods or a liquid diet
- mild nausea or dry retching
- malar or facial flushing, nightsweats
- sensation of heat in the palms and soles ('five hearts hot')

T slightly red and peeled in the centre, or red and dry with little or no coat; in severe or long standing cases the tongue may be so denuded of papillae as to resemble a piece of liver (mirror tongue) or have numerous surface cracks or a wide shallow central crack

P thready and rapid

Treatment principle

Nourish and supplement *yin* and moisten dryness
Strengthen the Spleen and disperse accumulation

Prescription

YI WEI TANG 益胃汤
(*Benefit the Stomach Decoction*) modified

sha shen (Radix Adenophorae seu Glehniae) 沙参 24-30g
mai dong (Tuber Ophiopogonis Japonici) 麦冬 12-15g
yu zhu (Rhizoma Polygonati Odorati) 玉竹 9-12g
sheng di (Radix Rehmanniae Glutinosae) 生地 9-12g
han lian cao (Herba Ecliptae Prostratae) 旱连草 12-15g
nu zhen zi (Fructus Ligustri Lucidi) 女贞子 12-15g
shan zhi zi (Fructus Gardeniae Jasminoides) 山栀子 9g
zhi shi (Fructus Immaturus Citri Aurantii) 枳实 9g
huo ma ren (Semen Cannabis Sativae) 火麻仁 6g

Method: Decoction. **Sha shen, mai dong, yu zhu** and **sheng di** nourish Stomach *yin*; **han lian cao** and **nu zhen zi** nourish Liver and Kidney *yin*; **zhi shi** regulates *qi*; **huo ma ren** moistens dryness and lubricates the Intestines. (Source: *Zhong Yi Nei Ke Shou Ce*)

Modifications

- With significant deficiency Heat, add **zhi mu** (Rhizoma Anemarrhenae Asphodeloides) 知母 9-12g and **xuan shen** (Radix Scrophulariae) 玄参 15-24g.
- With spasmodic or dull persistent pain, add **bai shao** (Radix Paeoniae Lactiflora) 白芍 12-18g and **gan cao** (Radix Glycyrrhizae Uralensis) 甘草 6g.
- With acid reflux, heartburn and nausea, add **wu zhu yu** (Fructus Evodiae Rutaecarpae) 吴茱萸 2g and **huang lian** (Rhizoma Coptidis) 黄连 6g.
- With poor appetite, add **mai ya** (Fructus Hordei Vulgaris Germinantus) 麦芽 15-30g and **ji nei jin** (Endothelium Corneum Gigeriae Galli) 鸡内金 9-12g.
- With excess gastric acid, add **duan wa leng zi** (calcined Concha Arcae) 煅瓦楞子 15g (or 3g as a powder washed down with the decoction).
- With hypoacidity, add **wu mei** (Fructus Pruni Mume) 乌梅 9-12g, **shi hu** (Herba Dendrobi) 石斛 12g and **shan zha** (Fructus Crataegi) 山楂 15g.
- With *qi* deficiency (swollen tongue with many surface cracks), add **tai zi shen** (Radix Pseudostellariae Heterophyllae) 太子参 15-24g and **wu wei zi** (Fructus Schizandrae Chinensis) 五味子 6g.
- With stagnant *qi*, add **mei gui hua** (Flos Rosae Rugosae) 玫瑰花 6g and **fo shou** (Fructus Citri Sarcodacylis) 佛手 9-12g, or consider **YI GUAN JIAN** (*Linking Decoction* 一贯煎, p.78).
- With stagnant Blood (intermittent stabbing pain, or a focal area that is

worse with pressure), add **dan shen** (Radix Salviae Miltiorrhizae) 丹参 12-18g and **tao ren** (Semen Persicae) 桃仁 9-12g.

- With severe constipation, add **sheng he shou wu** (unprocessed Radix Polygoni Multiflori) 生何首乌 12-15g and **xuan shen** (Radix Scrophulariae) 玄参 15-24g.
- For atrophy of the gastric mucosa, add **dan shen** (Radix Salviae Miltiorrhizae) 丹参 12-18g and **zhi huang qi** (honey fried Radix Astragali Membranacei) 炙黄芪 18-30g.
- If Kidney and/or Liver *yin* is also weakened (lower back ache, flushing, nightsweats and tinnitus) combine with **LIU WEI DI HUANG WAN** (*Rehmannia Six Formula* 六味地黄丸). Patent pills are usually sufficient.

Patent medicines

Gu Ben Wan 固本丸 (Gu Ben Wan, Ren Shen Ku Pen Wan)
- Stomach *qi* and *yin* deficiency

Liu Wei Di Huang Wan 六味地黄丸 (Liu Wei Di Huang Wan, Six Flavour Tea) - combine with the principal formula when there is Kidney *yin* deficiency

Zhi Bai Ba Wei Wan 知柏八味丸 (Zhi Bai Ba Wei Wan, Chih Pai Pa Wei Wan) - with lots of deficient Heat

Mai Wei Di Huang Wan 麦味地黄丸 (Mai Wei Di Huang Wan, Ba Xian Chang Shou Wan) - with Kidney *yin* deficiency

Luo Han Guo Chong Ji 罗汉果冲剂 (Luo Han Kuo Beverage)

Sheng Mai San Wan 生脉散丸 (Sheng Mai San Wan)
- *qi* and *yin* deficiency

Acupuncture (select from)

Ren.12 (*zhong wan* +) .... *mu* point of the Stomach, nourishes Stomach *yin*, regulates Stomach *qi*

St.25 (*tian shu*) .... *mu* point of the Large Intestine, regulates Intestinal function, alleviates abdominal distension

Ren.4 (*guan yuan* +) .... together these points supplement *yin*
Sp.6 (*san yin jiao* +) systemically, strengthen the Kidneys and regulate *qi*

St.36 (*zu san li* +) .... *he* sea point of the Stomach, powerfully strengthens the Spleen and Stomach, and supplements *qi* and *yin*

Bl.21 (*wei shu* +) .... *shu* point of the Stomach, supplements Stomach *qi* and *yin*

Bl.20 (*pi shu* +)................. *shu* point of the Spleen, supplements Spleen *qi* and *yin*

- with Heat, add St.44 (*nei ting* -) and Kid.2 (*ran gu* -)
- with Kidney *yin* deficiency, add Kid.6 (*zhao hai* +) and Kid.3 (*tai xi* +)
- *Ear points*: spleen, stomach, large intestine, small intestine, liver, abdomen

Clinical notes

- Stomach and Spleen *yin* deficiency type abdominal distension may be diagnosed biomedically as gastritis, chronic atrophic gastritis or peptic ulcer disease.
- This pattern responds reasonably well to prolonged treatment. Even though the distension may be alleviated within a relatively short period of weeks, treatment will need to continue so as to rebuild *yin*. In long standing cases, 6-9 months of treatment may be necessary for a satisfactory long term result.
- For dietary recommendations, see p.876.

SUMMARY OF GUIDING FORMULAE FOR ABDOMINAL AND EPIGASTRIC DISTENSION

Excess patterns
Food stagnation - *Bao He Wan* 保和丸
- with Damp Heat - *Zhi Shi Dao Zhi Wan* 枳实导滞丸
- with Spleen deficiency - *Jian Pi Wan* 健脾丸

Phlegm Damp - *Ping Wei San* 平胃散
- severe cases with *qi* deficiency - *Xuan Fu Dai Zhe Tang* 旋复代赭汤
- with Wind Cold - *Xiang Su San* 香苏散
- with *shao yang* symptoms - *Chai Hu Zhi Jie Tang* 柴胡枳桔汤

Liver *qi* stagnation - *Yue Ju Wan* 越鞠丸
- Liver invading the Spleen - *Chai Hu Shu Gan San* 柴胡疏肝散
- with constipation - *Liu Mo Tang* 六磨汤
- with food stagnation - *Mu Xiang Shun Qi Wan* 木香顺气丸

Lung *qi* accumulation - *Wu Ji San* 五积散

Damp Heat - *Lian Po Yin* 连朴饮
- severe cases - *Zhong Man Fen Xiao Wan* 中满分消丸

Deficient patterns
Spleen *qi* deficiency - *Bu Zhong Yi Qi Tang* 补中益气汤
- with Phlegm Damp - *Xuan Fu Dai Zhe Tang* 旋复代赭汤
- with Cold Damp and *qi* stagnation - *Xiang Sha Liu Jun Zi Tang*
- complex of Cold, Heat and deficiency - *Ban Xia Xie Xin Tang* 半夏泻心汤香砂六君子汤
- Spleen *yang* deficiency - *Zhi Shi Li Zhong Wan* 枳实理中丸

Stomach and Spleen *yin* deficiency - *Yi Wei Tang* 益胃汤

Table 1.2 *Differential diagnosis of abdominal and epigastric distension*

Pattern	Duration	Aggravated by	Ameliorated by	Other features	Nature of patient	Pulse and tongue
Food stagnation	acute or chronic	overindulgence, eating irregularly	eating less, eating slowly, eating regularly, defecation, belching, passing gas	flatulence, heartburn, bad breath, tendency to constipation	often overweight, may be robust	T: thick greasy white or yellow coat P: slippery, full
Phlegm Damp	acute or chronic, mostly chronic	consumption of dairy, sugar, greasy or rich foods	simple, bland diet	symptoms often worse in the morning, foggy-head, heaviness, nausea	sleepy, sluggish, may be overweight	T: thick greasy white coat P: slippery, wiry or moderate
Liver *qi* stagnation	chronic with acute exacerbations	emotional upset and stress	relaxation, contentment, following exercise	moodiness, depression, pre-menstrual symptoms, alternating bowel habits	nervy, tense, uptight, most common 20-50 yrs, F>M	T: unremarkable, thin white coat P: wiry
Accumulation of Lung *qi*	acute or chronic	eating, exposure to Wind and Cold		fatigue, spontaneous sweating, melancholy, cough	tends to frailness, hunched over posture, weak voice	T: pale, thin white coat P: weak in the Lung position, elevated in the Spleen position

Damp Heat	chronic or acute	tends to be worse in the afternoon, Damp or Heating substances		sluggish stools, afternoon feverishness, concentrated urine, nausea, bitter taste in the mouth	may have greasy skin, red complexion, strong body odour	T: thick greasy yellow coat P: slippery, soggy, rapid
Spleen and Stomach qi deficiency	chronic	cold or raw foods, cold medications	bland, light, well cooked food, small meals; application of warmth and pressure	poor appetite, early satiety, loose stools, fatigue	pale complexion, puffy eyes, poor muscle tone	T: pale, thin white coat P: weak, thready, deficient
Spleen and Stomach yang deficiency	chronic	cold or raw foods, cold medications, exertion	bland, light, well cooked food, small meals; application of warmth and pressure	diarrhoea with undigested food, cold intolerance, anorexia, early satiety	pale complexion, cold extremities, exhausted, low spirits, puffy face and eyes	T: pale and swollen, wet P: deep, weak, slow
Stomach yin deficiency	chronic	empty stomach, when tired, at night	bland or liquid diet	dryness of mouth, lips, stools, skin; malar flush, mild nausea	thin, flushed	T: slightly red and peeled centrally, or red and dry with no coat P: thready, rapid

2. Abdominal Pain

Excess Cold
Deficient Cold
Heat
Qi stagnation
Blood stagnation
Food stagnation
Worm accumulation

2 ABDOMINAL PAIN

fu tong 腹痛

For the purpose of analysing pain, the abdomen is divided into three sections, the hypochondriac region over the ribs and flanks, the epigastric region bounded by the hypochondriac region laterally and the abdominal region inferiorly and the remainder, the abdomen. The abdominal pain discussed in this chapter is pain below the epigastric and hypochondriac regions (Figure 2.1).

Abdominal pain is a common presenting symptom in the TCM clinic. The pain can be acute or chronic, diffuse or well localised. When acute and severe, surgical referral may be necessary. When analysing a patient with acute pain, it is important to keep in mind those conditions considered medical emergencies. Also note that textbook descriptions of pain are limited due to the different responses of individuals to pain. Obese and elderly patients tend to tolerate pain better than others, while in highly strung individuals the experience of pain may be magnified.

Patients with chronic pain are most likely to seek TCM treatment. As noted in Box 2.1, there are many biomedical causes of abdominal pain, many of which are amenable to TCM treatment.

Figure 2.1 *Regions of the abdomen (for the purpose of analysing pain)*

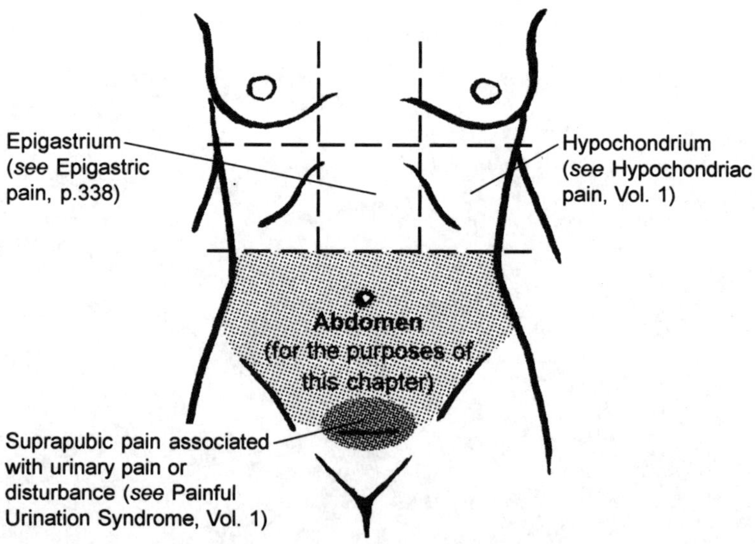

AETIOLOGY

Cold

Cold is an extremely common cause of both acute and chronic abdominal pain, as the nature of Cold is to 'freeze and constrict'. By freezing and constricting abdominal structures, the circulation of *qi* and Blood is retarded and pain is easily produced.

External Cold

Cold can be introduced into the body by association with Wind, by ingesting cold foods or drinks, or by direct exposure of the body to cold. A common example of the latter is invasion of the Uterus by cold while swimming during menstruation. Cold has an affinity with both the Intestines and the Uterus, and in both cases causes quite severe cramping or colicky pain that is significantly alleviated by application of heat. External Cold may be associated with Dampness, or may transform into a Heat pathogen once in the body.

Internal Cold

Internal Cold is the product of Spleen and/or Kidney *yang* deficiency patterns, where *yin* Cold becomes predominant relative to warming active *yang*. The manifestations of the pattern will vary depending on the degree of deficiency relative to the strength of the excess Cold. When the deficient aspects are dominant, the pain produced will be of a deficient Cold type (mild and dull, relieved by warmth and pressure). When *yin* Cold is ascendant, the pain will tend to be severe, relieved by warmth but worse for pressure.

The background *yang* deficiency patterns are chronic conditions. Spleen *yang* is primarily weakened by the diet (*see* p.50). Weak Kidney *yang* or *qi* may be an inherited condition, or may develop as a result of age, chronic illness, too much exposure to cold conditions, or excessive lifting or standing. Kidney *yang* or *qi* may also be damaged by excessive or premature sexual activity (especially in men, but also women), or specifically in women by many pregnancies, miscarriages and/or terminations.

Heat

Heat that causes abdominal pain includes invasion of external Heat, external and internally generated Damp Heat, Toxic Heat and Summerheat.

External Heat

External Heat can invade directly into the Intestines, or transform from a Cold invasion (also known as *yang ming fu* syndrome). The Heat parches the Intestine and stool causing constipation and pain.

External Damp Heat can invade the Intestines or Uterus. Damp Heat in

BOX 2.1 BIOMEDICAL CAUSES OF ABDOMINAL PAIN (# denotes most common and includes the TCM defined epigastric and hypochondriac pain, ! denotes medical emergencies)

ACUTE

Cardiovascular
- ruptured abdominal aortic aneurysm or dissecting aortic aneurysm !
- mesenteric artery occlusion !
- myocardial infarction !

Gastrointestinal
- acute gastroenteritis#
- acute appendicitis !
- peptic ulcer
- gastritis
- bowel obstruction, volvulus !
- perforated ulcer or diverticulum !
- diverticulitis
- irritable bowel syndrome#
- inflammatory bowel disease
- faecal impaction, constipation

Hepatobiliary
- hepatitis
- pancreatitis
- cholecystitis, cholelithiasis
- carcinoma

Genitourinary
- renal, ureteric colic
- pyelonephritis
- mittlesmerz#, dysmenorrhoea#
- endometriosis#
- ruptured ovarian cyst
- ectopic pregnancy !
- acute salpingitis
- ovarian or testicular torsion !

Other
- lactose intolerance
- shingles
- mesenteric adenitis (children)
- intussusception (children) !
- peritonitis !
- trigger points or myofacial tear in the abdominal wall
- splenic infarct or rupture !
- inguinal or femoral herniae
- vertebral lesions
- depression, stress
- atypical pneumonia

CHRONIC OR RECURRENT

Cardiovascular
- abdominal aortic aneurism
- mesenteric artery ischaemia

Gastrointestinal
- chronic appendicitis#
- mesenteric adenitis (children)
- peptic ulcer#
- gastritis
- reflux oesophagitis
- lactose intolerance
- food allergies#
- diverticulitis
- irritable bowel syndrome#
- inflammatory bowel disease
- faecal impaction, constipation
- carcinoma

Hepatobiliary
- chronic hepatitis
- cirrhosis
- chronic pancreatitis
- chronic cholecystitis, cholelithiasis
- carcinoma

Genitourinary
- mittlesmerz#, dysmenorrhoea#
- endometriosis#
- chronic PID
- ovarian cysts, fibroids

Drugs (acute pain also)
- alcohol
- antibiotics
- steroids
- iron
- nicotine (in cigarettes or gum)
- cytotoxic agents

Other
- trigger points or myofacial tear in the abdominal wall
- inguinal or femoral herniae
- vertebral lesions
- depression, stress
- lead poisoning
- adhesions (post surgical)

the Intestines can be a product of the season, commonly occurring during hot or humid weather, and more common in tropical climates. Damp Heat pathogens can also invade with spoiled food, or by sudden overindulgence in Damp Hot substances, such as alcohol, fats, and greasy rich foods.

Damp Heat in the Uterus can result from an external Damp Heat pathogen that invades through the *tai yang* (Urinary Bladder) channel, the leg *yin* channels or the local *luo* channels. In practice, transmission of Damp Heat through the *luo* channels is probably the most common mode of entry (especially in sexually active individuals). It also occurs in postpartum women due to their relative deficiency and thus their vulnerability to external invasion.

Internal Heat

Internally generated Heat or Damp Heat can also cause abdominal pain. Damp Heat generated in the middle *jiao* by overconsumption of rich, greasy or spicy foods and alcohol can simply sink and settle in the Intestines.

Damp Heat can also be generated in the lower *jiao* by any prolonged Heat in the system, such as the deficienct Heat arising from *yin* deficiency, the stagnant Heat from Liver *qi* stagnation, prolonged stagnation of Dampness or transformation of Cold.

Emotion

Liver *qi* stagnation is caused by repressed emotion, frustration, anger and resentment. These emotions, especially when chronically unexpressed, cause a low grade spasm and tension in the smooth muscle of the gut–a classical emotional 'holding pattern'. Patients with chronic *qi* stagnation type digestive problems will often note that their stress and tension is reflected in their gut and be aware of the consequences of stress–the knot in the stomach, cramps, loss of appetite, diarrhoea etc,. This type of abdominal pain tends to be intermittent and is clearly related to the emotional state.

Prolonged *qi* stagnation can contribute to several complications which also cause pain–Blood stagnation, stagnant Heat and Spleen deficiency with the eventual generation of internal Cold or Phlegm Damp. In addition, *qi* stagnation leads to a generalised hypertonicity of both skeletal and smooth muscle, further restricting the circulation of *qi* and Blood to the tissues.

Blood stagnation

Blood stagnation type abdominal pain may be acute or chronic. Acute pain may follow abdominal trauma or surgery. Chronic pain follows some other prolonged disorder affecting the abdomen. Any pathology, excess or deficient, if long lasting enough, may lead to Blood stasis or involve elements of Blood stasis. Some pathologies are particularly good at causing Blood stagnation. Cold pathologies (Cold and *yang* deficiency) can cause Blood stagnation by 'freezing and constricting' the vessels and slowing circulation of *qi* and Blood. Hot pathologies (Heat, Damp Heat, Phlegm Heat and *yin* deficiency) can cause stagnation by 'evaporating' Blood and increasing the viscosity and stickiness of Blood. Chronic Liver *qi* stagnation fails to lead the Blood and is a very common precursor to Blood stagnation.

Diet

The type of food consumed and the way it is consumed are important factors in the genesis of abdominal pain. Eating spoiled or contaminated food can produce acute pain, which in TCM terms may resemble an invasion of external Cold Damp or Damp Heat.

Too much cold natured or raw food can introduce Cold and weaken Spleen *qi* and *yang*. Some drugs weaken the Spleen and deplete Spleen *qi* and *yang*. These include purgative laxatives, antibiotics, nonsteroidal anti-inflammatory drugs (NSAIDs), and the antiretroviral drugs and protease inhibitors used to treat HIV infection. Reduced food intake as a result of strict dieting, or prolonged starvation and digestive insult, seriously damages Spleen *yang*. This can occur in patients with a history of anorexia nervosa, bulimia, or during famine.

Overconsumption in general, and excessive consumption of rich, heating or supplementing foods in particular, can lead to the accumulation of stagnant food and Heat or Damp Heat in the Stomach and Intestines. Food stagnation is a common precursor to a host of pathologies that may give rise to abdominal pain (*see* p.3). An excess of heating food, such as chillies, coffee, spirits, spices, fats and meat can introduce Heat and Damp, or damage *yin*. Sugar and dairy products create Dampness and Phlegm.

Figure 2.2 *Typical sites of some common biomedical causes of chronic abdominal pain*

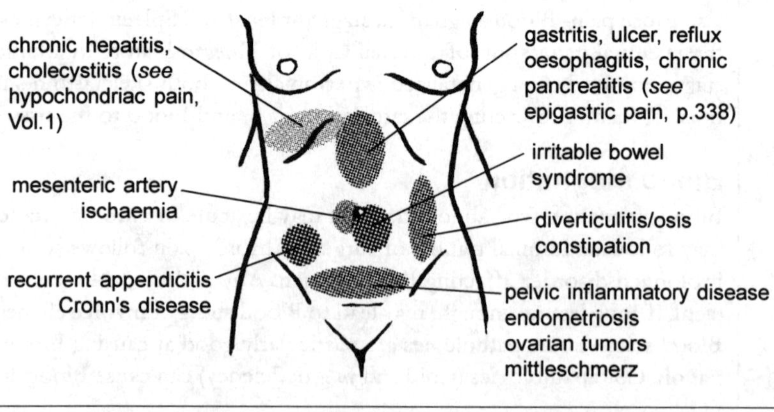

BOX 2.2 KEY DIAGNOSTIC POINTS

General

Careful questioning is necessary to clearly identify the nature and location of the pain.

- Ask the patient to point precisely to the pain, do not accept a vague wave of the hand.
- Do not assume that common terms like stomach, belly or tummy mean the same to everyone (for example, a common source of terminological confusion– patients often complain of 'stomach' pain when pointing to the lower abdomen).
- Rate the pain on a scale of severity (for example interference with sleep is classed as severe).
- Ask about diet, fluid intake and all drugs and medications
- Be aware that the intensity of physical signs may be reduced in the elderly or obese, and in patients taking steroids and analgesics.

Duration

- acute pain - excess
- chronic or recurrent - excess or deficient or mixed
- constant and progressive - severe Cold or Toxic Heat

Distribution

- focal, localised (points with a finger) - Blood stagnation
- vague, unlocalised (open hand indicates a wide area) - *qi* stagnation

Aggravation

- with pressure - excess
- with eating - excess

Amelioration

- with pressure - deficiency
- with heat - cold
- with rest - deficiency
- with activity - *qi* stagnation

Nature of the pain

- severe, cramping and continuous - Cold
- stabbing and fixed - Blood stagnation
- distension and variable intermittent mobile pain - *qi* stagnation
- dull, nagging - deficiency

Associations

- menstrual cycle - gynaecological
- eating, defecating - gastro-intestinal

PHYSIOLOGY OF PAIN

Pain in TCM terms is always due to some impediment to the circulation of *qi* and Blood, hence the adage **where there is obstruction there is pain, where there is no obstruction there is no pain** (*bu tong ze tong, tong ze bu tong* 不通则痛，通则不痛). This important principle provides a guide for the treatment of all types of pain. Pain can be broadly divided into two types–excess and deficient. *See also* p.343.

Excess pain is caused by the presence of a pathogen which physically obstructs *qi* and Blood flow. Any pathogen can hinder the flow of *qi* and Blood, but Cold, *qi* stagnation and Blood stagnation are the most likely to produce pain. The general principle of treatment for excess pain is to identify the obstructing pathogen and eliminate it.

Deficient pain is the result of insufficient motive force behind the circulation of low levels of *qi* and Blood, so that they become sluggish and begin to pool. This is likened to the stagnant pools that form in a riverbed as the water level drops during drought. Pain results, and the solution is to restore the *qi*, *yang* and Blood.

TCM DIFFERENTIAL DIAGNOSIS

- **Intestinal abscess** (*chang yong* 肠痈): An Intestinal abscess is a focal area of Heat (or Cold when chronic) and Blood stagnation causing pain in consistent areas of the abdomen, most commonly the right iliac fossa, but sometimes the left iliac fossa or suprapubic region. An Intestinal abscess is often acute and associated with fever, bowel disturbances, nausea and vomiting. Biomedical conditions such as acute and chronic appendicitis, diverticular disease and gynaecological infection, as well as abscesses in the intestinal tract may be included in this category.
- **Painful Urination syndrome** (*lin zheng* 淋证): Painful urination syndrome is a disorder characterised by suprapubic pain with dysuria, discomfort, and burning during urination. In biomedical terms, painful urination syndrome includes such diseases as urinary tract infections, urinary calculi, pyelonephritis, tumours of the urogenital system, prostatic diseases, chyluria and albuminuria. *See* Volume 1.
- ***Shan qi*** (疝气): *Shan qi* refers to pain and swelling in the lower abdomen, groin and external genitals, particularly the testicles and scrotum. It is usually related to dysfunction of the Liver and Liver channel. From a biomedical point of view, *shan qi* describes disorders such as herniae, varicocele, hydrocele, testicular torsion and orchitis. *See* Volume 1.

A note on abdominal palpation

Abdominal palpation is one of the key diagnostic features in deciding the nature of abdominal pain. Pain that is worse, and stays worse, when pressure is applied is considered excess, regardless of the deficient or otherwise weak state of the patient. Pain that is relieved with pressure (or at least not made worse), is considered deficient, regardless of the robust nature or appearance of the patient. Pain that is worse initially and then eases with continued pressure is associated with *qi* stagnation. When a pattern appears contradictory, the abdominal palpation findings should be regarded as the primary diagnostic finding. For example: a thin pale patient with obvious signs of *qi* deficiency complains of right iliac fossa pain which is definitely worse with palpation. Even though the patient is weak, the primary aim of therapy should be to clear the excess in the lower abdomen, with secondary support for *zheng qi*.

Abdominal palpation can also give information about the Heat or Cold nature of a pathogen. This should be done in two stages at the beginning of the examination, before any actual palpation is done. Firstly, a hand is held just above the surface of the abdomen to detect any areas of radiant Heat or Cold, and then lightly touches the surface of the abdomen. If the practitioner's hand rests too long in one place or too firmly, it will alter the temperature at that locus. Certain temperature findings are common and quite consistent from patient to patient. For example, patients with Spleen *qi* or *yang* deficiency digestive problems often feel cooler in the upper abdomen and epigastrium; patients with Kidney *yang* deficiency often feel cooler in the lower abdomen. Any locus of inflammation in the abdomen will be reflected in warmer tissues above, as any decrease in circulation, from Cold, Blood stagnation etc., will show in cooler areas above.

TREATMENT

TCM treatment of abdominal pain is frequently effective, however, practitioners should keep in mind the conditions that require emergency intervention (*see* Box 2.1 and 2.3). Because of the potential for complications in abdominal pain patterns, treatment should not proceed without a clear diagnosis, from both a biomedical and TCM perspective. Patients with acute abdominal pain patterns should be followed up every day, until the symptoms subside.

BOX 2.3 WHEN TO REFER FOR BIOMEDICAL INTERVENTION

- Acute severe abdominal pain with rigidity (perforated peptic ulcer, ruptured or dissecting aortic aneurysm, ruptured ectopic pregnancy, twisted ovarian cyst, acute peritonitis).
- Severe, progressive or projectile vomiting, faecal vomitus (intestinal obstruction).
- Progressive abdominal distension.
- When the patient is pale, sweating copiously and reluctant to move.

Figure 2.3 *Common locations of pain in certain biomedically defined diseases*

Diffuse abdominal pain–peritonitis, pancreatitis, leukaemia, sickle cell crisis, mesenteric adenitis/thrombosis, gastroenteritis, early appendicitis, colitis, intestinal obstruction

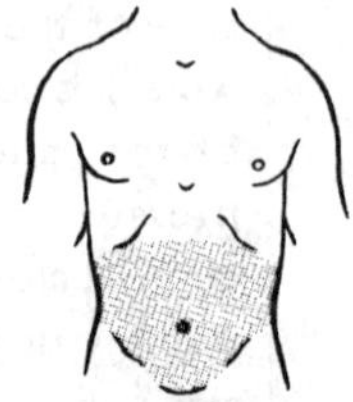

Right upper quadrant pain–gall bladder and biliary tract, hepatitis, hepatic abscess, hepatomegaly from congestive cardiac failure, peptic ulcer, pancreatitis, retrocecal appendicitis, renal colic, shingles

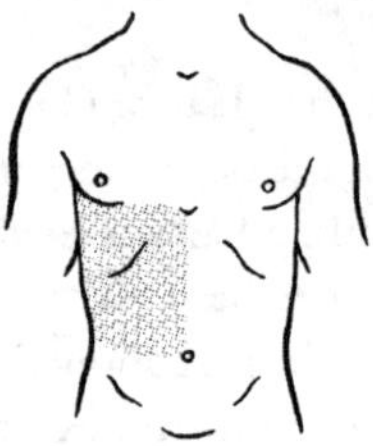

Left upper quadrant pain–splenic enlargement, gastritis, pancreatitis, infarct, aneurysm or rupture, renal colic, shingles, myocardial ischaemia

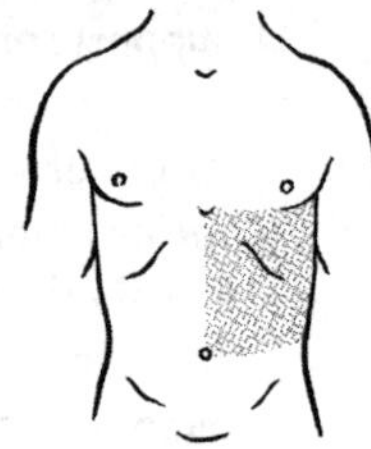

Right lower quadrant pain–appendicitis, intestinal obstruction, Crohn's disease, diverticulitis, perforated ulcer, leaking aneurysm, ectopic pregnancy, ovarian cyst, ovarian torsion, salpingitis, mittleschmerz, endometriosis, renal colic, urinary tract calculi, psoas abscess

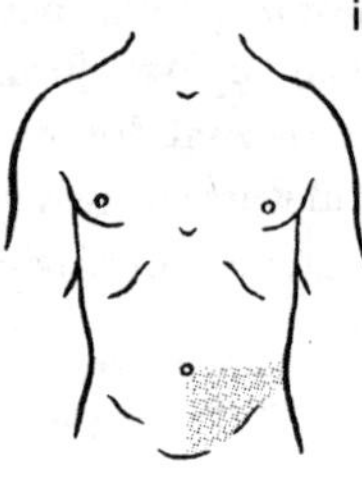

Left lower quadrant pain–diverticulitis, intestinal obstruction, ectopic pregnancy, mittleschmerz, ovarian cyst, ovarian torsion, salpingitis, endometriosis, psoas abscess, urinary tract calculi, renal colic, seminal vesiculitis

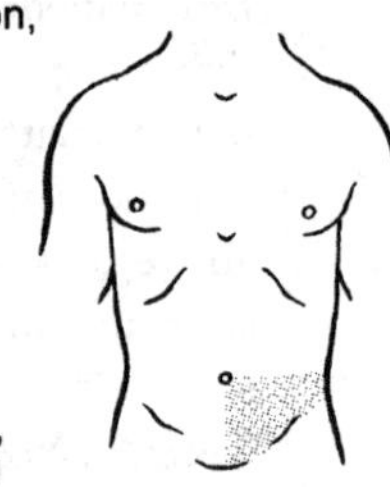

Myofacial trigger points in the abdominal muscles. These are included because they are a relatively common and frequently overlooked cause of chronic abdominal pain. The **X** represents common sites of trigger point activity, the shaded area the distribution of refered pain.

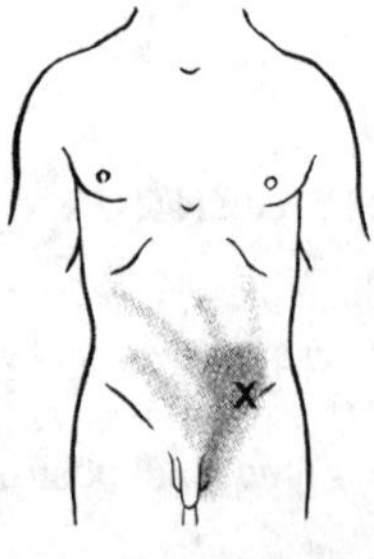

External oblique

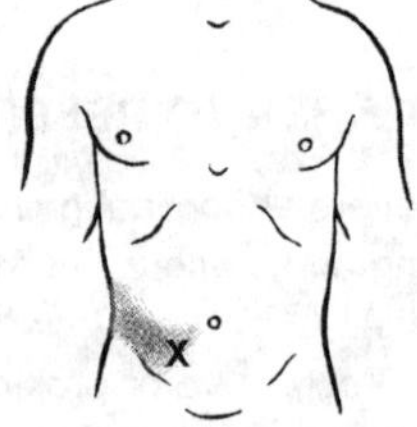

Rectus abdominus

Figure 2.4 *Diagnostic strategy for abdominal pain*

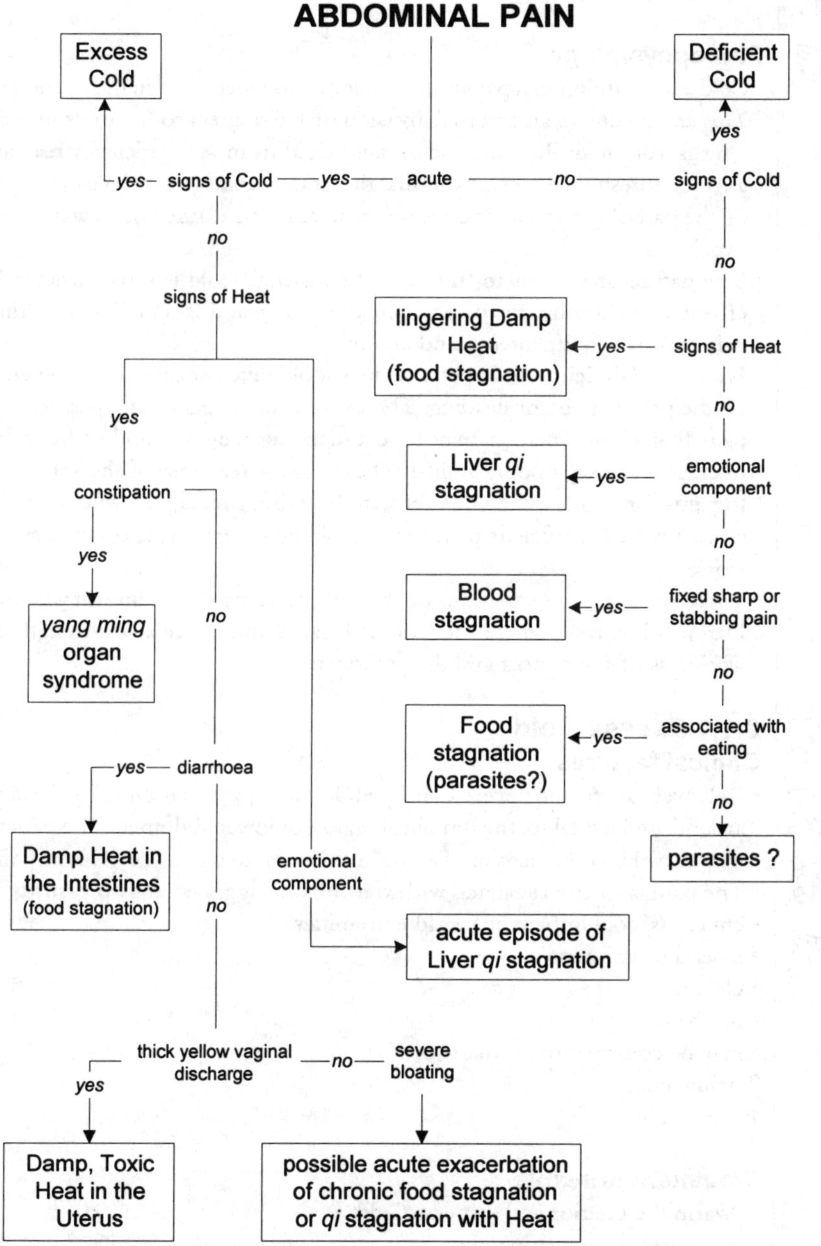

寒腹痛

2.1 COLD

2.1.1 Excess Cold
2.1.2 Deficient Cold

Pathophysiology

- Cold excess abdominal pain is the result of too much Cold in the abdomen. This can be due to an external invasion of Cold direct to the Intestines or Uterus. Alternatively, it may be because Cold from *yang* deficiency reaches a critical threshold of severity so that the Cold becomes the primary element of the pathology. In either case, the main aim of treatment is to warm and expel Cold.
- The nature of Cold is to 'freeze and constrict'. Cold is thus particularly effective in shutting down the circulation of *qi* and Blood. The resulting pain is usually quite intense and cramping.
- Excess and deficient Cold patterns may look quite similar and the severity of the pain may be misleading. The experience of pain is subjective, and pain that to one person may be excruciating may to another be quite tolerable. The key finding in difficult cases is the response of the abdomen to palpation–both will feel better with heat, but excess pain will be worse when pressed. Deficient pain may be better for pressure, or at least no worse.
- There are numerous variations of the Cold patterns, depending on whether Damp is involved, where the Cold is located and the relative strength or weakness of the patient and the pathogen.

寒实腹痛

2.1.1 Excess Cold

Clinical features

- Relatively acute and severe colicky abdominal pain that typically focuses around, and lateral to, the umbilical region or lower abdomen. The patient may draw his or her legs up, flexing at the waist to try to alleviate the pain. The pain is clearly alleviated with warmth and aggravated by pressure.
- chilliness, cold intolerance, cold extremities
- nausea or vomiting
- clear urine
- no thirst
- may be constipation or diarrhoea

T white coat
P wiry, tight

Treatment principle

Warm the interior and disperse Cold
Support *yang* and stop pain

Prescription

SI NI TANG 四逆汤
(*Frigid Extremities Decoction*)

This prescription is suitable for relatively severe cases. There may be underlying elements of *yang* deficiency. If there are no signs of recovery within 24 hours, or 2-3 doses, refer for further investigations.

zhi fu zi (Radix Aconiti Carmichaeli Praeparata) 制附子 9-12g
gan jiang (Rhizoma Zingiberis Officinalis) 干姜 9-12g
zhi gan cao (honey fried Radix Glycyrrhizae Uralensis)
炙甘草 6-9g

Method: Decoction. **Zhi fu zi** is cooked for 30 minutes before the other herbs (*xian jian* 先煎). **Zhi fu zi** powerfully warms and stimulates *yang qi*; it is supported by the **gan jiang** which warms the Spleen and Stomach and assists the **fu zi** in warming *yang*; **gan cao** protects the Stomach from the dispersing action of the main herbs.

Variations and additional prescriptions

Mild conditions

- In relatively mild conditions, a gentle approach is usually sufficient. This prescription is suitable for acute pain provoked by ingesting cold foods or fluids, or by an invasion of external Cold causing cramping pain. The bowels may be loose or normal. The aim of treatment is to warm the Spleen and Stomach and dispel Cold with **LIANG FU WAN** (*Galangal and Cyperus Pill* 良附丸).

gao liang jiang (Rhizoma Alpiniae Officinari) 高良姜 9-12g
xiang fu (Rhizoma Cyperi Rotundi) 香附 9-12g

Method: Decoction. **Gao liang jiang** warms the middle *jiao* and alleviates pain; **xiang fu** warms and regulates *qi*.

With constipation

- When Cold constrains all movement in the Intestines, abdominal pain with constipation, cold intolerance and cold extremities may result. The aim of treatment is to dispel Cold, unblock the bowels and stop pain with **DA HUANG FU ZI TANG** (*Rhubarb and Prepared Aconite Decoction* 大黄附子汤). If there is no bowel movement within 24 hours, referral for further investigation is recommended.

zhi fu zi (Radix Aconiti Carmichaeli Praeparata) 制附子 9-12g
da huang (Radix et Rhizoma Rhei) 大黄 6-9g
xi xin (Herba cum Radice Asari) 细辛 3-6g

Method: Decoction. **Zhi fu zi** is cooked for 30 minutes before the other herbs (*xian jian* 先煎). **Zhi fu zi** warms *yang* and dispels Cold; **da huang** is used to purge the Intestine, while its bitter coldness is balanced by the heat of the other herbs; **xi xin** dispels Cold.

With severe pain, add **bai shao** (Radix Paeoniae Lactiflorae) 白芍 15-24g and

gui zhi (Ramulus Cinnamomi Cassiae) 桂枝 9-12g; with abdominal distension, add **hou po** (Cortex Magnoliae Officinalis) 厚朴 9-12g and **mu xiang** (Radix Aucklandiae Lappae) 木香 6-9g; if the patient is weak or elderly, use **zhi da huang** (processed Radix et Rhizoma Rhei) 制大黄 and add **dang shen** (Radix Codonopsis Pilosulae) 党参 15-24g and **dang gui** (Radix Angelicae Sinensis) 当归 9-12g. (Source: *Shi Yong Zhong Yi Nei Ke Xue*)

With severe pain

- Severe abdominal pain and coldness which can't stand any pressure at all, incessant vomiting to the point of not being able to eat, borborygmus, a greasy white tongue coat and a thready, slow, wiry or tight pulse point to strong rebellious Cold in the abdomen, usually with deficiency of the middle *jiao*. The aim of treatment is to powerfully warm the interior, redirect *qi* downwards and stop pain, with **DA JIAN ZHONG TANG** (*Major Zanthoxylum Combination* 大建中汤). This prescription is used for excess accumulation of *yin* Cold with underlying Spleen *yang* deficiency. The main features here are associated with the dominance of the excess Cold. The underlying deficiency can be dealt with after alleviation of the pain and vomiting. If there are no signs of recovery within 24 hours, or 2-3 doses, refer for further investigations.

  chuan jiao (Pericarpium Zanthoxyli Bungeani) 川椒 6-9g
  gan jiang (Rhizoma Zingiberis Officinalis) 干姜 9-12g

Figure 2.5 *Variations of excess Cold abdominal pain*

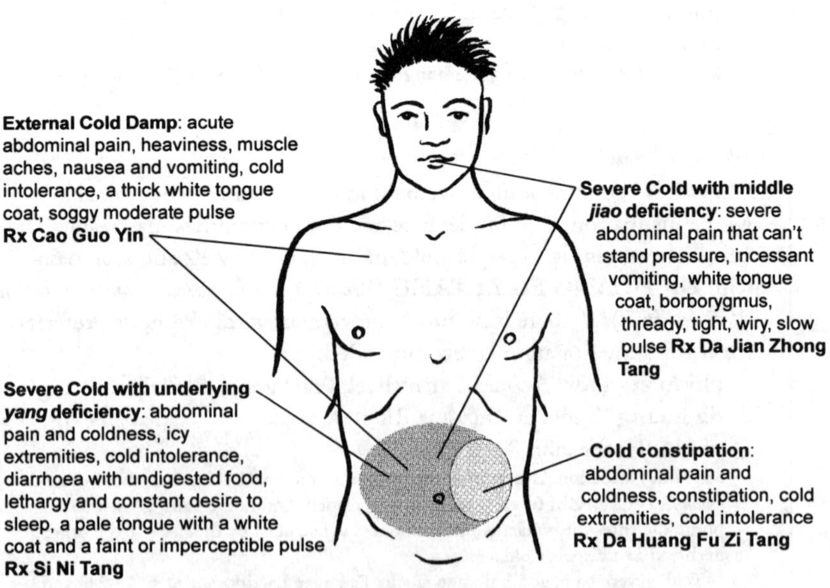

dang shen (Radix Codonopsis Pilosulae) 党参 15-24g
yi tang (Saccharum Granorum) 饴糖 30g

Method: Decoction. **Yi tang** is dissolved in the strained decoction (*yang hua* 烊化). **Chuan jiao** dispels Cold and stops pain; **gan jiang** warms the middle *jiao* and dispels Cold; **dang shen** and **yi tang** strengthen the Spleen and alleviate spasm.

With external Cold Damp invasion

- An invasion of external Cold Damp, may cause acute abdominal pain and distension that is worse for pressure, a very thick and greasy white tongue coat, cold intolerance, nausea and vomiting, loss of appetite, heaviness in the body, lethargy, muscle aches and a soggy, moderate pulse. The treatment is to warm the middle *jiao* and fragrantly disperse and dry Dampness with **CAO GUO YIN** (*Tsaoko Decoction* 草果饮).

cao guo (Fructus Amomi Tsao-ko) 草果 6g
gao liang jiang (Rhizoma Alpiniae Officinari) 高良姜 6g
qing pi (Pericarpium Citri Reticulatae Viride) 青皮 6g
huo xiang (Herba Agastaches seu Pogostemi) 藿香 9g
ban xia (Rhizoma Pinelliae Ternatae) 半夏 9g
hou po (Cortex Magnoliae Officinalis) 厚朴 6g
ding xiang (Flos Caryophylli) 丁香 6g
sheng jiang (Rhizoma Zingiberis Officinalis Recens) 生姜 3pce
da zao (Fructus Zizyphi Jujubae) 大枣 4pce

Method: Decoction. **Cao guo** and **hou po** dry Damp and disperse Cold; **gao liang jiang** and **ding xiang** warm the middle *jiao* and stop pain; **qing pi** and **hou po** regulate *qi*; **huo xiang** fragrantly transforms Damp, and with **ban xia** and **sheng jiang** directs *qi* downwards and stops nausea and vomiting; **da zao** and **sheng jiang** moderate spasms and ease the middle *jiao*. (Source: *Shi Yong Zhong Yao Xue*)

Patent medicines

Su He Xiang Wan 苏合香丸 (Liquid Styrax Pill)
- An extremely fragrant pill that powerfully disperses *qi* and Cold accumulation; usually used for acute abdominal and chest pain from Cold.

Fu Zi Li Zhong Wan 附子理中丸 (Fu Tzu Li Chung Wan, Carmichaeli Tea Pills, Li Chung Yuen Medical Pills)
- relatively severe Cold and/or *yang* deficiency pain.

Li Zhong Wan 理中丸 (Li Zhong Wan)

Xing Jun San 行军散 (Marching Powder, Five Pagodas Brand)

Huo Xiang Zheng Qi Pian 藿香正气片 (Huo Xiang Zheng Qi Pian, Huo Hsiang Cheng Chi Pien)
- The last two with exterior Cold Damp signs and symptoms. With severe or colicky spasmodic pain, wash the patent formula

selected down with a strong decoction of fresh ginger and cinnamon sticks.

Acupuncture (select from)

Ren.12 (*zhong wan* -▲) .... *mu* point of the Stomach, warms and regulates the Stomach, dispels Cold and directs Stomach *qi* downwards

St.25 (*tian shu* -▲) .... *mu* point of the Large Intestine, warms and regulates Intestinal function, dispels Cold

Ren.6 (*qi hai* ▲) .... dispels Cold, warms the abdomen

St.34 (*liang qiu* -) .... *xi* cleft point of the Stomach, stops acute pain

St.36 (*zu san li* ▲) .... *he* sea point of the Stomach, powerfully warms and strengthens the Spleen and Stomach, and supplements *qi*

St.37 (*shan ju xu* -) .... lower *he* point of the Large Intestine, regulates and eliminates Cold from the Stomach and Intestines

Sp.4 (*gong sun* -) .... *luo* point of the Spleen, master point of *chong mai*, regulates the Spleen and Stomach, stops pain

Sp.6 (*san yin jiao*) .... strengthens the Spleen, elevates Spleen *qi* and encourages turbid *qi* to descend

- with vomiting, add PC.6 (*nei guan*)
- with severe pain or diarrhoea, apply strong moxa on Ren.8 (*shen que*), usually on salt. Place a piece of thin cloth over the navel and fill it with salt. Burn large cones of moxa on the salt. The cloth enables quick removal of the salt and prevents burning.
- *Ear points*: abdomen, large intestine, small intestine, stomach, spleen, *shen men*, sympathetic

Clinical notes

- Excess Cold type abdominal pain may be diagnosed biomedically as intestinal spasm, intestinal obstruction, appendicitis, ulcerative colitis, stomach flu, viral illness or acute gastroenteritis.
- In mild cases, handy for those evening telephone consultations as most homes will have both ingredients, a strong decoction of fresh ginger and cinnamon sticks, 10-15 grams each boiled in 2-3 cups of water for 15 minutes, may suffice.

虚寒腹痛

2.1.2 Deficient Cold

There are numerous presentations of this common type of abdominal pain, depending on the location and nature of the deficiency, whether Intestinal or Uterine, and the degree of deficiency involved.

Clinical features

- Chronic, intermittent, spasmodic, dull abdominal pain which is alleviated by warmth and pressure, and by ingesting warm food and fluids.
- waxy pale or lustreless complexion
- cold intolerance, cold extremities
- lethargy and fatigue
- shortness of breath
- poor appetite, early satiety
- depression, low spirits

T pale and possibly swollen, with a white coat
P thready and weak

Treatment principle

Warm the interior and supplement *qi* and *yang*
Strengthen the Spleen and Stomach, and stop pain

Prescription

XIAO JIAN ZHONG TANG 小健中汤
(*Minor Cinnamon and Peony Combination*)

gui zhi (Ramulus Cinnamomi Cassiae) 桂枝 9-12g
bai shao (Radix Paeoniae Lactiflorae) 白芍 12-15g
sheng jiang (Rhizoma Zingiberis Officinalis Recens) 生姜 9-12g
zhi gan cao (honey fried Radix Glycyrrhizae Uralensis) 炙甘草 6-9g
da zao (Fructus Zizyphi Jujubae) 大枣 4pce
yi tang (Saccharum Granorum) 饴糖 30g

Method: Decoction. **Yi tang** is dissolved in the strained decoction (*yang hua* 烊化). **Gui zhi** warms the middle *jiao* and dispels Cold; **gui zhi** and **yi tang** combine pungent and sweet flavours to bolster *yang*; **bai shao**, **zhi gan cao** and **yi tang** moderate spasmodic pain; **sheng jiang** and **da zao** harmonise and warm the Stomach. (Source: *Shi Yong Zhong Yi Nei Ke Xue*)

Modifications

- With spontaneous sweating, low grade fever and frequent colds add **zhi huang qi** (honey fried Radix Astragali Membranacei) 炙黄芪 18-30g.
- For constant unlocalised abdominal pain and weakness following childbirth, add **dang gui** (Radix Angelicae Sinensis) 当归 9-12g. A tasty

and simple approach to this problem is to stew **dang gui** and **sheng jiang** (Rhizoma Zingiberis Officinalis Recens) 生姜 15-20g with mutton to warm and nourish Blood and stop pain.

Variations and additional prescriptions

With Spleen yang deficiency

- With Spleen *yang* deficiency, characterised by upper abdominal pain that is better for warmth and pressure, diarrhoea with undigested food (or occasionally constipation), copious clear urine, cold extremities, cold intolerance, a deep, slow and thready pulse and a pale swollen tongue, the aim of treatment is to warm and supplement Spleen *yang* with **FU ZI LI ZHONG WAN** (*Aconite, Ginseng and Ginger Formula* 附子理中丸, p.373).

With Spleen yang deficiency and constipation

- In patients with Spleen *yang* deficiency and resistant constipation, **WEN PI TANG** (*Warm the Spleen Decoction* 温脾汤) can be used to warm and supplement Spleen *yang* and purge Cold accumulation.

    zhi fu zi (Radix Aconiti Carmichaeli Praeparata)
    制附子 6-12g

Figure 2.6 *Variations of deficient Cold abdominal pain*

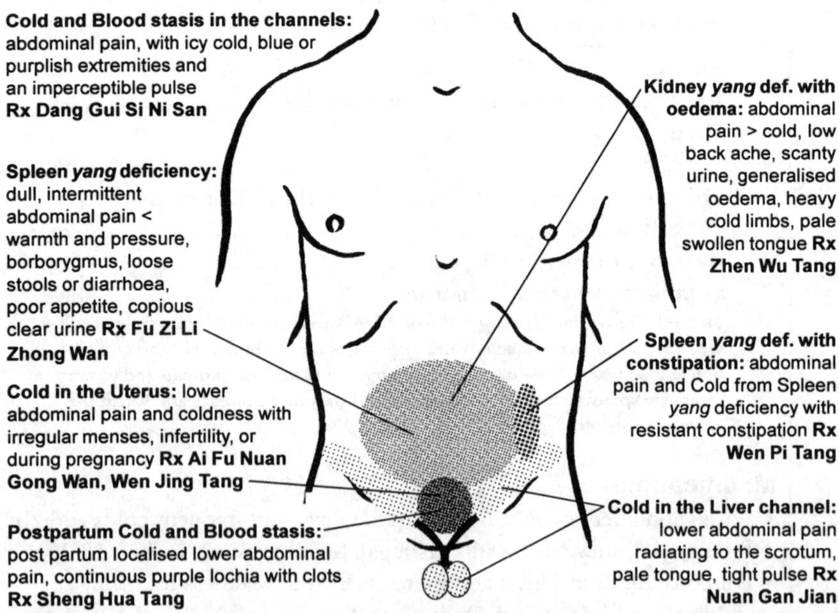

gan jiang (Rhizoma Zingiberis Officinalis) 干姜 6-9g
dang shen (Radix Codonopsis Pilosulae) 党参 15-24g
zhi gan cao (honey fried Radix Glycyrrhizae Uralensis)
炙甘草 6-9g
da huang (Radix et Rhizoma Rhei) 大黄 6-9g

Method: Decoction. **Zhi fu zi** is cooked for 30 minutes before adding the other herbs (*xian jian* 先煎). **Zhi fu zi** and **gan jiang** powerfully warm the middle *jiao* and dispel Cold, as well as stimulating Spleen and Stomach *yang qi* to promote correct functioning of the *qi* mechanism; **dang shen** and **zhi gan cao** support Spleen *qi* and protect the Stomach; **da huang** purges accumulation from the Intestines. Its bitter coldness is moderated by the hot herbs.

With Kidney yang deficiency and oedema

- With Kidney *yang* deficiency, causing abdominal pain that is worse for cold, scanty urination, oedema of the lower limbs, loose stools, dizziness, watery cough, heaviness and aching in the limbs and head, palpitations, a pale swollen tongue and a deep weak or imperceptible pulse, the aim of treatment is to warm *yang* and promote urination with **ZHEN WU TANG** (*True Warrior Decoction* 真武汤, p.911).

With Cold and Blood stagnation in the channels

- With Blood deficiency, stagnation of Cold internally and Cold lodged in the channels, the clinical features are abdominal pain accompanied by icy cold hands and feet that are blue or purplish and difficult to warm up, and a thready or imperceptible pulse. The aim of treatment is to warm the channels, disperse Cold, nourish the Blood and unblock the vessels with **DANG GUI SI NI TANG** (*Dang Gui Decoction for Frigid Extremities* 当归四逆汤). This type of pattern occurs in various peripheral vascular disorders, such as some connective tissue disorders with Raynaud's syndrome or peripheral neuropathies.

dang gui (Radix Angelicae Sinensis) 当归 9-12g
gui zhi (Ramulus Cinnamomi Cassiae) 桂枝 9-12g
bai shao (Radix Paeoniae Lactiflora) 白芍 12-18g
xi xin (Herba cum Radice Asari) 细辛 3-6g
mu tong (Caulis Mutong) 木通 3-6g
zhi gan cao (honey fried Radix Glycyrrhizae Uralensis)
炙甘草 6-9g
da zao (Fructus Zizyphi Jujubae) 大枣 4pce

Method: Decoction. **Dang gui** regulates Blood, and with **bai shao** supplements Blood; **gui zhi** and **xi xin** warm the channels and disperse Cold; **gui zhi** and **bai shao** harmonise the relationship between *ying* and *wei qi* and thus assist in warming the superficial tissues; **mu tong** promotes the flow of *qi* through the channels; **zhi gan cao** and **da zao** support the Spleen; **zhi gan cao** and **bai shao** alleviate spasmodic pain. (Source: *Shi Yong Zhong Yi Nei Ke Xue*)

With Cold accumulation in the Uterus

- If the abdominal pain is associated with Cold accumulation in the Uterus (lower abdomen pain alleviated by warmth and pressure, irregular and/or painful menstruation, infertility or pain of this type during the second or third trimester of pregnancy), the aim of treatment is to warm the Uterus, supplement the Blood (and calm the foetus) with **AI FU NUAN GONG WAN** (*Mugwort and Prepared Aconite Pill for Warming the Womb* 艾附暖宫丸).

  cu xiang fu (vinegar fried Rhizoma Cyperi Rotundi) 醋香附 180g
  ai ye (Folium Artemisiae Argyi) 艾叶 90g
  dang gui (Radix Angelicae Sinensis) 当归 90g
  zhi huang qi (honey fried Radix Astragali Membranacei) 炙黄芪 60g
  wu zhu yu (Fructus Evodiae Rutaecarpae) 吴茱萸 60g
  bai shao (Radix Paeoniae Lactiflorae) 白芍 60g
  chuan xiong (Radix Ligustici Chuanxiong) 川芎 60g
  xu duan (Radix Dipsaci Asperi) 续断 45g
  sheng di (Radix Rehmanniae Glutinosae) 生地 30g
  rou gui (Cortex Cinnamomi Cassiae) 肉桂 15g

  Method: Grind herbs to a powder and form into 9-gram pills with honey. The dose is one pill 2-3 times daily. May also be decocted with a 90% reduction in quantities. **Cu xiang fu** warms the Uterus, regulates *qi* and stops pain; **ai ye** warms the Uterus, dispels Cold and stops bleeding; **dang gui** and **zhi huang qi** powerfully supplement *qi* and Blood; **dang gui**, **bai shao**, **sheng di** and **chuan xiong** form **SI WU TANG**, the fundamental prescription for nourishing Blood; **rou gui** assists the transformation of *qi* into Blood, and with **wu zhu yu** warms *yang*; **xu duan** supplements Kidney *yang*, warms the Uterus and calms a restless foetus. (Source: *Shi Yong Zhong Yao Xue*)

With postpartum Cold and Blood stagnation

- Fixed lower abdominal pain and coldness in a postpartum woman, with incomplete expulsion of the placenta, continual discharge of purple clotted lochia and a pale purplish tongue is Cold and Blood stagnation in the Uterus. The aim of treatment is to invigorate the Blood, dispel Blood stasis, warm the Uterus and stop pain with **SHENG HUA TANG** (*Generation and Transformation Decoction* 生化汤). This prescription is frequently given to women for the first few days following childbirth to ensure complete expulsion of the placenta, or following incomplete miscarriage with continued bleeding and pain.

  dang gui (Radix Angelicae Sinensis) 当归 12-24g
  chuan xiong (Radix Ligustici Chuanxiong) 川芎 6-9g
  tao ren (Semen Persicae) 桃仁 6-9g

pao jiang (quick fried Rhizoma Zingiberis Officinalis)
炮姜 3-6g
zhi gan cao (honey fried Radix Glycyrrhizae Uralensis)
炙甘草 3-6g

Method: Decoction. Often taken with a little alcohol, such as yellow wine or vodka. **Dang gui** regulates and nourishes Blood; **chuan xiong** and **tao ren** invigorate Blood and eliminate stagnant Blood; **pao jiang** warms the Uterus, dispels Cold and stops bleeding and pain; **zhi gan cao** warms the middle *jiao* and eases spasmodic pain.

With Cold and qi stagnation in the genitals

- If Cold invades the Liver channel disrupting the movement of *qi*, it may cause lower abdominal pain (in men) radiating to the testicles, accompanied by a pale tongue and a deep tight pulse. The aim of treatment is to warm the Liver channel, move *qi* and stop pain, with **NUAN GAN JIAN** (*Warm the Liver Decoction* 暖肝煎).

rou gui (Cortex Cinnamomi Cassiae) 肉桂 6g
xiao hui xiang (Fructus Foeniculi Vulgaris) 小茴香 9-12g
fu ling (Sclerotium Poria Cocos) 茯苓 12-15g
wu yao (Radix Linderae Strychnifoliae) 乌药 6-9g
gou qi zi (Fructus Lycii) 枸杞子 9-12g
dang gui (Radix Angelicae Sinensis) 当归 9-12g
chen xiang (Lignum Aquilariae) 沉香 3-6g
sheng jiang (Rhizoma Zingiberis Officinalis Recens)
生姜 6-9g

Method: Decoction. **Rou gui** and **xiao hui xiang** warm the Liver channel and dispel Cold, **wu yao** and **chen xiang** regulate and warm *qi* and alleviate pain; **gou qi zi** and **dang gui** nourish Liver *yin* and Blood to relax the Tendons; **fu ling** strengthens the Spleen and leaches out Dampness; **sheng jiang** warms the Stomach.

With Cold and deficiency of chong and ren mai

- Lower abdominal pain, distension and coldness that are better for warmth, an irregular menstrual cycle (usually long, and either heavy or scant flow, with clotting), mild persistent uterine bleeding, lumbar and sacral pain which are worse following menstruation or when tired, profuse clear watery leucorrhoea, a pale tongue with a greasy white coat and deep slow pulse all point to Cold and deficiency of *chong* and *ren mai*. The aim of treatment is to warm the channels and disperse Cold, move *qi* and regulate Blood with **WEN JING TANG** (*Dang Gui and Evodia Combination* 温经汤) modified. This pattern may be associated with low grade chronic pelvic inflammatory disease and infertility.

wu zhu yu (Fructus Evodiae Rutaecarpae) 吴茱萸 3-6g
rou gui (Cortex Cinnamomi Cassiae) 肉桂 3-6g

dang gui (Radix Angelicae Sinensis) 当归 9-12g
bai shao (Radix Paeoniae Lactiflorae) 白芍 12-18g
chuan xiong (Radix Ligustici Chuanxiong) 川芎 6-9g
sheng jiang (Rhizoma Zingiberis Officinalis Recens)
生姜 6-9g
ban xia (Rhizoma Pinelliae Ternatae) 半夏 9-12g
gan cao (Radix Glycyrrhizae Uralensis) 甘草 6-9g
dang shen (Radix Codonopsis Pilosulae) 党参 12-15g
e jiao (Gelatinum Corii Asini) 阿胶 6-9g
xiao hui xiang (Fructus Foeniculi Vulgaris) 小茴香 9-12g
ai ye (Folium Artemisiae Argyi) 艾叶 9-12g

Method: Decoction. **E jiao** is melted in the hot strained decoction (*yang hua* 烊化). **Wu zhu yu** and **rou gui** warm the Uterus, dispel Cold, unblock the channels and invigorate the circulation of lower *jiao qi*; **dang gui**, **bai shao** and **chuan xiong** nourish and regulate Blood and menstruation; **e jiao** nourishes *yin* and Blood and stops bleeding; **ban xia** and **sheng jiang** warm and harmonise the Stomach and dry Dampness and Phlegm; **dang shen** and **gan cao** support the Spleen and supplement *qi*; **bai shao** and **gan cao** alleviate spasmodic pain; **xiao hui xiang** and **ai ye** warm the Uterus and dispel Cold. (Source: *Shi Yong Fang Ji Xue*)

Patent medicines

Fu Zi Li Zhong Wan 附子理中丸 (Carmichaeli Tea Pills, Fu Tzu Li Chung Wan, Li Chung Yuen Medical Pills)
- Spleen *yang* deficiency

Li Zhong Wan 理中丸 (Li Zhong Wan)

Jin Kui Shen Qi Wan 金匮肾气丸 (Sexoton Pills, Golden Book Tea, Fu Gui Ba Wei Wan)
- Kidney *yang* deficiency

Fu Ke Wu Jin Wan 妇科乌金丸 (Woo Garm Yuen Medical Pills)
- for Cold, deficiency and Blood stagnation in the Uterus

Shi Quan Da Bu Wan 十全大补丸 (Shi Quan Da Bu Wan, Ten Flavour Tea) - *qi* and Blood deficiency with Cold

Acupuncture (select from)

Ren.12 (*zhong wan* +▲) .. *mu* point of the Stomach, warms and regulates the Stomach, dispels Cold and directs Stomach *qi* downwards

St.25 (*tian shu* +▲) .... *mu* point of the Large Intestine, warms and regulates Intestinal function, dispels Cold

Ren.6 (*qi hai* +▲) .... these points warm the Kidneys and Uterus,
Ren.4 (*guan yuan* +▲) dispel Cold and warm the lower abdomen

Ren.7 (*yin jiao*) .... together these points regulate *chong* and *ren mai*
St.30 (*qi chong*)

St.36 (*zu san li* +▲) .... *he* sea point of the Stomach, powerfully warms and strengthens the Spleen and Stomach, and supplements *qi*
Sp.4 (*gong sun*) .... *luo* point of the Spleen, master point of *chong mai*, regulates the Spleen and Stomach, stops pain
Sp.6 (*san yin jiao* +▲) ...... strengthens the Spleen and Kidney, invigorates *qi* and Blood, removes obstruction from the *jing luo*
Kid.3 (*tai xi* +▲) .... *yuan* point of the Kidney, warms Kidney *yang*
LI.11 (*qu chi* +▲) .... *he* sea point of the Large Intestine, warms *yang ming* and stimulates *yang qi* in general when moxaed

- a moxa box over the abdomen, warm needle or strong non-scarring moxa cones over the main abdominal points is recommended.
- with nausea, add PC.6 (*nei guan*)
- the medicinal plaster *Gou Pi Gao* 狗皮膏 (Kou Pi Kao) can be applied to the abdomen over the site of the pain.
- With severe pain or diarrhoea, apply strong moxa on Ren.8 (*shen que*), usually on salt. Place a piece of thin cloth over the navel and fill it with salt. Burn large cones of moxa on the salt. The cloth enables quick removal of the salt and prevents burning.
- *Ear points*: abdomen, large intestine, small intestine, stomach, spleen, *shen men*, adrenal, sympathetic

Clinical notes

- Deficient Cold abdominal pain may be diagnosed biomedically as chronic colitis, chronic peptic ulcer disease, irritable bowel syndrome, postpartum pain, dysmenorrhoea, endometriosis, infertility, Raynaud's syndrome or hypothyroidism.
- Deficient Cold type abdominal pain generally responds well to correct treatment. The pain can often be alleviated quite quickly, but treatment of the underlying pathology will usually take some time. Three to twelve months of treatment is not unusual, depending on the degree of deficiency and any complications, such as Blood stagnation.
- For dietary recommendations, see the p.873.

实热腹痛

2.2 HEAT

- *yang ming* Heat
- Damp Heat
  - Intestines
  - Uterus
  - Bladder (see painful urination syndrome, Volume 1)

Pathophysiology

- Heat, in whatever form, causes pain by drying the Intestines and causing constipation, by 'scorching and burning' the Intestines or Uterus, or by simply obstructing the smooth and regular circulation of *qi* and Blood.
- There are numerous variations of Heat abdominal pain patterns. The Heat may be due to the invasion of an external pathogen (Heat, or another pathogen that becomes hot once in the body), or it may be generated internally. The basic features of Heat patterns are common to all types.

Common clinical features

- Abdominal pain, fullness and distension that is worse for pressure. With gentle touch, the skin over the pain may feel warmer than the surrounding skin, or a distinct sensation of heat may be perceived when palpating more firmly.
- fever, usually tidal but may be high and continuous
- dry mouth, thirst
- restlessness, irritability
- sweating, either whole body or hands and feet
- concentrated urine

T red or with red spots and a greasy or dry brown or yellow coat
P strong, bounding, rapid, slippery, or deep and strong

Particular features

- **Heat in the Intestines**: pain in the left or right iliac fossa, constipation or diarrhoea or both, or faecal impaction with foul green spurious diarrhoea, in which case there will a palpable mass and pain in the left iliac fossa, frequent flatulence.
- **Heat in the Uterus**: pain in the lower abdomen, thick yellow malodorous vaginal discharge (± constipation); in acute cases with chills or rigors.

Treatment principle(s)

Clear Heat, stop pain
- by purgation (Intestines)
- Dry Damp, clear Damp Heat and Toxic Heat (Uterus)

Prescription

DA CHENG QI TANG 大承气汤
(*Major Rhubarb Combination*)

This prescription is selected for pathogenic invasion (traditionally Cold which turns Hot) into the Stomach and Intestines (*yang ming fu* syndrome). The main feature is severe constipation or faecal impaction with watery diarrhoea, a painful and distended abdomen which feels worse for pressure especially over the site of the stool, a tense, firm abdomen, tidal fever, a thick, yellow or brown and dry tongue coat and a deep strong pulse. The treatment is to purge Heat (with the stool). Usually no more than a few doses are required.

da huang (Radix et Rhizoma Rhei) 大黄 9-12g
mang xiao (Mirabilitum) 芒硝 6-9g
zhi shi (Fructus Immaturus Citri Aurantii) 枳实 9-12g
hou po (Cortex Magnoliae Officinalis) 厚朴 12-15g

Method: Decoction. For powerful purgation **da huang** is added a few minutes before the end of cooking (*hou xia* 后下). **Mang xiao** is dissolved in the strained decoction (*yang hua* 烊化). **Da huang** is the main herb for purging accumulation from the Intestines and clearing Heat; it is assisted in this by **mang xiao** which softens hard dry stools, easing their passage; **zhi shi** and **hou po** regulate *qi* and direct *qi* downwards, and alleviate the cramps that **da huang** can sometimes cause.

Variations and additional prescriptions

With umbilical and right iliac fossa pain

- Abdominal pain that begins around the navel, then concentrates in the right iliac fossa, is worse with pressure and associated with rebound tenderness, abdominal guarding, fever, nausea, constipation and or diarrhoea, a greasy yellow tongue coat and slippery rapid pulse, is defined as an Intestinal abscess. The aim of treatment is to open the bowels to clear and purge Heat, move *qi* and eliminate Blood stagnation with **DA HUANG MU DAN PI TANG** (*Rhubarb and Moutan Decoction* 大黄牡丹皮汤, p.657).

With Damp or Toxic Heat in the Intestines

- Damp Heat or Toxic Heat can lodge in the Intestines causing dysenteric disorder with quite severe lateral or central abdominal pain, difficult defecation or diarrhoea with pus, mucus, blood and tenesmus, thirst, a red tongue with a yellow coat and a wiry rapid pulse. The aim of treatment is to clear Heat, eliminate Toxins and cool the Blood with **SHAO YAO TANG** (*Peony Decoction* 芍药汤, p.270).

Toxic Heat in the Uterus

- An acute invasion of Heat, or Cold that transforms into Heat, into the Uterus may intensify to form Toxic Heat. The main feature is acute lower abdominal or suprapubic pain that feels warm or hot to touch and is worse for pressure. The pain is associated with high fever, chills or rigors, thirst, copious malodorous vaginal discharge with blood and/or pus, constipation, concentrated urine, a thick greasy yellow tongue coat and a slippery or wiry rapid pulse. The aim of treatment is to clear Toxic Heat and invigorate the Blood with **YIN QIAO HONG JIANG JIE DU TANG** (*Lonicera, Forsythia, Sargentodoxae and Patrinia Decoction to Eliminate Toxin* 银翘红酱解毒汤).

jin yin hua (Flos Lonicerae Japonicae) 金银花 30g
lian qiao (Fructus Forsythia Suspensae) 连翘 30g
bai jiang cao (Herba cum Radice Patriniae) 败酱草 30g
hong teng (Caulis Sargentodoxae Cuneatae) 红藤 30g
yi ren (Semen Coicis Lachryma-jobi) 苡仁 12-18g
shan zhi zi (Fructus Gardeniae Jasminoides) 山栀子 9-12g
tao ren (Semen Persicae) 桃仁 9-12g
chi shao (Radix Paeoniae Rubrae) 赤芍 9-12g
mu dan pi (Cortex Moutan Radicis) 牡丹皮 9-12g
yan hu suo (Rhizoma Corydalis Yanhusuo) 延胡索 9-12g
chuan lian zi (Fructus Meliae Toosendan) 川楝子 9-12g
ru xiang (Gummi Olibanum) 乳香 6-9g
mo yao (Myrrha) 没药 6-9g

Method: Decoction. **Jin yin hua** and **lian qiao** clear Toxic Heat; **bai jiang cao** and **hong teng** clear Toxic Heat and dissipate inflammatory masses; **yi ren** aids the discharge of pus, **shan zhi zi** clears Damp Heat from the *san jiao*; **tao ren** invigorates Blood and eliminates stagnant Blood; **chi shao** and **mu dan pi** cool the Blood and eliminate stagnant Blood; **yan hu suo**, **chuan lian zi**, **ru xiang** and **mo yao**, invigorate *qi* and Blood and stop pain.

With severe pain, add **sheng pu huang** (Pollen Typhae) 生蒲黄 9g and **wu ling zhi** (Excrementum Trogopteri seu Pteromi) 五灵脂 9g; with symptoms of an exterior invasion, add **jing jie** (Herba seu Flos Schizonepetae Tenuifolia) 荆芥 12g, **fang feng** (Radix Ledebouriellae Divaricatae) 防风 9g and **bai zhi** (Radix Angelicae Dahuricae) 白芷 9g; with abdominal distension, add **xiang fu** (Rhizoma Cyperi Rotundi) 香附 9-12g, **mu xiang** (Radix Aucklandiae Lappae) 木香 6-9g and **sha ren** (Fructus Amomi) 砂仁 6g; with incessant leucorrhoea, add **huang bai** (Cortex Phellodendri) 黄柏 9g, **yin chen** (Herba Artemisiae Yinchenhao) 茵陈 9-12g and **chun gen pi** (Cortex Ailanthi Altissimae) 春根皮 9-12g; with palpable masses, add **san leng** (Rhizoma Sparganii Stoloniferi) 三棱 9g, **e zhu** (Rhizoma Curcumae Ezhu) 莪术 9g and **dan shen** (Radix Salviae Miltiorrhizae) 丹参 30g; with constipation, add **da huang** (Radix et Rhizoma Rhei) 大黄 6-9g and **mang xiao** (Mirabilitum) 芒硝 6-9g. (Source: *Shi Yong Zhong Yi Fu Ke Xue*)

Chronic Damp Heat and Blood stagnation following unresolved Toxic Heat

- If the previous pattern (Acute Toxic Heat in the Uterus) is unresolved, or becomes chronic, the result may be lingering Damp Heat and Blood stagnation in the Uterus. The main features are chronic or recurrent lower abdominal pain and distension, low grade or afternoon fever, lumbar and/or sacral soreness and pain which is worse after menstruation or when tired, prolonged menstrual cycle or heavy periods, profuse yellowish malodorous leucorrhoea, dry mouth but no desire to drink, constipation or diarrhoea, scanty dark urine, a red tongue with a greasy yellow coat and a wiry and rapid, or soft and rapid pulse. The aim of treatment is to clear Damp Heat from the Uterus and invigorate Blood with **QING RE JIE DU HUA YU TANG** (*Heat Clearing, Toxin Eliminating, Blood Stasis Transforming Decoction* 清热解毒化瘀汤)

    yu xing cao (Herba cum Radice Houttuyniae Cordatae) 鱼腥草 18-30g
    tu fu ling (Rhizoma Smilacis Glabrae) 土茯苓 18-30g
    ren dong teng (Ramus Lonicerae Japonicae) 忍冬藤 15-18g
    sheng yi ren (Semen Coicis Lachryma-jobi) 生苡仁 18-30g

Figure 2.7 *Variation of excess Heat abdominal pain pattern*

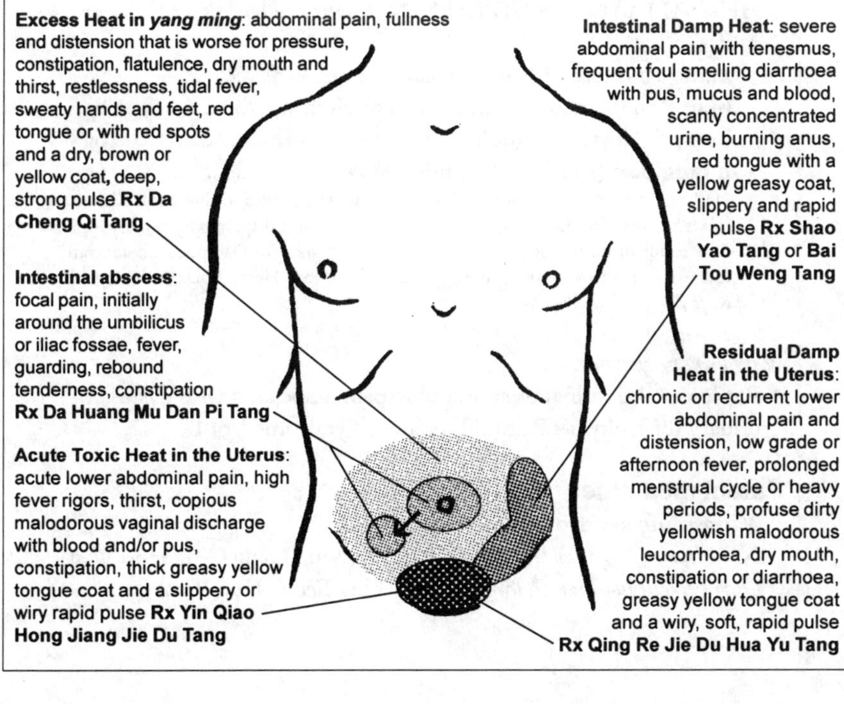

dang gui (Radix Angelicae Sinensis) 当归 9-12g
chi shao (Radix Paeoniae Rubrae) 赤芍 9-12g
xiang fu (Rhizoma Cyperi Rotundi) 香附 9-12g
lian qiao (Fructus Forsythia Suspensae) 连翘 9-12g
tao ren (Semen Persicae) 桃仁 9-12g
e zhu (Rhizoma Curcumae Ezhu) 莪术 9-12g
zhi ke (Fructus Citri Aurantii) 枳壳 6-9g
chuan xiong (Radix Ligustici Chuanxiong) 川芎 6-9g
gan cao (Radix Glycyrrhizae Uralensis) 甘草 3-6g

Method: Decoction. **Yu xing cao**, **tu fu ling**, **ren dong teng** and **lian qiao** clear Toxic and Damp Heat; **sheng yi ren** clears Damp Heat; **dang gui**, **chi shao**, **chuan xiong**, **tao ren** and **e zhu** regulate Blood and eliminate stagnant Blood; **xiang fu** and **zhi ke** regulate *qi*; **gan cao** supports the Spleen and harmonises the prescription.

With severe pain, add **yan hu suo** (Rhizoma Corydalis Yanhusuo) 延胡索 12g, **ru xiang** (Gummi Olibanum) 乳香 6g and **mo yao** (Myrrha) 没药 6g

With Summerheat

- If acute abdominal pain is associated with an invasion of Summerheat (acute abdominal pain, fever unrelieved by sweating, heaviness in the head and body, foggy-headedness, thirst, irritability, vomiting, diarrhoea, a floating pulse and a greasy, yellow tongue coat), the aim of treatment is to promote sweating to clear the exterior and expel Summerheat with **HUANG LIAN XIANG RU YIN** (*Coptis and Elsholtzia Decoction* 黄连香薷饮).

xiang ru (Herba Elsholtzia seu Moslae) 香薷 9g
bian dou (Semen Dolichos Lablab) 扁豆 9g
hou po (Cortex Magnoliae Officinalis) 厚朴 6g
huang lian (Rhizoma Coptidis) 黄连 6g

Method: Decoction. Do not cook longer than 15 minutes. Drink cool. **Xiang ru** clears the exterior, harmonises the *qi* mechanism and disperses Summerheat; **bian dou** and **hou po** harmonise the Stomach and transform Dampness to alleviate fullness and stop vomiting; **huang lian** clears Damp Heat. (Source: *Zhong Yi Nei Ke Ji Zheng Zheng Zhi*)

With urinary symptoms

- For lower abdominal or suprapubic pain associated with dysuria or urinary difficulty, *see* Painful Urination Syndrome Vol.1.

Patent medicines

Yang ming syndrome

Niu Huang Qing Huo Wan 牛黄清火丸 (Niu Huang Qing Huo Wan)
Qing Fei Yi Huo Pian 清肺抑火片 (Ching Fei Yi Huo Pien)

Damp (or Toxic) Heat in the Intestines

Huang Lian Jie Du Wan 黄连解毒丸 (Huang Lian Jie Du Wan)
- general Damp Heat or Toxic Heat patterns

Huang Lian Su Pian 黄连素片 (Huang Lien Su Tablets)

Chuan Xin Lian Kang Yan Pian 穿心连抗炎片 (Chuan Xin Lian Antiphlogistic Pills)

Long Dan Xie Gan Wan 龙胆泻肝丸 (Long Dan Xie Gan Wan, Lung Tan Xie Gan Wan)
- Damp Heat in the Liver system

Damp Heat in the Uterus

Chuan Xin Lian Kang Yan Pian 穿心连抗炎片 (Chuan Xin Lian Antiphlogistic Pills)

Huang Lian Jie Du Wan 黄连解毒丸 (Huang Lian Jie Du Wan)
- general Damp Heat or Toxic Heat patterns

Yu Dai Wan 愈带丸 (Yudai Wan [Leucorrhoea Pills])
- this patent can be combined with one of the previous patent medicines

Long Dan Xie Gan Wan 龙胆泻肝丸 (Long Dan Xie Gan Wan, Lung Tan Xie Gan Pill)
- Damp Heat in the Liver system

Acupuncture (select from)

Heat in the Intestines

St.25 (*tian shu* -) .... *mu* point of the Large Intestine, regulates Intestinal function and clears Heat

St.37 (*shang ju xu* -) .... lower *he* point of the Large Intestine, regulates and eliminates stagnation and accumulation from the Stomach and Intestines, clears Damp Heat

St.39 (*xia ju xu* -) .... lower *he* point of the Small Intestine, clears Heat and stagnation from the Intestines

St.44 (*nei ting* -) .... *rong* spring and Water point of the Stomach, clears Heat from *yang ming*, the Stomach and Stomach channel

Bl.25 (*da chang shu* -) .... *shu* point of the Large Intestine

ah shi points .... on the Urinary Bladder channel, between Bl.18 (*gan shu*) and Bl.28 (*pang guang shu*)

- with severe pain, add St.34 (*liang qiu* -)
- with fever, add Du.14 (*da zhui* -), LI.11 (*qu chi* -) and LI.4 (*he gu* -)
- with *shao yang* symptoms, add GB.39 (*xuan zhong* -), SJ.5 (*wai guan* -) and GB.34 (*yang ling quan* -)

- with constipation, add SJ.6 (*zhi gou* -)
- with diarrhoea, add LI.11 (*qu chi* -)
- *Ear points*: subcortex, abdomen, large intestine, small intestine, *shen men*, sympathetic

Heat in the Uterus

zi gong - (M-CA-18) .... extra point for the Uterus, clears Heat and stagnation

Ren.3 (*zhong ji* -) .... *mu* point of the Urinary Bladder, regulates the Uterus, clears Damp Heat

GB.26 (*dai mai* -) .... intersects the *dai* channel, clears Damp Heat from the lower abdomen

Sp.8 (*di ji* -) .... *xi* cleft point of the Spleen, regulates and invigorates Blood and clears Heat

Liv.5 (*li gou* -) .... *luo* point of the Liver, spreads Liver *qi*, clears Damp Heat from the genitals, clears the channels

Kid.7 (*fu liu* -) .... *jing* river and Metal point of the Kidney, clears Damp Heat from the lower abdomen

ah shi points .... between Bl.31 (*shang liao*) and Bl.34 (*xia liao*)

- with fever, add Du.14 (*da zhui* -), LI.11 (*qu chi* -) and LI.4 (*he gu* -)
- with *shao yang* symptoms, add GB.39 (*xuan zhong* -), SJ.5 (*wai guan* -) and GB.34 (*yang ling quan* -)
- with discharge and vaginal pruritus, add Sp.9 (*yin ling quan* -) and Liv.8 (*qu quan* -)
- with nausea, add PC.6 (*nei guan*)
- *Ear points*: abdomen, stomach, large intestine, small intestine, uterus, ovary, sympathetic, subcortex, *shen men*,

Clinical notes

- Abdominal pain of an excess Heat type often indicates an acute infection of the pelvic organs, and in severe cases may require antibiotic treatment to quickly clear Heat, in addition to TCM treatment to dispel the pathogen. In some cases surgery may be indicated. It may be diagnosed biomedically as acute appendicitis, diverticulitis, dysentery, ulcerative colitis, Crohn's disease, pelvic inflammatory disease, intestinal obstruction, mesenteric lymphadenitis, salpingitis, Trichomonas and nonspecific vaginitis.
- For dietary recommendations, see p.882.

2.3 LIVER QI STAGNATION

肝气滞满腹痛

Pathophysiology

- Abdominal pain of a Liver *qi* stagnation type can present in a number of ways depending on the location of the stagnation and the systems involved. The pain in this pattern may be acute or chronic. Acute cases can appear suddenly following some emotional event and last only a few hours. The patient feels normal before and after. More commonly seen in the clinic are the chronic patterns, where the patient is in circumstances that provoke ongoing *qi* stagnation, or has a personality which predisposes to *qi* stagnation.
- *Qi* stagnation patterns are typically complicated due to the numerous pathological relationships between the Liver and other systems. Because the Liver channel passes through the lower *jiao*, the reproductive system is frequently affected. Liver *qi* stagnation can affect the Spleen or Stomach or both, leading to Blood stagnation and Blood deficiency, Spleen deficiency, Dampness and the generation of Heat. In addition, *qi* stagnation patterns are frequently associated with a deficiency of either Liver Blood or *yin*.
- Liver *qi* stagnation patterns are associated with hypertonicity of smooth and skeletal muscle. This chronic hypertonicity restricts the circulation of *qi* and Blood, causing poor elasticity and nutrition of the tissues involved, predisposing them to further injury.
- The key feature of all Liver *qi* stagnation patterns is the relationship of symptoms to the emotional state of the patient.

Clinical features

- Abdominal or epigastric distension and pain, clearly related to the emotional state. The pain is intermittent, variable in intensity, moves around and may be vaguely localised, but tends to affect the lateral and lower abdomen, and is better for relaxation and the expulsion of gas. When identifying the site of the pain the patient may use the whole hand and indicate a large area.
- sluggish stools or alternating constipation and diarrhoea
- flatulence and/or belching, which relieve the pain
- tightness or stuffiness in the chest, difficulty getting a satisfying breath
- cold fingers and toes
- moodiness, depression, anxiety, irritability, tension

T normal or darkish or with reddish edges
P wiry

Treatment principle

Regulate Liver *qi* and soothe the Liver
Strengthen the Spleen and stop pain

Prescription

CHAI HU SHU GAN SAN 柴胡疏肝散
(Bupleurum and Cyperus Formula)

This prescription is best for predominantly excess cases with some Heat generated by constrained *qi*.

chai hu (Radix Bupleuri) 柴胡 9-12g
bai shao (Radix Paeoniae Lactiflorae) 白芍 12-18g
zhi shi (Fructus Immaturus Citri Aurantii) 枳实 9-12g
xiang fu (Rhizoma Cyperi Rotundi) 香附 9-12g
chuan xiong (Radix Ligustici Chuanxiong) 川芎 6-9g
chen pi (Pericarpium Citri Reticulatae) 陈皮 6-9g
zhi gan cao (honey fried Radix Glycyrrhizae Uralensis) 炙甘草 3-6g

Method: Decoction. **Chai hu** spreads Liver *qi*, **bai shao** softens the Liver, nourishes *yin* and Blood and assists **chai hu** in regulating and invigorating *qi* flow; **zhi shi** and **xiang fu** regulate *qi*; **chuan xiong** moves *qi* and Blood; **zhi gan cao** supports the Spleen and with **bai shao** alleviates cramping and spasmodic pain. (Source: *Shi Yong Zhong Yi Nei Ke Xue*)

Modifications

- With severe pain, increase the dose of **bai shao** to 30g, and add **yan hu suo** (Rhizoma Corydalis Yanhusuo) 延胡索 9-12g and **chuan lian zi** (Fructus Meliae Toosendan) 川楝子 9-12g, and substitute **chen pi** with **qing pi** (Pericarpium Citri Reticulatae Viride) 青皮 9-12g.
- With severe spasm and cramp, increase the dose of **bai shao** to 30g and the dose of **zhi gan cao** to 9g.
- If the pain radiates into the iliac fossae or genitals, add **li zhi he** (Semen Litchi Chinensis) 荔枝核 12g, **ju he** (Semen Citri Reticulatae) 橘核 9-12g and **xiao hui xiang** (Fructus Foeniculi Vulgaris) 小茴香 9-12g.
- With acid reflux, add **huang lian** (Rhizoma Coptidis) 黄连 6g, **wu zhu yu** (Fructus Evodiae Rutaecarpae) 吴茱萸 2g and **hai piao xiao** (Os Sepiae seu Sepiellae) 海螵蛸 15g.
- With flatulence or belching, add **hou po** (Cortex Magnoliae Officinalis) 厚朴 12g, **mu xiang** (Radix Aucklandiae Lappae) 木香 9g and **sha ren** (Fructus Amomi) 砂仁 6g.
- With nausea, add **huo xiang** (Herba Agastaches seu Pogostemi) 藿香 12g and **ban xia** (Rhizoma Pinelliae Ternatae) 半夏 9-12g.
- With Heat in the Stomach, add **huang qin** (Radix Scutellariae Baicalensis) 黄芩 9-12g and **huang lian** (Rhizoma Coptidis) 黄连 6g.
- With Heat in the Liver, add **mu dan pi** (Cortex Moutan Radicis) 牡丹皮 9-12g and **shan zhi zi** (Fructus Gardeniae Jasminoides) 山栀子 9-12g.

- With Spleen deficiency, add **dang shen** (Radix Codonopsis Pilosulae) 党参 12-15g and **bai zhu** (Rhizoma Atractylodes Macrocephalae) 白术 9-12g.
- With Cold, add **sheng jiang** (Rhizoma Zingiberis Officinalis Recens) 生姜 6-9g and **gui zhi** (Ramulus Cinnamomi Cassiae) 桂枝 6-9g.
- With Dampness, add **cang zhu** (Rhizoma Atractylodis) 苍术 9-12g and **hou po** (Cortex Magnoliae Officinalis) 厚朴 9-12g.
- For patients that are tense or depressed, add **he huan pi** (Cortex Albizziae Julibrissin) 合欢皮 15g and **yu jin** (Tuber Curcumae) 郁金 9-12g.

Variations and additional prescriptions

Qi stagnation with constipation

- When the stagnant *qi* is associated with a tendency to chronic constipation, a common situation in those in stressful sedentary occupations, **LIU MO TANG** (*Six Milled Herb Decoction 六磨汤*, p.183) may be used to move *qi* and aid the correct descent of *qi*. This is quite a strong *qi* invigorating prescription, and is suitable for robust patients with little or no deficiency. Once the bowels are moving and pain has been alleviated, the dose of **da huang** should be reduced or deleted.

With Spleen deficiency, pain and urgent diarrhoea

- When *qi* stagnation is complicated by Spleen deficiency, with cramping abdominal pain that may be associated with diarrhoea, borborygmus, bloating, poor appetite, flatulence, depression, irritability, a pale tongue and a wiry or soft pulse, the aim of treatment is to spread Liver *qi* and strengthen the Spleen with **TONG XIE YAO FANG** (*Important Formula for Painful Diarrhoea 痛泻要方*, p.239). In chronic cases, this prescription can be combined with the primary prescription.

Liver qi stagnation with Spleen qi and Blood deficiency

- Prolonged Liver *qi* stagnation is frequently complicated by Spleen *qi* deficiency and Blood deficiency, a mixture particularly common in women. The mixture of pathology is a common cause of premenstrual abdominal pain and breast tenderness, poor appetite, dizziness, occasional fatigue, tension headaches, tightness in the neck, shoulders and chest, pale edges on the tongue and a wiry thready pulse. The aim of treatment is to move Liver *qi*, nourish Blood and strengthen the Spleen with **XIAO YAO SAN** (*Bupleurum and Dang Gui Formula 逍遥散* see p.159). This is an excellent maintenance formula that may be used to regulate *qi* once the main symptoms have subsided; ideal for long term use in patients with a constitutional tendency to *qi* stagnation.

Liver qi stagnation with yin deficiency

- When Liver *qi* stagnation is complicated by Liver *yin* deficiency, strong *qi* moving herbs are not indicated as they can further deplete the already damaged *yin*. The abdominal pain of this pattern tends to be dull or cramping with occasional exacerbations, the pain is worse for stress and emotion. In addition there may be abdominal distension, dry mouth and throat, acid reflux, a red dry tongue with little or no coat and a thready, wiry pulse. The aim of treatment is to Nourish Liver *yin* and gently spread Liver *qi* with **YI GUAN JIAN** (*Linking Decoction* 一贯煎) modified.

sheng di (Radix Rehmanniae Glutinosae) 生地 18-45g
gou qi zi (Fructus Lycii) 枸杞子 9-18g
sha shen (Radix Adenophorae seu Glehniae) 沙参 9-12g
mai dong (Tuber Ophiopogonis Japonici) 麦冬 9-12g
dang gui (Radix Angelicae Sinensis) 当归 9-12g
chuan lian zi (Fructus Meliae Toosendan) 川楝子 9-12g
bai shao (Radix Paeoniae Lactiflorae) 白芍 12-18g
gan cao (Radix Glycyrrhizae Uralensis) 甘草 3-6g

Method: Decoction. **Sheng di**, **gou qi zi**, **sha shen** and **mai dong** nourish Liver and Stomach *yin*; **dang gui** regulates and supplements Blood; **chuan lian zi** regulates *qi* and stops pain; **bai shao** and **gan cao** combine sweet and sour flavours to create *yin*, ease cramps and alleviate spasmodic pain. (Source: *Formulas and Strategies*)

Affecting the Liver channel and genitals

- If Liver *qi* stagnation affects the Liver channel in the lower *jiao*, it can cause lower abdominal pain that radiates to the testicles, testicular pain and bilateral or unilateral swelling and distension of the scrotum that is provoked or initiated by anger, stress or emotional upset. The aim of treatment is to move Liver *qi*, disperse Cold and stop pain with **TIAN TAI WU YAO SAN** (*Top Quality Lindera Powder* 天台乌药散).

wu yao (Radix Linderae Strychnifoliae) 乌药 9-12g
qing pi (Pericarpium Citri Reticulatae Viride) 青皮 9-12g
gao liang jiang (Rhizoma Alpiniae Officinari) 高良姜 9-12g
mu xiang (Radix Aucklandiae Lappae) 木香 9-12g
chao xiao hui xiang (dry fried Fructus Foeniculi Vulgaris)
炒小茴香 9-12g
chuan lian zi (Fructus Meliae Toosendan) 川楝子 9-12g
bing lang (Semen Arecae Catechu) 槟榔 6-9g
ba dou (Semen Croton Tiglii) 巴豆 ....50 seeds

Method: **Chuan lian zi** and **ba dou** are dry fried together, the **ba dou** then discarded and the **chuan lian zi** ground to powder with the remaining herbs. Due to its toxicity **ba dou** is rarely used today. Take as a draft with yellow wine or sake. The dose is 3 grams, 2-3 times daily. May also be decocted with **ba dou** deleted. **Wu yao**, **gao liang jiang** and **chao xiao hui xiang** warm and regulate *qi* to stop pain; **qing pi** breaks up stagnant *qi*; **mu xiang** regulates *qi* and harmonises the Stomach; **chuan lian zi** regulates *qi* and stops pain; **bing lang** directs *qi* downwards and breaks up accumulation; when **ba dou** was used, its substance was deleted but its spirit retained to moderate the coldness of the **chuan lian zi** and to assist **bing lang** in leading the Cold out through the Intestine. (Source: *Shi Yong Zhong Yi Nei Ke Xue*)

Patent medicines

Shu Gan Wan 舒肝丸 (Shu Gan Wan, Shu Kan Wan)
- the best patent medicine for *qi* stagnation type pain

Chen Xiang Hua Qi Wan 沉香化气丸 (Chen Xiang Hua Qi Wan)
- with constipation

Chai Hu Shu Gan Wan 柴胡疏肝丸 (Chai Hu Shu Gan Wan)

Mu Xiang Shun Qi Wan 木香顺气丸 (Mu Xiang Shun Qi Wan)
- with sluggish bowels and food stagnation

Xiao Yao Wan 逍遥丸 (Xiao Yao Wan, Hsiao Yao Wan)
- with Spleen *qi* and Blood deficiency

Acupuncture (select from)

Ren.6 (*qi hai*) .... together these points regulate *qi* through the abdomen, strengthen the Spleen, improve digestion and promote Liver function
St.25 (*tian shu*)
St.21 (*liang men* -)
Liv.13 (*zhang men* -)

Figure 2.8 *Variations of qi stagnation abdominal pain patterns*

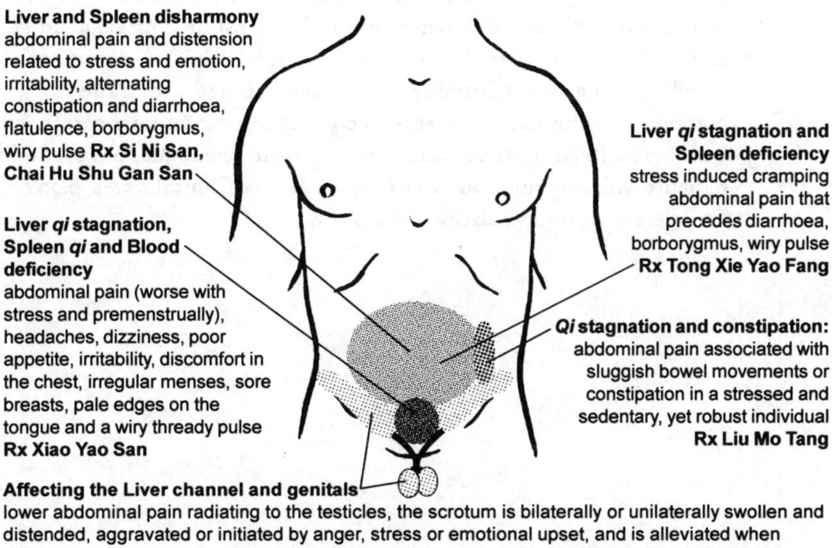

Liv.3 (*tai chong* -) .... together these points regulate, spread and
PC.6 (*nei guan* -) soothe Liver *qi*, harmonise the middle *jiao*, stop spasm and pain and calm the *shen*

GB.34 (*yang ling quan* -) ... together these points regulate *qi* in the
SJ.6 (*zhi gou* -) abdomen, invigorate Intestinal *qi* and moderate the influence of Liver *qi* stagnation on the Spleen and Stomach

St.36 (*zu san li*) .... *he* sea point of the Stomach, regulates *qi* and stops pain

- with Blood or *yin* deficiency, add Sp.6 (*san yin jiao* +), Bl.18 (*gan shu* +), Bl.23 (*shen shu* +)
- for severe pain, add Liv.5 (*li gou* -) and Sp.8 (*di ji* -)
- with testicular pain, add Liv.5 (*li gou* -)
- for nervous, anxious or tense patients, add *yin tang* (M-HN-3) and Ht.7 (*shen men*)
- *Ear points*: *shen men*, liver, abdomen, stomach, large intestine, small intestine, subcortex, endocrine, sympathetic

Clinical notes

- Liver *qi* stagnation type abdominal pain may be diagnosed biomedically as irritable bowel syndrome, chronic colitis, intestinal obstruction, chronic pelvic inflammatory disease, diverticulosis, chronic constipation, premenstrual syndrome, dysmenorrhoea or inguinal herniae.
- Acupuncture is often the treatment of choice for moving stagnant *qi* and if the pain is relatively recent, one course (or less) of acupuncture should effect a cure. Chronic pain that is associated with more complex patterns may need several courses of acupuncture combined with herbs. Relaxation and stress management techniques are useful in patients with ongoing sources of stress. *See also* Clinical notes, p.359.
- For dietary recommendations, see p.878.

血瘀腹痛

2.4 BLOOD STAGNATION

Pathophysiology

- Blood stagnation causes pain by physically obstructing the movement of *qi* and Blood. Because Blood stagnation is a substantial obstruction, it strongly blocks *qi* and Blood and thus causes quite intense, and usually fixed, pain.

Clinical features

- Relatively severe, sharp or stabbing abdominal pain, fixed in location and worse with pressure. The pain often occurs in the lower abdomen and iliac fossae.
- there may be palpable masses which may or may not be painful
- dark or purplish spider naevi or broken vessels on the trunk and around the inner ankle and knee
- dark, ashen, sallow or purplish complexion, dark or purplish lips and conjunctiva, dark rings around the eyes; in cases with significant underlying deficiency, the complexion is sallow or pale, and there may be dizziness.
- in women, the menses may be irregular, dark or purple and clotted

T purple or with brown or purple stasis spots; sublingual veins dark and distended

P thready and choppy or wiry

Treatment principle

Invigorate Blood circulation, eliminate stagnant Blood
Stop pain

Prescription

SHAO FU ZHU YU TANG 少腹逐瘀汤
(*Drive Out Blood Stasis in the Lower Abdomen Decoction*)

This formula is designed for Blood stagnation with Cold, especially in the lower abdomen..

dang gui (Radix Angelicae Sinensis) 当归 9-15g
chi shao (Radix Paeoniae Rubrae) 赤芍 9-12g
sheng pu huang (Pollen Typhae) 生蒲黄 9-12g
chao wu ling zhi (dry fried Excrementum Trogopteri seu Pteromi) 炒五灵脂 9-12g
yan hu suo (Rhizoma Corydalis Yanhusuo) 延胡索 9-12g
chuan xiong (Radix Ligustici Chuanxiong) 川芎 6-9g
xiao hui xiang (Fructus Foeniculi Vulgaris) 小茴香 9-12g
mo yao (Myrrha) 没药 6-9g
rou gui (Cortex Cinnamomi Cassiae) 肉桂 3g

pao jiang (quick fried Rhizoma Zingiberis Officinalis)
炮姜 3-6g

Method: Decoction. **Dang gui, chi shao, sheng pu huang, wu ling zhi, chuan xiong** and **mo yao** invigorate Blood and disperse stagnant Blood; **chuan xiong, xiao hui xiang** and **yan hu suo** warm and regulate *qi* and stop pain; **rou gui** and **pao jiang** warm *yang* and invigorate the circulation of *qi* and Blood; **rou gui** promotes generation of new Blood. (Source: *Shi Yong Zhong Yi Nei Ke Xue*)

Modifications

- With *qi* stagnation (abdominal distension, irritability), add **mu xiang** (Radix Aucklandiae Lappae) 木香 6-9g, **hou po** (Cortex Magnoliae Officinalis) 厚朴 9-12g and **bing lang** (Semen Arecae Catechu) 槟榔 9-12g.
- With masses, add **san leng** (Rhizoma Sparganii Stoloniferi) 三棱 9-12g and **e zhu** (Rhizoma Curcumae Ezhu) 莪术 9-12g.
- With *qi* deficiency, add **zhi huang qi** (honey fried Radix Astragali Membranacei) 炙黄芪 18-30g, **dang shen** (Radix Codonopsis Pilosulae) 党参 15-24g and **chao bai zhu** (dry fried Rhizoma Atractylodes Macrocephalae) 炒白术 9-12g.
- With Blood deficiency, add **zhi huang qi** (honey fried Radix Astragali Membranacei) 炙黄芪 18-30g and **shu di** (Radix Rehmanniae Glutinosae Conquitae) 熟地 15-18g.
- With Phlegm Damp, add **cang zhu** (Rhizoma Atractylodis) 苍术 12-15g, **yi ren** (Semen Coicis Lachryma-jobi) 苡仁 15-24g and **fu ling** (Sclerotium Poriae Cocos) 茯苓 12-15g.
- With signs of Heat, delete **pao jiang** and **rou gui**, increase the dose of **chi shao** to 15g and add **mu dan pi** (Cortex Moutan Radicis) 牡丹皮 9-12g and **da huang** (Radix et Rhizoma Rhei) 大黄 3-6g.
- With painful post surgical adhesions, add **hong hua** (Flos Carthami Tinctorii) 红花 9g and **ze lan** (Herba Lycopi Lucidi) 泽兰 9-12g.
- If the pain follows a traumatic injury add **san qi fen** (powdered Radix Notoginseng) 三七粉 6-9g and **wang bu liu xing** (Semen Vaccariae Segetalis) 王不留行 9-12g. Where there is extensive bruising, add **da huang** (Radix et Rhizoma Rhei) 大黄 6-9g, **gui zhi** (Ramulus Cinnamomi Cassiae) 桂枝 9-12g and **tao ren** (Semen Persicae) 桃仁 9-12g.

Variations and additional prescriptions

Liver qi and Blood stagnation

- Blood stagnation frequently follows years of Liver *qi* stagnation. Patients so afflicted may suffer chronic intermittent abdominal pain that gradually gets worse, with generalised signs of Blood stagnation and *qi* stagnation. There may be mobile pain intermingled with stabbing pain that is worse for pressure, spider vessels on the face and hypochondria, dark rings around the eyes, moodiness or chronic depression, purple patches on the tongue, chronic insomnia and heat at night. The aim of treatment is to move *qi* and Blood with a broad acting formula such as **XUE FU ZHU YU TANG** (*Achyranthes and Persica Combination* 血府逐瘀汤). This prescription is also useful for *qi* and Blood stagnation pain following an intense emotional trauma.

dang gui (Radix Angelicae Sinensis) 当归 9-12g
sheng di (Radix Rehmanniae Glutinosae) 生地 12-15g
chi shao (Radix Paeoniae Rubrae) 赤芍 9-12g
chuan xiong (Radix Ligustici Chuanxiong) 川芎 6-9g
tao ren (Semen Persicae) 桃仁 9-12g
hong hua (Flos Carthami Tinctorii) 红花 9-12g
chai hu (Radix Bupleuri) 柴胡 6-9g
zhi ke (Fructus Citri Aurantii) 枳壳 9-12g
gan cao (Radix Glycyrrhizae Uralensis) 甘草 3-6g
chuan niu xi (Radix Cyathulae Officinalis) 川牛膝 15-24g
jie geng (Radix Platycodi Grandiflori) 桔梗 3-6g

Method: Decoction. **Dang gui**, **sheng di**, **chuan xiong**, **chi shao**, **tao ren** and **hong hua** constitute **TAO HONG SI WU TANG**, a fundamental prescription to nourish, regulate and gently invigorate Blood; **chai hu**, **zhi ke**, **gan cao** and **chi shao** constitute **SI NI SAN**, the fundamental prescription to regulate Liver *qi* and move stagnant *qi*; **jie geng** opens up the movement of *qi* through the chest and diaphragm, and can direct *qi* to the upper body; the large dose of **niu xi** leads Blood downwards–together they seek to re-establish the correct ascent and descent of *qi* and Blood. (Source: *Xiao Hua Ke Zhuan Bing*)

Qi and Blood stagnation affecting shao yang

- Fixed pain that is not particularly severe, primarily affecting the lateral abdomen, or pain that radiates to the hypochondriac region and is associated with a confusing constellation of signs and symptoms (mostly Spleen deficiency, Liver *qi* stagnation and Damp or stagnant Heat), may be treated by focusing on moving *qi* and Blood at the *shao yang* level using **XIAO CHAI HU TANG** (*Minor Bupleurum Combination* 小柴胡汤) modified.

chai hu (Radix Bupleuri) 柴胡 9-12g
huang qin (Radix Scutellariae Baicalensis) 黄芩 9-12g
ban xia (Rhizoma Pinelliae Ternatae) 半夏 9-12g
dang shen (Radix Codonopsis Pilosulae) 党参 12-15g
sheng jiang (Rhizoma Zingiberis Officinalis Recens)
生姜 6-9g
zhi gan cao (honey fried Radix Glycyrrhizae Uralensis)
炙甘草 3-6g
da zao (Fructus Zizyphi Jujubae) 大枣 4pce
tao ren (Semen Persicae) 桃仁 9-12g
jiang huang (Rhizoma Curcumae Longae) 姜黄 9-12g

xiang fu (Rhizoma Cyperi Rotundi) 香附 9-12g
da huang (Radix et Rhizoma Rhei) 大黄 3-6g

Method: Decoction. **Chai hu** regulates the Liver and moves Liver *qi*; **huang qin** clears Damp Heat; together the two herbs vent pathogens from *shao yang*; **ban xia** transforms Phlegm and stops vomiting; **ren shen** and **zhi gan cao** strengthen the Spleen and supplement *qi*; **sheng jiang** and **da zao** harmonise the Stomach; **tao ren, jiang huang** and **da huang** invigorate Blood, eliminate stagnant Blood and stop pain; **xiang fu** regulates *qi*. (Source: *Shi Yong Zhong Yi Nei Ke Xue*)

Blood stagnation following trauma

- Localised or generalised abdominal pain following a physical trauma, such as a motor vehicle accident, should be treated with strong Blood moving herbs to swiftly metabolise the acute stagnation and bruising. **FU YUAN HUO XUE TANG** (*Revive Health by Invigorating the Blood Decoction* 复元活血汤) modified, is selected. This prescription is only used for one or two weeks, and the patient should experience dark diarrhoea as the bruising resolves.

jiu da huang (wine fried Radix et Rhizoma Rhei) 酒大黄 .. 9-12g
dang gui (Radix Angelicae Sinensis) 当归 9-12g
tian hua fen (Radix Trichosanthes Kirilowii) 天花粉 9-12g
tao ren (Semen Persicae) 桃仁 6-9g
hong hua (Flos Carthami Tinctorii) 红花 6-9g
chai hu (Radix Bupleuri) 柴胡 6-9g

Figure 2.9 *Variations of Blood stagnation abdominal pain patterns*

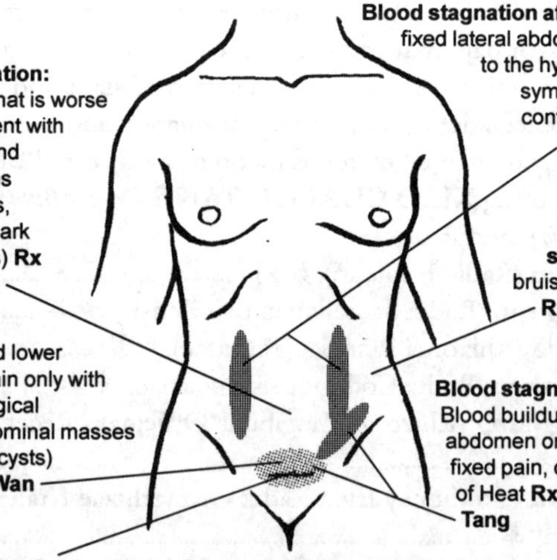

gan cao (Radix Glycyrrhizae Uralensis) 甘草 3-6g
wang bu liu xing (Semen Vaccariae Segetalis) 王不留行 ... 9-12g

Method: Decoction. Often taken with a little yellow wine or vodka. **Jiu da huang** breaks up and moves stagnant Blood, stimulates metabolism of old Blood and provides an outlet for it through the bile and the bowel; **dang gui**, **tao ren**, **hong hua** and **wang bu liu xing** invigorate Blood, reduce swelling, eliminate stagnant Blood and stop pain; **wang bu liu xing** unblocks the channels; **chai hu** regulates and moves *qi* to lead Blood; **tian hua fen** reduces swelling and stimulates healing; **gan cao** protects the Stomach and eases spasms. (Source: *Shi Yong Fang Ji Xue*)
NB: **Wang bu liu xing** is substituted for **chuan shan jia** (Squama Manitis) 穿山甲, the scales of the endangered pangolin that appeared in the original prescription.

Severe Blood stagnation in the Intestines or Uterus with Heat

- With Blood stagnation in the lower abdomen or left iliac fossa complicated by Heat (severe, fixed lower abdominal pain, dysmenorrhoea, amenorrhoea, fever at night, irritability, restlessness and thirst, urinary difficulty, hard to pass tarry stools or constipation and a choppy pulse) the aim of treatment is to drain Heat and break up Blood stasis with **TAO HE CHENG QI TANG** (*Major Rhubarb Combination* 桃核承气汤, p.507). This formula can be used for Blood stagnation in the reproductive system or in the Intestine (typically the left iliac fossa).

Benign gynaecological masses with mild pain

- If lower abdominal pain is relatively mild or only detected with palpation, and associated with immobile masses, persistent uterine bleeding of dark or purple blood, dysmenorrhoea, amenorrhoea and a choppy pulse, the treatment should invigorate Blood and reduce masses. **GUI ZHI FU LING WAN** (*Cinnamon and Hoelen Formula* 桂枝茯苓丸, p.909) is the formula of choice in treating mild Blood stasis giving rise to fibroids and other gynaecological cysts and benign tumours. To be effective it usually needs to be taken for at least 9-12 months.

Patent medicines

Xue Fu Zhu Yu Wan 血府逐瘀丸 (Xue Fu Zhu Yu Wan)
- strong general regulator of *qi* and Blood

Shi Xiao Wan 失笑丸 (Shi Xiao Wan)
- add to enhance analgesic action

Tong Jing Wan 痛经丸 (Tong Jing Wan)
- strong Blood regulator, especially for menstrual pain

Tao Hong Si Wu Wan 桃红四物丸 (Tao Hong Si Wu Wan)
- mild Blood stagnation with Blood deficiency

Fu Ke Wu Jin Wan 妇科乌金丸 (Woo Garm Yuen Medical Pills)
- especially for gynaecological Blood stasis, fibroids and other

benign masses with a degree of deficiency (mostly *yang* or *qi* deficiency)

Gui Zhi Fu Ling Wan 桂枝茯苓丸 (Cinnamon and Hoelen Formula)
- Suitable for mild Blood stagnation in the lower *jiao*. Generally needs to be taken for a long time for any result.

Yun Nan Bai Yao 云南白药 (Yunnan Paiyao)
- This famous patent medicine can be used prior to (but not within 24 hours) and following abdominal surgery to improve healing and reduce the likelihood of scarring and adhesions. It can also be used for pain and bruising following traumatic injury.

Zheng Gu Shui 正骨水 (Zheng Gu Shui)
- a liniment for external use only on bruising and traumatic pain

Acupuncture (select from)

Blood stagnation in the reproductive system

a shi points .... over the site of pain in the abdomen, reducing method

St.29 (*gui lai* -) .... these points regulate the movement of *qi* and
zi gong - (M-CA-18) Blood in the lower abdomen and reproductive
Ren.6 (*qi hai* -▲) system, and with Sp.8 (*di ji*) and Sp.6 (*san yin jiao*), eliminate Stagnant Blood

Sp.8 (*di ji* -) .... *xi* cleft point of the Spleen, for *qi* and Blood accumulation in the abdomen

Sp.6 (*san yin jiao* -) .... these points invigorate Blood circulation and
Sp.10 (*xue hai* -) eliminate stagnant Blood from the lower *jiao*
LI.4 (*he gu* -)

Liv.3 (*tai chong* -) .... *yuan*, *shu* and Earth point of the Liver, pacifies rising Liver *yang*, regulates *qi* and Blood, supplements Liver *yin* and Blood, regulates the channels, stops pain, extinguishes Wind, alleviates spasms; with LI.4 (*he gu*) forms the 'four gates' (see below)

Bl.17 (*ge shu* -) .... *hui* point for Blood, eliminates stagnant Blood

- Non-scarring moxa cones burnt over the *ren mai* points of the lower abdomen and *zi gong* are useful to activate Blood circulation.
- Bleeding the *ah shi* points of the *ba liao* (points over the sacral foramina) followed by strong cupping, can powerfully activate Blood in the reproductive system.
- *Ear points*: uterus, ovary, liver, heart, abdomen, sympathetic, *shen men*

Blood stagnation in the Intestines

ah shi points .... over the site of the lesion and distal points on the corresponding channel, usually the Stomach channel between St.36 (*zu san li*) and St.39 (*xia ju xu*).

St.25 (*tian shu* -) .... *mu* point of the Large Intestine, regulates Intestinal function and eliminates stagnation

Ren.6 (*qi hai* -) .... regulates *qi* and Blood in the lower *jiao*

Bl.25 (*da chang shu* -) .... these points invigorate Blood circulation and
Sp.10 (*xue hai* -) eliminate Blood stagnation from the Intestine
Sp.6 (*san yin jiao*)

Sp.4 (*gong sun*) .... *luo* point of the Spleen, master point of *chong mai*, regulates the Spleen and Stomach, stops pain

LI.4 (*he gu* -) .... the 'four gates', both *yuan* points, invigorate *qi*
Liv.3 (*tai chong*) and Blood, powerful sedative and calming action, relieve mental cloudiness, ease muscle spasm, stop pain

- *Ear points*: large intestine, small intestine, stomach, abdomen, distal segment rectum, sympathetic, *shen men*

Clinical notes

- Abdominal pain of a Blood stagnation type may be diagnosed biomedically as dysmenorrhoea, acute and chronic pelvic inflammatory disease (PID), fibroids, ovarian cysts, endometriosis, postpartum placental retention, prostatitis, prostate cancer, urinary bladder cancer, intestinal obstruction or adhesions and trauma.
- TCM treatment for this pattern should not proceed without a thorough medical evaluation.
- In general, Blood stagnation patterns are chronic and will take some time to resolve well, often 6-18 months depending on the duration and severity of the problem. Herbs are usually required for the chronic and systemic patterns, although acupuncture is excellent for localised Blood stagnation.
- For dietary recommendations, see p.886.

食积腹痛

2.5 FOOD STAGNATION

Pathophysiology

- Under normal circumstances Spleen *qi* should ascend and Stomach *qi* should descend. When blocked by accumulated and fermenting food, normal movement of *qi* through the middle *jiao* is constrained causing pain and distension. Food stagnation occurs due to overeating or because a weak Spleen is unable to adequately digest food. Food stagnation patterns are frequently complicated by, or are a complication of, other patterns, particularly *qi* stagnation, internal Heat, Damp, Phlegm or Phlegm Heat and *qi* and *yang* deficiency.
- Clinically, food stagnation can be pure excess, or a mixture of excess and Spleen deficiency. As the pattern progresses, the deficiency may become more and more prominent.

Clinical features

- abdominal and epigastric pain, fullness and distension, alleviated by belching, vomiting or bowel movement and worse for pressure and eating
- sour foul belching, flatulence
- loss of appetite, aversion to food
- acid reflux, heartburn
- vomiting of sour, undigested food
- constipation, sluggish foul stools, or diarrhoea

T thick greasy coat

P slippery and strong

Treatment principle

Relieve food stagnation and harmonise the Stomach
Strengthen digestion and stop pain

Prescription

BAO HE WAN 保和丸
(*Citrus and Crategus Formula*) modified

chao shan zha (dry fried Fructus Crataegi) 炒山楂 18-24g
fu ling (Sclerotium Poriae Cocos) 茯苓 12-15g
chao shen qu (dry fried Massa Fermentata) 炒神曲 12-15g
ban xia (Rhizoma Pinelliae Ternatae) 半夏 9-12g
chen pi (Pericarpium Citri Reticulatae) 陈皮 9-12g
lai fu zi (Semen Raphani Sativi) 莱服子 9-12g
lian qiao (Fructus Forsythia Suspensae) 连翘 6-9g
qing pi (Pericarpium Citri Reticulatae Viridae) 青皮 9-12g
yan hu suo (Rhizoma Corydalis Yanhusuo) 延胡索 9-12g

Method: Grind herbs to a powder and form into 9-gram pills with water. The dose is 1 pill twice daily. May also be decocted with the quantities as shown. **Shan zha, shen qu** and **lai fu zi** improve digestion and alleviate food stagnation; **ban xia** and **chen pi** eliminate Phlegm; **lian qiao** disperses accumulation and clears Heat; **fu ling** strengthens the Spleen; **qing pi** breaks up *qi* accumulation; **yan hu suo** regulates *qi* and Blood and stops pain. (Source: *Shi Yong Zhong Yi Nei Ke Xue*)

Modifications

- With severe pain and distension, add **e zhu** (Rhizoma Curcumae Ezhu) 莪术 9-12g, **san leng** (Rhizoma Sparganii Stoloniferi) 三棱 9-12g and **mu xiang** (Radix Aucklandiae Lappae) 木香 6-9g.
- With nausea or vomiting, add **sheng jiang** (Rhizoma Zingiberis Officinalis Recens) 生姜 9-12g.
- If excessive meat was consumed, use large doses of **shan zha** (Fructus Crataegi) 山楂 (up to 30g).
- If pain occurs after eating starchy, carbohydrate rich foods, such as noodles or grains, increase the dose of **lai fu zi** to 15g.
- With constipation, add **da huang** (Radix et Rhizoma Rhei) 大黄 6-9g **bing lang** (Semen Arecae Catechu) 槟榔 9-12g and **zhi shi** (Fructus Immaturus Citri Aurantii) 枳实 9-12g.
- With Heat in the Stomach, add **lu gen** (Rhizoma Phragmitis Communis) 芦根 15-24g and **huang lian** (Rhizoma Coptidis) 黄连 3-6g.
- With Cold in the Stomach, delete **lian qiao**, and add **gan jiang** (Rhizoma Zingiberis Officinalis) 干姜 6-9g and **sha ren** (Fructus Amomi) 砂仁 6-9g.

Variations and additional prescriptions

Food stagnation with Damp Heat

- For more chronic cases, with significant digestive disruption and the generation of Damp Heat, with severe abdominal pain, foul diarrhoea or constipation, excessive flatulence, scanty concentrated urine, a red tongue with a greasy yellow coat and a deep strong pulse, the aim of treatment is to guide stagnation downward, clear Heat and dispel Damp with **ZHI SHI DAO ZHI WAN** (*Immature Bitter Orange Pill to Guide out Stagnation* 枳实导滞丸, p.9).

Purging the stagnation

- If the patient is really uncomfortable and distended, a few doses of a mild purge, such as **TIAO WEI CHENG QI TANG** (*Regulate the Stomach and Order the Qi Decoction* 调胃承气汤, p.468) may be employed to first clear the stagnation from the Intestines.

Food stagnation with Spleen deficiency

- Some chronic cases are likely to proceed towards greater deficiency, wherein the Spleen and Stomach are increasingly weakened and more and more unable to deal with the digestive demands placed upon them. In these cases, the patient experiences pain, bloating and early satiety with a small intake of food. In addition, there will be signs of *qi* deficiency–pallor, weakness and fatigue. Initial treatment should strengthen the Spleen and resolve food stagnation with **JIAN PI WAN** (*Strengthen the Spleen Pill* 健脾丸, p.10). Once the digestion is stronger, a more supplementing prescription (for example, **LIU JUN ZI TANG** *Six Major Herbs Combination* 六君子汤, p.769) may be used for longer term strengthening of the digestive system.

Patent medicines

Bao He Wan 保和丸 (Bao He Wan)
Mu Xiang Shun Qi Wan 木香顺气丸 (Mu Xiang Shun Qi Wan)
Shen Qu Cha 神曲茶 (Shen Chu Cha)
Liu He Bao He Wan 六合保和丸 (Bo Wo Yuen Medical Pills)
Jian Pi Wan 健脾丸 (Jian Pi Wan)
- Spleen deficiency with food stagnation

Acupuncture (select from)

Ren.12 (*zhong wan*) .... *mu* point of the Stomach, alleviates stagnation in the Stomach
St.25 (*tian shu*) .... *mu* point of the Large Intestine, regulates Intestinal function
Ren.6 (*qi hai*) .... regulates *qi* and alleviates distension
St.36 (*zu san li*) .... *he* sea point of the Stomach, regulates and strengthens the Stomach, strengthens digestion
St.40 (*feng long* -) .... *luo* point of the Stomach, transforms Phlegm and clears stagnant food, Heat and Phlegm from the Stomach
LI.10 (*shou san li*) .... benefits digestion and regulates gastro-intestinal function
St.44 (*nei ting* -) .... *rong* spring and Water point of the Stomach, clears Heat from the Stomach, alleviates food stagnation

- with severe pain, add Sp.4 (*gong sun* -), St.34 (*liang qiu* -), Sp.8 (*di ji* -) and St.21 (*liang men* -)
- with nausea, add PC.6 (*nei guan* -)
- with borborygmus, add Sp.5 (*shang qiu* -)
- with constipation, add St.37 (*shang ju xu* -) and SJ.6 (*zhi gou* -)

- with Spleen deficiency, add Sp.6 (*san yin jiao* +) and Bl.20 (*pi shu* +)
- with Liver *qi* stagnation, add GB.34 (*yang ling quan* -)
- *Ear points*: stomach, spleen, abdomen, small intestine, pancreas, *shen men*, sympathetic

Clinical notes

- A liquid or semiliquid diet, or total fasting should be maintained for the first few days of the treatment, and smaller meals, perhaps more frequently, considered afterwards. Because this is largely a disorder of overindulgence and irregular dietary habits, the patient should be counselled accordingly, and, in uncomplicated cases, this is usually enough to cure the problem.
- The Chinese have long known the benefits of sipping small amounts of certain teas while eating. The action of such teas helps assist digestion, especially of fats, and reduces the risk of food stagnation. European cultures use table wine in much the same way, hence 'a little wine for thy stomach's sake'. Similarly, 'bitters', combinations of bitter herbs and alcohol, are a common accompaniment to food, either as a digestive aid following a meal, or as an aperitive. The bitterness of the herbs assists the descent of Stomach *qi* and dries Damp.

虫积

2.6 WORM ACCUMULATION

2.6.1 True worms (pin, tape, thread, round, hook)
2.6.2 Other unwanted lodgers (*gu* syndrome)

蛊证

Pathophysiology

- Intestinal worms are an often overlooked cause of abdominal pain and may contribute to numerous other, often baffling, symptoms in the Western world. Worms and other parasites appear to be quite common even in developed societies, especially in warmer climates.
- The term 'worm' (*chong* 虫) has several connotations in TCM. It can refer to the large and visible variety of worm, such as round, tape, pin or thread worms that inhabit the intestines, or blood parasites such as schistosomes. It can also refer to the 'invisible' variety, manifesting in conditions which we may describe as 'candidiasis', *gu* syndrome, or any of a number of patterns due to the lingering persistence of some obstinate pathogenic influence (*fu xie* 伏邪). These may be chronic viral, bacterial or fungal infections.
- Depending on the type of *chong* infestation, the approach will be different. For the large and visible variety, vermicidal herbs can be used for a relatively short period of time to kill the worms, perhaps then followed by a Spleen strengthening prescription to restore the digestion. For the invisible variety, treatment needs to be prolonged and flexible, slowly altering the internal environment to make it hostile to the lodger, while gently strengthening *zheng qi*. This can be a complex business, as too much supplementation can strengthen the pathogen, and too much pathogen clearing can damage *zheng qi*.

2.6.1 True worms

Clinical features

The features will vary depending on the type of infestation, however the following are a selection of common signs and symptoms.

- intermittent abdominal pain of variable intensity, usually around the umbilicus
- persistent abdominal distension, flatulence
- ravenous hunger or loss of appetite
- itchy anus or nose
- tooth grinding at night
- dark rings under the eyes, blue or purple spots or lines in the sclera
- scaly white spots on the face and neck (*chong ban* 虫斑), small red papules on the inside of the lips and upper surface of the tongue
- lethargy

- there will often be some objective evidence–worms or worm parts or eggs in the stools
- in chronic cases there will be signs of *qi* and Blood deficiency–emaciation, sallow complexion, fatigue, dizziness, insomnia, pale tongue and weak pulse

Treatment principle

Kill worms

Prescription

ZHUI CHONG WAN 追虫丸
(*Pursue Parasites Pill*) modified

This prescription is a broad spectrum vermicide. It should not be used for more than a week or two, and then always followed by an appropriate Spleen strengthening prescription.

bing lang (Semen Arecae Catechu) 槟榔 12g
ku lian gen pi (Cortex Meliae Radicis) 苦楝根皮 12g
zhi ke (Fructus Citri Aurantii) 枳壳 12g
lei wan (Sclerotium Omphaliae Lapidescens) 雷丸 9g
shi jun zi (Fructus Quisqualis Indicae) 使君子 9g
mu xiang (Radix Aucklandiae Lappae) 木香 9g
qian niu zi (Semen Pharbitidis) 牵牛子 9g
hou po (Cortex Magnoliae Officinalis) 厚朴 9g

Method: Decoction. **Bing lang**, **lei wan**, **shi jun zi** and **ku lian gen pi** kill worms; **mu xiang** regulates *qi* and stops pain; **bing lang**, **qian niu zi**, **zhi ke** and **hou po**, direct *qi* and the worms downwards to be expelled. (Source: *Zhong Yi Nei Ke Ji Zheng Zheng Zhi*)

QU TAO TANG 驱绦汤
(*Expel Tapeworm Decoction*)

This prescription is suitable for tapeworms. It is contraindicated during pregnancy. The smaller dose is for children, the larger dose is for adults.

nan gua zi (Semen Cucurbitae Moschatae) 南瓜子 60-120g
bing lang (Semen Arecae Catechu) 槟榔 30-60g

Method: Powder and swallow the **nan gua zi** (pumpkin seeds) on an empty stomach with water. Follow this two hours later with a concentrated decoction of the **bing lang**. Within 4-5 hours this should produce diarrhoea that contains the tapeworms. If not, follow with 9 grams of **mang xiao** (Mirabilitum) 芒硝 dissolved in water. If there are no tapeworm heads (scolex) present, repeat the treatment in two weeks. **Nan gua zi** kills tapeworms; **bing lang** guides the sick or dying worms down and out.

If symptoms of Damp Heat are obvious, add **huang bai** (Cortex Phellodendri) 黄柏 9g and **huang lian** (Rhizoma Coptidis) 黄连 9g to the decoction. (Source: *Shi Yong Fang Ji Xue*)

WU MEI WAN 乌梅丸
(*Mume Pill*)

This prescription is selected for intermittent periumbilical pain associated with infestation by intestinal roundworms. This interesting prescription, with its mix of hot and cold herbs, treats a variety or complex patterns characterised by Heat, Cold and *qi* deficiency. It may be used for chronic gastro-intestinal conditions with apparent contradictory presentations, for example chronic dysentery with abdominal pain that is relieved by warmth in a patient with a red tongue. In the absence of actual worms, this prescription is also useful for some presentations of the primary pathological triad (*see* p.912).

wu mei (Fructus Pruni Mume) 乌梅 .... 48 (24)g
huang lian (Rhizoma Coptidis) 黄连 .... 48 (9)g
huang bai (Cortex Phellodendri) 黄柏 .... 18 (9)g
gan jiang (Rhizoma Zingiberis Officinalis) 干姜 .... 30 (9)g
dang gui (Radix Angelicae Sinensis) 当归 .... 12 (9)g
ren shen (Radix Ginseng) 人参 .... 18 (9)g
zhi fu zi (Radix Aconiti Carmichaeli Praeparata)
制附子 .... 18 (6)g
gui zhi (Ramulus Cinnamomi Cassiae) 桂枝 .... 18 (6)g
chuan jiao (Pericarpium Zanthoxyli Bungeani) 川椒 .... 12 (3)g
xi xin (Herba cum Radice Asari) 细辛 .... 18 (3)g

Method: Grind the herbs to a fine powder and form into 9-gram pills with honey. The dose is one pill 2-3 times daily. May also be decocted with the quantities shown in brackets, in which case **zhi fu zi** is cooked for 30 minutes before adding the other herbs (*xian jian* 先煎). **Wu mei** eliminates roundworms; **chuan jiao** and **xi xin** assist the **wu mei** in stunning the roundworms while warming the interior; **huang lian** and **huang bai** attack the worms by making the environment hostile, and drain downwards with their bitter coldness; **gan jiang**, **zhi fu zi** and **gui zhi** warm *yang* and dispel Cold and balance the bitter coldness of the previous two herbs; **dang gui** and **ren shen** supplement *qi* and Blood.

Patent medicines

Fei Zi San 肥仔散 (Baby Fat Powder)

- This medicine is a specific vermicide and is designed for infants and children. It can also be used for adults with up to four times the child's dose.

Acupuncture

Acupuncture is a second choice of treatment for true worms, but a Spleen strengthening and *qi* mechanism correcting strategy is recommended following the expulsion of the worms. *See* p.96 for suggestions.

- roundworms in the bile duct: St.2 (*si bai*), St.25 (*tian shu*), Ren.4 (*qi hai*), *dan nang xue* (M-LE-23)

Clinical notes

- Some consider that the most practical approach in cases of pin, thread, hook, tape or roundworms is to use a pharmaceutical vermicide such as Combantrin or Vermox. These medicines are usually single dose and practical for children. The whole family (including animals) should be treated to eliminate carriers. The advantage of the herbal approach is its mildness and the fact that small children can easily tolerate the medicine.
- Once the worms have been eliminated, always follow up with an appropriate Spleen strengthening prescription.

2.6.2 Gu syndrome (蛊证)

Pathophysiology

- *Gu* syndrome describes a state of chronic infection by fungi, bacteria or viruses. G*u* syndrome is thought to be a complex type of systemic infection involving a host with a weakened constitution in a pathological equilibrium with an unwelcome guest. Fruehauf (1998) notes that *gu* toxins are like 'oil seeping into flour–it is everywhere and cannot be separated out' He also notes that treatment of *gu* syndrome is lengthy, requiring months or even years.
- Because of its interwoven complexity, the treatment of *gu* syndrome is also quite complicated. A large percentage of patients however, present with variations of the primary pathological triad (p.912), and depending on where the patient maps on the triad (p.914), the primary treatment strategy will vary. The treatment strategy has two components, the rectification of the underlying pathology that allows the *gu* to flourish, and specific targeting and dispersal of the *gu* itself.

Clinical features

- abdominal pain, cramping and/or distension
- chronic diarrhoea or alternating constipation and diarrhoea
- nausea and vomiting
- loss of appetite, ravenous hunger or odd food craving
- muscle soreness, heaviness or weakness, wandering pains
- physical and mental exhaustion
- depression, mood swings, easy anger, confusion, restlessness, disordered thought patterns
- fluid retention

T variable, likely possibilities include thick white or yellow coat, dark or pale with toothmarks, or with redder edges

P variable

Treatment principle

Strengthen the Spleen and supplement *qi*
Clear Damp, Damp Heat or stagnant Heat
Regulate Liver *qi*
Fragrantly disperse *gu* parasites

Prescription

In practice, a flexible approach to treatment is necessary and the primary prescription will vary as the currents of the patient's pathology ebb and flow. Depending on where the patient is mapped on the pathological triad the guiding formula and the thrust of treatment will be different. See p.912 for a discussion.

Modifications

- According to Fruehauf, the specific pathogen, the *gu*, is adequately dispersed with a trio of fragrant herbs, **zi su ye** (Folium Perillae Frutescentis) 紫苏叶, **bo he** (Herba Mentha Haplocalycis) 薄荷 and **bai zhi** (Radix Angelicae Dahuricae) 白芷. These may be added to the appropriate primary prescription. See Fruehauf H (1998): *Journal of Chinese Medicine, Gu syndrome* 蛊证, 57:10-17 for more detail on approaches to this interesting topic.

Patent medicines

Zhui Feng Su He Wan 追风苏合丸 (So Hup Yuen Medical Pills)
Fei Zi San 肥仔散 (Baby Fat Powder)
- This medicine is a specific vermicide and is designed for infants and children. It can also be used for adults with up to four times the child's dose.

Xing Jun San 行军散 (Marching Powder, Five Pagodas Brand)
- a small dose of this extremely fragrant medicine can be useful over a long period of time, in combination with an appropriate constitutional prescription

Acupuncture (select from)

Treatment is focused on strengthening the Spleen and Stomach, clearing Damp and Damp Heat and easing the Liver so as to make the environment hostile to the invader.

Ren.12 (*zhong wan* +▲) .. *mu* point of the Stomach, strengthens the Spleen and Stomach, directs Stomach *qi* downwards and harmonises the Stomach
St.25 (*tian shu*) .... *mu* point of the Large Intestine, regulates Intestinal function

Sp.15 (*da heng*) .... strengthens the Spleen and resolves Damp
Ren.6 (*qi hai*) .... strengthens the Kidneys, regulates *qi* and alleviates distension
St.36 (*zu san li* +▲) .... *he* sea point of the Stomach, powerfully strengthens the Spleen and Stomach, supplements *qi*
Sp.3 (*tai bai*) .... *yuan*, *shu* stream and Earth point of the Spleen, strengthens the Spleen and transforms Dampness
St.40 (*feng long* -) .... *luo* point of the Stomach, transforms Phlegm and clears Dampness, with Sp.3 (*tai bai*)
Sp.6 (*san yin jiao*) .... strengthens the Spleen, regulates Liver *qi*, benefits the Kidneys
Bl.20 (*pi shu* +) .... *shu* point of the Spleen, strengthens Spleen *qi*
Bl.21 (*wei shu* +) .... *shu* point of the Stomach, regulates the *qi* mechanism

- with nausea, add PC.6 (*nei guan* -)
- with abdominal bloating, add Sp.4 (*gong sun* -) or Sp.5 (*shang qiu* -)
- with Spleen deficiency, add Sp.6 (*san yin jiao* +) and Bl.20 (*pi shu* +)

Clinical notes

- *Gu* syndrome may be diagnosed biomedically as leaky gut syndrome, candidiasis, giardiasis or a variety of unnamed chronic viral, fungal, amoebic or bacterial gastro-intestinal disorders.
- *Gu* syndrome is a complex situation with no simple solution. However the general approach described above can be applied to some of the more mysterious and difficult ailments we see in the clinic, for example chronic fatigue syndrome and candidiasis.
- Dietary recommendations are usually based on avoidance of Damp and Damp Heat promoting elements, and Spleen *qi* strengthening. See p.870 and 880.

SUMMARY OF GUIDING FORMULAE FOR ABDOMINAL PAIN

Excess Cold - *Si Ni Tang* 四逆汤
- in mild cases - *Liang Fu Wan* 良附丸
- with constipation - *Da Huang Fu Zi Tang* 大黄附子汤
- with severe pain - *Da Jian Zhong Tang* 大建中汤
- with external Cold Damp invasion - *Cao Guo Yin* 草果饮

Deficient Cold - *Xiao Jian Zhong Tang* 小健中汤
- with Spleen *yang* deficiency - *Fu Zi Li Zhong Wan* 附子理中丸
- with Kidney *yang* deficiency - *Zhen Wu Tang* 真武汤
- with Spleen *yang* deficiency and constipation - *Wen Pi Tang* 温脾汤
- with icy cold or purple extremities and an imperceptible pulse - *Dang Gui Si Ni Tang*
- with menstrual disorder - *Ai Fu Nuan Gong Wan* 艾附暖宫丸, *Wen Jing Tang* 温经汤, *Sheng Hua Tang* 生化汤
- with postpartum Cold and Blood stagnation - *Sheng Hua Tang* 生化汤
- with Cold and *qi* stagnation in the genitals - *Nuan Gan Jian* 暖肝煎
- with Cold and deficiency of *chong* and *ren mai* - *Wen Jing Tang* 温经汤

Heat - *Da Cheng Qi Tang* 大承气汤
- with intestinal abscess - *Da Huang Mu Dan Pi Tang* 大黄牡丹皮汤
- Damp Heat in the intestines - *Shao Yao Tang* 芍药汤
- acute Damp Heat in the Uterus - *Yin Qiao Hong Jiang Jie Du Tang* 银翘红酱解毒汤
- chronic Damp Heat in the Uterus - *Qing Re Jie Du Hua Yu Tang* 清热解毒化瘀汤
- Summerheat - *Huang Lian Xiang Ru Yin* 黄连香薷饮

Liver *qi* stagnation - *Chai Hu Shu Gan San* 柴胡疏肝散
- with chronic constipation - *Liu Mo Tang* 六磨汤
- with diarrhoea and cramping pain - *Tong Xie Yao Fang* 痛泻要方
- with Spleen deficiency and Blood deficiency - *Xiao Yao San* 逍遥散
- with Liver *yin* deficiency - *Yi Guan Jian* 一贯煎
- lower abdominal pain or testicular pain and coldness - *Tian Tai Wu Yao San* 天台乌药散

Blood stagnation - *Shao Fu Zhu Yu Tang* 少腹逐瘀汤
- with *qi* and Blood stagnation - *Xue Fu Zhu Yu Tang* 血府逐瘀汤
- with *shao yang* involvement - *Xiao Chai Hu Tang* 小柴胡汤
- mild cases with gynaecological masses - *Gui Zhi Fu Ling Wan* 桂枝茯苓丸

- with Heat - *Tao He Cheng Qi Tang* 桃核承气汤
- following trauma - *Fu Yuan Huo Xue Tang* 复元活血汤

Food stagnation - *Bao He Wan* 保和丸
- with severe Damp Heat - *Zhi Shi Dao Zhi Wan* 枳实导滞丸
- with Spleen deficiency - *Jian Pi Wan* 健脾丸

Worm accumulation - *Zhui Chong Wan* 追虫丸
- tapeworms - *Qu Tao Tang* 驱绦汤
- roundworms - *Wu Mei Wan* 乌梅丸

Table 2.1 *Differential diagnosis of abdominal pain*

Pattern	Duration	Aggravated by	Ameliorated by	Nature of pain	Nature of patient	Pulse and tongue
Excess Cold	mostly acute	ingesting cold substances, pressure on the abdomen	warmth on the abdomen	violent, cramping, colicky, may come in spasmodic waves	may be robust, young or otherwise in good health	T: white coat P: wiry, tight
Deficient Cold	mostly chronic, with occasional acute exacerbations	ingesting cold substances, exposure to cold, when fatigued, raw cold food	pressure and warmth applied to abdomen	dull, nagging, intermittent	pale, run down, cold intolerant possibly overweight or tends to oedema, cold intolerance, F>M	T: pale and swollen P: deep, slow, weak
Heat	acute	pressure, heat	application of cold to abdomen, evacuation of bowels	pain, especially in the left iliac fossa, with a very tense abdomen	all ages	T: dry yellow coat P: deep, strong
Damp Heat	mostly acute, may be chronic	pressure, heat	application of cold to abdomen, evacuation of bowels	lower abdominal pain with either diarrhoea or copious yellow vaginal discharge	all ages (Uterine D/H F>18)	T: greasy yellow coat P: slippery, rapid

Liver *qi* stagnation	mostly chronic	emotion and stress	relaxation, expulsion of gas	cramping, intermittent	tense, uptight, nervy, most common 20-50 yrs F>M	T: normal or dark or with red edges P: wiry
Blood stagnation	chronic, although may be acute after surgery or trauma	pressure		stabbing, fixed, in location, often severe	adults, mostly older 40+	T: purple or with brown or purple spots P: choppy, wiry
Food stagnation	acute or chronic	eating, pressure	vomiting, belching, defecation, expulsion of gas	distending, focal	adults, sedentary occupation, business lunches	T: thick greasy yellow coat P: full, slippery
Worm accumulation	chronic	cold or raw food sugar, dairy		intermittent, umbilical	all ages, particularly children	

3. Acid Reflux (Heartburn)

Liver *qi* invading the Stomach
Stomach and Liver Heat
Phlegm Damp
Food stagnation
Spleen and Stomach *qi*/*yang* deficiency
Stomach and Liver *yin* deficiency

3 ACID REFLUX (Heartburn)

tu suan 吐酸

Acid reflux[1] and heartburn (also known as gastro-oesophageal reflux disease, or GERD), are conditions in which gastric acids ascend from the stomach to the oesophagus or mouth. Acid reflux, incorporating heartburn, is sour gastric acid that can be detected in the mouth or throat. Heartburn specifically refers to a sensation of retrosternal burning that spreads upwards to the throat.

Acid reflux and heartburn often occur in association with other gastrointestinal 'disease symptoms' like epigastric pain, abdominal distension and discomfort, nausea and indeterminate gnawing hunger, but may occur alone.

In Chinese medicine, reflux is generally associated with rebellious Stomach *qi*. Stomach *qi* should descend, carrying the waste by-products of digestion through the Intestines to the exterior of the body. Stomach *qi* will rise if it is blocked and unable to descend, or it is forced to rise by Heat, or if it is too weak to descend. The descent of Stomach *qi* can be blocked by disruption to the *qi* mechanism as a result of *qi* stagnation, or by pathogens such as Phlegm Damp or stagnant food.

Chronic acid reflux and heartburn can contribute to a number of other problems depending on where the acid ends up. If gastric contents are aspirated into the lungs, as may occur during sleep, bronchitis and asthma may result. If the throat is affected it can cause hoarseness and sore throat. If the oesophagus is scarred, dysphagia and regurgitation may result.

AETIOLOGY

Diet

Diet plays a major role in the production of acid reflux and heartburn. Perhaps the most common is eating large quantities of foods that heat the Stomach and Liver. These include substances like chilli and spices, alcohol, coffee and chocolate. Once Heat is resident in the Stomach its natural tendency to rise can carry acid up through the oesophagus to the mouth. In addition, there are certain groups of food that are particularly problematic to people prone to heartburn. These include acid foods like the citrus family, tomatoes, uncooked peppers and capsicums, radishes, onions and garlic.

Eating at odd hours, too late at night, while rushing or in times of stress can disrupt the function of the Stomach, contributing to food stagnation (*see* p.3), and the eventual weakening of the Spleen and Stomach. Eating more food than the Spleen and Stomach can cope with, either because of

[1]Wiseman's 'Acid Vomiting'

simple overeating or because the Spleen is already weak, will obstruct the *qi* mechanism and thus the descent and ascent of middle *jiao qi*. Once the *qi* mechanism is obstructed by unprocessed and accumulated food, various complications can arise to further aggravate the disordered movement of Stomach *qi*, most typically the generation of Dampness and Phlegm and/or constipation.

BOX 3.1 SOME BIOMEDICAL CAUSES OF ACID REFLUX

- peptic ulcer disease
- acute and chronic gastritis
- alcohol and tobacco excess
- dyspepsia
- cardiac sphincter scarring
- hiatus hernia
- pregnancy
- obesity

Drugs
- anticholinergics
- calcium channel blockers
- theophylline

In addition to the heat inducing aspects of the diet, those that weaken the Spleen and Stomach can also contribute to acid reflux and heartburn by causing failure of the *qi* mechanism. Cold raw foods weaken Spleen *qi* and *yang*. Medications to clear Heat, including herbs and antibiotics, weaken the Spleen and contribute to Dampness. Reduced food intake as a result of strict dieting, or prolonged starvation or digestive insult, such as occurs in patients with a history of anorexia nervosa, bulimia or during famine, serious damages Spleen *yang*. Digestive inefficiency may then contribute to the clogging of the *qi* mechanism by Dampness and increase the potential for complicating food stagnation.

Emotion

Liver *qi* stagnation is a common cause of reflux and heartburn. Liver *qi* stagnation impacts on the abdomen in numerous ways. Liver *qi* can invade the Spleen and Stomach and disrupt the *qi* mechanism. It can impair the Spleen's ability to efficiently extract all the goodness from ingested material, leaving a clogging residue of Damp. Damp can also result from the retardation of fluid movement by the reluctant *qi*. *Qi* stagnation can slow the passage of food through the Intestines, causing constipation and a backing up of *qi* through the gastro-intestinal system, in turn causing Stomach *qi* to rise.

Liver *qi* stagnation is most commonly produced by repression of emotion, the buried frustrations of everyday life, the suppressed anger and resentments. These unexpressed feelings cause a low grade spasm and tension in the smooth muscle of the gut. Patients with chronic *qi* stagnation type digestive problems will often note that stress and tension are stored in the gut and be aware of the consequences of stress, the knot in the stomach, heartburn, loss of appetite, etc. This type of reflux tends to be episodic and is clearly related to the patient's emotional state.

BOX 3.2 KEY DIAGNOSTIC POINTS

Aggravation
- with stress - *qi* stagnation
- with heating foods (alcohol, coffee, chocolate) - Stomach and Liver Heat
- with bending or lying - Spleen deficiency
- with a cold or flu - Lung *qi* accumulation
- with eating - food stagnation, Phlegm Damp, Damp Heat
- with emotions and stress - Liver qi stagnation, *yin* (Blood) deficiency
- with palpation - Blood stagnation, Damp Heat, *qi* stagnation (up to a point)

Amelioration
- belching, release of gas - food stagnation, *qi* stagnation

In addition to the emotional factors that upset the Liver, worry, obsessive thinking and prolonged concentration, in combination with a sedentary or studious lifestyle and poor diet, will weaken Spleen *qi*. The weakened Spleen is predisposed to invasion by Liver *qi* resulting in further damage, as well as primarily disrupting the *qi* mechanism. Spleen *qi* naturally ascends, creating the appropriate equilibrium for the descent of turbid waste materials, so it is said the Spleen governs 'the raising of the clear and descent of the turbid'. If this activity fails, the *qi* and 'clear and turbid' (turbid here implying Dampness as well as waste materials) intermingle and accumulate in the middle *jiao*, further preventing the descent of Stomach *qi*.

TREATMENT

The first aspect of treatment is to rigorously assess the patient's diet for possible aggravating elements, and then remove them.

There are two aspects to consider when planning the treatment strategy, the patient's symptoms and constitution. Constitutional treatment is always applied. Depending on the severity of the symptoms, the weight given to treatment of symptoms (the *biao*) can vary. In severe cases, the focus of treatment may be to first swiftly alleviate reflux, then when the symptoms are under control, deal with the underlying pattern (the *ben*).

A note on antacid medications

There are numerous antacid medications available over the counter. These drugs are heavily advertised and their use is widespread, and in general they are effective at symptomatically alleviating acid reflux and heartburn. Most are based on a metal ion (calcium, magnesium, aluminium or sodium) linked to an alkali (hydroxide, bicarbonate, trisilicate) which neutralises the hydrochloric acid of the stomach.

BOX 3.3 SPECIFIC ASPECTS OF MANAGEMENT

These are some common behaviours and foods that aggravate a tendency to acid reflux and heartburn. The advice below may be offered in the appropriate situation.

Behaviour

- lose weight
- exercise regularly
- do not eat late at night, and leave several hours between the evening meal and bed
- avoid overeating or eating too fast
- chew food thoroughly
- avoid overly tight or restrictive clothing, belts, support garments or corsets
- take medications with plenty of water while sitting upright
- elevate the bed by putting a 10-20cm wooden block under the head of the bed
- keep bowel habits regular
- practise stress management

Food

- reduce intake of coffee, chocolate, cola drinks, orange and other citrus juices and tomatoes
- reduce or avoid tobacco and alcohol
- avoid foods that produce gas or are hard to digest, such as onions and garlic, beans and pulses, cucumbers, radishes, capsicum and cabbage; in some people wheat products
- avoid excessive carbohydrates (bread, pasta, rice etc.) in the evening
- reduce dairy products

There are two negative aspects associated with prolonged use of antacids. First, the underlying cause of the reflux is generally not addressed and second, they have side effects including constipation, diarrhoea, belching, flatulence and nausea. More worrying are the consequences of accumulation of metal ions, and electrolyte disturbances such as alkalosis and hypercalcaemia.

Table 3.1 *Herbs and substances specific for hyperacidity and heartburn*

<table>
<tr><th>Herb</th><th colspan="2">Characteristics</th></tr>
<tr><td>Huang Lian 黄连 (Rhizoma Coptidis)

Wu Zhu Yu 吴茱萸 (Fructus Evodiae Rutaecarpae)</td><td colspan="2">This pair of herbs constitutes ZUO JIN WAN (Left Metal Pill 左金丸), one of the most important combinations for heartburn and hyperacidity. Although classically indicated for Heat in the Liver and Stomach, they can be added to most prescriptions to give symptomatic relief. They appear in most prescriptions for excess patterns in this chapter. An interesting feature is the unusual proportion of the herbs- a large dose of huang lian (usually 3-6 fold) relative to wu zhu yu. They can be used alone for Liver and Stomach Heat type heartburn, but are more commonly incorporated into an appropriate constitutional formula.</td></tr>
<tr><td>Hai Piao Xiao 海螵蛸 (Os Speiae seu Sepiellae)</td><td rowspan="4">These substances are largely composed of calcium carbonate and are used powdered to neutralise gastric acid. Each has its own characteristics and specific clinical uses. They are used for controlling symptoms in the short term and are generally not suitable for long term use. Can be decocted or taken as a powder and followed by a strained decoction.</td><td>Cuttle fish bone. Astringent for leakage of various fluids- bleeding, diarrhoea, leucorrhoea.</td></tr>
<tr><td>Wa Leng Zi 瓦楞子 (Concha Arcae)</td><td>Cockle shell. Softens hardness , invigorates Blood and disperses Phlegm. Good when there is a mass or focal pain.</td></tr>
<tr><td>Mu Li 牡蛎 (Concha Ostrea)</td><td>Oyster shell. Astringent, calms the shen. Best when there is emotional or shen disturbance- insomnia, anxiety, panic attacks.</td></tr>
<tr><td>Hai Ge Ke 海蛤壳 (Concha Cyclinae Sinensis)</td><td>Clam shell. Clears Heat, softens hardness and dissipates nodules. Best for Heat patterns and those with Phlegm.</td></tr>
</table>

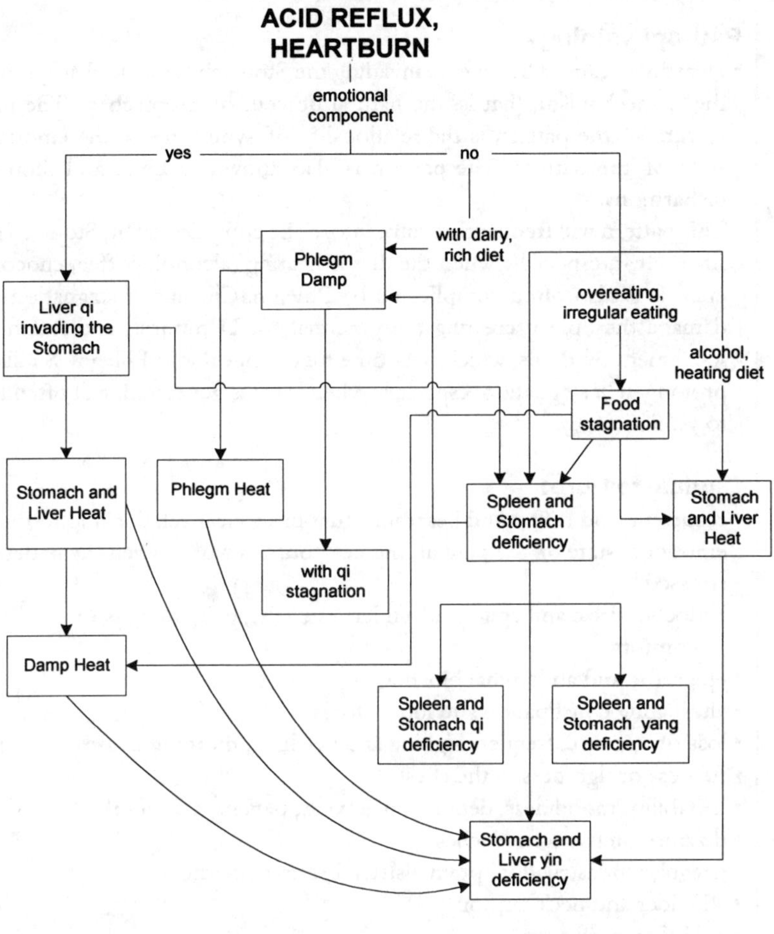

Figure 3.1 *Diagnostic strategy for acid reflux and heartburn*

肝胃不和

3.1 LIVER QI INVADING THE STOMACH

Pathophysiology

- Heartburn caused by Liver *qi* invading the Stomach is due to disruption of the *qi* mechanism, that is, the natural descent of Stomach *qi*. The main feature of the pattern is the relationship of symptoms to the emotional state of the patient. The pattern is also known as Liver and Stomach disharmony.
- This pattern will frequently evolve into, or be complicated by, Stomach and Liver Heat, especially when the diet is heating (alcohol, coffee, chocolate etc.). It is also often complicated by Phlegm. Chronic *qi* stagnation will damage the Spleen creating the potential for Dampness, and retard the movement of fluids, which over time may congeal into Phlegm. Similarly, prolonged *qi* stagnation, especially when Heat is generated, will often lead to *yin* deficiency.

Clinical features

- recurrent acid reflux and heartburn that has a clear relationship to the emotional state of the patient; the heartburn is worse when the patient is stressed
- hypochondriac and epigastric tenderness, ache, pain, fullness or discomfort
- epigastric and abdominal bloating
- alternating constipation and loose stools
- loss of appetite, frequent sighing and belching, morning nausea
- fullness or tightness in the chest
- irritability, moodiness, depression, anxiety, patient 'a worrier'
- dizziness, tension headaches
- irregular menstruation, premenstrual breast tenderness
- shoulder and neck tension
- cold fingers and toes

T unremarkable or darkish, with a thin white coat
P wiry

Treatment principle

Regulate *qi*, harmonize the Liver and Stomach
Redirect Stomach *qi* downwards

Prescription

SI NI SAN 四逆散
(*Bupleurum and Zhi Shi Formula*) modified

chai hu (Radix Bupleuri) 柴胡 9-12g

zhi shi (Fructus Immaturus Citri Aurantii) 枳实 9-12g
bai shao (Radix Paeoniae Lactiflora) 白芍 12-18g
zhi gan cao (honey fried Radix Glycyrrhizae Uralensis)
炙甘草 6-9g
hai piao xiao (Os Sepiae seu Sepiellae) 海螵蛸 15g
huang lian (Rhizoma Coptidis) 黄连 3-6g
wu zhu yu (Fructus Evodiae Rutaecarpae) 吴茱萸 1-2g

Method: Decoction. **Chai hu** regulates and invigorates Liver *qi* and clears Heat; **zhi shi** breaks up stagnant *qi*, directs *qi* downwards and alleviates distension, it's descending action neatly balances the ascending nature of **chai hu** thus facilitating the correct functioning of the *qi* mechanism; **bai shao** softens the Liver and nourishes *yin* and Blood, thus preventing excessive dispersal of, and damage to, *qi* and Liver *yin* by **chai hu; gan cao** harmonises the Stomach and strengthens the Spleen, and with **bai shao** eases spasms, thereby alleviating cramping pain; **hai piao xiao** alleviates gastric acidity; **huang lian** clears Heat from the Liver and Stomach; **wu zhu yu** is pungent and warm and promotes movement of *qi*, together these last two herbs clear Heat and direct Stomach *qi* downward. (Source: *Shi Yong Zhong Yi Nei Ke Xue*)

Modifications

- In severe cases, add **duan wa leng zi** (calcined Concha Arcae) 煅瓦楞子 15g and **zhe bei mu** (Bulbus Fritillariae Thunbergii) 浙贝母 12g.
- With a severe retrosternal sharp burning sensation, add **pu gong ying** (Herba Taraxaci Mongolici) 蒲公英 18-30g.
- With epigastric pain, add **yan hu suo** (Rhizoma Corydalis Yanhusuo) 延胡索 9-12g and **yu jin** (Tuber Curcumae) 郁金 9-12g.
- With nausea, add **ban xia** (Rhizoma Pinelliae Ternatae) 半夏 9-12g and **sheng jiang** (Rhizoma Zingiberis Officinalis Recens) 生姜 9-12g.
- With vomiting, add **dai zhe shi** (Haematitum) 代赭石 15g and **shi di** (Calyx Diospyri Kaki) 柿蒂 9-12g.
- If the patient is irritable, tense and uptight, add **he huan pi** (Cortex Albizziae Julibrissin) 合欢皮 15g and **shan zhi zi** (Fructus Gardeniae Jasminoides) 山栀子 9-12g.
- With insomnia or restlessness at night, add **mu li** (Concha Ostreae) 牡蛎 15-30g, **zhen zhu mu** (Concha Margaritiferae) 珍珠母 15g and **yu jin** (Tuber Curcumae) 郁金 9-12g.
- With gallstones, add **jin qian cao** (Herba Lysimachiae) 金钱草 30g, **yin chen** (Herba Artemisiae Yinchenhao) 茵陈 12g and **ji nei jin** (Endothelium Corneum Gigeriae Galli) 鸡内金 12g.

Variations and additional prescriptions

Qi stagnation in the Spleen and Stomach

- When the patient presents with general symptoms of Stomach and Spleen (middle *jiao*) *qi* stagnation, with a lesser element of Liver *qi* stagnation (the focus of symptoms is in the epigastrium and oesophagus, the emotional component is not so clear, and there is a clear dietary relationship), a general *qi* moving and stagnation clearing approach is appropriate. The aim of treatment is to move *qi* and clear the 'six stagnations' (*qi*, Damp, Fire, Food, Blood and Phlegm–modify the prescription accordingly) with **YUE JU WAN** (*Escape Restraint Pill* 越鞠丸) modified.

xiang fu (Rhizoma Cyperi Rotundi) 香附 100g
cang zhu (Rhizoma Atractylodis) 苍术 100g
chuan xiong (Radix Ligustici Chuanxiong) 川芎 100g
shan zhi zi (Fructus Gardeniae Jasminoides) 山栀子 100g
shen qu (Massa Fermentata) 神曲 100g
huang lian (Rhizoma Coptidis) 黄连 60g
wu zhu yu (Fructus Evodiae Rutaecarpae) 吴茱萸 20g

Method: Grind the herbs to powder and form into 6-gram pills with water. The dose is one pill 2-3 times daily. May also be decocted with a 90% reduction in quantities. **Xiang fu** is the main herb and disperses stagnant Liver *qi*; **cang zhu** dries Dampness and Phlegm, and works with **xiang fu** to improve Spleen and Stomach function; **chuan xiong** invigorates *qi* and Blood and reinforces the *qi* moving function of **xiang fu**; **shan zhi zi** clears Heat from all three *jiao*; **shen qu** alleviates food stagnation, aids digestion and harmonises the Stomach; **huang lian** clears Heat from the Liver and Stomach; **wu zhu yu** is pungent and warm and promotes movement of *qi*, together these last two herbs clear Heat and direct Stomach *qi* downward. For other modifications see Abdominal distension, p.18).

With Phlegm

- *Qi* stagnation is frequently complicated by Phlegm due to the general inhibition of fluid movement and damage to the Spleen that results. Once Phlegm has been generated, it aggravates the obstruction in the middle *jiao* and the various structures of the digestive tract. This pattern may occur relatively late in the course of chronic reflux as the oesophagus is scarred and sclerosed. The main features are recurrent heartburn, acid reflux or regurgitation, an intermittent sensation of something lodged in the throat ('plum stone *qi*'), occasional difficulty swallowing, fullness in the chest and epigastrium, belching, nausea or vomiting, a dry mouth and throat, a greasy white tongue coat and a slippery/wiry pulse. The main symptoms are worse for stress and alleviated when the patient is relaxed. The aim of treatment is to regulate *qi*, transform Phlegm and redirect *qi* downwards with **QI GE SAN** (*Open the Diaphragm Powder* 启膈散) modified.

sha shen (Radix Adenophorae seu Glehniae) 沙参 24g
dan shen (Radix Salviae Miltiorrhizae) 丹参 18g
quan gua lou (Fructus Trichosanthes) 全瓜蒌 15g
fu ling (Sclerotium Poriae Cocos) 茯苓 15g

xuan fu hua (Flos Inulae) 旋复花 15g
ban xia (Rhizoma Pinelliae Ternatae) 半夏 12g
yu jin (Tuber Curcumae) 郁金 12g
zi su geng (Rhizoma Perilla) 紫苏梗 9g
sha ren (Fructus Amomi) 砂仁 6g
zhi gan cao (honey fried Radix Glycyrrhizae Uralensis) 炙甘草 6g

Method: Decoction. **Xuan fu hua** is usually decocted in a bag (*bao jian* 包煎). **Sha shen** and **fu ling** nourish *yin*, transform Phlegm and dissipate accumulations; **dan shen** and **yu jin** transform stagnant Blood and Phlegm, regulate and alleviate constraint of *qi*; **sha ren** fragrantly transforms Damp and harmonises the Stomach; **zi su geng** and **gua lou** open up *qi* flow through the chest; **ban xia** transforms Phlegm; **xuan fu hua** directs *qi* downwards; **zhi gan cao** harmonises the other herbs and protects the Stomach. (Source: *Xiao Hua Ke Zhuan Bing*).

With stagnant Heat, premenstrual heartburn

- If *qi* stagnation generates a degree of stagnant Heat, the main features are acid reflux and heartburn that are initiated or aggravated by stress or before menstruation, restlessness, irritability, insomnia, temporal headaches, feeling hot during episodes, a tendency to constipation, red edges on the tongue and a wiry rapid pulse. The aim of treatment is to clear stagnant Liver Heat with **DAN ZHI XIAO YAO SAN** (*Bupleurum and Paeonia Formula* 丹栀逍遥散) modified.

chai hu (Radix Bupleuri) 柴胡 9-12g
bai shao (Radix Paeoniae Lactiflora) 白芍 12-18g
fu ling (Sclerotium Poriae Cocos) 茯苓 12-15g
shan zhi zi (Fructus Gardeniae Jasminoidis) 山栀子 9-12g
dang gui (Radix Angelicae Sinensis) 当归 9-12g
bai zhu (Rhizoma Atractylodes Macrocephalae) 白术 9-12g
mu dan pi (Cortex Moutan Radicis) 牡丹皮 9-12g
zhi gan cao (honey fried Radix Glycyrrhizae Uralensis) 炙甘草 3-6g
huang lian (Rhizoma Coptidis) 黄连 6-9g
wu zhu yu (Fructus Evodiae Rutaecarpae) 吴茱萸 2-3g

Method: Decoction. **Chai hu** and **bai shao** regulate and move Liver *qi*; **fu ling**, **bai zhu** and **zhi gan cao** strengthen the Spleen; **fu ling** leaches out Damp and promotes urination; **bai zhu** dries Damp; **dang gui** and **bai shao** nourish Blood and soften the Liver; **shan zhi zi** and **mu dan pi** cool the Liver and clear stagnant Heat; **huang lian** and **wu zhu yu** clear Heat from the Liver and Stomach and alleviate heartburn.

Patent medicines

Chai Hu Shu Gan Wan 柴胡疏肝丸 (Chai Hu Shu Gan Wan)
- Liver invading the Stomach and Spleen

Shu Gan Wan 舒肝丸 (Shu Gan Wan, Shu Kan Wan)
- with epigastric pain

Xiao Yao Wan 逍遥丸 (Xiao Yao Wan, Hsiao Yao Wan, Bupleurum Sedative Pills)
- with Spleen and Blood deficiency

Jia Wei Xiao Yao Wan 加味逍遥丸 (Jia Wei Xiao Yao Wan, Dan Zhi Xiao Yao Wan)
- with stagnant Heat

Wei Te Ling 胃特灵 (Wei Te Ling Stomach Sedative)
- an antacid formula that can be combined with the appropriate constitutional formula for symptomatic relief

Xiang Lian Wan 香莲丸 (Xiang Lian Wan)
- this patent can be combined with the appropriate constitutional formula for symptomatic relief

Acupuncture (select from)

Ren.12 (*zhong wan*) .... these points direct rising Stomach *qi*
Ren.13 (*shang wan*) downwards and stimulate the *qi* mechanism

Ren.17 (*shan zhong*) .... upper sea of *qi*, helps direct *qi* downwards
PC.6 (*nei guan*) .... *luo* point of the Pericardium, master point of *yin wei mai*, spreads Liver *qi*, regulates the middle *jiao* and stimulates the *qi* mechanism
Liv.3 (*tai chong* -) ....*yuan*, *shu* and Earth point of the Liver, regulates and spreads Liver *qi* and Blood, pacifies rising *yang*
St.36 (*zu san li*) .... *he* sea point, powerfully regulates and supplements *qi* and corrects the *qi* mechanism
LI.10 (*shou san li*) .... good for regulating *qi* in the epigastrium, often tender in Stomach disorders

Bl.18 (*gan shu*) .... *shu* points of the Liver, Gallbladder and
Bl.19 (*dan shu*) Stomach respectively, move Liver *qi* and
Bl.21 (*wei shu*) correct the *qi* mechanism

- with lateral headaches and neck tension, add GB.34 (*yang ling quan*)
- with hypochondriac pain, add Liv.14 (*qi men* -)
- with Gallbladder involvement, add GB.24 (*ri yue*), GB.40 (*qiu xu* -), and *dan nang xue* (M-LE-23)
- with Heat in the Liver, add Liv.2 (*xing jian* -)
- with Spleen deficiency, add Bl.20 (*pi shu* +)
- with Phlegm or plum stone throat, add PC.5 (*jian shi* -), St.40 (*feng long* -) and Sp.3 (*tai bai*)

- with dizziness, add GB.20 (*feng chi* -)
- In most cases, points to calm the *shen* should be added: select one or two points from Ht.7 (*shen men*), *yin tang* (M-HN-3), Du.19 (*hou ding*), Du. 24 (*shen ting*)
- *Ear points*: oesophagus, pylorus, liver, spleen, stomach, *shen men*, subcortex, sympathetic

Clinical notes

- Liver *qi* invading the Stomach type acid reflux and heartburn may be diagnosed biomedically as reflux oesophagitis, gastro-oesophageal reflux, chronic gastritis, peptic ulcer disease, nervous stomach, functional dyspepsia or hiatus hernia.
- This is a common pattern of acid reflux, and one that often requires diligence to resolve completely. Identification and, if possible, rectification of the emotional and stress triggers is essential to long term success, as are suitable strategies designed to minimise their impact. These tools include, meditation, yoga, active relaxation and exercise. They are important components of treatment for all *qi* stagnation disorders.
- Acupuncture and herbs are among the best and most reliable treatments for curing this condition. Treatment often needs to be prolonged (3 months+) to effect long term change. Acupuncture, given regularly, can facilitate 'physiological retaining', modifying the way the patient responds to the stress triggers that cause the reflux.
- For dietary recommendations, see p.878.

肝胃郁热

3.2 STOMACH AND LIVER HEAT

Pathophysiology

- Stomach and Liver Heat may evolve from the previous pattern (Liver invading the Stomach), or may be associated with overconsumption of heating foods, or both. The emotional aspects, if any, will generally be overshadowed by the influence of the diet, so the main feature will often be the relationship between the time of eating and the onset or aggravation of the heartburn. When chronic, Stomach and Liver Heat will often be complicated by *yin* deficiency.

Clinical features

- recurrent or relentless acid reflux and heartburn, aggravated or initiated by certain foods (especially chocolate, coffee and alcohol) or stress; the patient may wake in the middle of the night, often around 1-2am, with discomfort and reflux
- sour or bitter belching
- epigastric discomfort or burning sensation
- indeterminate gnawing hunger
- foul stools
- dry mouth, thirst
- irritability, easy anger, hot temper

T red or with red edges and a thick yellow coat
P wiry and/or slippery, possibly rapid

Treatment principle

Clear Heat from the Stomach and Liver
Harmonise the Stomach and direct Stomach *qi* downwards

Prescription

HUA GAN JIAN 化肝煎
(*Transform the Liver Decoction*) modified

mu dan pi (Cortex Moutan Radicis) 牡丹皮 9-12g
shan zhi zi (Fructus Gardeniae Jasminoides) 山栀子 9-12g
bai shao (Radix Paeoniae Lactiflora) 白芍 9-12g
fo shou (Fructus Citri Sarcodacylis) 佛手 9-12g
ba yue zha (Fructus Akebiae) 八月扎 9-12g
xiang yuan pi (Pericarpium Citri Medica) 香橼皮 9-12g
ban xia (Rhizoma Pinelliae Ternatae) 半夏 9-12g
huang lian (Rhizoma Coptidis) 黄连 6-9g
wu zhu yu (Fructus Evodiae Rutaecarpae) 吴茱萸 2-3g

Method: Decoction. **Mu dan pi** and **shan zhi zi** cool the Liver and clear stagnant

Heat; **bai shao** calms and softens the Liver and assists the Liver in spreading *qi*; **fo shou, ba yue zha** and **xiang yuan pi** gently regulate *qi* without damaging and dispersing *qi* and *yin*; **ban xia** directs *qi* downward and harmonises the Stomach; **huang lian** and **wu zhu yu** combine bitter cold descent with pungent warm dispersal to clear stagnant Heat and correct the *qi* mechanism–these herbs have a special effect on clearing Heat and alleviating heartburn. (Source: *Zhong Yi Zhi Liao Yi Nan Za Bing Mi Yao*).

Modifications

- To enhance the general antacid effect of the prescription (especially in the early stages of treatment or in severe or resistant cases) add **hai piao xiao** (Os Sepiae seu Sepiellae) 海螵蛸 15g and **duan wa leng zi** (calcined Concha Arcae) 煅瓦楞子 15g.
- With lots of Heat in the Liver (red eyes, flushing, red neck, irritability), add **pu gong ying** (Herba Taraxaci Mongolici) 蒲公英 30g.
- With constipation, add **da huang** (Radix et Rhizoma Rhei) 大黄 6-9g and **zhi shi** (Fructus Immaturus Citri Aurantii) 枳实 9-12g.

Variations and additional prescriptions

In severe cases

- When reflux is severe the possibility of damage and scarring of the oesophagus is increased. The focus of treatment should aim to quickly settle down the reflux and prevent damage with **ZUO JIN WAN** (*Left Metal Pill* 左金丸) modified.

huang lian (Rhizoma Coptidis) 黄连 15g
wu zhu yu (Fructus Evodiae Rutaecarpae) 吴茱萸 3g
hai piao xiao (Os Sepiae seu Sepiellae) 海螵蛸 15g
duan wa leng zi (calcined Concha Arcae) 煅瓦楞子 15g

Method: Decoction. **Hai piao xiao** and **wa leng zi** can be decocted or powdered and washed down with the strained decoction. **Huang lian** and **wu zhu yu** combine the opposing natures of bitter descending and acid warming to dissipate accumulated Heat and lead it downwards–these herbs have a special effect on clearing Heat and alleviating heartburn; **hai piao xiao** and **wa leng zi** neutralise gastric acid.

With Stomach Heat

- When Stomach Heat is primary, the aetiology typically involves an overly heating diet and the heartburn is aggravated by certain foods. The influence of the patient's emotional state on the development of symptoms is negligible, or at least minor relative to that of diet. The features of classic Stomach Heat include acid reflux and heartburn, halitosis, swollen inflamed gums, mouth ulcers, dry mouth and lips, thirst, a red tongue (or red centrally) and a rapid, slippery pulse. The aim of treatment is to clear Heat from the Stomach and cool the Blood with **QING WEI TANG** (*Clear the Stomach Decoction* 清胃汤) modified.

shi gao (Gypsum) 石膏 15-30g
huang qin (Radix Scutellariae Baicalensis) 黄芩 9-12g
sheng di (Radix Rehmanniae Glutinosae) 生地 12-18g
mu dan pi (Cortex Moutan Radicis) 牡丹皮 9-12g
dang gui (Radix Angelicae Sinensis) 当归 6-9g
huang lian (Rhizoma Coptidis) 黄连 6-9g
sheng ma (Rhizoma Cimicifugae) 升麻 3-6g
hai piao xiao (Os Sepiae seu Sepiellae) 海螵蛸 15g

Method: Decoction. **Shi gao** is decocted for 30 minutes prior to the other herbs (*xian jian* 先煎). **Shi gao** clears Heat from the Stomach; **huang qin** and **huang lian** clear Heat from the Lungs, Heart and Stomach; **sheng di** cools the Blood and nourishes Stomach *yin*; **mu dan pi** cools the Blood; **sheng ma** raises and disperses Heat, and enables the other cooling herbs to more thoroughly access and clear the Heat; the rising nature of **sheng ma** is nicely balanced with the descending nature of the cooling herbs, thus enabling Heat to be cleared and dispersed without causing damage to *qi* or *yin*; **hai piao xiao** neutralises gastric acid.

Damp Heat in the Stomach and Spleen

- When Damp Heat affects the Spleen and Stomach, the aetiology is usually related to consumption of Damp and Heating substances, in particular alcohol and rich greasy food. The features are recurrent acid reflux and heartburn, epigastric distension and discomfort, dry mouth, a thick greasy yellow tongue coat and slippery rapid pulse. In addition, patients often have acne problems or a tendency to boils and sores, greasy skin, and strong body odour. The aim of treatment is to clear Damp Heat, regulate *qi* and harmonise the Stomach with **XIE XIN TANG** (*Coptis and Rhubarb Combination* 泻心汤) modified.

huang qin (Radix Scutellariae Baicalensis) 黄芩 9-12g
huang lian (Rhizoma Coptidis) 黄连 6-9g
da huang (Radix et Rhizoma Rhei) 大黄 6-9g
pu gong ying (Herba Taraxaci Mongolici) 蒲公英 15-30g
fo shou (Fructus Citri Sarcodacylis) 佛手 9-12g
zhi shi (Fructus Immaturus Citri Aurantii) 枳实 9-12g
hou po (Cortex Magnoliae Officinalis) 厚朴 9-12g
hai piao xiao (Os Sepiae seu Sepiellae) 海螵蛸 12-15g
zhe bei mu (Bulbus Fritillariae Thunbergii) 浙贝母 9-12g

Method: Decoction. **Huang qin**, **huang lian** and **da huang** clear Heat from the upper body and eliminate it through the bowel; **pu gong ying** clears Toxic Heat and cools the Liver; **fo shou** regulates *qi* without dispersing *yin*; **zhi shi** and **hou po** direct *qi* downwards; **hai piao xiao** and **zhe bei mu** neutralise gastric acid.

With nausea or vomiting, add **zhu ru** (Caulis Bambusae in Taeniis) 竹茹 15g and **ban xia** (Rhizoma Pinelliae Ternatae) 半夏 12g; with epigastric pain, add **yan hu suo** (Rhizoma Corydalis Yanhusuo) 延胡索 12g; with food stagnation, add **shen qu** (Massa Fermentata) 神曲 15g, **mai ya** (Fructus Hordei Vulgaris Germinantus) 麦芽 30g and **gu ya** (Fructus Oryzae Sativae Germinatus) 谷芽 30g. (Source: *Xiao Hua Ke Zhuan Bing*)

A complex of Heat, Cold and deficiency

- A common, yet somewhat more complex situation, occurs where both Heat and Cold accumulate in the middle *jiao* against a background of Spleen and Stomach deficiency. The main features are heartburn with a sensation of blockage, distension, fullness and discomfort in the epigastrium, which, when palpated, feels soft and without pain. In addition, there may be nausea, gnawing hunger, borborygmus with diarrhoea, poor appetite, a thin greasy yellow tongue coat and a soft, slippery, slightly wiry and possibly rapid pulse. This pattern is often associated with the mixed pathology of the primary pathological triad (PPT, p.912). The treatment is to harmonise the Stomach, direct *qi* downwards, clear Damp Heat and support the Spleen with **BAN XIA XIE XIN TANG** (*Pinellia Combination* 半夏泻心汤) modified.

ban xia (Rhizoma Pinelliae Ternatae) 半夏 9-12g
huang qin (Radix Scutellariae Baicalensis) 黄芩 9-12g
huang lian (Rhizoma Coptidis) 黄连 6-9g
gan jiang (Rhizoma Zingiberis Officinalis) 干姜 6-9g
zhi gan cao (honey fried Radix Glycyrrhizae Uralensis)
炙甘草 6-9g
dang shen (Radix Codonopsis Pilosulae) 党参 15-18g
da zao (Fructus Zizyphi Jujubae) 大枣 4pce
wu zhu yu (Fructus Evodiae Rutaecarpae) 吴茱萸 2-3g

Method: Decoction. **Ban xia** transforms Phlegm, dries Damp, directs rising Stomach *qi* downwards and stops nausea; **gan jiang**, pungent and hot, warms Spleen and Stomach *yang* and dispels Cold; **huang qin** and **huang lian**, bitter and cold, clear Heat; the hot dispersing action of **gan jiang** and **wu zhu yu** neatly balances the bitter cold descending action of **huang qin** and **huang lian**, assisting the correct flow of *qi* and repairing the *qi* mechanism; **dang shen** and **da zao** strengthen the Spleen, supplement *qi* and prevent the dispersing action of the principal herbs from injuring the Spleen and Stomach *qi* and *yin*; **zhi gan cao** strengthens the Spleen and harmonises the Stomach; **wu zhu yu** warms the Stomach and Liver, and with **huang lian** forms **ZUO JIN WAN**, to reinforce the antacid action.

With Phlegm Heat

- With Phlegm Heat (reflux and heartburn, nausea or vomiting, indeterminate gnawing hunger, insomnia, anxiety, a greasy yellow tongue coat and a slippery, rapid pulse) the aim of treatment is to resolve Hot Phlegm, direct *qi* downwards and stop reflux with **WEN DAN TANG** (*Bamboo and Hoelen Combination* 温胆汤) modified. Reflux associated with this pattern may also occur in the recovery phase of an acute febrile illness like *yang ming* syndrome, in which case it typically persists for up to six weeks after the fever has abated.

zhu ru (Caulis Bambusae in Taeniis) 竹茹 12-15g
zhi shi (Fructus Immaturus Citri Aurantii) 枳实 9-12g

ban xia (Rhizoma Pinelliae Ternatae) 半夏 9-12g
chen pi (Pericarpium Citri Reticulatae) 陈皮 9-12g
fu ling (Sclerotium Poria Cocos) 茯苓 12-15g
gan cao (Radix Glycyrrhizae Uralensis) 甘草 3-6g
sheng jiang (Rhizoma Zingiberis Officinalis Recens)
生姜 6-9g
huang lian (Rhizoma Coptidis) 黄连 3-6g
wu zhu yu (Fructus Evodiae Rutaecarpae) 吴茱萸 2-3g

Method: Decoction. **Zhu ru** clears Phlegm Heat from the Stomach and Gallbladder and directs Stomach *qi* downwards; **zhi shi** breaks up stagnant *qi*, directs *qi* downwards and alleviates distension; **ban xia** transforms Phlegm, dries Damp and directs rising Stomach *qi* downwards; **chen pi** transforms Phlegm and dries Damp, regulates middle *jiao qi* and corrects the *qi* mechanism; **fu ling** strengthens the Spleen and leaches out Damp; **gan cao** strengthens the Spleen and harmonises the Stomach; **sheng jiang** assists the other herbs in harmonising the Stomach and correcting the *qi* mechanism; **huang lian** and **wu zhu yu** combine bitter cold descent with pungent warm dispersal to clear stagnant Heat and correct the *qi* mechanism–these herbs have a special effect on clearing Heat and alleviating heartburn. (Source: *Shi Yong Zhong Yi Nei Ke Xue*)

Patent medicines

Jia Wei Xiao Yao Wan 加味逍遥丸 (Jia Wei Xiao Yao Wan, Dan Zhi Xiao Yao Wan) - Liver *qi* stagnation with stagnant Heat

Wen Dan Wan 温胆丸 (Wen Dan Wan)
- Phlegm Heat

Huang Lian Jie Du Wan 黄连解毒丸 (Huang Lian Jie Du Wan)
- Damp Heat, Stomach Heat

Wei Te Ling 胃特灵 (Wei Te Ling Stomach Sedative)
- an antacid formula that can be combined with the appropriate constitutional formula for symptomatic relief

Xiang Lian Wan 香莲丸 (Xiang Lian Wan)
- this patent can be combined with the appropriate constitutional formula for symptomatic relief

Acupuncture (select from)

Ren.12 (*zhong wan*) .... these points direct rising Stomach *qi*
Ren.13 (*shang wan*) downwards and stimulate the *qi* mechanism

Ren.17 (*shan zhong*) .... upper sea of *qi*, helps direct *qi* downwards
PC.8 (*lao gong* -) .... *rong* spring and Fire point of the Pericardium, drains Heat from the Stomach channel and cools the Blood and Heart Fire
St.44 (*nei ting* -) .... *rong* spring and Water point of the Stomach, clears Heat from *yang ming*, the Stomach and Stomach channel

Liv.2 (*xing jian* -) .... *rong* spring and Fire point of the Liver, drains Fire from the Liver, spreads stagnant *qi*, clears the lower *jiao*, subdues Wind

GB.34 (*yang ling quan* -) ... *he* sea point of the Gallbladder, cools the Liver (with Liv.2) and subdues rising *yang*

St.36 (*zu san li* -) .... *he* sea point of the Stomach, powerfully regulates and supplements *qi* and corrects the *qi* mechanism

LI.11 (*qu chi* -) .... *he* sea point of the Large Intestine, clears Heat and Dampness from *yang ming*

- with severe Heat, add St.45 (*li dui* ↓) and SJ.2 (*ye men* -)
- with constipation, add SJ.6 (*zhi gou* -) and St.25 (*tian shu* -)
- with Lung and Stomach Heat, add Lu.5 (*chi ze* -)
- with nausea, add PC.6 (*nei guan*)
- *Ear points*: oesophagus, pylorus, liver, spleen, stomach, *shen men*, subcortex, sympathetic

Clinical notes

- Stomach and Liver Heat type acid reflux and heartburn may be diagnosed biomedically as acute or chronic gastritis, gastro-oesophageal reflux, reflux oesophagitis, hepatitis, cholecystitis, gallstones or excessive intake of alcohol.
- This is a common pattern causing acid reflux and heartburn, and in combination with modifications in diet, responds well to correct treatment. Depending on the longevity of the pattern, the patient should expect reasonable symptomatic relief within a week or two, but will often need to continue treatment for several months to consolidate the result and achieve long term relief.
- For dietary recommendations, see p.882.

痰湿阻滞

3.3 PHLEGM DAMP

Pathophysiology

- Phlegm Damp obstructs the *qi* mechanism and blocks the descent of Stomach *qi* which rebels upwards taking Stomach acid up to the mouth.
- Phlegm Damp patterns often involve elements of other patterns, especially *qi* stagnation and, in chronic cases, Spleen deficiency.

Clinical features

- acid reflux, heartburn
- epigastric and abdominal distension and fullness
- loss of appetite, decreased sense of taste
- tendency to loose stools or diarrhoea
- nausea, vomiting
- tired, heavy limbs, generalised sensation of heaviness in the body
- variable fatigue–may feel better for activity and exertion
- poor concentration, foggy-headedness
- may tend to be overweight or pear shaped
- maybe chronic mucus production from the sinuses and lungs
- dizziness, headaches that can be triggered by strong smells
- greasy skin, musty body odour

T thick white tongue coat, possibly swollen
P slippery, moderate

Treatment principle

Dry Dampness and transform Phlegm
Invigorate Spleen function and *qi* movement, harmonise the Stomach

Prescription

PING WEI SAN 平胃散
(*Magnolia and Ginger Formula*) modified

cang zhu (Rhizoma Atractylodis) 苍术 12-15g
hou po (Cortex Magnoliae Officinalis) 厚朴 9-12g
chen pi (Pericarpium Citri Reticulatae) 陈皮 9-12g
sheng jiang (Rhizoma Zingiberis Officinalis Recens) 生姜 6-9g
da zao (Fructus Zizyphi Jujubae) 大枣 2pce
zhi gan cao (honey fried Radix Glycyrrhizae Uralensis) 炙甘草 3-6g
wu zhu yu (Fructus Evodiae Rutaecarpae) 吴茱萸 3g

Method: Grind the herbs into powder and take 9-grams as a draft on an empty stomach. May also be decocted. **Cang zhu** powerfully parches and dries

Dampness, thereby liberating the Spleen and improving its function; **hou po** regulates *qi*, transforms Dampness and directs *qi* downwards; **ban xia** and **chen pi** transform Phlegm and dry Dampness, regulate middle *jiao qi* and correct the *qi* mechanism; **zhi gan cao** strengthens the Spleen and harmonises the Stomach; **sheng jiang** and **da zao** harmonise the Stomach; **wu zhu yu** warms the Stomach and directs Stomach *qi* downwards. (Source: *Shi Yong Zhong Yi Nei Ke Xue*)

Modifications

- With Cold, add **gan jiang** (Rhizoma Zingiberis Officinalis) 干姜 9g.
- With food stagnation add **mai ya** (Fructus Hordei Vulgaris Germinantus) 麦芽 15-30g and **gu ya** (Fructus Oryzae Sativae Germinatus) 谷芽 15-30g.
- With severe Dampness (thick greasy tongue coat, heaviness, distension etc.) add **huo xiang** (Herba Agastaches seu Pogostemi) 藿香 12-15g and **pei lan** (Herba Eupatorii Fortunei) 佩兰 9-12g.
- With foggy-headedness and poor concentration, add **yuan zhi** (Radix Polygalae Tenuifoliae) 远志 6-9g and **shi chang pu** (Rhizoma Acori Graminei) 石菖蒲 6-9g.
- With nausea, add **ban xia** (Rhizoma Pinelliae Ternatae) 半夏 9-12g.
- If prolonged stagnation of Dampness generates a degree of Heat, giving rise to a greasy yellow tongue coat, yellow urine, irritability and a rapid pulse, add **huang qin** (Radix Scutellariae Baicalensis) 黄芩 6-9g, **shan zhi zi** (Fructus Gardeniae Jasminoides) 山栀子 6-9g, **tong cao** (Medulla Tetrapanacis Papyriferi) 通草 3-6g and **yi ren** (Semen Coicis Lachryma-jobi) 苡仁 15-24g.
- With Spleen deficiency (loss of appetite, pale tongue, weak pulse), add **huang qi** (Radix Astragali Membranacei) 黄芪 12-18g, **bai zhu** (Rhizoma Atractylodis Macrocephalae) 白术 9-12g and **shan yao** (Radix Dioscoreae Oppositae) 山药 12-15g.

Patent medicines

Ping Wei San 平胃散 (Ping Wei San, Tabellae Pingwei)

Xiang Sha Liu Jun Zi Wan 香砂六君子丸 (Xiang Sha Liu Jun Wan, Aplotaxis-Ammomum Pills, Six Gentlemen Tea Pills)
- with Spleen deficiency

Xiang Sha Yang Wei Wan 香砂养胃丸 (Xiang Sha Yang Wei Wan, Hsiang Sha Yang Wei Wan)
- with *qi* and Damp stagnation

Wei Te Ling 胃特灵 (Wei Te Ling Stomach Sedative)
- an antacid formula that can be combined with the appropriate constitutional formula for symptomatic relief

Xiang Lian Wan 香莲丸 (Xiang Lian Wan)
- this patent can be combined with the appropriate constitutional formula for symptomatic relief

Acupuncture (select from)

Ren.12 (*zhong wan* -) .... *mu* point of the Stomach, clears Phlegm Damp, directs Stomach *qi* downwards and harmonises the Stomach

Ren.17 (*shan zhong*) .... upper sea of *qi*, directs *qi* downward

Sp.3 (*tai bai*) .... *yuan luo* pair with a powerful Phlegm and
St.40 (*feng long* -) Damp transforming action, especially good for Phlegm Damp in the Stomach blocking the *qi* mechanism

PC.5 (*jian shi* -) .... *jing* river point of the Pericardium, transforms Phlegm and harmonises the Stomach

PC.6 (*nei guan* -) .... *luo* point of the Pericardium, master point of *yin wei mai*, regulates the middle *jiao* and stimulates the *qi* mechanism and stops nausea

- with Spleen deficiency, add St.36 (*zu san li* +) and Liv.13 (*zhang men* +)
- with Liver *qi* stagnation, add Liv.3 (*tai chong*)
- with foggy-headedness, add GB.20 (*feng chi*) and Bl.62 (*shen mai*)
- with Cold Phlegm, apply moxa cones to Bl.20 (*pi shu* ▲) and Bl.21 (*wei shu* ▲)
- with muscle aches and heaviness, add Sp.21 (*da bao*)
- with fluid retention and oedema, add Sp.9 (*yin ling quan* -) and Sp.6 (*san yin jiao*)
- with somnolence, add Kid.6 (*zhao hai*) and Bl.62 (*shen mai*)
- with severe abdominal bloating, add St.25 (*tian shu*) and Sp.15 (*da heng*)
- *Ear points*: oesophagus, pylorus, spleen, stomach, *shen men*, subcortex, sympathetic

Clinical notes

- This pattern is a relatively common cause of acid reflux and heartburn. In association with dietary modification, it usually responds well to correct treatment, but, depending on the degree of Phlegm Damp accumulation, will generally require some months of treatment for complete resolution.
- For dietary recommendations, see p.880.

饮食积滞

3.4 FOOD STAGNATION

Pathophysiology

- Food stagnation type reflux is directly related to overeating or irregular eating. In the developed world, where people consistently overeat and are often sedentary, the pattern combines with weakness of Spleen and Stomach *qi*. Clinically, this pattern is usually a mixture of excess and deficiency. As the pattern progresses the deficiency will become more and more prominent.
- Food stagnation is also frequently complicated by, or is the by-product of, other excess accumulations such as Liver *qi* stagnation, Phlegm Damp or Phlegm Heat.

Clinical features

- acid reflux, heartburn usually associated with eating a large meal or hard to digest foods
- epigastric distension, fullness, discomfort and pain which is relieved by vomiting and belching, and worse for pressure and eating
- sour, foul belching
- halitosis
- nausea and vomiting with undigested food
- constipation, or diarrhoea that relieves the pain

T thick greasy coat
P slippery and full

Treatment principle

Eliminate stagnant food, regulate digestion
Harmonise the Stomach and direct *qi* downwards

Prescription

BAO HE WAN 保和丸
(*Citrus and Crategus Formula*) modified

chao shan zha (dry fried Fructus Crataegi) 炒山楂 18-24g
chao shen qu (dry fried Massa Fermentata) 炒神曲 12-15g
chao lai fu zi (dry fried Semen Raphani Sativi)
炒莱服子 9-12g
ban xia (Rhizoma Pinelliae Ternatae) 半夏 9-12g
fu ling (Sclerotium Poriae Cocos) 茯苓 12-15g
chen pi (Pericarpium Citri Reticulatae) 陈皮 6-9g
lian qiao (Fructus Forsythia Suspensae) 连翘 6-9g
qing pi (Pericarpium Citri Reticulatae Viridae) 青皮 6-9g
huang lian (Rhizoma Coptidis) 黄连 3-6g
wu zhu yu (Fructus Evodiae Rutaecarpae) 吴茱萸 2-3g

Method: Grind herbs to a powder and form into 9-gram pills with water. The dose is 1 pill twice daily. May also be decocted with the quantities as shown. **Chao shan zha, chao shen qu** and **chao lai fu zi** improve digestion and alleviate food stagnation; **ban xia** and **chen pi** eliminate Phlegm; **lian qiao** disperses accumulation and clears Heat; **fu ling** strengthens the Spleen; **qing pi** breaks up stagnant *qi* and alleviates accumulation; **huang lian** and **wu zhu yu** combine bitter coldness with pungent warmth with the aim of dispersing accumulation and assisting descent of Stomach *qi*, and correcting the *qi* mechanism to alleviate acid reflux. (Source: *Shi Yong Zhong Yi Nei Ke Xue*)

Modifications

- With constipation, add **bing lang** (Semen Arecae Catechu) 槟榔 9-12g and **da huang** (Radix et Rhizoma Rhei) 大黄 6-9g.
- With Spleen deficiency add **bai zhu** (Rhizoma Atractylodis Macrocephalae) 白术 12-15g.

Patent medicines

Bao He Wan 保和丸 (Bao He Wan)
Mu Xiang Shun Qi Wan 木香顺气丸 (Mu Xiang Shun Qi Wan)
- with sluggish stools

Zi Sheng Wan 资生丸 (Zi Sheng Wan, Zi Sheng Stomachic Pills)
Jian Pi Wan 健脾丸 (Jian Pi Wan)
- with Spleen deficiency

Xiang Sha Yang Wei Wan 香砂养胃丸 (Xiang Sha Yang Wei Wan, Hsiang Sha Yang Wei Wan)
- with *qi* stagnation

Wei Te Ling 胃特灵 (Wei Te Ling Stomach Sedative)
- an antacid formula that can be combined with the appropriate constitutional formula for symptomatic relief

Xiang Lian Wan 香莲丸 (Xiang Lian Wan)
- this patent can be combined with the appropriate formula for symptomatic relief

Acupuncture (select from)

Ren.12 (*zhong wan* -) .... *mu* point of the Stomach, directs *qi* downwards and alleviates food stagnation
St.21 (*liang men* -) .... promotes the function of the Spleen and Stomach
PC.6 (*nei guan* -) .... *luo* point of the Pericardium, master point of *yin wei mai*, regulates the middle *jiao* and directs rising Stomach *qi* downward
LI.10 (*shou san li* -) .... benefits digestion and regulates gastro-intestinal function, improves digestion

St.36 (*zu san li* -) .... *he* sea point of the Stomach, regulates and strengthens the Spleen and Stomach and corrects the *qi* mechanism

St.40 (*feng long* -) .... *luo* point of the Stomach, transforms Phlegm, clears Heat and stagnant food from the Stomach

St.44 (*nei ting* -) .... *rong* spring and water point of the Stomach, clears Heat from the Stomach, alleviates food stagnation

- with Spleen deficiency, add Sp.6 (*san yin jiao*) and Bl.20 (*pi shu* +)
- with constipation, add St.37 (*shang ju xu* -) and SJ.6 (*zhi gou* -)
- *Ear points*: oesophagus, stomach, spleen, small intestine, abdomen

Clinical notes

- This is a common cause of acute acid reflux and heartburn. Simple regulation of the diet (regular eating, smaller meals) will generally clear up food stagnation patterns. Chronic cases and those that are complicated by deficiency and/or Phlegm will take longer and require diligence in treatment and dietary discipline.
- The Chinese have long known the benefits of sipping small amounts of certain teas while eating. The action of such teas helps assist digestion, especially of fats, and reduces the risk of food stagnation. European cultures use table wine in much the same way, hence 'a little wine for thy stomach's sake'. Similarly, 'bitters', combinations of bitter herbs and alcohol, are a common accompaniment to food, either as a digestive aid following a meal, or as an aperitive. The bitterness of the herbs assists the descent of Stomach *qi* and dries Damp.

脾胃虚弱

3.5 SPLEEN AND STOMACH QI/YANG DEFICIENCY

Pathophysiology

- Spleen *qi* (*yang*) deficiency reflux is a chronic disorder that is associated with a disturbance of the *qi* mechanism (failure of Stomach *qi* descent and Spleen *qi* ascent due to weakness). The basic deficiency pattern is often complicated and compounded by *qi* blockage caused by accumulated Dampness, Phlegm or pathological fluids. *Qi* blockage can be exacerbated when Cold from *yang* deficiency freezes and constricts *qi* movement through the middle *jiao*.

Clinical features

- Intermittent chronic acid reflux and heartburn which tend to be worse with hard to digest or raw foods and with bending or any increase in abdominal pressure. Waking during the night with heartburn is typical.
- mild epigastric discomfort or pain that is better for warmth and pressure
- feeling of a blockage at the level of the epigastrium; bloating after eating
- hypersalivation, drooling
- sour belching
- poor appetite
- fatigue, weakness, tired limbs, poor muscle tone
- tendency to loose stools or diarrhoea
- cold intolerance, cold extremities

T pale and swollen with tooth marks, thin white coat
P deep, slow, thready or weak

Treatment principle

Warm and strengthen the Spleen and harmonise the Stomach
Redirect *qi* downwards and alleviate reflux

Prescription

XIANG SHA LIU JUN ZI TANG 香砂六君子汤
(*Saussurea and Cardamon Combination*) modified

dang shen (Radix Codonopsis Pilosulae) 党参 15-24g
bai zhu (Rhizoma Atractylodis Macrocephalae) 白术 12-15g
fu ling (Sclerotium Poriae Cocos) 茯苓 12-15g
ban xia (Rhizoma Pinelliae Ternatae) 半夏 9-12g
chen pi (Pericarpium Citri Reticulatae) 陈皮 9-12g
mu xiang (Radix Aucklandiae Lappae) 木香 6-9g
sha ren (Fructus Amomi) 砂仁 6-9g
zhi gan cao (honey fried Radix Glycyrrhizae Uralensis)
炙甘草 3-6g

gan jiang (Rhizoma Zingiberis Officinalis) 干姜 6-9g
wu zhu yu (Fructus Evodiae Rutaecarpae) 吴茱萸 3-6g
Method: Decoction. **Sha ren** is added towards the end of cooking time (*hou xia* 后下). **Dang shen** and **zhi gan cao** supplement *qi* and strengthen the Spleen; **chao bai zhu** strengthens the Spleen and dries Dampness; **fu ling** strengthens the Spleen and leaches out Dampness through the urine; **ban xia** transforms Phlegm, dries Damp, regulates *qi* and directs rising Stomach *qi* downwards; **chen pi** transforms Phlegm and dries Damp, regulates middle *jiao qi* and corrects the *qi* mechanism; **sha ren** and **mu xiang** regulate and mobilise *qi* in the middle *jiao*, alleviate distension and stimulate the appetite; **gan jiang** and **wu zhu yu** warm Spleen *yang* dispel Cold and harmonise the Stomach. (Source: *Shi Yong Zhong Yi Nei Ke Xue*)

Modifications

- With severe heartburn, add **hai piao xiao** (Os Sepiae seu Sepiellae) 海螵蛸 15g and **zhe bei mu** (Bulbus Fritillariae Thunbergii) 浙贝母 12g.
- With Cold or *yang* deficiency, add **ding xiang** (Flos Caryophylli) 丁香 3-6g and **xiao hui xiang** (Fructus Foeniculi Vulgaris) 小茴香 9-12g.
- With Dampness (thick greasy tongue coat, heaviness, distension etc.) add one or two of the following herbs: **cang zhu** (Rhizoma Atractylodis) 苍术 12-15g, **hou po** (Cortex Magnoliae Officinalis) 厚朴 9-12g, **huo xiang** (Herba Agastaches seu Pogostemi) 藿香 12-15g or **pei lan** (Herba Eupatorii Fortunei) 佩兰 9-12g.
- With poor muscle tone (and possible hiatus hernia), add a relatively small dose of **huang qi** (Radix Astragali Membranacei) 黄芪 12-15g. Be careful with this addition however, as **huang qi** can cause *qi* to rise.
- With food stagnation add **chao mai ya** (dry fried Fructus Hordei Vulgaris Germinantus) 炒麦芽 15-30g and **chao gu ya** (dry fried Fructus Oryzae Sativae Germinatus) 炒谷芽 15-30g.

Patent medicines

Xiang Sha Liu Jun Zi Wan 香砂六君丸 (Xiang Sha Liu Jun Wan)
Xiang Sha Yang Wei Wan 香砂养胃丸 (Xiang Sha Yang Wei Wan, Hsiang Sha Yang Wei Wan)
- with *qi* stagnation

Li Zhong Wan 理中丸 (Li Zhong Wan)
- with *yang* deficiency

Wei Te Ling 胃特灵 (Wei Te Ling Stomach Sedative)
- an antacid formula that can be combined with the appropriate constitutional formula for symptomatic relief

Xiang Lian Wan 香莲丸 (Xiang Lian Wan)
- this patent can be combined with the appropriate constitutional formula for symptomatic relief

Acupuncture (select from)

Ren.12 (*zhong wan* +▲) .. these points warm and strengthen the Stomach
Ren.13 (*shang wan* +▲) and middle *jiao*, and direct Stomach *qi* downwards

Ren.17 (*shan zhong*) .... upper sea of *qi*, helps direct *qi* downwards
St.36 (*zu san li* +▲) .... *he* sea point of the Stomach, powerfully warms and strengthens the Spleen and Stomach, regulates and supplements *qi* and stimulates the *qi* mechanism
Sp.6 (*san yin jiao*) .... strengthens and regulates the Spleen and supplements *qi*
PC.6 (*nei guan* -) .... *luo* point of the Pericardium, regulates the middle *jiao* and stimulates the *qi* mechanism, directs *qi* downwards

Bl.20 (*pi shu* +▲) .... *shu* points of the Spleen and Stomach, warm
Bl.21 (*wei shu* +▲) and strengthen middle *jiao qi* function

- with Phlegm Damp, add PC.5 (*jian shi*), St.40 (*feng long* -) and Sp.3 (*tai bai*)
- a moxa box over the epigastrium is excellent, especially for *yang* deficiency
- *Ear points*: spleen, stomach, oesophagus, pylorus, *shen men*, adrenal, subcortex, sympathetic

Clinical notes

- Spleen deficiency type acid reflux and heartburn may be diagnosed as hiatus hernia, functional dyspepsia, gastro-oesophageal reflux, chronic gastritis, peptic ulcer disease or reflux oesophagitis.
- This is quite a common cause of acid reflux and heartburn, although the patterns complicated by Phlegm Damp appear to be more likely to produce acid reflux than uncomplicated ones. In combination with dietary modification, Spleen and Stomach deficiency patterns respond well to correct treatment. Symptomatic relief can usually be achieved within a week or two, but depending on the degree of deficiency, treatment will usually need to persist for at least 3-6 months for satisfactory resolution.
- For dietary recommendations, see p.870-873.

胃肝阴虚

3.6 STOMACH AND LIVER YIN DEFICIENCY

Pathophysiology

- Stomach and Liver *yin* deficiency is a result of chronic excess Heat in the Liver and Stomach, which in turn is often a result of chronic Liver *qi* invading the Spleen. The reflux and heartburn are associated with the combined effects of the weakness of the Stomach and the failure of it's *qi* to descend correctly, and the rising nature of any Heat present.

Clinical features

- chronic acid reflux, hyperacidity and heartburn; the heartburn may be worse with stress and in the evening; the patient may wake during the night (often around 1-4am) with reflux and discomfort which may be temporarily relieved by eating
- mild, dull epigastric and/or hypochondriac discomfort or pain
- loss of appetite or indeterminate gnawing hunger
- dry mouth and throat
- tendency to dry stools or constipation

T red and dry with little or no coat, or red and peeled in the centre or on the edges

P thready and wiry, possibly rapid

Treatment principle

Nourish and supplement Stomach and Liver *yin*
Regulate *qi*, redirect *qi* downwards and harmonise the Stomach

Prescription

YI GUAN JIAN 一贯煎
(*Linking Decoction*) modified

sheng di (Radix Rehmanniae Glutinosae) 生地 18-30g
gou qi zi (Fructus Lycii) 枸杞子 12-15g
sha shen (Radix Adenophorae seu Glehniae) 沙参 12-15g
mai dong (Tuber Ophiopogonis Japonici) 麦冬 12-15g
dang gui (Radix Angelicae Sinensis) 当归 9-12g
chuan lian zi (Fructus Meliae Toosendan) 川楝子 6-9g
bai shao (Radix Paeoniae Lactiflora) 白芍 12-18g
hai piao xiao (Os Sepiae seu Sepiellae) 海螵蛸 15g
zhe bei mu (Bulbus Fritillariae Thunbergii) 浙贝母 12g

Method: Decoction. **Sheng di, gou qi zi, sha shen** and **mai dong** nourish and supplement Stomach and Liver *yin*; **dang gui, bai shao** and **gou qi zi** nourish and supplement Liver Blood, and soften the Liver; **chuan lian zi** regulates *qi* and stops pain; **hai piao xiao** and **zhe bei mu** neutralise gastric acid. (Source: *Xiao Hua Ke Chuan Bing*)

Modifications

- With severe *yin* deficiency, add **shi hu** (Herba Dendrobi) 石斛 12-15g.
- With a degree of excess Stomach Heat (bitter taste in the mouth, slippery wiry pulse), add a small dose of **huang lian** (Rhizoma Coptidis) 黄连 1-3g.
- With constipation, add **gua lou ren** (Semen Trichosanthis) 瓜蒌仁 12-18g.
- With distension and loss of appetite, add **mai ya** (Fructus Hordei Vulgaris Germinantus) 麦芽 15-30g.
- With dull or nagging pain, include herbs that gently move *qi* without damaging *yin*, such as **fo shou** (Fructus Citri Sarcodacylis) 佛手 9-12g, **ba yue zha** (Fructus Akebiae) 八月扎 9-12g, **mei gui hua** (Flos Rosae Rugosae) 玫瑰花 6-9g or **xiang yuan pi** (Pericarpium Citri Medica) 香橼皮 9-12g.
- With *qi* deficiency, add **dang shen** (Radix Codonopsis Pilosulae) 党参 15-18g, **huang jing** (Rhizoma Polygonati) 黄精 12-15g and **shan yao** (Radix Dioscoreae Oppositae) 山药 15-18g.

Patent medicines

Gu Ben Wan 固本丸 (Gu Ben Wan, Ren Shen Ku Pen Wan)
- Stomach *qi* and *yin* deficiency

Wei Te Ling 胃特灵 (Wei Te Ling Stomach Sedative)
- an antacid formula that can be combined with the appropriate constitutional formula for symptomatic relief

Xiang Lian Wan 香莲丸 (Xiang Lian Wan)
- this patent can be combined with the appropriate constitutional formula for symptomatic relief

Acupuncture (select from)

Ren.12 (*zhong wan* +) .... *mu* point of the Stomach, nourishes Stomach *yin*, regulates the Stomach and directs Stomach *qi* downwards

Liv.13 (*zhang men* +) .... *mu* point of the Spleen and *hui* point of the *zang*, strengthens the Spleen, supplements *qi* and *yin*, harmonises the Liver and Stomach/ Spleen and promotes Liver function

Bl.20 (*pi shu* +) .... *shu* points of the Spleen and Stomach,
Bl.21 (*wei shu* +) supplement *yin* and *qi* and regulate middle *jiao* *qi* function

St.36 (*zu san li* +) .... *he* sea point of the Stomach, powerfully strengthens the Spleen and Stomach, supplements *qi* and *yin* and stimulates the *qi* mechanism

PC.6 (*nei guan*) .... *luo* point of the Pericardium and master point of *yin wei mai*, regulates the middle *jiao* and directs Stomach *qi* downwards

Kid.9 (*zhu bin* +) .... *xi* point of *yin wei mai*, with PC.6 (*nei guan*) can direct weak Stomach *qi* downwards

- *Ear points*: oesophagus, pylorus, liver, spleen, stomach, *shen men*, subcortex, sympathetic

Clinical notes

- Stomach and Liver *yin* deficiency type acid reflux and heartburn may be diagnosed biomedically as gastro-oesophageal reflux, chronic atrophic gastritis, chronic gastritis, peptic ulcer disease or reflux oesophagitis.
- This is a relatively common cause of chronic acid reflux and heartburn, and can be difficult to treat. It will often take some weeks before adequate symptomatic relief is obtained with herbs and acupuncture alone, and the underlying pattern usually requires 6-9 months of treatment for satisfactory results. Getting the patient to continue with pharmaceutical antacids until the treatment takes effect is appropriate. Mucilaginous substances that put a lining on the oesophageal and gastric walls, such as slippery elm powder, are also useful.
- For dietary recommendations, see p.876.

SUMMARY OF GUIDING FORMULAE FOR ACID REFLUX AND HEARTBURN

Excess patterns

Liver *qi* invading the Stomach - *Si Ni San* 四逆散
- with Phlegm - *Qi Ge San* 启隔散
- with stagnant Heat - *Dan Zhi Xiao Yao San* 丹栀逍遥散

Stomach and Liver Heat - *Hua Gan Jian* 化肝煎
- in severe cases - *Zuo Jin Wan* 左金丸
- with Stomach Heat - *Qing Wei Tang* 清胃汤
- with Damp Heat - *San Huang Xie Xin Tang* 三黄泻心汤
- mixed with Cold and deficiency - *Ban Xia Xie Xin Tang* 半夏泻心汤
- with Phlegm Heat - *Wen Dan Tang* 温胆汤

Phlegm Damp - *Ping Wei San* 平胃散

Food stagnation - *Bao He Wan* 保和丸

Deficient patterns

Spleen and Stomach *qi* deficiency - *Xiang Sha Liu Jun Zi Tang* 香砂六君子汤

Stomach and Liver *yin* deficiency - *Yi Guan Jian* 一贯煎

Table 3.1 *Differential diagnosis of acid reflux and heartburn*

Pattern	Duration	Aggravated by	Ameliorated by	Other features	Nature of patient	Pulse and tongue
Liver *qi* invading the Stomach	chronic with acute exacerbations	emotional upset and stress	relaxation, contentment, following exercise	moodiness, depression, headaches, general muscle tension, alternating bowel habits	nervy, tense, uptight, most common 20-50 yrs, F>M	T: unremarkable, thin white coat P: wiry
Liver and Stomach Heat	chronic with acute exacerbations	spicy foods, alcohol, coffee, chocolate, stress	simple diet, avoidance of aggravating foods and fluids	often wakes around 1-2am with reflux, irritable	flushed, tense, may tend to binge when stressed or emotional	T: red or with red edges, thick yellow coat P: wiry, slippery, rapid
Phlegm Damp	acute or chronic, mostly chronic	consumption of dairy, sugar, greasy or rich foods	simple, bland diet	symptoms often worse in the morning, foggy-head, heaviness, nausea	sleepy, sluggish, may be overweight	T: thick greasy white coat P: slippery, wiry or moderate
Food stagnation	acute or chronic	overindulgence, eating irregularly	eating less, eating slowly, eating regularly, belching	flatulence, distension, bad breath, tendency to constipation	often overweight, may be robust	T: thick greasy white or yellow coat P: slippery, full

Spleen qi/yang deficiency	chronic	cold or raw foods, cold medications, bending, increased abdominal pressure	bland, light, well cooked food, small meals; application of warmth and pressure	poor appetite or anorexia, early satiety, loose stools, fatigue, cold intolerance, hypersalivation	pale complexion, puffy eyes, poor muscle tone; mostly >40 years, F>M	T: pale, thin or thick white coat P: weak, thready, deficient, slow, deep
Stomach yin deficiency	chronic	empty stomach, when tired, at night, stress	bland or liquid diet, eating something during episodes	dryness of mouth, lips, stools, skin; malar flush, indeterminate gnawing hunger	thin, flushed, anxious	T: slightly red and peeled centrally, or red and dry with no coat P: thready, rapid

4. Anorexia, Loss of Appetite

Lingering external pathogens
- Damp Heat
- *shao yang* syndrome
- Phlegm Heat

Spleen *qi/yang* deficiency
Phlegm Damp in the Stomach
Liver *qi* stagnation

4 ANOREXIA, LOSS OF APPETITE

shi yu bu zhen 食欲不振

Anorexia, or loss of appetite is a commonly encountered complaint in the clinic. The difference between anorexia and loss of appetite for the purposes of this chapter is one of degree. Anorexia is the more severe manifestation in which a patient has no desire to eat at all. Loss of appetite reflects a reduction of the appetite, although the patient may still pick at food.

A good appetite is indicative of healthy Spleen function, and demonstrates the integrity of the *hou tian zhi qi*, the ability to acquire the *qi* from food and drink necessary for daily functioning. All anorexia and loss of appetite is ultimately due to weakness of, or obstruction to, Spleen and Stomach function.

Anorexia or diminished appetite can have significant repercussions on health. There is nothing more fundamental to the restoration and maintenance of good health than eating properly. If there is no *qi* being acquired, none of the other organ systems will function efficiently. If acquired *qi* is not being gathered, the reserves of *yuan qi* located in the Kidney organ system are plundered and drained to support essential physiological functions. These deep reserves of inherited *qi* cannot be replaced, and because their quantity determines life-span and quality of life, significant loss is potentially catastrophic.

The restoration of appetite during convalescence from serious illness, chemotherapy or surgery is of primary importance, regardless of what other physical processes are going on. Return of appetite following a major illness is considered the primary sign of recovery.

The patterns discussed in this chapter reflect those that can present with anorexia. Many causes of illness will have anorexia as a component, however most will present with another TCM disease symptom. For example, patients with acute external Damp Heat affecting the Liver will experience anorexia, but will usually present with jaundice or fever.

Other appetite disorders

Anorexia as discussed in this chapter should be distinguished from anorexia nervosa, a psychological disorder characterised by a refusal to eat or an aberration in eating patterns, rather than a true lack of appetite.

Anorexia and loss of appetite should also be distinguished from symptoms that can look similar. There are three appetite disorders in addition to true loss of appetite. These are an aversion to food, a relatively normal appetite but early satiety so the patient spontaneously reduces the quantity of food consumed so as to feel more comfortable, and no desire to eat despite a sense of hunger.

Aversion to food
With an aversion to food, the patient feels like eating but is made nauseous by certain foods, or the thought of eating them. It generally applies only to certain foods at certain times. Aversion to food is usually associated with an excess accumulation in the Stomach as occurs in food stagnation, Phlegm Damp accumulation or Damp Heat. Food aversions may also be a characteristic of pregnancy.

Early satiety
A patient with uncomfortable abdominal or epigastric bloating associated with eating will often adjust the quantities of food consumed to compensate. When inquiring about diet, it can appear that they eat very little. This may be erroneously interpreted as loss of appetite, when in fact the appetite may be quite normal.

No desire to eat despite a sensation of hunger
This sensation is described as Indeterminate Gnawing Hunger (*see* chapter 16) and is an uncomfortable sensation in the epigastric region that mimics hunger without the patient actually wanting to eat. Patients will often wake in the middle of the night with a nagging discomfort in the pit of their stomach, feeling that they need to eat something but not knowing what they want, or eating a little something that then relieves the discomfort.

BOX 4.1 SOME BIOMEDICAL CAUSES OF ANOREXIA AND LOSS OF APPETITE

Acute infection
- many bacterial and viral infections, including hepatitis, glandular fever, tuberculosis, rheumatic fever, influenza

Gastro-intestinal
- oral or dental disease
- gastritis
- appendicitis
- Crohn's disease
- cirrhosis
- pancreatitis
- carcinoma

Metabolic
- glomerulonephritis
- uraemia

Drugs
- amphetamines
- ephedrine
- chemotherapy

Other
- malignancy, leukaemia
- depression
- fad diets
- old age
- social isolation
- stress

AETIOLOGY

External pathogens

Invasion by external pathogens commonly causes a loss of appetite, and in most cases this is normal and appropriate. The diminishment of the appetite frees up the *qi* that is consumed by digestion and distribution, making it available to support *wei* and *zheng qi* to repel the invader.

In certain circumstances, however, a pathogen can overcome and breach the body's defences and get deeper into the body. Once in the body the pathogen may induce pathological changes or reach an equilibrium with the *zheng qi* whereby it is 'contained' in the *shao yang* level.

The common residual effects of external invasion are lingering Damp Heat in *yang ming* following a Damp, Damp Heat or Summerheat invasion, creation of Phlegm Heat after a vigorous *qi* level fever, or penetration, hiding and containment of a *wei* level pathogen in the *shao yang* level.

Spleen and Stomach deficiency

Any factor that weakens Spleen function can lead to a loss of appetite. Overwork, excessive worry or mental activity, irregular dietary habits or prolonged illness can weaken Spleen *qi*.

Chronic retention of Dampness following an unresolved external invasion or from a damp environment will eventually drain Spleen *qi* and cause deficiency. Patterns that are initially Cold Damp excess patterns often end up as Spleen deficiency when untreated or in susceptible patients. Damp Heat patterns that are treated too enthusiastically with bitter cold herbs or medications can also damage the Spleen. Excessive mental strain or prolonged concentration may deplete Spleen *qi*. The damage is aggravated when an irregular diet is combined with sustained mental activity and too much sitting.

Spleen *yang* is weakened by excessive consumption of cold raw food and irregular eating habits, or by too many cold natured herbs or antibiotics in the treatment of a febrile or other Hot disease. It may develop from deterioration of Spleen *qi* deficiency. Additional factors are prolonged or serious illness, gastro-intestinal surgery or excessive ingestion of very cold substances. Prolonged starvation or digestive insult, such as occurs in anorexia nervosa, bulimia and famine conditions, seriously damages Spleen *yang*.

Emotion

Frustration, anger, resentment, prolonged emotional turmoil, repressed emotions and stress disrupt the circulation of Liver *qi*. These emotions, especially when chronically unexpressed, cause a low grade spasm and tension in the smooth muscle of the gut. When the smooth movement of Liver *qi* is impeded, it finds alternative pathways. In this case the stagnant *qi* is discharged sideways (or overcontrols Earth through the *ke* cycle), disrupting the function of the Spleen, weakening it and contributing to the development deficiency, and Dampness and Phlegm. Loss of appetite associated with *qi* stagnation tends initially to be intermittent, and has a direct relationship to the patient's emotional state. As the condition develops, however, the deficiency elements induced by the repeated invasion come to the fore and Spleen *qi* deficiency or Phlegm Damp type anorexia and loss of appetite may intervene.

With serious depression associated with Liver *qi* stagnation, complete loss of appetite or anorexia may occur.

TREATMENT

Chinese medicine is very effective at restoring and stimulating the appetite. In addition to any herbal or acupuncture treatment, a bland, easily assimilated yet nutritious diet is recommended while the patient's appetite recovers. Particularly good are the various types of rice porridge popular with the Chinese (*jook* or *zhou* 粥), usually cooked in chicken stock, with small amounts of nutritious and easily digested titbits added.

外邪内留

4.1 LINGERING EXTERNAL PATHOGENS

Pathophysiology

- External pathogenic invasion usually causes an acute loss of appetite, which in general is self limiting and appropriate for the duration of the illness. There are many acute illnesses that can cause a loss of appetite and in almost all cases, the loss of appetite itself is benign and needs no treatment. Patients with acute pathogenic illness that have loss of appetite as a feature will usually present with something else, for example jaundice, vomiting, diarrhoea or headache.
- In certain circumstances, however, a pathogenic invasion can lead to a prolonged loss of appetite, beyond the usefulness of a fast, sometimes lasting weeks or even months after the initial illness has resolved. Specific treatment in these circumstances is clearly warranted and this section addresses loss of appetite due to lingering, rather than acute, pathogens. There are three common patterns that can lead to prolonged loss of appetite.

湿热

4.1.1 Lingering Damp Heat

Patients with this pattern will be able to recall an acute disorder, usually characterised by nausea, vomiting and/or diarrhoea. Due to the inherent sticky nature of Damp Heat or Summerheat, it is often incompletely cleared from the body and lingers at a low level, sometimes for weeks or even months. Its retention can be facilitated by improper treatment (such as purging, diaphoresis, antibiotics), by not resting sufficiently during convalescence or by a pre-existing Spleen deficiency. When anorexia is a major feature, it is the Dampness that predominates.

Clinical features

- loss of appetite
- sensation of heaviness in the body, lethargy, listlessness
- muscle aches, foggy-headedness, headaches (like being 'wrapped in a damp towel')
- fullness and discomfort in the chest
- tendency to loose stools or diarrhoea
- sallow complexion
- no thirst
- low grade afternoon feverishness
- in general all symptoms are worse around mid afternoon

T greasy white or yellowish coat
P soggy, thready or wiry

Treatment principle

Clear Damp Heat from the *qi* level by facilitating the descent and distribution of Lung *qi*, promoting urination and liberating the *qi* mechanism

Prescription

SAN REN TANG 三仁汤
(*Three Nut Decoction*)

xing ren (Semen Pruni Armeniacae) 杏仁 12-15g
bai dou kou (Fructus Amomi Kravanh) 白豆蔻 6-9g
yi ren (Semen Coicis Lachryma-jobi) 苡仁 18-30g
ban xia (Rhizoma Pinelliae Ternatae) 半夏 9-12g
hou po (Cortex Magnoliae Officinalis) 厚朴 6-9g
dan zhu ye (Herba Lophatheri Gracilis) 淡竹叶 6-9g
hua shi (Talcum) 滑石 18g
tong cao Medulla Tetrapanacis Papyriferi) 通草 6g

Method: Decoction. **Bai dou kou** is added towards the end of cooking (*hou xia* 后下). **Xing ren** directs Lung *qi* downwards, facilitating correct functioning of the 'upper source of water' thus promoting urination and providing an outlet for the Damp Heat; **bai dou kou** fragrantly transforms Damp and releases the Spleen to invigorate the *qi* mechanism; **yi ren** leaches Damp Heat from the lower *jiao* and promotes urination; **ban xia** and **hou po** are bitter warm and drying, and assist **xing ren** and **bai dou kou** in moving *qi* and freeing up the *qi* mechanism; **dan zhu ye, hua shi** and **tong cao** promote urination to clear Damp Heat. (Source: *Zui Xin Fang Ji Shou Ce*)

Modifications

- With severe Dampness (very thick tongue coat, nausea, epigastric distension, muscle aches), add **huo xiang** (Herba Agastaches seu Pogostemi) 藿香 12-15g and **shi chang pu** (Rhizoma Acori Graminei) 石菖蒲 6-9g.
- With more Heat (yellow tongue coat, irritability, some thirst) add **shan zhi zi** (Fructus Gardeniae Jasminoides) 山栀子 9-12g and **huang lian** (Rhizoma Coptidis) 黄连 3-6g.
- With residual exterior symptoms, add **zi su ye** (Folium Perillae Frutescentis) 紫苏叶 12g.

Patent medicines

Xing Jun San 行军散 (Marching Powder, Five Pagodas Brand)
- a small dose (¼ - ½ teaspoon) several times daily will help to dry Damp

Huo Xiang Zheng Qi Pian 藿香正气片 (Huo Xiang Zheng Qi Pian, Huo Hsiang Cheng Chi Pien)

Acupuncture (select from)

Lu.6 (*kong zui*) .... *xi* cleft point of the Lungs, facilitates dispersal and descent of Lung *qi*, directs Lung *qi* downwards and dispels pathogens

LI.4 (*he gu* -) .... *yuan* point of the Large Intestine, activates the dispersing function of the Lungs, dispels pathogens and clears the exterior

Ren.12 (*zhong wan* -) .... *mu* point of the Stomach, clears pathogens, directs Stomach *qi* downwards and harmonises the Stomach

Sp.9 (*yin ling quan* -) .... together these points promote urination to
Sp.5 (*shang qiu* -) drain and transform Damp

St.36 (*zu san li*) .... *he* sea point of the Stomach, regulates the Spleen and Stomach and the *qi* mechanism and invigorates Spleen's digestion and distribution function

- *Ear points*: spleen, stomach, lung, *shen men*, sympathetic

Clinical notes

- It is recommended to continue treatment for at least a few days after the patient has recovered to consolidate the result and ensure all Damp has been cleared.
- For dietary recommendations, see p.884.

4.1.2 Shao yang syndrome

少阳伏邪

The *shao yang* level is neither internal nor external, but represents a transitional zone between the surface and the interior of the body. Pathogens can hide there and get locked away, sometimes for prolonged periods. *Shao yang* patterns usually follow an ignored or unresolved Wind (*wei* or *tai yang* level) invasion.

The principle of treatment described by the *Shang Han Lun* is to harmonise the *shao yang*, which essentially means closing the space available to the pathogen, thus evicting it. Harmonising also refers to the fact that because the disorder is no longer external and not yet internal, diaphoresis and purging are inappropriate.

Clinical features

- reduced appetite or anorexia
- alternating fever and chills
- nausea
- hypochondriac pain, distension or tenderness

- fullness in the chest
- dizziness
- irritability
- bitter taste in the mouth

T often unremarkable, or coated only on the left side, or slightly red on the edges

P wiry

Treatment principle

Harmonise *shao yang*

Prescription

XIAO CHAI HU TANG 小柴胡汤
(*Minor Bupleurum Combination*) modified

chai hu (Radix Bupleuri) 柴胡 9-12g
huang qin (Radix Scutellariae Baicalensis) 黄芩 9-12g
ban xia (Rhizoma Pinelliae Ternatae) 半夏 9-12g
sheng jiang (Rhizoma Zingiberis Officinalis Recens) 生姜 6-9g
dang shen (Radix Codonopsis Pilosulae) 党参 12-15g
zhi gan cao (honey fried Radix Glycyrrhizae Uralensis) 炙甘草 3-6g
da zao (Fructus Zizyphi Jujubae) 大枣 4pce
sha ren (Fructus Amomi) 砂仁 6-9g

Method: Decoction. **Chai hu** harmonises and closes off the *shao yang* level to lingering pathogens, as well as regulating *qi*; **huang qin** clears Heat from the Liver, Gallbladder and *shao yang*. Together these two herbs are the main synergistic pair for dispersing pathogens residing in the *shao yang* level. **Ban xia** and **sheng jiang** harmonise the Stomach and stop nausea; **dang shen** and **gan cao** support *zheng qi* and assist in preventing the pathogen from penetrating further; **sheng jiang** and **da zao** support **ban xia** in harmonising the Stomach and stopping nausea and vomiting; **sha ren** fragrantly transforms Damp, stimulates the Spleen and the appetite.

Modifications

- With lingering Dampness in *shao yang* (relatively severe anorexia, muscle aches, chills greater than fever, heaviness in the body, in addition to the *shao yang* symptoms), add **cang zhu** (Rhizoma Atractylodis) 苍术 12-15g, **hou po** (Cortex Magnoliae Officinalis) 厚朴 9-12g and **chen pi** (Pericarpium Citri Reticulatae) 陈皮 9-12g.

Patent medicines

Xiao Chai Hu Wan 小柴胡丸 (Xiao Chai Hu Wan)

Acupuncture (select from)

SJ.5 (*wai guan* -) .... these points harmonise *shao yang*, closing
GB.39 (*xuan zhong* -) the space available to any lurking pathogen,
GB.41 (*zu lin qi* -) and regulate Liver *qi*
GB.34 (*yang ling quan* -)

Bl.19 (*dan shu* -) .... *shu* point of the Gallbladder, regulates *qi*
Bl.21 (*wei shu*) .... *shu* point of the Stomach, regulates Stomach *qi* and eliminates stagnation
Bl.22 (*san jiao shu* -) .... regulates transformation of *qi*, eliminates Damp and promotes urination

- with Spleen deficiency, add St.36 (*zu san li* +) and Liv.13 (*zhang men* +)
- *Ear points*: liver, *san jiao*, spleen, stomach, *shen men*, sympathetic

Clinical notes

- *Shao yang* syndrome is a relatively common pattern in patients presenting with loss of appetite. Typically patients will have had an acute exterior Wind Cold, Wind Heat or Wind Damp pattern that was for some reason unresolved. The initial symptoms of the acute exterior disorder give way to fatigue, feelings of heat and cold and loss of appetite. Patients may harbour lurking pathogens in the *shao yang* for weeks, months or even years.
- When correctly identified, *shao yang* patterns respond extremely well to treatment, indeed, patterns that have persisted for months can often be resolved in a few weeks.

痰热

4.1.3 Residual Phlegm Heat

Phlegm Heat can sometimes remain after a febrile disease has run its course. The initial Heat cooks and congeals body fluids into Phlegm. In general, it takes a relatively high fever (*qi* level, affecting the Lungs, Stomach or both), to thicken fluids sufficiently into Phlegm. The Phlegm may persist for some time following resolution of the initial illness, obstructing the Spleen, Stomach and the *qi* mechanism, thus reducing the appetite.

Clinical features

- loss of appetite, or appetite yet to return following a febrile illness
- nausea, vomiting, belching, acid reflux, bitter taste in the mouth
- insomnia or fitful sleep with much dreaming, or waking in the early hours of the morning (typically around 4am), unable to fall back to sleep
- palpitations with anxiety and nervousness
- irritability and restlessness
- dizziness and vertigo

- heavy or foggy-headedness
- fullness and discomfort in the chest, possibly with residual Phlegm or cough

T thick greasy yellow coat
P wiry or slippery and rapid

Treatment principle

Clear Heat and transform Phlegm
Harmonise the Stomach and calm the *shen*

Prescription

WEN DAN TANG 温胆汤
(*Bamboo and Hoelen Combination*)

zhu ru (Caulis Bambusae in Taeniis) 竹茹 12-15g
zhi shi (Fructus Immaturus Citri Aurantii) 枳实 9-12g
ban xia (Rhizoma Pinelliae Ternatae) 半夏 9-12g
fu ling (Sclerotium Poriae Cocos) 茯苓 12-15g
chen pi (Pericarpium Citri Reticulatae) 陈皮 9-12g
sheng jiang (Rhizoma Zingiberis Officinalis Recens) 生姜 3-6g
gan cao (Radix Glycyrrhizae Uralensis) 甘草 3-6g

Method: Decoction. **Zhu ru** clears Phlegm Heat from the Stomach and Gallbladder and directs Stomach *qi* downwards; **zhi shi** breaks up stagnant *qi*, directs *qi* downwards and alleviates distension; **ban xia** transforms Phlegm, dries Damp and directs rising Stomach *qi* downwards; **chen pi** transforms Phlegm and dries Damp, regulates middle *jiao qi* and corrects the *qi* mechanism; **fu ling** strengthens the Spleen and leaches out Damp; **gan cao** strengthens the Spleen and harmonises the Stomach; **sheng jiang** assists the other herbs in transforming the Phlegm.

Modifications

- With severe Phlegm Heat (thick yellow greasy tongue coat, dizziness, foggy-headedness, congested Lungs), add **tian zhu huang** (Concretio Silicea Bambusae Textillis) 天竺黄 9-12g, **zhu li** (Succus Bambusae) 竹沥 12-15g and **dan nan xing** (Pulvis Arisaemae cum Felle Bovis) 胆南星 6-9g.
- With food stagnation, belching or reflux, add two or three of the following herbs: **jiao shen qu** (baked Massa Fermentata) 焦神曲 15g, **jiao shan zha** (baked Fructus Crataegi) 焦山楂 15g, **chao mai ya** (dry fried Fructus Hordei Vulgaris Germinantus) 炒麦芽 15-30g or **chao lai fu zi** (dry fried Semen Raphani Sativi) 炒莱服子 15g.
- With constipation, add **da huang** (Radix et Rhizoma Rhei) 大黄 6-9g and **gua lou ren** (Semen Trichosanthis) 栝楼仁 12-18g.

Patent medicines

Wen Dan Wan 温胆丸 (Wen Dan Wan)

Acupuncture (select from)

Ren.12 (*zhong wan* -) .... *mu* point of the Stomach, clears pathogens, directs Stomach *qi* downwards and harmonises the Stomach

PC.6 (*nei guan* -) .... *luo* point of the Pericardium, master point of *yin wei mai*, regulates the middle *jiao*, stops vomiting, calms the Heart and *shen*, spreads Liver *qi*

St.40 (*feng long* -) .... *luo* point of the Stomach, transforms Phlegm and clears Heat and Phlegm from the Stomach

St.36 (*zu san li*) .... *he* sea point of the Stomach, regulates the Spleen and Stomach and the *qi* mechanism, and invigorates Spleen's digestion and distribution function

St.43 (*xiang gu* -) .... *shu* and Wood point of the Stomach, clears Heat from the Stomach

- with severe Heat, add PC.8 (*lao gong* -) and St.45 (*li dui* ↓)
- with Stomach discomfort, add St.34 (*liang qiu* -)
- with dizziness, add GB.43 (*xia xi* -)
- with anxiety, add Du.19 (*hou ding*) and Du.24 (*shen ting*)
- with foggy-headedness, add Du.20 (*bai hui*) and PC.5 (*jian shi*)
- *Ear points*: spleen, stomach, heart, *shen men*, sympathetic

Clinical notes

- Loss of appetite of this type responds well to treatment although treatment needs to continue until all signs of Phlegm are cleared, in particular, until the tongue coat becomes normal. Herbs may be more efficient at clearing entrenched Phlegm although acupuncture itself often starts to improve the appetite quickly, especially on the day of treatment.
- For dietary recommendations, see p.885.

脾气阳虚

4.2 SPLEEN QI/YANG DEFICIENCY

Pathophysiology

- Spleen *qi* and/or *yang* deficiency patterns are the most common presentations of diminished appetite or anorexia. Adequate Spleen *yang qi* is the 'Fire' of the digestive process, and just as Kidney *yang* is the basis of sexual desire, so too is Spleen *yang qi* the basis of the desire to eat.
- The degree of appetite loss accurately reflects the degree of deficiency; the closer to *yang* deficiency the patient is the greater the loss of appetite.

Clinical features

- diminished appetite (*qi* deficiency) or anorexia (*yang* deficiency)
- epigastric and abdominal distension
- loose stools or diarrhoea
- nausea or vomiting, often in the morning
- waxy pale or lustreless complexion
- tiredness, lethargy and fatigue, tired weak limbs
- shortness of breath, reluctance to speak, low voice
- oedema, particularly in the eyelids and fingers
- if *yang* is deficient: cold extremities, cold intolerance, undigested food in the stools, abdominal pain which is better for warmth and pressure

T pale and swollen with toothmarks; the coat will vary from thin (in pure deficiency) to thick and greasy (with accumulated Damp)

P deep and thready or deficient, big and weak (especially right middle position)

Treatment principle

Strengthen the Spleen, supplement *qi* and *yang*
Harmonise the Stomach, warm the middle *jiao*

Prescription

XIANG SHA LIU JUN ZI TANG 香砂六君子汤
(*Saussurea and Cardamon Combination*)

This prescription is selected for Spleen *qi* deficiency with a degree of Phlegm Damp.

dang shen (Radix Codonopsis Pilosulae) 党参 15-24g
chao bai zhu (dry fried Rhizoma Atractylodis Macrocephalae) 炒白术 12-15g
fu ling (Sclerotium Poriae Cocos) 茯苓 12-15g
ban xia (Rhizoma Pinelliae Ternatae) 半夏 9-12g
chen pi (Pericarpium Citri Reticulatae) 陈皮 9-12g
sha ren (Fructus Amomi) 砂仁 6-9g
mu xiang (Radix Aucklandiae Lappae) 木香 6-9g

zhi gan cao (honey fried Radix Glycyrrhizae Uralensis) 炙甘草 3-6g

Method: Decoction. **Sha ren** is added towards the end of cooking time (*hou xia* 后下). **Dang shen** supplements *qi* and strengthens the Spleen; **chao bai zhu** strengthens the Spleen, supplements *qi* and dries Dampness; **fu ling** strengthens the Spleen and leaches out Dampness through the urine; **ban xia** transforms Phlegm, dries Damp, directs rising Stomach *qi* downwards and stops nausea and vomiting; **chen pi** transforms Phlegm and dries Damp, regulates middle *jiao qi* and corrects the *qi* mechanism; **zhi gan cao** strengthens the Spleen and harmonises the Stomach; **sha ren** and **mu xiang** regulate *qi* and correct the *qi* mechanism.

LI ZHONG WAN 理中丸
(*Ginseng and Ginger Formula*)

This prescription is selected for Spleen and Stomach *yang* deficiency. In this case the patient tends to anorexia.

gan jiang (Rhizoma Zingiberis Officinalis) 干姜 9-12g
dang shen (Radix Codonopsis Pilosulae) 党参 15-24g
chao bai zhu (dry fried Rhizoma Atractylodes Macrocephalae) 炒白术 12-15g
zhi gan cao (honey fried Radix Glycyrrhizae Uralensis) 炙甘草 3-9g

Method: Decoction. **Gan jiang**, the main herb, warms Spleen and Stomach *yang* and dispels Cold; **dang shen** supplements *qi* and strengthens the Spleen; **chao bai zhu** strengthens the Spleen and dries Dampness; **zhi gan cao** supplements *qi* and harmonises the Stomach.

Variations and additional prescriptions

With Blood deficiency

- When the patient does not eat sufficient to create good quality Blood, or requirements of *qi* and Blood are high (as in pregnancy or breast-feeding), Blood deficiency will complicate the *qi* deficiency. Most patients with prolonged *qi* deficiency will eventually become Blood deficient as well. *Qi* and Blood supplementing prescriptions are recommended, in particular **SHI QUAN DA BU TANG** (*Ginseng and Dang Gui Ten Combination* 十全大补汤, p.729). Also effective are the popular patent medicines **DANG GUI JI JING** 当归鸡精 (Tangkwei Essence of Chicken) and **WU JI BAI FENG WAN** 乌鸡白凤丸 (Wu Chi Pai Feng Wan).

With a tendency to food stagnation

- A very simple, elegant and effective prescription for *qi* deficiency with a degree of food stagnation is **ZHI ZHU WAN** (*Immature Bitter Orange and Atractylodes Macrocephala Pill* 枳术丸).

bai zhu (Rhizoma Atractylodes Macrocephalae) 白术 60g
zhi shi (Fructus Immaturus Citri Aurantii) 枳实 30g

Method: Grind the herbs into a fine powder and form into 9-gram pills with water. The dose is one pill 2-3 times daily. May also be decocted with a 60% reduction in quantities. **Bai zhu** strengthens the Spleen and dries Dampness; **zhi shi** directs *qi* downward and reduces distension.

Other Spleen strengthening prescriptions

- Although we find the above prescriptions to be the most effective in stimulating a poor appetite, most other Spleen *qi* supplementing prescriptions will have good results (as by strengthening the Spleen the appetite naturally revives). When Spleen deficiency is the diagnosis, an appropriate Spleen supplementing prescription may be chosen on the basis of the specific aspect of Spleen function that is weak. For example, with easy bruising or heavy menstrual periods, **GUI PI TANG** (*Ginseng and Longan Combination* 归脾汤, p.728) may be selected; if accompanied by diarrhoea or loose stools, select **SHEN LING BAI ZHU SAN** (*Ginseng and Atractylodes Formula* 参苓白术散, p.243); with prolapse, haemorrhoids, poor muscle tone select **BU ZHONG YI QI TANG** (*Ginseng and Astragalus Combination* 补中益气汤, p.502).

Patent medicines

Xiang Sha Liu Jun Zi Wan 香砂六君子丸 (Xiang Sha Liu Jun Wan, Aplotaxis-Ammomum Pills, Six Gentlemen Tea Pills)
- *qi* deficiency with Phlegm Damp

Xiang Sha Yang Wei Wan 香砂养胃丸 (Xiang Sha Yang Wei Wan, Hsiang Sha Yang Wei Wan)
- *qi* deficiency with *qi* stagnation

Fu Zi Li Zhong Wan 附子理中丸 (Fu Tzu Li Chung Wan, Carmichaeli Tea Pills, Li Chung Yuen Medical Pills)

Li Zhong Wan 理中丸 (Li Zhong Wan)
- Spleen *yang* deficiency

Dang Gui Ji Jing 当归鸡精 (Tangkwei Essence of Chicken)
- postpartum, with *qi* and Blood deficiency

Chong Cao Ji Jing 虫草鸡精 (Cordyceps Essence of Chicken)
- excellent following chemotherapy or radiotherapy

Shi Quan Da Bu Wan 十全大补丸 (Shi Quan Da Bu Wan, Ten Flavour Tea) - *qi* and Blood deficiency

Wu Ji Bai Feng Wan 乌鸡白凤丸 (Wu Chi Pai Feng Wan)
- *qi* and Blood deficiency

Jian Pi Wan 健脾丸 (Jian Pi Wan)
- Spleen deficiency with food stagnation

Acupuncture (select from)

Ren.12 (*zhong wan* +▲) .. *mu* point of the Stomach, warms and regulates the Stomach, directs Stomach *qi* downwards

St.36 (*zu san li* +▲) .... *he* sea point of the Stomach, powerfully warms and strengthens the Spleen and Stomach, and supplements *qi*

Sp.6 (*san yin jiao* +) .... strengthens the Spleen, regulates Liver *qi*, benefits the Kidneys, invigorates *qi* and Blood

LI.11 (*qu chi* +▲) .... *he* sea point of the Large Intestine, warms and strengthens *yang ming*

Bl.20 (*pi shu* +▲) .... *shu* point of the Spleen, warms and supplements Spleen *qi* and *yang*

Bl.21 (*wei shu* +▲) .... *shu* point of the Stomach, warms and strengthens the Stomach

- a moxa box over the upper abdomen is useful
- with Phlegm Damp, add PC.6 (*nei guan*) and Sp.3 (*tai bai*)
- with diarrhoea, add St.25 (*tian shu* +▲) and St.37 (*shan ju xu*)
- with abdominal distension, add Sp.3 (*tai bai*) and Sp.15 (*da heng*)
- *Ear points*: spleen, stomach, lung, adrenal, pancreas *shen men*, sympathetic

Clinical notes

- Spleen deficiency patterns respond well to correct treatment, but the more chronic or profound, the more time required for lasting results. With *yang* deficient patterns, some months of treatment are usually required to restore the Spleen and appetite completely.
- For dietary recommendations, see pp.870-873.

痰湿阻胃

4.3 PHLEGM DAMP IN THE STOMACH

Pathophysiology

• Phlegm Damp causes loss of appetite by obstructing the *qi* mechanism and the ascent of Spleen *qi* to the mouth. This pattern may be associated with a history of unrestrained dietary intake of substances that generate Phlegm Damp, or be a complication of Liver *qi* stagnation, or Spleen *qi* or *yang* deficiency.

Clinical features

• anorexia or reduced appetite, loss of sense of taste
• epigastric and abdominal distension and fullness
• nausea or vomiting, often in the morning
• acid reflux, belching
• loose stools or diarrhoea
• fatigue, lethargy, sluggishness, heaviness in the body and limbs, frequent desire to sleep, after which the patient often feels worse or more sluggish
• poor concentration, heavy or foggy-headedness
• copious salivation
• dizziness, palpitations or headaches that can be triggered by strong smells
• stuffiness in the chest
• may be chronic mucus production from the sinuses and lungs
• greasy skin, musty body odour
• tendency to obesity, pear shape

T thick, greasy, white coat, possible swollen or flabby tongue body
P slippery, wiry, moderate

Treatment principle

Dry and transform Phlegm Damp
Invigorate digestion and distribution of *qi* and fluids
Harmonise the Stomach

Prescription

PING WEI SAN 平胃散
(*Magnolia and Ginger Formula*)

cang zhu (Rhizoma Atractylodis) 苍术 12-15g
hou po (Cortex Magnoliae Officinalis) 厚朴 9-12g
chen pi (Pericarpium Citri Reticulatae) 陈皮 9-12g
gan cao (Radix Glycyrrhizae Uralensis) 甘草 3-6g
sheng jiang (Rhizoma Zingiberis Officinalis) 生姜 6-9g
da zao (Fructus Zizyphi Jujubae) 大枣 4pce

Method: Grind the herbs into powder and take 9-grams as a draft on an empty stomach 2-3 times daily. May also be decocted. **Cang zhu** powerfully parches and dries Damp, thereby liberating the Spleen and allowing it to function correctly; **hou po** regulates *qi*, transforms Damp and alleviates distension; **ban xia** and **chen pi** transform Phlegm and dry Damp, regulate middle *jiao qi* and correct the *qi* mechanism; **zhi gan cao** strengthens the Spleen and harmonises the Stomach; **fu ling** strengthens the Spleen and leaches out Damp. (Source: *Shi Yong Zhong Yi Nei Ke Xue*)

Modifications

- With Spleen deficiency, reduce the dose of **cang zhu** by half, and add **chao bai zhu** (dry fried Rhizoma Atractylodes Macrocephalae) 炒白术 9-12g, **chao shan yao** (dry fried Radix Dioscoreae Oppositae) 炒山药 12-15g and **zhi huang qi** (honey fried Radix Astragali Membranacei) 炙黄芪 18-30g.
- With Cold, add **rou gui** (Cortex Cinnamomi Cassiae) 肉桂 3g and **gan jiang** (Rhizoma Zingiberis Officinalis) 干姜 6-9g.
- With foggy-headedness, add **shi chang pu** (Rhizoma Acori Graminei) 石菖蒲 6-9g and **yuan zhi** (Radix Polygalae Tenuifoliae) 远志 6-9g.

Variations and additional prescriptions

With qi stagnation

- The presence of Phlegm and/or Damp in the middle *jiao* can easily obstruct the movement of *qi* and disrupt the *qi* mechanism, leading to combined *qi* and Phlegm Damp stagnation. The main features are reduced appetite, persistent epigastric bloating, indigestion, borborygmus, flatulence, nausea, acid reflux and an epigastrium that feels soft or flaccid with palpation. The aim of treatment is to dry Dampness, transform Phlegm and regulate *qi* with **XIANG SHA YANG WEI TANG** (*Nourish the Stomach Decoction with Aucklandia and Ammomum* 香砂养胃汤).

    bai zhu (Rhizoma Atractylodes Macrocephalae) 白术 30g
    ban xia (Rhizoma Pinelliae Ternatae) 半夏 30g
    chen pi (Pericarpium Citri Reticulatae) 陈皮 30g
    fu ling (Sclerotium Poria Cocos) 茯苓 30g
    sha ren (Fructus Amomi) 砂仁 20g
    xiang fu (Rhizoma Cyperi Rotundi) 香附 20g
    zhi shi (Fructus Immaturus Citri Aurantii) 枳实 20g
    cao dou kou (Semen Alpiniae Katsumadai) 草豆蔻 20g
    huo xiang (Herba Agastaches seu Pogostemi) 藿香 20g
    hou po (Cortex Magnoliae Officinalis) 厚朴 20g
    gan cao (Radix Glycyrrhizae Uralensis) 甘草 10g

    Method: Grind the herbs into powder and take 9-grams as a draft on an empty stomach, 2-3 times daily. May also be decocted with a 60% reduction in quantities. **Bai zhu** strengthens the Spleen and dries Dampness; **ban xia** and **chen pi** transform Phlegm, dry Dampness and regulate middle *jiao qi*; **fu ling** strengthens the Spleen and leaches out Dampness; **huo xiang** fragrantly revives the Spleen, dissipates Dampness and releases the Stomach from it's viscous grasp; **xiang fu, mu xiang, chen pi, hou po, sha ren** and **cao dou kou**, regulate *qi* and stimulate the *qi* mechanism, transform Dampness and warm the middle *jiao*; **zhi shi** regulates and directs *qi* downward; **gan cao** protects the Stomach and harmonises the action of the other herbs. (Source: *Zui Xin Fang Ji Shou Ce*)

With obesity and Spleen yang deficiency

- Patients with constitutional Phlegm Damp are often overweight and may attempt, often serially, various types of weight loss programme. Many modern forms of weight loss treatment are based on raw food diets, or practices that can severely injure Spleen *yang*. People with Phlegm Damp constitutions, when subjected to this regimen, may find that they can eat virtually nothing, yet not only not lose weight, but even gain weight. The additional weight is usually accumulated pathogenic water from severe deterioration of the ability of Spleen *yang* to metabolise fluids. At the same time the patient feels the effect of the *yang* depletion–anorexia, cold intolerance, fatigue, oedema, loose stools or diarrhoea and a pale swollen tongue. The initial aim of treatment is to vigorously warm and re-invigorate Spleen *yang* and mobilise fluids with a formula such as **SHI PI YIN** (*Magnolia and Atractylodes Combination* 实脾饮).

zhi fu zi (Radix Aconiti Carmichaeli Praeparata) 制附子 6-12g
gan jiang (Rhizoma Zingiberis Officinalis) 干姜 9-12g
fu ling (Sclerotium Poria Cocos) 茯苓 12-15g
bai zhu (Rhizoma Atractylodes Macrocephalae) 白术 9-12g
mu gua (Fructus Chaenomelis) 木瓜 6-9g
hou po (Cortex Magnoliae Officinalis) 厚朴 6-9g
mu xiang (Radix Aucklandiae Lappae) 木香 6-9g
da fu pi (Pericarpium Arecae Catechu) 大腹皮 6-9g
cao guo (Fructus Amomi Tsao-ko) 草果 6-9g
zhi gan cao (honey fried Radix Glycyrrhizae Uralensis)
炙甘草 3-6g
sheng jiang (Rhizoma Zingiberis Officinalis) 生姜 6-9g
da zao (Fructus Zizyphi Jujubae) 大枣 3pce

Method: Decoction. **Zhi fu zi** is cooked for 30 minutes prior to the other herbs (*xian jian* 先煎). **Zhi fu zi** warms Spleen and Kidney *yang*, dispels Cold, promotes movement and transformation of *qi* and fluids and unblocks all channels; **gan jiang** warms Spleen *yang*, and invigorates the Spleen's ability to transform and distribute food and fluids–as the main herbs they powerfully warm Spleen *yang*, dispel Cold, stimulate digestion, mobilise fluids and improve fluid metabolism; **bai zhu** and **fu ling** strengthen the Spleen, dry Dampness and promote urination; **mu gua, hou po, mu xiang, da fu pi** and **cao guo** direct *qi* downwards, alleviate stagnation, transform Dampness and promote urination; **gan cao, sheng jiang** and **da zao** harmonise the middle *jiao* and the actions of the other herbs.

Once the *yang* has been restored, a more general Spleen *qi* strengthening, Phlegm Damp resolving approach, such as **XIANG SHA LIU JUN ZI TANG** (*Saussurea and Cardamon Combination* 香砂六君子汤, p.149) may be adopted.

Patent medicines

Ping Wei San 平胃散 (Ping Wei San)

Xiang Sha Liu Jun Zi Wan 香砂六君子丸 (Xiang Sha Liu Jun Wan, Aplotaxis-Ammomum Pills, Six Gentlemen Tea Pills)
- with Spleen deficiency

Xiang Sha Yang Wei Wan 香砂养胃丸 (Xiang Sha Yang Wei Wan, Hsiang Sha Yang Wei Wan)
- with *qi* stagnation

Fu Zi Li Zhong Wan 附子理中丸 (Fu Tzu Li Chung Wan, Carmichaeli Tea Pills, Li Chung Yuen Medical Pills)
- Spleen *yang* deficiency

Bao Ying Dan 保婴丹 (Bo Ying Compound)
- for infants

Acupuncture (select from)

Ren.12 (*zhong wan* -) .... *mu* point of the Stomach, clears pathogens, directs Stomach *qi* downwards and harmonises the Stomach

St.21 (*liang men* -) .... promotes the function of the Spleen and Stomach

Sp.3 (*tai bai*) ....*yuan luo* couple, these two points are a special
St.40 (*feng long* -) combination for transforming Phlegm Damp, unhindering and invigorating the Spleen and piquing the appetite

St.36 (*zu san li* +▲) .... *he* sea point of the Stomach, powerfully warms and strengthens the Spleen and Stomach, regulates the *qi* mechanism and invigorates Spleen's digestion and distribution function

Sp.5 (*shang qiu* -)..............*jing* river point of the Spleen, transforms Dampness

PC.5 (*jian shi*) ....*jing* river point of the Pericardium, transforms Phlegm, harmonises the Stomach

- with fluid retention and oedema, add Ren.9 (*shui fen* ▲), St.28 (*shui dao* -), Sp.9 (*yin ling quan* -) and Sp.6 (*san yin jiao*)
- with sluggish stools or constipation, add SJ.6 (*zhi gou* -), St.37 (*shang ju xu* -) and St.41 (*jie xi* -)

- with *qi* stagnation, add Liv.3 (*tai chong*) and PC.6 (*nei guan*)
- with foggy-headedness, add GB.20 (*feng chi*) and Bl.62 (*shen mai*)
- with Cold Phlegm, apply moxa cones to Bl.20 (*pi shu* ▲) and Bl.21 (*wei shu* ▲)
- with somnolence, add Kid.6 (*zhao hai*) and Bl.62 (*shen mai*)
- *Ear points*: spleen, stomach, *shen men*, sympathetic

Clinical notes

- In contrast to the residual Phlegm Heat pattern that follows a febrile illness, Phlegm Damp in the Stomach generally tends to be a more chronic and slow to resolve condition. In addition to dietary modification, Phlegm Damp patterns usually require substantial and persistent treatment for satisfactory results.
- As the Phlegm Damp resolves the treatment strategy changes to strengthening the Spleen and regulating digestion. It can take 6-9 months to restore healthy Spleen function in chronic cases.
- For dietary recommendations, see p.880.

肝郁气滞

4.4 LIVER QI STAGNATION

Pathophysiology

- Stagnation of Liver *qi* can impact on the function of the Spleen and Stomach upsetting the normal *qi* mechanism and interfering with the appetite.

Clinical features

- reduced appetite which is related to the patient's emotional state
- epigastric and abdominal distension, sense of knotting in the epigastrium
- hypochondriac discomfort, ache or tightness
- belching, frequent sighing
- early satiety
- borborygmus, indigestion, acid reflux
- irritability, moodiness, depression
- 'plumstone' throat, sense of tightness in the throat, difficulty swallowing
- tendency to loose stools, or alternating constipation and diarrhoea

T thin white coat
P wiry

Treatment principle

Soothe the Liver and regulate *qi*
Harmonise the Liver and Spleen, strengthen the Spleen

Prescription

YUE JU WAN 越鞠丸
(*Escape Restraint Pill*)

This prescription is selected when the predominant effect of the *qi* stagnation is expressed in the Stomach. The main features in addition to the reduced appetite are epigastric distension, indigestion, belching and acid reflux.

xiang fu (Rhizoma Cyperi Rotundi) 香附 9-15g
cang zhu (Rhizoma Atractylodis) 苍术 9-15g
shen qu (Massa Fermentata) 神曲 9-15g
chuan xiong (Radix Ligustici Chuanxiong) 川芎 6-12g
shan zhi zi (Fructus Gardeniae Jasminoides) 山栀子 6-12g

Method: Decoction. **Xiang fu** is the main herb and disperses stagnant *qi*; **cang zhu** dries Dampness and Phlegm, and works with **xiang fu** to improve Spleen and Stomach function; **chuan xiong** invigorates *qi* and Blood and reinforces the *qi* moving function of **xiang fu**; **shan zhi zi** clears Heat from all three *jiao*; **shen qu** alleviates food stagnation, aids digestion and harmonises the Stomach.

XIAO YAO SAN 逍遥散
(*Bupleurum and Dang Gui Formula*)

This prescription is designed for Liver *qi* stagnation complicated by Spleen *qi* and Blood deficiency, a common pattern, especially in women. The main features, in addition to the reduced appetite, include premenstrual symptoms such as breast tenderness and irritability, irregular menstruation, tension headaches, variable energy levels, fatigue that improves with activity, pale edges on the tongue and a thready wiry pulse.

chai hu (Radix Bupleuri) 柴胡 9-12g
dang gui (Radix Angelicae Sinensis) 当归 9-12g
bai shao (Radix Paeoniae Lactiflorae) 白芍 12-18g
bai zhu (Rhizoma Atractylodis Macrocephalae) 白术 9-12g
fu ling (Sclerotium Poria Cocos) 茯苓 12-15g
zhi gan cao (honey fried Radix Glycyrrhizae Uralensis)
炙甘草 3-6g
wei jiang (roasted Rhizoma Zingiberis Officinalis) 煨姜 ... 3-6g
bo he (Herba Mentha Haplocalycis) 薄荷 3-6g

Method: Decoction. **Bo he** is added a few minutes before the end of cooking (*hou xia* 后下). **Chai hu** moves Liver *qi*; **dang gui** and **bai shao** nourish Liver Blood and soften the Liver; **bai zhu** and **fu ling** strengthen the Spleen and dry and leach out Dampness respectively; **zhi gan cao** supplements *qi* and, with **bai shao**, eases muscle spasms; **wei jiang** warms and harmonises the Stomach; **bo he** assists **chai hu** in moving Liver *qi*.

Modifications

- With a degree of Heat, add **shan zhi zi** (Fructus Gardeniae Jasminoides) 山栀子 6-9g and **mu dan pi** (Cortex Moutan Radicis) 牡丹皮 6-9g.
- Liver *qi* stagnation is frequently complicated by Phlegm Damp. In such cases, treatment incorporates *qi* regulation and Phlegm transformation. *See* **XIANG SHA YANG WEI TANG** (*Nourish the Stomach Decoction with Aucklandia and Ammomum* 香砂养胃汤, p.154).

Patent medicines

Xiao Yao Wan 逍遥丸 (Xiao Yao Wan, Hsiao Yao Wan, Bupleurum Sedative Pills) - best for constitutional treatment of Liver *qi* stagnation in women and those with Blood deficiency

Jia Wei Xiao Yao Wan 加味逍遥丸 (Jia Wei Xiao Yao Wan, Dan Zhi Xiao Yao Wan) - Liver *qi* stagnation with stagnant Heat

Chai Hu Shu Gan Wan 柴胡疏肝丸 (Chai Hu Shu Gan Wan) - good for robust patients

Xiang Sha Yang Wei Wan 香砂养胃丸 (Xiang Sha Yang Wei Wan)
- with Spleen and Stomach deficiency

Acupuncture (select from)

Ren.12 (*zhong wan* -) .... *mu* point of the Stomach, clears pathogens, directs Stomach *qi* downwards and harmonises the Stomach
Liv.13 (*zhang men*) .... *mu* point of the Spleen, regulates and harmonises the Liver and Spleen
St.36 (*zu san li* +▲) .... *he* sea point of the Stomach, powerfully warms and strengthens the Spleen and Stomach, regulates the *qi* mechanism and invigorates Spleen's digestion and distribution function
GB.34 (*yang ling quan* -) ... *he* sea point of the Gallbladder, regulates *qi* and subdues exuberant Liver *yang*
Liv.3 (*tai chong* -) ....*yuan*, *shu* and Earth point of the Liver, regulates Liver *qi*
Sp.4 (*gong sun*) .... *luo* point of the Spleen, master point of *chong mai*, regulates the Spleen and Stomach, invigorates Spleen's digestion and distribution function
PC.6 (*nei guan* -) .... *luo* point of the Pericardium, master point of *yin wei mai*, regulates the middle *jiao*, spreads Liver *qi*

- In most cases, points to calm the *shen* should be added: select one or two points from *yin tang* (M-HN-3), Du.19 (*hou ding*), Du. 24 (*shen ting*)
- with Blood or *yin* deficiency, add Sp.6 (*san yin jiao* +), St.36 (*zu san li* -), Bl.18 (*gan shu* +) and Bl.23 (*shen shu* +)
- with Phlegm or 'plum stone' throat, add PC.5 (*jian shi* -), St.40 (*feng long* -) and Sp.3 (*tai bai*)
- *Ear points*: liver, stomach, spleen, endocrine, sympathetic, *shen men*

Clinical notes

- *Qi* stagnation type diminished appetite may be diagnosed biomedically as nervous stomach, irritable bowel syndrome or a stress related loss of appetite.
- Acupuncture is often the treatment of choice for moving stagnant *qi* and if the loss of appetite is relatively recent, one course (or less) of acupuncture should effect a cure. When deficiency patterns intervene, herbs should be added. Relaxation and stress management techniques are useful in patients with ongoing sources of stress.
- For dietary recommendations, see p.878.

SUMMARY OF GUIDING FORMULAE FOR ANOREXIA AND LOSS OF APPETITE

Residual pathogens
- lingering Damp Heat - *San Ren Tang* 三仁汤
- *shao yang* syndrome - *Xiao Chai Hu Tang* 小柴胡汤
- Phlegm Heat - *Wen Dan Tang* 温胆汤

Spleen and Stomach *qi* deficiency - *Xiang Sha Liu Jun Zi Tang* 香砂六君子汤
- *yang* deficiency - *Li Zhong Wan* 理中丸
- with Blood deficiency - *Shi Quan Da Bu Tang* 十全大补汤
- mild cases with a tendency to food stagnation - *Zhu Zhu Wan* 枳术丸

Phlegm Damp - *Ping Wei San* 平胃散
- with *qi* stagnation - *Xiang Sha Yang Wei Wan* 香砂养胃丸
- with Spleen deficiency and oedema - *Shi Pi Yin* 实脾饮

Liver *qi* stagnation - *Yue Ju Wan* 越鞠丸
- with Spleen and Blood deficiency - *Xiao Yao San* 逍遥散
- with Phlegm Damp - *Xiang Sha Yang Wei Wan* 香砂养胃丸

Table 4.1 *Differential diagnosis of anorexia and loss of appetite*

Pattern	Duration	Aggravated by	Other features	Pulse and tongue
Lingering Damp Heat	relatively short duration (weeks)	humid weather	low grade afternoon fever, muscle aches, foggy-headedness, heaviness	T: greasy white or yellow coat P: soggy, thready, wiry
Shao yang syndrome	usually relatively short duration, but can be prolonged	fatigue, being run down	dizziness, nausea, alternating fever and chills, bitter taste, irritability	T: unremarkable P: wiry
Phlegm Heat	relatively short duration (weeks)	humid weather, strong smells	heartburn, belching, dizziness, insomnia, palpitations, foggy-headedness	T: thick greasy yellow coat P: slippery, rapid
Spleen qi/yang deficiency	mostly chronic, but may be acute following surgery or certain medications	cold or raw food, cold medications	fatigue, weakness, morning nausea, puffy face and fingers, cold intolerance, pale complexion, often worse towards the end of the day	T: pale and swollen P: deep, thready, weak
Phlegm Damp in the Stomach	mostly chronic	dairy, sugar, raw food, greasy food	heartburn, distension, morning nausea, heaviness, foggy-headedness, often worse in the morning	T: thick greasy white coat, flabby body P: slippery, wiry
Liver qi stagnation	chronic with acute exacerbations	emotional stress	irritability, depression, alternating bowel habits, sighing	T: unremarkable, or dark P: wiry

5. Constipation

Excess patterns

Heat

Food stagnation

Qi stagnation

Phlegm accumulation

Deficient patterns

Blood deficiency

Qi deficiency

Yin deficiency

Yang deficiency with Cold accumulation

5 CONSTIPATION

bian bi 便秘

Constipation is difficulty in passing stools, prolonged intervals between stools, or a desire to defecate without the ability to do partially or completely. The stools may be hard, dry and pebble like, or essentially normal (that is, moist and well formed).

People have widely varying ideas as to what constitutes a normal bowel pattern, and it must be established what the patient means when describing bowel movements. To some individuals, one motion per week is normal, while others consider themselves constipated if they defecate only once daily. In TCM the baseline for 'normal' is at least one unforced stool every day or second day. Establishing precisely what a patient means by constipation, in terms of frequency, sensation and the nature of the stools is essential.

Constipation is a common problem, and in the Western world appears to be largely related to diet and sedentary habits. Constipation can also be an acute event associated with other primary illnesses, typically those characterised by fever or dehydration. In these situations however, the constipation itself is unlikely to be the presenting problem, although it will certainly be considered in the treatment strategy. More commonly in the Western clinic, constipation is a chronic problem, often of many years duration.

Constipation can be broadly divided into two types, excess and deficient. The excess patterns are characterised by the presence of a pathogen (typically Heat or Phlegm) or by pathological accumulation of *qi* that blocks the *qi* mechanism and the descent of Large Intestine *qi*.

The deficient patterns are characterised by dryness from insufficient fluid lubrication in the form of body fluids, Blood or *yin*, or lack of propulsion through the digestive tract from deficiency of *qi* or *yang*.

AETIOLOGY

Heat

Heat causing constipation can be of external or internal origin. When external Heat causes constipation, it may be systemic Heat (as in Heat in the Blood), or more commonly, Heat in the *qi* level, that is, Heat invasion of the Lungs and/or Stomach and Intestines.

External Heat

Heat in the Lungs

Invasion of an external Heat pathogen, or other pathogen which transforms into heat once in the body, will dry body fluids and parch those parts of the body most sensitive to dryness, the Lungs and Intestines. A Heat pathogen in the Lungs, for example Phlegm Heat or Lung Fire, will dry both the Lungs and Intestines (through their *yin yang* relationship) and obstruct the descent of Lung *qi*. Indeed, other pathogens may also contribute to constipation by obstructing the descent of Lung *qi*, thus impeding Large Intestine *qi* movement. The drying power of Heat makes it by far the most common external pathogen to cause constipation. This is the type of constipation that frequently accompanies upper respiratory tract infections such as bronchitis and pneumonia. In these cases however, the constipation is unlikely to be the presenting disease symptom; much more likely the presenting disease will be cough, fever or wheezing.

Heat in the Stomach and Intestines (yang ming fu *syndrome, and variations*)
Heat invasion of the Stomach and Large Intestine is described as *yang ming* syndrome. The earliest description, by Zhang Zhong-Jing, circa 200 AD, relates to an invasion of Cold through the most exterior of the six levels (*liu jing* 六经) into either the *yang ming* channels or organs. The Cold transforms into Heat once through the surface and then lodges in the interior. These *yang ming* patterns are acute disorders that usually follow an unresolved or powerful Wind Cold or Wind Heat surface invasion, and are characterised by the 'four bigs'–big fever, thirst, sweat and pulse. When the *yang ming* organs are affected, constipation is the main additional feature, and it is the purging of the constipation that is the key to eliminating the Heat (through the 'big exit'). Pathogens may overlap two or more levels, for example the *shao yang* and *yang ming* levels, or all three *yang* levels. Specific formulae have been developed to treat these variations.

Internal Heat

The most common cause of internal Heat type constipation is diet (*see* below).

Internal Heat can also be generated by prolonged frustration, resentment, or other emotional turmoil that impedes the movement of Liver *qi*. The transformation of stagnant *qi* into Heat is aided by consumption of heating foods and beverages, especially alcohol, rich, fatty or supplementing foods. In addition, cigarette smoking, or working in a very dry or dehumidified environment can dry the Lungs, and by extension, the Large Intestine.

Diet

The type of food consumed and the way it is consumed are important factors in the genesis of constipation. The western diet is, for the most part, heavy in protein and fat, and light on dietary fibre. Dietary fibre, from the cell walls of grains, vegetables and fruits is largely composed of cellulose, and is indigestible in humans. Fibre acts as a bulking agent, increasing the volume

BOX 5.1 KEY DIAGNOSTIC POINTS

Nature of the stool
- Dry stool - Heat or *yin* or Blood deficiency
- Pebble or button like stools - Heat
- Neither dry nor hard - *qi* or *yang* deficiency, *qi* stagnation
- Moist stools with mucus - Phlegm accumulation

of a stool, thus triggering the stretch receptors in the intestinal wall. This in turn stimulates intestinal peristalsis and decreases transit time of waste material through the intestines. Insufficient fibre and a high proportion of fat, which slows transit time, contribute significantly to sluggish movement of waste material through the bowel, and thus constipation. This tendency to sluggishness is compounded by the lack of physical activity and hours of sitting, common in todays office environment.

In TCM terms, the typical western diet is heating and overly supplementing. People often overeat as well, leading to food stagnation (*see* p.3). An excess of heating and drying foods, such as chillies, coffee and bitter substances, can dry the Intestines and damage *yin*. Large quantities of diuretic substances, such as coffee and cola drinks, can promote excessive urination and an uneven distribution of fluids, causing dryness in the Intestines.

Yang deficiency usually gives rise to diarrhoea, however, in some patients chronic constipation may result. This type of constipation is due to the combined effects of the constricting Cold and lack of *yang* propulsion through the Intestines. Cold natured or raw foods can introduce Cold and weaken Spleen *qi* and *yang*. Some drugs weaken the Spleen and deplete Spleen *qi* and *yang*. Prolonged use of purgative laxatives, such as senna or cascara, will eventually weaken *yang*. Antibiotics and the antiretroviral drugs and protease inhibitors used to treat HIV infection are also Cold in nature and weaken the Spleen. Reduced food intake as a result of strict dieting, or prolonged starvation or digestive insult, serious damages Spleen *yang*.

Emotion

The Stomach and Intestines rely on the smooth passage of Liver *qi* for their orderly function, and to some extent on the unimpeded descent of Lung *qi*. A combination of stress, which disrupts Liver *qi*, and inactivity or a sedentary occupation which weakens Lung *qi* and causes a general sluggishness of *qi*, can lead to a general derangement of gastro-intestinal function and sluggishness of *qi* movement through the Intestines.

Liver *qi* stagnation is a frequent cause of internal stagnant Heat, as the pressure buildup of the stagnant *qi* can easily transform to Heat, especially if the diet is rich in heating foods.

Prolonged Liver *qi* stagnation can also contribute to the generation of Phlegm which can accumulate in the Intestines and contribute to the constipation. The Phlegm can be generated by Liver *qi* invading and weakening the Spleen, or by the retarded movement and distribution of fluids, which over time congeal into Phlegm.

Failure of Lung *qi* to descend properly can also contribute to constipation by not assisting Large Intestine *qi* descent. This can be seen in the constipation that often accompanies or follows an upper respiratory tract infection and cigarette smoking. The emotions experienced following the death or absence of a parent or loved one, a sudden change from a comfortable routine to an unfamiliar one, can obstruct Lung *qi*. The Lung system, which incorporates the Large Intestine, is affected and *qi* begins to knot, causing a tendency to constipation.

Similarly, if Lung *qi* has been weakened for some reason, such as lack of exercise or postural problems, the feeble Lung *qi* may not descend, contributing to a failure of Large Intestine *qi* descent.

Anxiety, embarrassment or denial associated with bowel habits can contribute to constipation. Children unwilling to have a bowel movement at school, for example, may ignore the natural urges to such an extent that the stretch receptors in the bowel wall are reset. As a consequence, the intestines fail to respond to the presence of a stool. The peristaltic response and

BOX 5.2 BIOMEDICAL CAUSES OF CONSTIPATION

Most common
- low fibre diet, poor bowel habits, sedentary lifestyle, lack of exercise
- travel

Medications
- chronic laxative abuse
- analgesics
- aluminium containing antacids
- diuretics
- opiates
- iron supplements
- tricyclic antidepressants
- anticholinergic agents
- antidiarrhoeal agents

Mental emotional
- irritable bowel syndrome
- depression
- anorexia nervosa
- anxiety, embarrassment

Endocrine
- hypothyroidism
- hyperkalaemia

Neoplastic
- carcinoma or polyps of the colon, sigmoid or rectum
- tumours of structures outside the colon, exerting pressure on the colon

Megacolon
- congenital (Hirschsprung's disease) - in infants
- acquired

Anal lesions (usually associated with hesitance to defecate due to anticipated pain)
- stenosis
- fissure
- thrombosed haemorrhoid
- ischiorectal abscess
- diverticulosis

urge to defecate diminish. This habitual behaviour can lead to chronic and difficult to rectify constipation.

Phlegm

Phlegm can contribute to constipation because its sticky glutinous nature easily clogs the *qi* mechanism and disrupts the descent of Stomach and Large Intestine *qi*. When Phlegm is implicated in constipation, it is frequently associated with Liver *qi* stagnation, and it is usually the *qi* stagnation that weakens the Spleen and slows the distribution of fluids, encouraging them to congeal into Phlegm.

Phlegm can also be generated by chronic food stagnation, that is, an ongoing tendency to overeating, in particular overeating rich or otherwise congesting and Phlegm generating foods. It is common for patients with Phlegm type constipation to be overweight. Phlegm type constipation can have a constitutional component and may run in families. When constitutional, the tendency to constipation or sluggish stools will probably be evident from childhood.

Yin, Blood and fluid deficiency

Yin, Blood and fluid deficiency patterns are very common causes of chronic constipation and are due to insufficient lubrication of the bowel by *yin* fluids, including Blood. *Yin* and Blood deficiency patterns frequently occur in elderly patients, whose *yin* is naturally depleted by ageing, and in postpartum women. *Yin* deficiency constipation can also follow a febrile illness, such as the *yang ming* syndrome above, or Lung Heat, which has consumed and damaged *yin* fluids in general. Damage to *yin* fluids can also result from fluid loss or excessive drying following over-enthusiastic treatment for some other disorder. Typical examples include causing excessive sweating for an external pathogenic surface invasion, excess diuresis for oedema, or the use of too many or inappropriate bitter parching or warming herbs.

Blood deficiency occurs following haemorrhage, prolonged breast-feeding, excessive sweating or if there is insufficient protein in the diet. It frequently complicates Spleen *qi* deficiency.

Qi and yang deficiency

Qi and *yang* deficiency types of constipation are due to a lack of *qi* movement in the Intestines, compounded in the case of *yang* deficiency by Cold which 'freezes and constricts' movement through the Intestines, further slowing the passage of stools. The stools of *qi* and *yang* deficiency constipation are usually moist and loosely formed; the main characteristic is the lack of desire to defecate. *Qi* deficiency, usually of the Lung and Spleen, can arise from lack of exercise or excessive exercise, overwork, overconsumption of cold, raw or Damp inducing foods, excessive worry or mental activity. Lung *qi* deficiency may result from a combination of poor posture, shallow breathing, or unexpressed or prolonged grief or sadness. *Qi* deficiency can also result from consumption of *qi* following a prolonged illness. Smoking cigarettes may in the short term assist in opening the bowels by dispersing Lung *qi* and therefore Large Intestine *qi*, but will eventually weaken Lung *qi* and introduce Heat that will dry the Lungs and Intestines, contributing to constipation.

The aetiology of *yang* deficiency is similar to *qi* deficiency, however it is more frequent in older patients whose *yang* is in natural decline. Spleen *yang* is weakened by excessive consumption of cold raw foods or cold drugs. It may develop from deterioration of Spleen *qi* deficiency. Additional factors are prolonged or serious illness, gastro-intestinal surgery or excessive ingestion of very cold substances. Fad dieting and prolonged starvation, seriously damages Spleen *yang*. Kidney *yang* declines with age, exposure to cold, multiple pregnancies and chronic illness.

Lack of exercise

Insufficient physical activity can contribute to constipation. People who sit all day tend to have systemically sluggish *qi*, which impedes movement of *qi* and thus waste materials through the Intestines. Similarly, lack of exercise weakens the Spleen and Lungs. When the Spleen is weak, the *qi* mechanism is easily disrupted, Stomach *qi* fails to descend properly and *qi* movement through the abdomen slows. Weak Lung *qi* may fail to assist the normal descent of Large Intestine *qi*.

Medications

Certain medications are frequently implicated in constipation. The most notorious are the opiates, including codeine. Some more commonly used substances may also cause constipation, and can be easily overlooked during diagnosis. These include iron supplements, diuretics and antidepressants. *See also* Box 5.2, p.167.

DIAGNOSIS

Of the excess patterns, the most frequent cause of constipation in the western world is insufficient dietary fibre, with consequent lack of bulk in the stool. With rich, high density, supplementing foods, like fats and meat, colonic transit time is slowed and food stagnates. As noted previously, this type of diet can lead to accumulation of food, Dampness and Heat, in the Liver, Spleen, Stomach and Intestines. Damp Heat affecting the Liver can also aggravate any tendency to Liver *qi* stagnation, which in turn can generate more Heat and so on. Herbs and acupuncture can be useful in speeding recovery, but the main treatment is to reduce the excess by modifying the diet.

The deficient patterns are characterised by lack of moisture and intestinal lubrication ('not enough water to float the boat'), or weakened intestinal propulsion.

There are several traps to be avoided in the analysis and treatment of constipation. Firstly, it is important to clearly establish that the patient is truly constipated and without unreal expectation of what regularity implies.

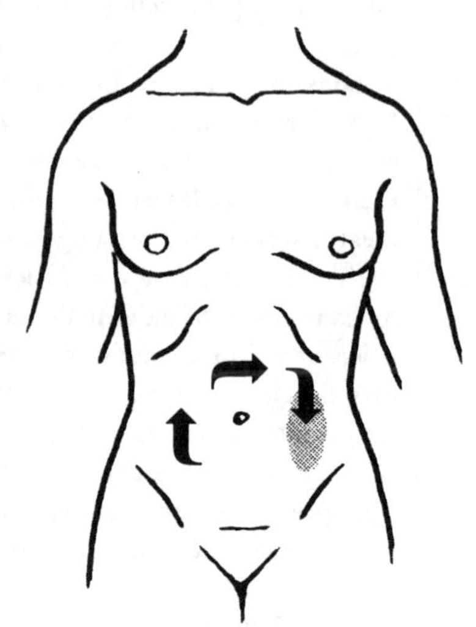

Figure 5.1 *Direction of palpation and common location of constipated stool in descending colon*

Always palpate the abdomen to see if any masses can be detected. Patients with impacted faeces may present with diarrhoea ('spurious'). Abdominal palpation is also useful when a patient presents with a confusing or complicated pattern or mixture of patterns. The abdominal findings can guide the initial treatment priority in such cases. A patient with an abdomen that is tense, firm or tight, and that resists the palpating hand, i.e. is worse for pressure, most likely has an excess pattern. This is consistent even in a patient who may otherwise appear deficient or weak. On the other hand, a patient with an abdomen that is flabby or soft, and that likes, or at least does not dislike pressure on the abdomen most likely has a deficient pattern as the main feature, regardless of the robust nature or excess appearance of the patient.

TREATMENT

Acute constipation is easy to treat and will generally resolve satisfactorily within a few days. Chronic constipation is more difficult and often requires prolonged treatment for adequate results. The situation is complicated by the fact that many patients will have been using laxatives, frequently inappropriately. For example, patients with deficiency types of constipation, such as Blood or *yin* deficiency which need to be nourished and moistened, often take bitter cold purgative herbs like senna or cascara, as they are freely available over the counter in pharmacies and drug stores and are recommended for all types of constipation. Prolonged use of these substances weakens the Spleen, Stomach and Intestines and can significantly inhibit the patient's response to the treatment. Patients taking these laxative substances have to be weaned off them slowly as the appropriate treatment takes effect. In all the chronic types, however, persistence is the key to success, and prolonged treatment will usually be successful. Our aim of treatment should not be to keep treating or medicating patients *ad infinitum*, but to re-establish normal functioning. In practice, dietary and life changes are usually necessary to maintain long term results, in both the excess and deficiency patterns.

Therefore it is important to educate as well as provide treatment. The two free therapies, diet and exercise, can be introduced and encouraged, and these will, in many cases, be successful alone in alleviating constipation.

Diet

Diet is such an important part of maintaining a healthy bowel habit and preventing constipation that it should be considered the primary treatment for many people. The foods and approaches outlined in Chapter 26 are suitable for the dietary treatment of constipation.

Exercise

Moderate exercise stimulates the Spleen and Stomach, strengthens the Lungs, and improves the functioning of the *qi* mechanism. This in turn has a stimulating effect on the harvesting of *qi* from food and the movement of the residue through the Intestines. Regular daily exercise, 30 minutes of sustained walking is often enough, is beneficial for everyone, except those in extreme debility. Exercise is especially beneficial for patients with *qi* stagnation and Spleen deficiency patterns. In fact, for patients with *qi* stagnation patterns, often increasing exercise levels alone will encourage regular bowel habits.

CAUTIONS

Recent onset of constipation in middle aged and elderly people may suggest neoplasms of the bowel. Extrinsic malignancy invading or compressing the bowel, lymphoma or carcinoma in the genito-urinary system, should be considered.

Depression and purgative abuse are often unrecognised as factors in chronic constipation.

Changes in the shape of the stools, or slender or ribbon like stools, may suggest a physical obstruction in the bowel.

Figure 5.2 *Diagnostic strategy for constipation*

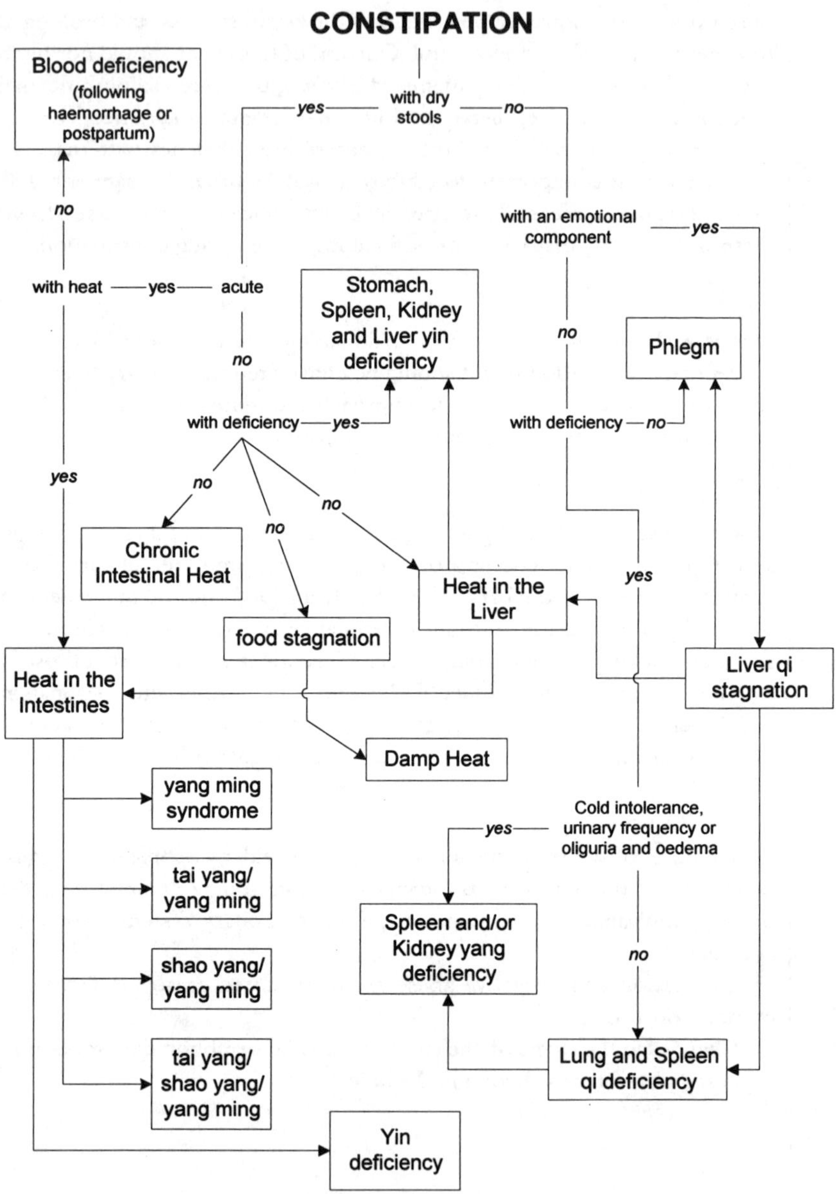

热秘

5.1 HEAT

- Chronic Heat (internally generated)
  - Heat in the Large Intestine
  - Liver Heat
  - Damp Heat (usually associated with food stagnation, p.181)
- Acute Heat (external invasion with fever)

Pathophysiology

- Heat causes constipation by drying the Intestines and the stool. Without sufficient 'water to float the boat' the parched stools come to a halt and obstruct the descent of Stomach and Intestinal *qi*. Patients with Heat type constipation will have the urge to move their bowels, but be unable to do so without some laxative aid. The key feature in all cases is the hard, dry, pellet like stools.
- The Heat may be from an external pathogen, in which case the constipation is usually acute. More commonly in the Western clinic, however, Heat constipation is of internal origin and chronic, often of months or years duration.
- The three common presentations are:
  - Chronic Heat in the Stomach and Intestines–primarily related to a diet, and often associated with food stagnation.
  - Chronic Heat in the Liver–related to chronic stress combined with a rich diet and alcohol.
  - Acute accumulation of Heat in *yang ming* due to transmission of pathogens from the surface.

5.1.1 Chronic Heat

Clinical features

- chronic constipation with hard, dry, pellet like stools
- red complexion
- bad breath
- concentrated urine
- dry mouth, thirst
- with Heat in the Liver: temporal headaches, dizziness, irritability, short temper, sore red eyes, hypochondriac pain

T red with a dry yellow coat; with Liver Heat, redder on the edges
P slippery and rapid; with Liver Heat, wiry, rapid and strong

Treatment principle

Clear Heat, moisten dryness and lubricate the Intestines
Promote bowel movement

Prescription

MA ZI REN WAN 麻子仁丸
(*Apricot Seed and Linum Formula*)

This prescription is appropriate for chronic low grade Heat accumulation in the Large Intestine, best taken in pill form. Ideally, it should not be used unmodified for lengthy periods of time as patients may habituate to the **da huang**. As the patient's diet is adjusted and the Heat clears, the formula should be gradually withdrawn.

huo ma ren (Semen Cannabis Sativae) 火麻仁 300g
zhi da huang (processed Radix et Rhizoma Rhei)
制大黄 300g
zhi shi (Fructus Immaturus Citri Aurantii) 枳实 150g
hou po (Cortex Magnoliae Officinalis) 厚朴 150g
bai shao (Radix Paeoniae Lactiflorae) 白芍 150g
chao xing ren (dry fried Semen Pruni Armeniacae)
炒杏仁 150g

Method: Grind herbs to powder and form into 9-gram pills with honey. The dose is one pill 2-3 times daily with warm water. When the patient has a smooth bowel movement every day, the dose can be reduced until the minimum required is found. May also be decocted with a 90-95% reduction in quantities. If taken as a decoction, **da huang** (3-9g) is added towards the end of cooking (*hou xia* 后下). **Huo ma ren** and **xing ren** lubricate and moisten the bowel; **zhi da huang** opens the bowels and clears Heat; **zhi shi** and **hou po** regulate and direct *qi* downwards and alleviate the cramping that may occur with **da huang**; **bai shao** nourishes Blood, softens the Liver and assists the regulating herbs in preventing abdominal cramps. **Huo ma ren** may be unavailable in some countries. An alternative herb is **hu ma ren** (Semen Lini) 胡麻仁. (Source: *Shi Yong Zhong Yi Nei Ke Xue*)

Modifications

- If the constipation is severe and the stools are hard and dry add **mang xiao** (Mirabilitum) 芒硝 150g to soften the stools.
- With damage to body fluids and obvious dryness (dry tongue, lips and throat), add **sheng di** (Radix Rehmanniae Glutinosae) 生地 100g**, xuan shen** (Radix Scrophulariae) 玄参 100g and **shi hu** (Herba Dendrobii) 石斛 100g.
- With intestinal parasites, add **bing lang** (Semen Arecae Catechu) 槟榔 150g.
- With haemorrhoids and bleeding of fresh blood, add **huai hua mi** (Flos Sophora Japonicae Immaturus) 槐花米 150g and **di yu** (Radix Sanguisorbae Officinalis) 地榆 150g. *See also* Variations and additional prescriptions.
- With residual Phlegm Heat in the Lungs, usually in the convalescent phase of an upper respiratory tract infection, add **huang qin** (Radix Scutellariae Baicalensis) 黄芩 150g and **gua lou ren** (Semen Trichosanthis) 栝楼仁 150g. *See also* Lung abscess, Volume 1.

DANG GUI LONG HUI WAN 当归龙荟丸
(*Tangkuei, Gentiana Longdancao, and Aloe Pill*) modified

This prescription clears Heat and Fire from the Liver and opens the bowels. It is selected when *qi* stagnation impedes movement of Intestinal *qi* and generates Heat, which dries the Intestines.

dang gui (Radix Angelicae Sinensis) 当归 30g
long dan cao (Radix Gentianae Longdancao) 龙胆草 30g
huang qin (Radix Scutellariae Baicalensis) 黄芩 30g
huang lian (Rhizoma Coptidis) 黄连 30g
huang bai (Cortex Phellodendri) 黄柏 30g
shan zhi zi (Fructus Gardeniae Jasminoides) 山栀子 30g
da huang (Radix et Rhizoma Rhei) 大黄 15g
lu hui (Herba Aloes) 芦荟 15g
qing dai (Indigo Pulverata Levis) 青黛 15g
mu xiang (Radix Aucklandiae Lappae) 木香 6-9g

Method: Grind herbs to a powder and form into 6-gram pills with honey. The dose is one pill 2-3 times daily. **Long dan cao** and **qing dai** cool the Liver and clear Fire; **huang qin**, **huang lian**, **huang bai** and **shan zhi zi** powerfully clear Damp and Toxic Heat; **da huang** and **lu hui** purge the Intestines and clear Heat; **dang gui** prevents excessive drying and damage to *yin* and Blood by the bitter cold herbs; **mu xiang** regulates *qi*.

NB: The original prescription contained the glandular secretion, **she xiang** (Secretio Moschus) 麝香, of the endangered musk deer.

As the Heat clears and the patient's *qi* is regulated, the formula should be gradually withdrawn, perhaps being replaced by a *qi* regulating formula, such as **CHAI HU SHU GAN SAN** (*Bupleurum and Cyperus Formula* 柴胡疏肝散, p.76), or **XIAO YAO SAN** (*Bupleurum and Dang Gui Formula* 逍遥散, p.159).

Variations and additional prescriptions

With haemorrhoids

- A useful prescription for chronic Heat type constipation with haemorrhoids and bleeding of fresh blood (Intestinal Wind) is the modern Japanese formula **YI ZI TANG** (*Cimicifuga Combination* 乙字汤). Available in powder form, this popular prescription, clears Heat, opens the Intestines and elevates *qi*, while moistening and restoring the Intestinal lining.

dang gui (Radix Angelicae Sinensis) 当归 12-15g
huang qin (Radix Scutellariae Baicalensis) 黄芩 6-9g
da huang (Radix et Rhizoma Rhei) 大黄 3-6g
sheng ma (Rhizoma Cimicifugae) 升麻 3-6g
chai hu (Radix Bupleuri) 柴胡 6-9g
gan cao (Radix Glycyrrhizae Uralensis) 甘草 3-6g

Method: Decoction or as powder. When decocted, **da huang** is added towards the end of cooking (*hou xia* 后下). **Dang gui** moistens the Intestines, regulates

Blood and with **gan cao** alleviates pain and promotes smooth bowel movements; **huang qin** clears Heat from the Intestine; the small dose of **da huang** gently opens the Intestines and clears Heat; **chai hu** regulates *qi* flow and with **sheng ma** elevates *yang qi*, while assisting in clearing Heat.

Spurious diarrhoea around an impacted stool

- A not uncommon variation of the Heat pattern occurs in patients with pre-existing *qi* and/or *yin* and/or Blood deficiency, typically elderly or bedridden patients. The patient presents with green, watery, foul smelling diarrhoea and abdominal pain that increases with pressure. There will be masses palpable in the left iliac fossa. Signs of deficiency include shortness of breath, fatigue, dry mouth and throat, a deficient pulse and a dry yellow or black tongue coat. The aim of treatment is to purge Heat from the interior and support *zheng qi* with **HUANG LONG TANG** (*Yellow Dragon Decoction 黄龙汤*).

zhi da huang (processed Radix et Rhizoma Rhei) 制大黄 6-12g
mang xiao (Mirabilitum) 芒硝 6-12g
zhi shi (Fructus Immaturus Citri Aurantii) 枳实 9-12g
hou po (Cortex Magnoliae Officinalis) 厚朴 9-12g
dang shen (Radix Codonopsis Pilosulae) 党参 12-15g
dang gui (Radix Angelicae Sinensis) 当归 9-12g
jie geng (Radix Platycodi Grandiflori) 桔梗 3-6g
sheng jiang (Rhizoma Zingiberis Officinalis Recens) 生姜 6-9g
da zao (Fructus Zizyphi Jujubae) 大枣 2pce
gan cao (Radix Glycyrrhizae Uralensis) 甘草 3-6g

Method: Decoction. **Mang xiao** is dissolved in the strained decoction (*chong fu* 冲服). **Zhi da huang, mang xiao, zhi shi** and **hou po** form **Da Cheng Qi Tang**, the premier prescription for purging Heat and accumulated stool from *yang ming*. **Zhi da huang** is less violent than unprocessed **da huang**. **Dang shen** and **dang gui** supplement and protect *qi* and Blood; **jie geng** unblocks Lung *qi* thereby facilitating the downward movement of Large Intestine *qi*; **sheng jiang, da zao** and **gan cao** support and protect the Stomach and Spleen from the bitter cold purgatives.

With *yin* deficiency combine with **ZENG YE TANG** (*Increase the Fluids Decoction 增液汤*, p.200).

Patent medicines

Ma Zi Ren Wan 麻子仁丸 (Ma Zi Ren Wan)
Dang Gui Long Hui Wan 当归龙荟丸 (Dang Gui Long Hui Wan)
- Liver Heat

Chen Xiang Hua Qi Wan 沉香化气丸 (Chen Xiang Hua Qi Wan)
- with *qi* deficiency

Acupuncture (select from)

SJ.6 (*zhi gou* -) .... *jing* river and Fire point of the *san jiao*, spreads *qi*, disperses accumulation from the Intestines and promotes bowel movement

St.25 (*tian shu* -) .... together these points regulate Intestinal
Sp.15 (*da heng* -) function, clear Heat and promote bowel movement

St.44 (*nei ting* -) .... together these points clear Heat from
LI.4 (*he gu* -) *yang ming*

St.36 (*zu san li* -) .... *he* sea point of the Stomach, regulates Stomach and Intestine function, strengthens the Spleen and Stomach and supplements *qi*
St.37 (*shang ju xu* -) .... lower *he* point of the Large Intestine, clears Heat and regulates the Intestines
St.40 (*feng long* -) .... *luo* point of the Stomach, transforms Phlegm and clears Heat and Phlegm from the Stomach

- with fever add LI.11 (*qu chi*) and Du.14 (*da zhui*)
- with Heat in the Liver, add Liv.2 (*xing jian* -)
- *Ear points*: constipation area, large intestine, lungs, distal segment rectum, *san jiao*, *shen men*

Clinical notes

- Heat clearing, purgative herbs should not be used for too long as the bowel become habituated to their stimulus and over time requires increasing doses. Once the bowels are moving, dietary and other changes made, the focus of treatment should be altered to more nourishing and moistening of the bowel, to promote a healthy intestinal wall and flora. For dietary recommendations, see p.882.

5.1.2 Acute Heat (in a disease with fever)

There are several presentations of acute Heat type constipation depending on which of the six levels are involved. These patterns generally follow an unresolved or powerful external pathogenic invasion, usually beginning as a Wind Cold or Wind Heat attack. Most commonly, patients will not present with constipation, but with fever or an acute exterior disorder. However treatment of the constipation by vigorously purging the bowel, thus clearing the Heat with the constipated stool, will often resolve the disorder. The patterns are therefore summarised here (Table 5.1, p.179). For more detail *see* the appendices to Chapter 1 in Volume 1 of this series.

Constipation is a common accompaniment to the strong fevers of childhood, and an important part of the treatment is to move the bowel to take the Heat out. This can often be achieved, especially in infants, by firmly massaging the abdomen in a clockwise direction to physically shift the constipated stool. Once the bowels have moved the fever will often break.

Acupuncture (select from)

Yang ming syndrome (base prescription for all variants)

St.25 (*tian shu* -) .... together these points regulate Intestinal
Sp.15 (*da heng* -) function, clear Heat and promote bowel movement

SJ.6 (*zhi gou* -) .... *jing* river and Fire point, spreads *qi*, disperses accumulation in the Intestines and promotes bowel movement

St.37 (*shang ju xu* -) .... lower *he* point of the Large Intestine, clears Heat and regulates the Intestines

- with fever, add LI.11 (*qu chi* -), LI.4 (*he gu* -)
- with *tai yang* Wind Cold, add Lu.7 (*lie que* -) and LI.4 (*he gu* -)
- with *tai yang* Wind Heat, add LI.11 (*qu chi* -), LI.4 (*he gu* -) and Du.14 (*da zhui* -)
- with *shao yang* symptoms, add GB.39 (*xuan zhong* -), SJ.5 (*wai guan* -) and GB.34 (*yang ling quan* -)
- *Ear points*: constipation area, lungs, large intestine, distal segment rectum, *san jiao*, *shen men*

Clinical notes

- Heat type constipation may be diagnosed biomedically as habitual constipation, diet and lifestyle related constipation, post febrile disease constipation, a variety of diseases with fever, cholecystitis, pancreatitis and intestinal obstruction.
- For dietary recommendations, see p.882.

Table 5.1 *Acute patterns that may be accompanied by constipation*

Pattern	Clinical features	Prescription, Patent medicine
Tai yang (Wind Cold) - yang ming overlap syndrome	simultaneous high fever and chills or rigors, cough, no sweating, occipital headache, muscle aches, thirst, irritability, sore throat, constipation; floating, tight pulse	Da Qing Long Tang
Tai yang (Wind Heat) - yang ming overlap syndrome	simultaneous high fever and chills, dizziness, headache, red sore eyes, concentrated urine, halitosis, constipation, bitter taste in the mouth, sore throat, cough, pyogenic skin sores; floating, strong, full, slippery pulse; red tongue with a dry, yellow coat	Fang Feng Tong Sheng Tang Niu Huang Jie Du Pien
Shao yang - yang ming overlap syndrome	alternating fever and chills, hypochondriac pain, nausea and vomiting, pounding headache, epigastric fullness and pain, constipation, irritability, bitter taste in the mouth; rapid, strong, wiry pulse; red tongue with a dry, yellow coat	Da Chai Hu Tang Niu Huang Jie Du Pien
Tai yang - shao yang - yang ming overlap syndrome	fullness in the chest, palpitations, irritability, constipation, heaviness in the body, inability to rotate at the waist, confusion; wiry pulse; a red tongue with a dry, yellow coat	Chai Hu Jia Long Gu Mu Li Tang
Yang ming syndrome	constipation or faecal impaction with foul spurious diarrhoea, a tense painful abdomen, tidal fever, sweating, thirst; big, full, strong, bounding pulse; red tongue with a dry, yellow coat	Da Cheng Qi Tang Ching Fei Yi Huo Pien Niu Huang Qing Huo Pian

食秘

5.2 FOOD STAGNATION

Pathophysiology

- Food stagnation type constipation is related to overindulgence combined with a sedentary occupation. In the West the pattern is often combined with weakness of Spleen and Stomach *qi*, so the onset may be gradual, rather than manifesting as an acute event. As the pattern progresses the deficiency will become more and more prominent.
- Chronic food stagnation will often be complicated by Damp Heat (or Phlegm Heat) in the Large Intestine. This a common disorder in the western world, when consumption of too much food relative to the energetic output is the norm.
- This type of constipation occurs commonly in infants and small children as 'accumulation disorder'.

Clinical features

- constipation or sluggish bowel movements, possibly alternating with loose foul smelling stools
- nausea and vomiting, acid reflux, indigestion
- epigastric and abdominal fullness and distension
- foul belching and flatulence
- aversion to food

T thick greasy coat
P slippery

Treatment principle

Relieve food stagnation and harmonise the Stomach
Redirect Stomach *qi* downward, promote bowel movement

Prescription

BAO HE WAN 保和丸
(*Citrus and Crataegus Formula*) modified

chao shan zha (dry fried Fructus Crataegi) 炒山楂 180g
chao shen qu (dry fried Massa Fermentata) 炒神曲 60g
fu ling (Sclerotium Poriae Cocos) 茯苓 90g
ban xia (Rhizoma Pinelliae Ternatae) 半夏 90g
chen pi (Pericarpium Citri Reticulatae) 陈皮 30g
lian qiao (Fructus Forsythia Suspensae) 连翘 30g
lai fu zi (Semen Raphani Sativi) 莱服子 30g
bing lang (Semen Arecae Catechu) 槟榔 60g
da huang (Radix et Rhizoma Rhei) 大黄 30g

Method: Grind herbs to a powder and form into 9-gram pills with water. The dose is one pill 2-3 times daily until a regular movement is achieved, then reduced to the minimum required for maintenance. Pills are best for this pattern, however, the prescription may also be decocted with a 90% reduction in quantities. **Chao shan zha** and **chao shen qu** improve digestion and alleviate food stagnation; **lai fu zi** improves digestion, transforms Phlegm and directs *qi* downwards; **ban xia, chen pi** and **fu ling** transform Dampness and harmonise the Stomach; **lian qiao** clears Heat and disperses accumulations; **bing lang** encourages the downwards movement of *qi*; **da huang** purges accumulations from the Intestines and clears Heat. (Source: *Shi Yong Zhong Yi Nei Ke Xue*)

Modifications

- With Heat in the Stomach add **lu gen** (Rhizoma Phragmitis Communis) 芦根 120g and **huang lian** (Rhizoma Coptidis) 黄连 30g.
- With Cold in the Stomach, delete **lian qiao**, and add **gan jiang** (Rhizoma Zingiberis Officinalis) 干姜 60g and **sha ren** (Fructus Amomi) 砂仁 60g.

Variations and additional prescriptions

With Damp Heat

- Chronic food stagnation, by disrupting Spleen function and generating Heat, often leads to accumulation of Damp Heat in the Intestines. The main features are constipation or sluggish difficult bowel movements which may or may not be dry, and which feel incomplete. In addition there is relatively severe abdominal distension, concentrated urine, lethargy and heaviness worse in the afternoon, possible nightsweats, a greasy yellow tongue coat and slippery, full pulse. The aim of treatment is to guide stagnation downward, clear Heat and dispel Damp with **ZHI SHI DAO ZHI WAN** (*Immature Bitter Orange Pill to Guide out Stagnation* 枳实导滞丸).

  da huang (Radix et Rhizoma Rhei) 大黄 30g
  zhi shi (Fructus Immaturus Citri Aurantii) 枳实 15g
  chao shen qu (dry fried Massa Fermentata) 炒神曲 15g
  huang qin (Radix Scutellariae Baicalensis) 黄芩 9g
  huang lian (Rhizoma Coptidis) 黄连 9g
  fu ling (Sclerotium Poriae Cocos) 茯苓 9g
  bai zhu (Rhizoma Atractylodes Macrocephalae) 白术 9g
  ze xie (Rhizoma Alismatis Orientalis) 泽泻 6g

  Method: Grind the herbs to powder and form into 9-gram pills with water. The dose is one pill 2-3 times daily. May also be decocted with the **da huang** reduced to 6-9 grams, added towards the end of cooking (*hou xia* 后下). **Da huang** clears Damp Heat, food accumulation and constipated stool from the Intestines by purging; **zhi shi** regulates *qi* and directs *qi* downwards; **chao shen qu** alleviates food stagnation and improves digestion; **huang qin** and **huang lian** clear Damp Heat; **fu ling** strengthens the Spleen and with **ze xie** promotes urination to provide another outlet for the Damp Heat; **bai zhu** strengthens the Spleen and dries Damp. (Source: *Shi Yong Zhong Yi Nei Ke Xue*)

Patent medicines

Mu Xiang Shun Qi Wan 木香顺气丸 (Mu Xiang Shun Qi Wan)
Bao He Wan 保和丸 (Bao He Wan)
Zi Sheng Wan 资生丸 (Zi Sheng Wan, Zi Sheng Stomachic Pills)
Jian Pi Wan 健脾丸 (Jian Pi Wan)
- Spleen deficiency with food stagnation

Acupuncture (select from)

St.25 (*tian shu* -) .... together these points regulate Intestinal
Sp.15 (*da heng* -) function, clear Heat and promote bowel movement

SJ.6 (*zhi gou* -) .... together these points regulate *qi* in the *san jiao*,
GB.34 (*yang ling quan* -) soothe the Liver and encourage *qi* movement through the Intestine to promote bowel movement

St.37 (*shang ju xu* -) .... lower *he* point of the Large Intestine, clears Heat and regulates the Intestines
Bl.25 (*da chang shu* -) .... *shu* point of the Large Intestine, regulates Intestinal function and promotes bowel movement
St.44 (*nei ting* -) .... *rong* spring and Water point of the Stomach, clears Heat from the Stomach and alleviates food stagnation

- with nausea, add PC.6 (*nei guan* -)
- with Phlegm accumulation, add St.40 (*feng long* -)
- with Damp Heat, add St.45 (*li dui* ↓) and St.40 (*feng long* -)
- with Spleen deficiency, add Sp.6 (*san yin jiao*) and St.36 (*zu san li*)
- with abdominal pain, add Sp.8 (*di ji* -) and Sp.4 (*gong sun* -)
- *Ear points*: constipation area, stomach, spleen, abdomen, large intestine, small intestine, *shen men*, sympathetic

Clinical notes

- Because this is largely a disorder of overindulgence and irregular dietary habits, the patient should change eating habits, and generally this is enough to prevent the problem recurring. *See also* comments in Clinical notes, p.127.
- This is a common pattern of constipation in demand fed babies. Their immature digestive systems are easily overloaded, thus overfeeding, or feeding too frequently, before the previous meal has been digested, can lead to constipation.

气秘

5.3 QI STAGNATION

Pathophysiology

- *Qi* stagnation, particularly Liver *qi* stagnation, disrupts the correct movement and descent of Stomach and Intestinal *qi*, which reduces the peristaltic activity of the Intestine. This pattern is common in people with sedentary occupations, particularly those working in stressful situations. It may also follow a traumatic injury or abdominal surgery, which can cause adhesions. In some cases this type of constipation is associated with intestinal parasites or worms.
- Lung *qi* stagnation may be a contributing factor, as descent of Lung *qi* is required for descent of Large Intestine *qi*. This situation may be associated with an event that causes grief or a sense of loss in the patient, such as the sudden death of a loved one, family break up or change from the familiar to the unfamiliar.

Clinical features

- Constipation with difficulty in passing stools, feelings of incomplete evacuation and sluggishness, or normal stools with little or no urge to defecate. In general, the stools tend to be pebble like, or thin, and are usually not especially dry or hard, but may be if Heat has been generated. The constipation is worse when the patient is stressed or upset, and in women will often be worse premenstrually.
- abdominal distension, discomfort or pain which is alleviated following a bowel movement
- irritability, depression, moodiness
- fullness or tightness in the chest and hypochondria
- poor appetite, frequent belching, flatulence and sighing
- stiffness and tightness of the neck and upper back
- premenstrual syndrome, irregular menstruation, breast tenderness

T unremarkable or dark; thin coat
P wiry

Treatment principle

Regulate and move Liver *qi* and Large Intestine *qi*
Eliminate stagnation and promote downward movement of *qi*

Prescription

LIU MO TANG 六磨汤
(*Six Milled Herb Decoction*)

This formula is selected when constipation is habitual, that is, the patient tends to be constipated all the time. It should not be used unmodified for prolonged periods, as patients may habituate to the **da huang**. Once the bowels are moving the **da huang** should be gradually eliminated.

chen xiang (Lignum Aquilariae) 沉香 6g
bing lang (Semen Arecae Catechu) 槟榔 9g
wu yao (Radix Linderae Strychnifoliae) 乌药 9g
zhi shi (Fructus Immaturus Citri Aurantii) 枳实 9g
mu xiang (Radix Aucklandiae Lappae) 木香 9g
da huang (Radix et Rhizoma Rhei) 大黄 6g

Method: The herbs are usually ground to a fine powder, stored in an airtight container, then steeped in hot water before use. The dosage varies depending on the individual. Generally a larger dose should be given at first (1-2 teaspoons, 3 times daily, or more) until the bowels move, then the dose is reduced to the minimum required for a smooth evacuation. **Chen xiang**, **bing lang**, **wu yao**, **zhi shi** and **mu xiang** regulate *qi* and direct *qi* downwards; **da huang** purges the Intestines. (Source: *Shi Yong Zhong Yi Nei Ke Xue*)

Modifications

- With Heat (dry stools and throat, bitter taste in the mouth, red edges on the tongue and a yellow coat) add **long dan cao** (Radix Gentianae Longdancao) 龙胆草 6g, **shan zhi zi** (Fructus Gardeniae Jasminoides) 山栀子 6-9g and **huang qin** (Radix Scutellariae Baicalensis) 黄芩 6-9g.
- For depression and melancholy add **chai hu** (Radix Bupleuri) 柴胡 9g, **bai shao** (Radix Paeoniae Lactiflorae) 白芍 9-12g and **he huan pi** (Cortex Albizziae Julibrissin) 合欢皮 12-15g.
- With parasites or worms, increase the dose of **bing lang** and add **lei wan** (Sclerotium Omphaliae Lapidescens) 雷丸 9g, **fei zi** (Semen Torreyae Grandis) 榧子 9g and **shi jun zi** (Fructus Quisqualis Indicae) 使君子 9g.
- With severe abdominal bloating, increase the dose of **zhi shi** to 12g and add **sha ren** (Fructus Amomi) 砂仁 9g.
- With food stagnation, add **shan zha** (Fructus Crataegi) 山楂 12g, **chao shen qu** (dry fried Massa Fermentata) 炒神曲 12g and **ji nei jin** (Endothelium Corneum Gigeriae Galli) 鸡内金 9g.
- If the condition occurs following trauma or surgery (with possible adhesions) add herbs to invigorate Blood, such as **tao ren** (Semen Persicae) 桃仁 9g, **hong hua** (Flos Carthami Tinctorii) 红花 9g and **chi shao** (Radix Paeoniae Rubrae) 赤芍 12g.
- With fluid accumulation in the intestine (may occur following surgery with residual adhesions), take **jiao zao jiao** (baked Fructus Gleditsiae Sinensis) 焦皂角 1g and **gan sui** (Radix Euphorbiae Kansui) 甘遂 0.5g as powder along with the draft until the fluid is expelled.

TONG XIE YAO FANG 痛泻要方
(*Important Formula for Painful Diarrhoea*) modified

This prescription is selected when Liver *qi* invades the Stomach and Spleen, inhibiting the *qi* mechanism and disrupting the descent of Large Intestine *qi*. The features are intermittent constipation and abdominal pain aggravated or initiated by stress, or constipation interspersed with episodes of diarrhoea. This is the primary formula to moderate the effects of stress on the Intestines. It eases spasm, softens the Liver and is suitable for long term use. Excellent for those who suffer from constipation when in an unfamiliar situation or when travelling.

chao bai shao (dry fried Radix Paeoniae Lactiflorae) 炒白芍 12-24g
chao bai zhu (dry fried Rhizoma Atractylodes Macrocephalae) 炒白术 12-15g
chen pi (Pericarpium Citri Reticulatae) 陈皮 9-12g
fang feng (Radix Ledebouriellae Divaricatae) 防风 9-12g
da fu pi (Pericarpium Arecae Catechu) 大腹皮 9-12g
fo shou (Fructus Citri Sarcodactylis) 佛手 9-12g
zhi shi (Fructus Immaturus Citri Aurantii) 枳实 9-12g

Method: Decoction. **Chao bai shao** softens the Liver and regulates *qi*; **chao bai zhu** strengthens the Spleen against the incursions of the Liver; **chen pi** regulates *qi*; **fang feng** expels Wind, regulates Intestinal *qi* and with **bai shao** alleviates cramping; **da fu pi** regulates *qi*, promotes urination and directs *qi* downwards; **fo shou** and **zhi shi** regulate *qi* and alleviate distension. (Source: *Zhong Yi Nei Ke Lin Chuang Shou Ce*)

Modifications

- With severe irritability and stagnant *qi*, add **chai hu** (Radix Bupleuri) 柴胡 9-12g, **qing pi** (Pericarpium Citri Reticulatae Viridae) 青皮 9-12g and **xiang fu** (Rhizoma Cyperi Rotundi) 香附 9-12g.
- With *qi* deficiency, fatigue and pallor, add **dang shen** (Radix Codonopsis Pilosulae) 党参 15-18g.
- With colicky abdominal pain, increase the dose of **bai shao** (Radix Paeoniae Lactiflorae) 白芍 to 30g, and add **yan hu suo** (Rhizoma Corydalis Yanhusuo) 延胡索 9-12g and **gan cao** (Radix Glycyrrhizae Uralensis) 甘草 6-9g.
- With bleeding, add **di yu** (Radix Sanguisorbae Officinalis) 地榆 9-12g and **san qi fen** (powdered Radix Notoginseng) 三七粉 3-6g.
- With mucus in the stools, add **cang zhu** (Rhizoma Atractylodis) 苍术 12-15g.
- With food stagnation (epigastric and abdominal fullness, foul belching, a thick tongue coat), add **chao mai ya** (dry fried Fructus Hordei Vulgaris Germinantus) 炒麦芽 15-30g, **jiao shan zha** (baked Fructus Crataegi) 焦山楂 15-18g and **jiao shen qu** (baked Massa Fermentata) 焦神曲 15-

18g.

- With mild signs of stagnant Blood (occasional sharp focal pain), add **dan shen** (Radix Salviae Miltiorrhizae) 丹参 12-18g, **yu jin** (Tuber Curcumae) 郁金 9-12g and **yan hu suo** (Rhizoma Corydalis Yanhusuo) 延胡索 9-12g.
- For patients who are nervous or anxious, add **he huan pi** (Cortex Albizziae Julibrissin) 合欢皮 15g, **wu wei zi** (Fructus Schizandrae Chinensis) 五味子 6g and **fu xiao mai** (Semen Tritici Aestivi Levis) 浮小麦 30g.

Variations and additional prescriptions

Follow up treatment

- Once the bowels are moving regularly and smoothly, a more general *qi* regulating formula may be selected for long term constitutional therapy. Generally patent medicines are sufficient, and suitable formulae include *Xiao Yao Wan* 逍遥丸 (Xiao Yao Wan, Hsiao Yao Wan), *Shu Gan Wan* 舒肝丸 (Shu Gan Wan, Shu Kan Wan) and *Xiang Sha Yang Wei Wan* 香砂养胃丸 (Xiang Sha Yang Wei Wan, Hsiang Sha Yang Wei Wan).

Lung qi stagnation with accumulation of Cold Phlegm

- A variation involving *qi* stagnation is associated with stagnant Lung *qi* and consequent accumulation of Cold Phlegm Fluids. The failure of Lung *qi* to descend disrupts the downwards movement of Large Intestine *qi*. The features are constipation with stools that are not dry, a chronic cough and wheeze with watery sputum, shortness of breath, fullness in the chest, oedema and a greasy white tongue coat. The correct treatment is to redirect Lung *qi* downwards with **SU ZI JIANG QI TANG** (*Perilla Fruit Combination* 苏子降气汤) modified.

  su zi (Fructus Perillae Fructescentis) 苏子 9-12g
  ban xia (Rhizoma Pinelliae Ternatae) 半夏 9-12g
  qian hu (Radix Peucedani) 前胡 9-12g
  dang gui (Radix Angelicae Sinensis) 当归 6-9g
  chen pi (Pericarpium Citri Reticulatae) 陈皮 6-9g
  hou po (Cortex Magnoliae Officinalis) 厚朴 6-9g
  zhi gan cao (honey fried Radix Glycyrrhizae Uralensis)
  炙甘草 3-6g
  rou gui (Cortex Cinnamomi Cassiae) 肉桂 3g
  wei ling xian (Radix Clematidis) 威灵仙 6-9g
  huo ma ren (Semen Cannabis Sativae) 火麻仁 9-12g

  Method: Grind the herbs to a fine powder and take 6-grams as a draft, 2-3 times daily. May also be decocted. **Su zi** transforms Phlegm and directs Lung *qi* downwards; **ban xia**, **hou po** and **qian hu** expel Phlegm, direct *qi* downward and stop cough; **chen pi** transforms Phlegm and regulates *qi*; **rou gui** dispels Cold; **dang gui** is used here to protect the *qi* and *yin* from the pungent drying properties of the other herbs; **wei ling xian** transforms Phlegm; **huo ma ren** moistens the Intestines. **Huo ma ren** may be unavailable in some countries. An alternative herb is **hu ma ren** (Semen Lini) 胡麻仁. (Source: *Shi Yong Zhong Yi Nei Ke Xue*)

Patent medicines

Chen Xiang Hua Qi Wan 沉香化气丸 (Chen Xiang Hua Qi Wan)
Mu Xiang Shun Qi Wan 木香顺气丸 (Mu Xiang Shun Qi Wan)
- designed for *qi* and food stagnation causing constipation

Xiao Yao Wan 逍遥丸 (Xiao Yao Wan, Hsiao Yao Wan)
- particularly good for women with premenstrual or intermittent *qi* stagnation constipation

Shu Gan Wan 舒肝丸 (Shu Gan Wan, Shu Kan Wan)
- with pain

Xiang Sha Yang Wei Wan 香砂养胃丸 (Xiang Sha Yang Wei Wan, Hsiang Sha Yang Wei Wan)
- *qi* stagnation with Spleen deficiency

Su Zi Jiang Qi Wan 苏子降气丸 (Su Zi Jiang Qi Wan)
- Lung *qi* stagnation

Run Chang Wan 润肠丸 (Fructus Persica Compound Pills)
- This mild laxative formula may be combined with any of the above patent medicines to enhance the laxative effect if required; suitable in a small dose, 6-12 pills per day, when the primary patent formula selected needs a little 'kick along' in moving the bowel.

Acupuncture (select from)

St.25 (*tian shu* -) .... *mu* point of the Large Intestine, regulates Intestinal function, alleviates stagnation and promotes bowel movement

Ren.6 (*qi hai* -) .... regulates and moves *qi* in the lower abdomen

SJ.6 (*zhi gou* -) ....
GB.34 (*yang ling quan* -) together these points regulate *qi* in the *san jiao*, soothe the Liver and encourage *qi* movement through the Intestine and promotes bowel movement

St.37 (*shang ju xu* -) .... lower *he* point of the Large Intestine, regulates Intestinal *qi* and clears stagnation

Liv.3 (*tai chong* -) ....*yuan*, *shu* and Earth point of the Liver, pacifies rising Liver *yang*, regulates and moves *qi* and Blood and alleviates spasm

Liv.5 (*li gou* -) .... *luo* point of the Liver, regulates *qi*, good for abdominal pain from *qi* stagnation

- with abdominal distension, add Sp.15 (*da heng* -)
- with Phlegm, add St.40 (*feng long* -) and Sp.3 (*tai bai* -)
- with Spleen deficiency, add St.36 (*zu san li* +)
- with nausea, acid reflux and indigestion, add PC.6 (*nei guan*), Bl.18 (*gan shu*) and Bl.20 (*pi shu*)
- with insomnia or lateral headaches, add SJ.5 (*wai guan*) and GB.39 (*xuan zhong*)
- with signs of Heat, add Liv.2 (*xing jian* -) and LI.11 (*qu chi* -)
- with extreme tension, anxiety or nervousness, add PC.6 (*nei guan*), Ht.7 (*shen men*), *yin tang* (M-HN-3) and Du.24 (*shen ting*)
- with Lung *qi* stagnation, add Lu.7 (*lie que*) and Bl.42 (*po hu*)
- Add *a shi* points along the lower Stomach channel as appropriate. Tender points will usually be found around St.37 (*shang ju xu*) or St.39 (*xia ju xu*).
- *Ear points*: constipation area, liver, large intestine, abdomen, *shen men*, subcortex, sympathetic

Clinical notes

- *Qi* type constipation may be diagnosed biomedically as irritable bowel syndrome and the general effects of stress, travel or change on the bowel, nervous stomach and habitual constipation.
- Exercise is an essential component of treatment. Particularly useful is walking, swimming, yoga or *tai ji chuan*, although all exercise is beneficial. Thirty minutes of walking every day is often sufficient.
- Overall, the prognosis is variable and chronic *qi* stagnation constipation can be difficult. Recent cases, however, generally respond well to correct treatment and 3-6 weeks may be sufficient. If a patient has a constitutional tendency to *qi* stagnation, or suffers from deep insecurities or is in an unresolvable stressful situation, the treatment must be persistent, (3-6 months+) and combined with appropriate relaxation and stress management techniques.
- Gentle and regular massage, particularly of the abdomen, neck and mid thoracic region is also useful.
- For dietary recommendations, see p.878.

痰秘

5.4 PHLEGM ACCUMULATION

Pathophysiology

- Phlegm contributes to constipation by congesting and obstructing the *qi* mechanism of the digestive system, preventing the natural descent of Stomach and Large Intestine *qi*.
- Phlegm is frequently complicated by, or is a complication of, Liver *qi* stagnation and/or food stagnation, and treatment should take account of all mechanisms.
- The diagnosis of Phlegm constipation may be arrived at by a process of elimination, especially when the Phlegm is deep seated and few if any clear Phlegm signs and symptoms are apparent. When moistening laxative or purgative treatments either have no effect or make the patient feel worse, a tentative diagnosis of Phlegm accumulation may be made.

Clinical features

- Chronic constipation or sluggish stools which are not dry and may contain mucus. There may be tenesmus. After evacuation the patient feels much lighter and clear headed.
- abdominal distension and discomfort
- foggy-headedness, poor concentration, poor memory
- tendency to sleepiness, lethargy, heaviness in the body
- may be chronic mucus production from the sinuses and lungs
- greasy skin, musty body odour
- dizziness, headaches that can be triggered by strong smells
- tendency to obesity, pear shape

T flabby swollen tongue with a greasy white coat, thicker on the root
P deep and slippery or wiry

Treatment principle

Transform and eliminate Phlegm and open the bowels
Elevate *yang* to facilitate descent of turbid *yin*, regulate Liver *qi*
Strengthen the Spleen

Prescription

TAN BI TANG 痰秘汤
(*Phlegm Constipation Decoction*)

bai zhu (Rhizoma Atractylodes Macrocephalae) 白术 12-15g
lai fu zi (Semen Raphani Sativi) 莱服子 12-15g
ban xia (Rhizoma Pinelliae Ternatae) 半夏 12-15g
fang feng (Radix Ledebouriellae Divaricatae) 防风 9-12g
chai hu (Radix Bupleuri) 柴胡 9-12g

qiang huo (Rhizoma et Radix Notopterygii) 羌活 9-12g
bai zi ren (Semen Biotae Orientalis) 柏子仁 9-12g
zhi shi (Fructus Immaturus Citri Aurantii) 枳实 9-12g
bing lang (Semen Arecae Catechu) 槟榔 9-12g
hou po (Cortex Magnoliae Officinalis) 厚朴 9-12g
gan cao (Radix Glycyrrhizae Uralensis) 甘草 3-6g

Method: Decoction. **Bai zhu**, the main herb, neatly performs the necessary tasks of strengthening the Spleen to stop Phlegm production and drying Phlegm Damp; **lai fu zi** and **ban xia** transform Phlegm and direct *qi* downwards; **fang feng**, **chai hu** and **qiang huo** elevate *yang qi* and disperse stagnant Liver *qi* thus assisting the *qi* mechanism; **zhi shi** and **ban xia** regulate and direct *qi* downwards, thus balancing the ascending nature of the previous herbs, so assisting the *qi* mechanism; **bing lang** alleviates accumulation, directs *qi* downwards, promotes urination, eliminates pathological fluids and assists bowel movements; **gan cao** assists **bai zhu** in strengthening the Spleen. (Source: *Zhong Yi Tan Bing Xue*)

Modifications

- In resistant cases, take **jiao zao jiao** (blackened Fructus Gleditsiae Sinensis) 焦皂角 3g as powder, washed down by the decoction.
- With Cold, add **gan jiang** (Rhizoma Zingiberis Officinalis) 干姜 6-9g and **rou gui** (Cortex Cinnamomi Cassiae) 肉桂 3g.
- With Heat, add **gua lou ren** (Semen Trichosanthis) 栝楼仁 15-18g and **zhu ru** (Caulis Bambusae in Taeniis) 竹茹 9-12g.
- With foggy-headedness, add **shi chang pu** (Rhizoma Acori Graminei) 石菖蒲 6-9g and **yuan zhi** (Radix Polygalae Tenuifoliae) 远志 6-9g.
- With anxiety or palpitations, add **zhen zhu mu** (Concha Margaritaferae) 珍珠母 15-30g and **mu li** (Concha Ostreae) 牡蛎 15-30g.
- With food stagnation, add **jiao shen qu** (baked Massa Fermentata) 焦神曲 15g, **jiao shan zha** (baked Fructus Crataegi) 焦山楂 15g, **chao mai ya** (dry fried Fructus Hordei Vulgaris Germinantus) 炒麦芽 15g.

Patent medicines

Er Chen Wan 二陈丸 (Er Chen Wan)
Ping Wei San 平胃散 (Ping Wei San, Tabellae Pingwei)
Qing Qi Hua Tan Wan 清气化痰丸 (Qing Qi Hua Tan Wan, Pinellia Expectorant Pills)
- Phlegm Heat

Wen Dan Wan 温胆丸 (Wen Dan Wan)
- Phlegm Heat

Bao He Wan 保和丸 (Bao He Wan)
- add with food stagnation

Xiang Sha Liu Jun Zi Wan 香砂六君子丸 (Xiang Sha Liu Jun Wan, Aplotaxis-Ammomum Pills, Six Gentlemen Tea Pills)
- with Spleen deficiency

Acupuncture (select from)

St.25 (*tian shu* -) .... together these points regulate Intestinal
Sp.15 (*da heng* -) function, clear stagnation from the Intestines and promote bowel movement

SJ.6 (*zhi gou* -) .... together these points regulate *qi* in the *san jiao*,
GB.34 (*yang ling quan* -) soothe the Liver and encourage *qi* movement through the Intestine and promotes bowel movement

St.40 (*feng long* -) .... together, this *yuan luo* pair strengthen the
Sp.3 (*tai bai* -) Spleen and supplement *qi* to transform Phlegm and improve fluid metabolism

St.41 (*jie xi* -) .... *jing* river and Fire point of the Stomach, clears Dampness and regulates the Spleen and Stomach

Ren.12 (*zhong wan*) .... *mu* point of the Stomach, strengthens digestion and improves fluid metabolism with St.36 and LI.4

St.36 (*zu san li*) .... *he* sea point of the Stomach, regulates and strengthens the Spleen and Stomach to transform Phlegm

LI.4 (*he gu*) .... stimulates the dispersing function of the Lungs and thus the descent of Large Intestine *qi*, relieves stagnation in the Intestines

Liv.3 (*tai chong* -) .... regulates Liver *qi* to assist in shifting and processing fluids so as to stop production of Phlegm

- with foggy-headedness, fullness in the chest, anxiety or nausea, add PC.5 (*jian shi*) or PC.6 (*nei guan*)
- with Spleen deficiency, add Bl.20 (*pi shu*)
- with abdominal pain, add Sp.4 (*gong sun* -) and Liv.5 (*li gou* -)
- *Ear points*: constipation area, large intestine, small intestine, spleen, stomach, lungs, sympathetic

Clinical notes

- Phlegm type constipation is often associated with a constitutional tendency towards Phlegm, and lifelong problems with bowel habits. Persistent treatment, as well as lifestyle and dietary modification, is required for a satisfactory result.
- For dietary recommendations, see p.880.

血虛便秘

5.5 BLOOD DEFICIENCY

Pathophysiology

- Blood moistens and nourishes all parts of the body, so Blood deficiency can lead to a general drying up of normally moist surfaces, in this case the mucous lining of the Intestines.
- This pattern is common in postpartum women, following haemorrhage, in elderly patients and following chronic diseases which damage the Blood.

Clinical features

- constipation with dry stools that may be pellet or button like
- generalised dryness–skin, hair, eyes, mucous membranes
- generalised pallor–face, lips, nails, conjunctiva
- palpitations, anxiety
- poor memory, forgetfulness
- postural dizziness, blurring vision
- insomnia
- numbness or tingling in the limbs

T pale with a thin coat
P thready and weak

Treatment principle

Nourish and supplement the Blood
Moisten the Intestines and promote bowel movement

Prescription

RUN CHANG WAN 润肠丸
(*Moisten the Intestines Pill*)

dang gui (Radix Angelicae Sinensis) 当归 30g
sheng di (Radix Rehmanniae Glutinosae) 生地 30g
tao ren (Semen Persicae) 桃仁 30g
huo ma ren (Semen Cannabis Sativae) 火麻仁 30g
zhi ke (Fructus Citri Aurantii) 枳壳 30g

Method: Grind herbs to a powder and form into 9-gram pills with honey. The dose is one pill 2-3 times daily. Pills are the best for this condition, however, the herbs may also be decocted with a 50% reduction in quantities. **Dang gui** and **sheng di** effectively lubricate and moisten the bowel while nourishing Blood and *yin*; **tao ren** and **huo ma ren** moisten and lubricate the bowel; **zhi ke** regulates and promotes the downward movement of *qi*. **Huo ma ren** may be unavailable in some countries. An alternative herb is **hu ma ren** (Semen Lini) 胡麻仁. (Source: *Shi Yong Zhong Yi Nei Ke Xue*)

Modifications

- With Heat (thirst, irritability, restlessness, red cheeks and a peeled tongue) add **xuan shen** (Radix Scrophulariae) 玄参 15-24g, **sheng he shou wu** (Radix Polygoni Multiflori) 生何首乌 12-15g and **zhi mu** (Rhizoma Anemarrhenae Asphodeloides) 知母 9-12g.

- For recalcitrant constipation, add two or three of the following herbs: **chao xing ren** (dry fried Semen Pruni Armeniacae) 炒杏仁 9-12g, **bai zi ren** (Semen Biotae Orientalis) 柏子仁 9-12g, **yu li ren** (Semen Pruni) 郁李仁 9-12g or **song zi ren** (Semen Pini) 松子仁 9-12g.
- With *qi* deficiency, add **huang jing** (Rhizoma Polygonati) 黄精 12-18g and **tai zi shen** (Radix Pseudostellariae Heterophyllae) 太子参 12-18g.

Patent medicines

Dang Gui Ji Jing 当归鸡精 (Tang Kuei Essence of Chicken)
- especially good postpartum with quite severe (and acute) Blood deficiency

Gui Pi Wan 归脾丸 (Gui Pi Wan, Angelicae Longana Tea, Kwei Be Wan)
- especially good when there are *shen* disturbances

Ba Zhen Wan 八珍丸 (Ba Zhen Wan, Women's Precious Pills)
- for *qi* and Blood deficiency

Run Chang Wan 润肠丸 (Run Chang Wan, Fructus Persica Compound Pills) - This is a mild laxative formula containing **da huang**. A small dose, 6-12 pills per day, may be combined with one of the above patent formulae if necessary, but should be reduced as soon as possible as **da huang** is not suitable for prolonged use in deficient patterns.

Acupuncture (select from)

Ren.12 (*zhong wan* +) .... these points strengthen the Spleen and
St.36 (*zu san li* +▲) Stomach, and the promote production of *qi*
Sp.6 (*san yin jiao* +▲) and Blood

St.25 (*tian shu* -) .... *mu* point of the Large Intestine, regulates Intestinal function and promotes bowel movement

Ren.6 (*qi hai* +) .... these points regulate *qi* in the lower abdomen,
Ren.4 (*guan yuan* +) and with Sp.6 supplement *yin* and Blood

Bl.18 (*gan shu* +) .... *shu* points of the Liver, Spleen and Kidney,
Bl.20 (*pi shu* +) supplement and regulate Blood and stimulate
Bl.23 (*shen shu* +▲) Blood production

Bl.17 (*ge shu*) .... *hui* point of the Blood, regulates and assists production of Blood

Sp.10 (*xue hai*) .... regulates and nourishes Blood

- In general, acupuncture is not as effective as diet and herbal therapy for Blood deficiency type constipation
- *Ear points*: constipation area, spleen, heart, lungs, large intestine, distal segment rectum, *san jiao*, *shen men*, sympathetic

Clinical notes

- Blood deficiency type constipation may be diagnosed biomedically as habitual constipation, postpartum constipation and constipation in the elderly.
- Chronic constipation of this type can take a long time to cure, especially if the patient has been taking bitter stimulant laxatives, like senna and cascara. In cases of shorter duration, for example, following fever, haemorrhage or childbirth, some weeks to a couple of months be sufficient; in elderly patients and those with chronic problems, one to two years may be required to restore health and enable an easy bowel movement without the use of a laxative formula.
- Increasing the consumption of *yin* and Blood moistening foods is helpful. These include black sesame seeds, walnuts, pine nuts, honey, apricots, prunes and bananas. The Chinese like to mix a variety of these foods together in cakes and biscuits for prolonged use. These foods are suitable for all chronic dry types of constipation.
- For more dietary recommendations see p.874.

气虚便秘

5.6 QI DEFICIENCY

Pathophysiology

- *Qi* deficiency constipation involves weakness of the Lungs and Spleen. In chronic cases the Kidneys may be involved as well. The mechanism of the constipation may be twofold. Weakness of Lung *qi* may fail to aid the natural descent of Large Intestine *qi*. Weakness of Spleen *qi* may compromise the *qi* mechanism, causing a failure of Stomach *qi* descent and thus Large Intestine *qi* descent.
- The main feature of *qi* deficiency constipation is weak propulsion of the stools; peristalsis is feeble and insufficient to move the stool through the Intestines.

Clinical features

- Constipation with stools that are difficult to pass but are generally not dry or hard. The stools tend to be soft, large and thick. There is a desire to defecate but the patient must strain. The patient feels tired following a bowel movement, and may experience sweating and shortness of breath while trying to have a bowel movement. There may be distension but no discomfort in the abdomen, even after days of not emptying the bowel.
- waxy pale complexion
- lethargy and fatigue
- soft voice, reluctance to speak
- spontaneous sweating

T swollen and pale with tooth marks and a thin white coat
P weak and deficient

Treatment principle

Strengthen the Spleen and Stomach and supplement *qi*
Promote movement of *qi* and stimulate the *qi* mechanism

Prescription

HUANG QI TANG 黄芪汤
(*Astragalus Decoction*)

zhi huang qi (honey fried Radix Astragali Membranacei) 炙黄芪 30-60g
dang shen (Radix Codonopsis Pilosulae) 党参 15-24g
chao bai zhu (dry fried Rhizoma Atractylodes Macrocephalae) 炒白术 12-15g
chen pi (Pericarpium Citri Reticulatae) 陈皮 9-12g
huo ma ren (Semen Cannabis Sativae) 火麻仁 15g
feng mi (honey) 蜂蜜 1spoon

Method: Decoction. The honey is added to the strained decoction (*chong fu* 冲服). **Zhi huang qi**, **dang shen** and **chao bai zhu** strengthen the Spleen and supplement *qi*; the large dose of **huang qi** powerfully mobilises *qi* movement and stimulates peristalsis; **bai zhu** dries any complicating Dampness; **huo ma ren** lubricates the Intestines; **chen pi** regulates *qi*; **honey** moistens the Intestines and benefits *qi*. **Huo ma ren** may be unavailable in some countries. An alternative herb is **hu ma ren** (Semen Lini) 胡麻仁. (Source: *Zhong Yi Nei Ke Lin Chuang Shou Ce*)

Modifications

- With abdominal distension after eating, add **sha ren** (Fructus Amomi) 砂仁 6-9g and **bai dou kou** (Fructus Amomi Kravanh) 白豆蔻 6-9g.
- To stimulate the *qi* mechanism, add **zhi shi** (Fructus Immaturus Citri Aurantii) 枳实 9-12g, **mu xiang** (Radix Aucklandiae Lappae) 木香 6-9g and **sha ren** (Fructus Amomi) 砂仁 6-9g.
- If Spleen *qi* sinks downwards causing heaviness in the lower *jiao*, haemorrhoids or prolapse of the rectum, bladder or uterus, add **sheng ma** (Rhizoma Cimicifugae) 升麻 9-12g, **chai hu** (Radix Bupleuri) 柴胡 6-9g and **jie geng** (Radix Platycodi Grandiflori) 桔梗 6-9g, or consider **BU ZHONG YI QI TANG** (*Ginseng and Astragalus Combination* 补中益气汤, p.502) as the guiding formula.
- With a chronic cough, add **wu wei zi** (Fructus Schizandrae Chinensis) 五味子 6g, **zi wan** (Radix Asteris Tatarici) 紫菀 9-12g and **bai qian** (Radix et Rhizoma Cynanchi Baiqian) 白前 9-12g.
- Blood deficiency frequently complicates *qi* deficiency. If so, add **dang gui** (Radix Angelicae Sinensis) 当归 6-9g and **tao ren** (Semen Persicae) 桃仁 6-9g.
- With weak Kidney *qi* (lower back ache, nocturia, weak proximal pulses), add **rou cong rong** (Herba Cistanches Deserticolae) 肉苁蓉 18-30g and **suo yang** (Herba Cynomorii Songarici) 锁阳 12-18g or consider **DA BU YUAN JIAN** (*Great Tonify the Basal Decoction* 大补元煎, p.791) as guiding formula.

Patent medicines

Bu Zhong Yi Qi Wan 补中益气丸 (Bu Zhong Yi Qi Wan, Central Qi Pills) - Lung and Spleen *qi* deficiency

Ren Shen Yang Ying Wan 人参养营丸 (Ginseng Tonic Pills)
- Lung, Spleen and Kidney *qi* deficiency

Xiang Sha Liu Jun Zi Wan 香砂六君子丸 (Xiang Sha Liu Jun Wan, Aplotaxis-Ammomum Pills, Six Gentlemen Tea Pills)
- with *qi* stagnation and Phlegm Damp

Cong Rong Bu Shen Wan 从容补肾丸 (Cong Rong Bu Shen Wan)
- These pills are a specific laxative formula for *qi* or *yang* deficiency atonic constipation. They can be combined with one of the constitutional formulae above.

Acupuncture (select from)

St.25 (*tian shu* ▲) .... together these points regulate Intestinal
Sp.15 (*da heng*) function and support the function of Spleen *qi*
Ren.6 (*qi hai* +▲) to encourage *qi* movement

Ren.12 (*zhong wan* +▲) .. warms and strengthens the Spleen and Stomach and stimulates movement of *qi* through the Intestines, especially in combination with St.36 and Sp.6

St.36 (*zu san li* +▲) .... *he* sea point of the Stomach, powerfully warms and strengthens the Spleen and Stomach and supplements *qi*

Sp.6 (*san yin jiao* +▲)...... strengthens the Spleen, regulates Liver *qi*, benefits the Kidneys and invigorates *qi* and Blood

Bl.13 (*fei shu* +▲)............ *shu* points of the Lung, Spleen and Large
Bl.20 (*pi shu* +▲) Intestine respectively, supplement and
Bl.25 (*da chang shu* +▲) strengthen *qi* and the movement of *qi* through the Intestines

- with prolapse or haemorrhoids, add Du.20 (*bai hui* ▲)
- with a chronic cough, add Lu.9 (*tai yuan* +) and Lu.1 (*zhong fu*)
- with Kidney deficiency, add Bl.23 (*shen shu* +▲)
- to strengthen Lung *qi*, add Du.14 (*da zhui* ▲)
- to aid the Lung's dispersing function, add LI.4 (*he gu*)
- *Ear points*: constipation area, spleen, lungs, large intestine, distal segment rectum, *san jiao*, *shen men*, sympathetic

Clinical notes

- *Qi* deficiency constipation may be diagnosed biomedically as chronic constipation in the elderly or frail, or constipation following a severe illness, abdominal surgery or emotional trauma (such as the sudden death of a spouse).
- Chronic *qi* deficiency constipation can take a long time to cure, especially if the patient has been taking stimulant laxatives, such as senna or cascara.
- Exercise is an essential component of treatment to strengthen the Lungs and Spleen and rebuild *qi*. Particularly useful is walking, swimming, yoga or *tai ji chuan*.
- Regular abdominal massage in a clockwise direction can help to stimulate peristalsis.
- For dietary recommendations see p.870.

阴虚便秘

5.7 YIN DEFICIENCY

Pathophysiology

- *Yin* deficiency constipation can develop in two ways. It may occur gradually with a general weakening of *yin* associated with factors such as ageing, drug use, shift work, a heating diet or prolonged dehydration. Alternatively, *yin* depletion can progress more rapidly, following a Hot disease. The mechanism of the constipation is dryness of the Intestines from lack of *yin* fluids. The dryness may be compounded by deficient Heat, if present.
- There are two degrees of *yin* deficiency to consider. The most superficial is that involving the Stomach (and Spleen), which in the early stages is associated with dryness and a lack of *yin* fluids, and may lack the Heat of deeper *yin* deficiency. As *yin* deficiency deepens, it begins to affect the fundamental *yin*, that is, the Liver and Kidney, with the classic signs of deficiency Heat and a more prolonged course.

Clinical features

- constipation with dry stools, like sheep or rabbit droppings
- general dryness of the skin, eyes, mucous membranes and hair, thirst
- Liver and Kidney *yin*: facial and malar flushing, nightsweats, sensation of heat in the palms and soles ('five hearts hot'), dizziness, tinnitus, lower back and knees sore and weak
- Stomach *yin*: indeterminate gnawing hunger, epigastric discomfort or burning, morning nausea

T Liver and Kidney *yin:* red, thin and dry with little or no coat, or cracked surface
Stomach *yin*: normal or red body, peeled or cracked centrally

P thready and rapid

Treatment principle

Nourish *yin*, moisten the Intestines, promote bowel movement
Supplement the Liver and Kidney, (and/or Spleen and Stomach)

Prescription

LIU WEI DI HUANG WAN 六味地黄丸
(*Rehmannia Six Formula*) modified

This prescription is most suitable for chronic Kidney and Liver *yin* deficiency constipation, and generally needs to be taken for lengthy periods to achieve a result.

shu di (Radix Rehmanniae Glutinosae Conquitae) 熟地 240g
chao shan yao (dry fried Radix Dioscoreae Oppositae)
炒山药 120g

shan zhu yu (Fructus Corni Officinalis) 山茱萸 120g
mu dan pi (Cortex Moutan Radicis) 牡丹皮 90g
fu ling (Sclerotium Poriae Cocos) 茯苓 90g
ze xie (Rhizoma Alismatis Orientalis) 泽泻 90g
huo ma ren (Semen Cannabis Sativae) 火麻仁 90g
xuan shen (Radix Scrophulariae) 玄参 90g
yu zhu (Rhizoma Polygonati Odorati) 玉竹 90g

Method: Grind herbs to a powder and form into 9-gram pills with honey. The dose is one pill 2-3 times daily. May also be decocted with a 90% reduction in quantities. **Shu di** and **shan zhu yu** nourish Liver and Kidney *yin*; **shan yao** strengthens the Spleen and nourishes *yin*, **fu ling, ze xie** and **mu dan pi** moderate the cloying tendency of the *yin* supplementing herbs; **fu ling** strengthens the Spleen; **ze xie** promotes urination and balances fluids; **mu dan pi** cools and invigorates the Blood; **huo ma ren** moistens the Intestines; **xuan shen** nourishes *yin*, cools the Blood and softens hardness; **yu zhu** moistens and nourishes Stomach *yin*. **Huo ma ren** may be unavailable in some countries. An alternative herb is **hu ma ren** (Semen Lini) 胡麻仁. (Source: *Shi Yong Zhong Yi Nei Ke Xue*)

YI WEI TANG 益胃汤
(Benefit the Stomach Decoction)

This prescription is selected for Spleen and Stomach *yin* deficiency. In general, the dryness aspects are prominent and there are few Heat signs.

sheng di (Radix Rehmanniae Glutinosae) 生地 15-24g
sha shen (Radix Adenophorae seu Glehniae) 沙参 12-18g
mai dong (Tuber Ophiopogonis Japonici) 麦冬 12-15g
yu zhu (Rhizoma Polygonati Odorati) 玉竹 12-15g
bing tang (rock sugar) 冰糖 6-9g

Method: Decoction. **Sheng di, sha shen, mai dong**, and **yu zhu** nourish Stomach *yin*; **bing tang** moistens dryness. (Source: *Shi Yong Zhong Yi Nei Ke Xue*)

Modifications

- With Blood deficiency in the elderly, add **sang shen** (Fructus Mori Albae) 桑椹 12-15g and **sang ji sheng** (Ramulus Sangjisheng) 桑寄生 12-15g.
- With epigastric pain, add **bai shao** (Radix Paeoniae Lactiflora) 白芍 12-18g and **gan cao** (Radix Glycyrrhizae Uralensis) 甘草 6-9g.
- With acid reflux and heartburn, add **hai piao xiao** (Os Sepiae seu Sepiellae) 海螵蛸 15g (or 3g as a powder washed down with the decoction).

Variations and additional prescriptions

Yin deficiency following a febrile disease

- When *yin* deficiency is acute, and follows a severe or prolonged febrile disease (typically a disorder affecting the Large Intestine, such as dysentery) the aim of treatment is to replenish fluids, moisten dryness and open the bowels with **ZENG YE TANG** (*Increase the Fluids Decoction* 增液汤).

xuan shen (Radix Scrophulariae) 玄参 30g
mai dong (Tuber Ophiopogonis Japonici) 麦冬 24g
sheng di (Radix Rehmanniae Glutinosae) 生地 24g

Method: Decoction. The quantities of the herbs can be reduced as the bowels become more regular. **Xuan shen** nourishes *yin*, cools the Blood and softens hardness; **mai dong** moistens dryness and nourishes Stomach, Lung and Intestinal *yin*; **sheng di** nourishes *yin*, cools the Blood and moistens dryness. (Source: *Shi Yong Zhong Yi Nei Ke Xue*)

- In hard to shift cases, a honey enema may be useful in the initial stages of treatment. Two or three tablespoons of honey mixed with 100-200 mls of warm water (37^{0}C) and a teaspoon of sesame oil can be retained for 20 minutes. A warm soapy enema will achieve a similar result.
- A teaspoon of the osmotic laxative Epsom salts (**mang xiao**) dissolved in water and taken before bed may also be useful in the early stages of treatment to get the bowels moving.

Patent medicines

Liu Wei Di Huang Wan 六味地黄丸 (Liu Wei Di Huang Wan, Six Flavour Tea)

Zhi Bai Ba Wei Wan 知柏八味丸 (Zhi Bai Ba Wei Wan, Chih Pai Pa Wei Wan) - with lots of deficient Heat

Gu Ben Wan 固本丸 (Gu Ben Wan, Ren Shen Ku Pen Wan)
- Spleen and Stomach *yin* deficiency

Sheng Mai San Wan 生脉散丸 (Sheng Mai San Wan)
- Lung and Stomach *qi* and *yin* deficiency

Run Chang Wan 润肠丸 (Fructus Persica Compound Pills)
- This is a laxative formula containing **da huang**. It may be combined with one of the above formulae if necessary, but should be reduced as soon as possible as **da huang** is not suitable for prolonged use in deficient patterns.

Acupuncture (select from)

St.25 (*tian shu* -) .... *mu* point of the Large Intestine, regulates Intestinal function, benefits Intestinal *yin* and promotes bowel movement

Ren.4 (*guan yuan*) .... meeting point of the *yin*, supplements *yuan qi* and *yin*, especially with Sp.6

Ren.12 (*zhong wan* +)....... *mu* point of the Stomach, supplements Stomach *yin* and stimulates movement of *qi* through the Intestines, especially in combination with St.36 and Sp.6

St.36 (*zu san li* +) .... *he* sea point of the Stomach, powerfully strengthens the Spleen and Stomach and supplements *qi* and *yin*

Sp.6 (*san yin jiao* +) .... strengthens the Spleen and Kidney to moisten and supplement *yin* and regulates *qi* in the digestive system

Bl.25 (*da chang shu*) .... *shu* point of the Large Intestine, regulates movement of *qi* through the Intestines and promotes bowel movement

Bl.20 (*pi shu* +)................. these points supplement Stomach and Kidney *yin*
Bl.21 (*wei shu* +)
Bl.23 (*shen shu* +)

Kid.6 (*zhao hai* +)............ these points nourish the source of *yin*, the Kidneys
Kid.3 (*tai xi* +)

- acupuncture alone is not especially effective for this pattern
- *Ear points*: constipation area, kidney, stomach, large intestine, distal segment rectum, *san jiao*, *shen men*, sympathetic

Clinical notes

- *Yin* deficiency constipation may be diagnosed biomedically as constipation following a febrile illness or dehydration, the chronic constipation of the elderly and menopausal women.
- Chronic *yin* deficiency constipation can be quite difficult to treat satisfactorily and usually takes a long time to cure, especially if the patient has been taking stimulant laxatives, like senna or cascara. One or two years of treatment may be required to rebuild Intestinal *yin* to enable a healthy bowel movement without a laxative formula.
- Increasing the consumption of *yin* moistening foods may be helpful. These include black sesame seeds, walnuts, pine nuts, honey, apricots, prunes and bananas. The Chinese like to mix a variety of these foods together in cakes and biscuits for prolonged use. These foods are suitable for all chronic dry type constipations. For more dietary recommendations, see p.876.

冷秘

5.8 YANG DEFICIENCY WITH COLD ACCUMULATION

Pathophysiology

- *Yang* deficiency constipation involves weakness of Spleen and Kidney *yang* and is chronic and most common in the elderly. Kidney *yang* and/or Spleen *yang* may dominate. The constipation can be due to several factors–
  1. Failure of *yang* propulsion through the intestines–the main problem is simply insufficient force behind the stool. The stools are normal in appearance and moisture, albeit large.
  2. Cold accumulation which 'freezes and constricts', further impedes *yang* movement through the Intestine.
  3. Disordered fluid metabolism. If there is insufficient *yang* to transform and mobilize fluids, they may be poorly distributed, either pouring out as frequent urination or nocturia, or sitting in the tissues as oedema. In both cases, fluids that would normally lubricate the passage of the stool are unavailable, so in addition to the weak propulsion, the Intestines (and stools) will be dry.

Clinical features

- constipation with hard to expel stools that may or may not be dry; the patient may be exhausted following an attempted or successful defecation
- copious clear urine, nocturia, or scanty urination and pitting oedema
- cold extremities, cold intolerance
- abdominal pain which is better for warmth; the abdomen feels cool when palpated
- waxy pale complexion
- lower back ache, knees cold and sore

T pale, swollen and moist, with tooth marks and a white coat
P deep and slow

Treatment principle

Warm and strengthen *yang*, promote peristalsis and bowel movement
Improve fluid metabolism to redistribute fluids

Prescription

JI CHUAN JIAN 济川煎
(*Benefit the River Decoction*) modified

This prescription is suitable for all types of *yang* deficiency constipation. Once the bowels are moving, a specific Spleen and/or Kidney *yang* strengthening formula should be selected. This formula is suitable whether or not the stools are dry.

rou cong rong (Herba Cistanches Deserticolae) 肉苁蓉 30g
dang gui (Radix Angelicae Sinensis) 当归 9-12g
niu xi (Radix Achyranthis Bidentatae) 牛膝 9-12g
zhi ke (Fructus Citri Aurantii) 枳壳 6-9g
ze xie (Rhizoma Alismatis Orientalis) 泽泻 6-9g
sheng ma (Rhizoma Cimicifugae) 升麻 3-6g
rou gui (Cortex Cinnamomi Cassiae) 肉桂 3g

Method: Decoction. **Rou cong rong** requires substantial cooking for best effect, so this prescription should be cooked for at least one hour. **Rou gui** is added towards the end of cooking (*hou xia* 后下). **Rou cong rong** warms *yang*, stimulates peristalsis and opens the bowels; **dang gui** moistens and lubricates the Intestines; **niu xi** strengthens the Kidneys and facilitates downward movement of *qi*; **zhi ke** directs *qi* downward and regulates *qi*; **sheng ma** elevates *qi* and balances **zhi ke** and **niu xi** to 'elevate the clear to promote descent of the turbid'; **ze xie** promotes urination to correct fluid imbalance; **rou gui** warms *yang* and promotes transformation of *qi*. (Source: *Zhong Yi Nei Ke Lin Chuang Shou Ce*)

Modifications

- With *qi* deficiency, add **huang qi** (Radix Astragali Membranacei) 黄芪 15-24g.
- With copious urination and dry stools, delete **ze xie** and add **suo yang** (Herba Cynomorii Songarici) 锁阳 15g and **huo ma ren** (Semen Cannabis Sativae) 火麻仁 15g (or **hu ma ren** [Semen Lini] 胡麻仁).
- With lower back ache and coldness, add **gou qi zi** (Fructus Lycii) 构杞子 12g and **du zhong** (Cortex Eucommiae Ulmoidis) 杜仲 12g.

Variations and additional prescriptions

With Kidney yang deficiency

- When Kidney *yang* deficiency is prominent and the stools are not dry, the aim of treatment is to warm Kidney *yang* with **JIN KUI SHEN QI WAN** (*Rehmannia Eight Formula* 金匮肾气丸) modified.

zhi fu zi (Radix Aconiti Carmichaeli Praeparata) 制附子 60g
rou gui (Cortex Cinnamomi Cassiae) 肉桂 60g
shu di (Radix Rehmanniae Glutinosae Conquitae) 熟地 240g
shan zhu yu (Fructus Corni Officinalis) 山茱萸 120g
shan yao (Radix Dioscoreae Oppositae) 山药 120g
fu ling (Sclerotium Poriae Cocos) 茯苓 90g
ze xie (Rhizoma Alismatis Orientalis) 泽泻 90g
mu dan pi (Cortex Moutan Radicis) 牡丹皮 90g
rou cong rong (Herba Cistanches Deserticolae) 肉苁蓉 180g
suo yang (Herba Cynomorii Songarici) 锁阳 150g
dang gui (Radix Angelicae Sinensis) 当归 90g

Method: Grind herbs to powder and form into 9-gram pills with honey. The dose is one pill 2-3 times daily with warm water. May also be decocted with a 80-90% reduction in quantities. When decocted **zhi fu zi** and **rou cong rong** are cooked for 30 minutes before the other herbs (*xian jian* 先煎). **Rou gui** is added towards the end of cooking (*hou xia* 后下). **Zhi fu zi** and **rou gui** warm Kidney *yang* and stimulate transformation of *qi* to mobilise *yang qi* and fluids; **shu di**, **shan zhu yu** and **shan yao** nourish the Kidneys and Liver; **fu ling**, **ze xie** and **mu dan pi** alleviate the supplementing herbs' cloying tendency; **rou cong rong** and **suo yang** warm *yang* and open the Intestines; **dang gui** moistens and lubricates the Intestines. (Source: *Shi Yong Zhong Yi Nei Ke Xue*)

Spleen yang deficiency

- When Spleen *yang* deficiency is primary, the aim of treatment is to warm and supplement Spleen *yang* with **FU ZI LI ZHONG WAN** (*Aconite, Ginseng and Ginger Formula* 附子理中丸) modified.

zhi fu zi (Radix Aconiti Carmichaeli Praeparata) 制附子 6-12g
gan jiang (Rhizoma Zingiberis Officinalis) 干姜 9-12g
dang shen (Radix Codonopsis Pilosulae) 党参 15-24g
chao bai zhu (dry fried Rhizoma Atractylodis Macrocephalae) 炒白术 12-15g
zhi gan cao (honey fried Radix Glycyrrhizae Uralensis) 炙甘草 6-9g
rou cong rong (Herba Cistanches Deserticolae) 肉苁蓉 30g
suo yang (Herba Cynomorii Songarici) 锁阳 15g

Method: Grind herbs into powder and form into 3-gram pills with honey. The dose is one pill 2-3 times daily. May also be prepared as a decoction, in which case **zhi fu zi** and **rou cong rong** are cooked for 30 minutes prior to the other herbs (*xian jian* 先煎). **Zhi fu zi** and **gan jiang** warms Spleen and Kidney *yang*; **dang shen**, **bai zhu** and **zhi gan cao** strengthen the Spleen and supplement *qi*; **rou cong rong** and **suo yang** warm *yang* and open the Intestines.

With copious or frequent urination and dry stools

- Some patients with Kidney *yang* deficiency type constipation, are constipated because the fluids which should lubricate the bowel are escaping as excessive urination. The main features are chronic constipation with dry stools, frequent urination and nocturia, cold intolerance, a pale swollen tongue and a deep pulse. The treatment should aim to warm the *yang*, strengthen Kidney function and improve fluid metabolism. This can be achieved with a combination of **JIN KUI SHEN QI WAN** (*Rehmannia Eight Formula* 金匮肾气丸, p.203) and **JIN SUO GU JING WAN** (*Metal Lock Pill to Stabilize the Essence* 金锁固精丸, p.909).

In the elderly with severe Cold

- In elderly patients with severe Cold, combine with **BAN LIU WAN** (*Pinellia and Sulphur Pill* 半硫丸), a pill made from **liu huang** (Sulphur)

硫黄 and **ban xia** (Rhizoma Pinelliae Ternatae) 半夏, or 1-2 grams of **liu huang** can be taken as a powder (in capsules) with the decoction. Only the purest sulphur is appropriate. Not suitable for prolonged use.

Patent medicines

Jin Kui Shen Qi Wan 金匮肾气丸 (Fu Gui Ba Wei Wan, Sexoton Pills, Golden Book Tea)
- Kidney *yang* deficiency

Fu Zi Li Zhong Wan 附子理中丸 (Fu Tzu Li Chung Wan, Carmichaeli Tea Pills, Li Chung Yuen Medical Pills)
- Spleen *yang* deficiency

Cong Rong Bu Shen Wan 从容补肾丸 (Cong Rong Bu Shen Wan)
- specific for *yang* deficiency constipation, can be combined with one of the above formulae

Acupuncture (select from)

St.25 (*tian shu* +▲) .... these points warm and regulate Intestinal
Sp.15 (*da heng* +▲) function to promote *qi* movement and stimulate persistalsis

Ren.4 (*guan yuan* +▲) ..... warms Kidney and stimulates *yuan qi* to promote the movement of *yang* though the abdomen and persistalsis
Bl.20 (*pi shu* +▲) .... *shu* point of the Spleen, warms and supplements Spleen *yang*
Bl.23 (*shen shu* +▲) .... *shu* point of the Kidney, warms and supplements Kidney *yang*
Du.4 (*ming men* +▲) .... warms and stimulates the movement of *yang qi*
Bl.25 (*da chang shu* +▲) .. *shu* point of Large Intestine, warms and stimulates Intestinal function and persistalsis
St.36 (*zu san li* +▲) .... *he* sea point of the Stomach, powerfully warms and strengthens the Spleen and Stomach and supplements *qi*
Sp.6 (*san yin jiao* +▲) ...... strengthens the Spleen and Kidneys and invigorates movement of *qi* and Blood
Kid.3 (*tai xi* +▲) .... *yuan* point of the Kidneys, warms and supplements Kidney *yang*

- a moxa box over the low abdomen or back is effective
- with frequent urination, add Kid.7 (*fu liu* -) and Ren.3 (*zhong ji*)
- *Ear points*: constipation area, kidney, spleen, stomach, large intestine, *san jiao*, *shen men*, adrenal

Clinical notes

- *Yang* deficiency constipation may be diagnosed biomedically as the chronic constipation of the elderly or debilitated, atonic constipation, paralytic ileus, constipation associated with hypothyroidism, or constipation following abdominal surgery.
- Chronic *yang* deficiency constipation can be quite difficult and take a long time to cure, especially if the patient has been taking bitter cold stimulant laxatives, such as senna or cascara. These substances especially damage the *yang* of the Intestines. Nine to twelve months of treatment (or even more) may be required to sufficiently rebuild *yang* to enable a smooth unassisted bowel movement.
- For dietary recommendations see p.873.

SUMMARY OF GUIDING FORMULAE FOR CONSTIPATION

Chronic Heat accumulation - *Ma Zi Ren Wan* 麻子仁丸
- with Heat in the Liver - *Dang Gui Long Hui Wan* 当归龙荟丸
- with Damp Heat - *Huang Long Tang* 黄龙汤
- with haemorrhoids - *Yi Zi Tang* 乙字汤

Acute external Heat invasion
- *yang ming* syndrome - *Da Cheng Qi Tang* 大承气汤
- Wind Cold/*yang ming* overlap - *Da Qing Long Tang* 大青龙汤
- Wind Heat/*shao yang*/*yang ming* overlap - *Fang Feng Tong Sheng Tang* 防风通圣汤
- *shao yang*/*yang ming* overlap - *Da Chai Hu Tang* 大柴胡汤
- *tai yang*/ *shao yang*/*yang ming* overlap - *Chai Hu Jia Long Gu Mu Li Tang* 柴胡加龙骨牡蛎汤

Food stagnation - *Bao He Wan* 保和丸
- with Damp Heat - *Zhi Shi Dao Zhi Wan* 枳实导滞丸

Liver *qi* stagnation
- in sedentary patients - *Liu Mo Tang* 六磨汤
- with Spleen *qi* and Blood deficiency - *Xiao Yao San* 逍遥散
- with alternating constipation and diarrhoea - *Tong Xie Yao Fang* 痛泻要方

Phlegm - *Tan Bi Tang* 痰秘汤

Blood deficiency - *Run Chang Wan* 润肠丸

Qi deficiency - *Huang Qi Tang* 黄芪汤

Yin deficiency
- Liver and Kidney *yin* deficiency - *Liu Wei Di Huang Wan* 六味地黄丸
- Spleen and Stomach *yin* deficiency - *Yi Wei Tang* 益胃汤
- following a febrile disease - *Zeng Ye Tang* 增液汤

Yang deficiency - *Ji Chuan Jian* 济川煎
- Kidney *yang* deficiency - *Jin Kui Shen Qi Wan* 金匮肾气丸
- Spleen *yang* deficiency - *Fu Zi Li Zhong Wan* 附子理中丸

Table 5.2 *Differential diagnosis of constipation*

Pattern		Duration	Nature of stool	Associated symptoms	Nature of patient	Pulse and tongue
Heat	Large Intestine	chronic	dry, hard, pellet like	bad breath, dry mouth, thirst	red complexion	T: red with a dry yellow coat P: slippery, rapid
	Liver	mostly chronic but may be acute	dry, hard, pellet like	red sore eyes, headaches, high blood pressure, irritability	angry, tense, red complexion	T: red edges, yellow coat P: wiry, rapid
	Damp Heat	mostly chronic	difficult or sluggish stools, may or may not be dry, feeling of incomplete evacuation	abdominal distension, heaviness and lethargy in the afternoon, nightsweats	red complexion, may have oily skin, musty body odour	T: greasy yellow coat P:slippery, full
	acute external	acute	dry, hard	variable depending on pathogen and location		
Food stagnation		chronic or acute	sluggish, foul, may alternate with diarrhoea	abdominal distension, foul belching, flatulence, nausea, acid reflux	well fed, possibly overweight	T: thick greasy coat P: slippery
Qi stagnation		mostly chronic but may be acute	pebble like or thin, may or may not be dry	moodiness, depression, loss of appetite, muscle tension	irritable, tense, uptight, stressed	T: unremarkable or dark; thin coat P: wiry

Phlegm	chronic	sluggish, incomplete, not dry, with mucus	foggy-headedness, heaviness in the body, bloating	tends to obesity, greasy skin, phlegmatic, musty body odour	T: flabby with a greasy coat P: deep, slippery, wiry
Blood deficiency	chronic, but may be acute after haemorrhage	dry, pebble like	postural dizziness, insomnia, anxiety, insufficient lactation	generalised pallor and dryness	T: pale P: thready
Yin deficiency	chronic, but may be acute after fever	dry, pebble like	general dryness of skin, mucous membranes, flushing, nightsweats, thirst, gnawing hunger	thin, warm, dry	T: red, dry, cracked P: thready, rapid
Qi deficiency	chronic	moist, large	tiredness following bowel movement, no urge to defecate, poor muscle tone, poor appetite	weak, fatigued, short of breath, low voice	T: pale P: weak
Yang deficiency with Cold accumulation	chronic	dry or moist, large	tired following bowel movement, sleepiness, frequent urination, low back ache, aching legs	weak, fatigued, cold intolerant	T: pale, swollen P: deep, slow

6. Diarrhoea

Excess patterns

Summerdamp, Summerheat
Damp Heat
Cold Damp
Food stagnation
Blood stagnation

Deficient patterns

Liver *qi* invading the Spleen
Spleen and Stomach *qi* deficiency
Spleen and Kidney *yang* deficiency
Fluid retention in the Intestines

6 DIARRHOEA

xie xie 泄泻

Diarrhoea is defined as the frequent passage of loose or watery stools. The basic features are an increase in the softness or fluidity of the stool, and an increase in frequency of bowel motion. Diarrhoea causes distress and embarrassment, and in some diseases and in the developing world is a significant contributor to morbidity and mortality. Diarrhoea is still one of the biggest causes of infant mortality. In TCM terms diarrhoea is frequently associated with the presence of Dampness and thus most commonly involves the Spleen, either as the primary source of the Damp, or as the target of external Damp.

There are three main mechanisms that give rise to diarrhoea (Table 6.1). The first is the presence of a pathogen of some kind, most commonly Damp with or without Cold or Heat. The pathogen, once lodged in the Spleen and Stomach, disrupts digestive function and enables more Damp to accumulate. The Damp sinks through the bowel and appears as diarrhoea. This type of diarrhoea is mostly acute and self limiting, although it can become more entrenched and chronic if the patient is run down or has inappropriate treatment. There are two sub-types of pathogenic diarrhoea which are not acute and do not involve Dampness, at least not as a primary pathogen. These are Blood stagnation and food stagnation.

The second mechanism is the generation of Dampness by a weakened and poorly functioning Spleen. In this situation, Spleen deficiency is the primary factor, and Dampness secondary. This is a chronic situation, characterised by signs and symptoms of deficiency. Once a patient has a degree of Spleen deficiency, he/she is more prone to invasion by external

Table 6.1 *TCM mechanisms of diarrhoea*

Mechanism	Pattern
Presence of a pathological entity that the body tries to eject (excess patterns)	Summer Damp Summer Heat Cold Damp Damp Heat Blood stagnation
Weakness of gastro-intestinal function (deficiency patterns)	Spleen *qi* deficiency Spleen and Kidney *yang* deficiency Fluid retention in the Intestines (mixed)
Hypersensitivity and hypertonicity of the gut (excess pattern)	Liver *qi* invading the Spleen

pathogens and the potential complications of a mixed deficiency and excess pattern.

The third mechanism involves hypersensitivity and hypertonicity of the gut as the result of long term Liver *qi* stagnation. The gastro-intestinal system is responsive to emotional stress and the low grade spasticity that results causes chronic dysfunction. This is a common cause of diarrhoea and is often found in combination with Spleen deficiency, as the Liver 'overcontrols' the Spleen, or with Dampness.

AETIOLOGY

External pathogens

Diarrhoea as a result of invasion by external pathogens is common and occurs in all climates. Both adults and children are susceptible, but children are particularly vulnerable due to the fragility of the immature Spleen. Indeed, acute pathogenic diarrhoea is still one of the most common causes of infant mortality in the developing world.

The primary pathogen is always Dampness, in association with other seasonal factors. Indeed it is noted that 'without Dampness there is no diarrhoea'. The reason for this is the Spleen's digestive activity is easily clogged (the 'Spleen likes dryness') and weakened by Dampness. When weakened, a cycle is created whereby the Spleen produces more Dampness, and so on. The Dampness, being heavy and turbid by nature, sinks downwards to appear as diarrhoea.

An invasion by external pathogens can produce systemic symptoms, such as fever, chills, malaise and myalgia, or may involve only the digestive system. There are four common types of external pathogenic diarrhoea:

- Damp Heat type
  - with external symptoms (by convention Summerheat)
  - without external symptoms.
- Damp or Cold Damp type
  - with external symptoms (by convention Summerdamp)
  - without external symptoms

In general, the Summer disorders are a species of pathogen that are seasonal, often occurring during humid or wet weather. Dampness is implicit in the Summer patterns, but the degree of Heat associated with the pathogen varies considerably, from none to extreme. In this chapter, Summer disorders are defined by their systemic effects, as much as by their effects on the digestive system. Thus patients afflicted by Summer pathogens will have surface signs and symptoms in addition to digestive symptoms. A sub-type of the Summerheat pattern (with the same name, *shu re* 暑热), is associated with severe heatstroke, dehydration and disturbance of consciousness.

On the other hand, Cold Damp and Damp Heat pathogens can invade through the mouth directly into the Spleen and Intestines, bypassing the exterior. This commonly occurs late in Summer when the days are warm but the evenings are cool and people eat unwisely, are too lightly dressed for the change, or are subject to unseasonable cold snaps. Cold Damp can also invade following direct exposure, for example from living in a cold damp house, or remaining in wet clothes after walking in rain or perspiring heavily.

Damp Heat can be a product of the season, commonly occurring during hot or humid weather, and tends to be more common in tropical climates. Damp Heat pathogens can also invade with spoiled food, or by overindulgence in Damp Hot substances, such as alcohol, fats, spices or chilli.

Diet

Numerous dietary factors can cause diarrhoea. Eating spoiled or contaminated food is a common cause of acute and often violent diarrhoea, which in TCM terms may resemble an attack of Summerdamp, Summerheat, Cold Damp or Damp Heat. Changes in dietary routine, such as occur while travelling, easily upsets digestive function and may cause diarrhoea in some people.

Too much cold natured or raw food can introduce Cold into the Stomach and Intestines and weaken Spleen *qi* and *yang*. Some drugs weaken the Spleen and deplete

BOX 6.1 SOME BIOMEDICAL CAUSES OF DIARRHOEA (# denotes most common)

Acute

Infection
- acute gastroenteritis#
- bacterial
- viral#
- protozoal

Food poisoning (non microbial)
- mushrooms, toadstools, fava beans, immature potatoes

Medications (may also cause chronic diarrhoea)
- antibiotics#
- laxatives, purgatives
- thyroxine
- digitalis
- alcohol
- vitamin C
- protease inhibitors, anti-retrovirals

Chronic
- irritable bowel syndrome#
- malabsorption syndrome
- lactose intolerance, milk or food allergy
- chronic enteric infection such as amoebiasis, giardia#, and cryptosporidium
- diverticular disease
- intussusception (in children)
- post gastro-intestinal surgery
- pelvic abscess
- carcinoma of the bowel
- ischaemic colitis (elderly)
- faecal impaction with spurious diarrhoea
- Coeliac disease

Inflammatory
- Crohn's disease
- ulcerative colitis
- pseudomembranous colitis

Endocrine
- hyperthyroidism
- diabetes
- Addison's disease

Spleen *qi* and *yang* or create Dampness. These include purgative laxatives, Heat clearing herbs, antibiotics, and the antiretroviral drugs and protease inhibitors used to treat HIV infection. Inappropriate fad diets, based on fruit, single food items or unsound nutritional theories are a common cause of Spleen *qi* and *yang* deficiency, or accumulation of Dampness. Prolonged starvation or digestive insult, such as occurs in patients with a history of anorexia nervosa, bulimia or during famine, serious damages Spleen *yang*.

Eating irregularly, missing meals, eating at odd hours, or late at night weakens Spleen and Stomach *qi* and leads to food stagnation (*see* p.3). Overconsumption in general, and excessive consumption of rich, heating or supplementing foods in particular, can lead to the accumulation of food and Damp Heat in the Intestines. An excess of heating food, such as chillies, coffee, spirits, spices, fats and meat can introduce Heat and Dampness, or damage *yin*.

Eating while stressed or upset makes the Spleen and Stomach vulnerable to invasion by pent up Liver *qi*.

Dairy products and excessive quantities of sugar or sweet foods create Dampness and Phlegm.

Emotion

Emotional stress is an important cause of a variety of digestive complaints, and a common cause of diarrhoea. The gastro-intestinal tract is sensitive to, and easily disturbed by, emotional stress. This sensitivity frequently has a familial component, and is often found in several members of the same family.

The emotions most usually implicated in causing *qi* stagnation are frustration, anger, resentment, hatred, repressed emotions and stress. As *qi* accumulates, it builds up behind the obstruction. At a certain point, the pent up *qi* can escape and invade the Spleen and Stomach via the controlling (*ke* 克) cycle (Figure 6.1). Living or working in an emotionally stressful, high pressure or unfulfilling situation can cause the Liver to invade the Spleen and Stomach. Tension at meal times, or fighting around the dinner

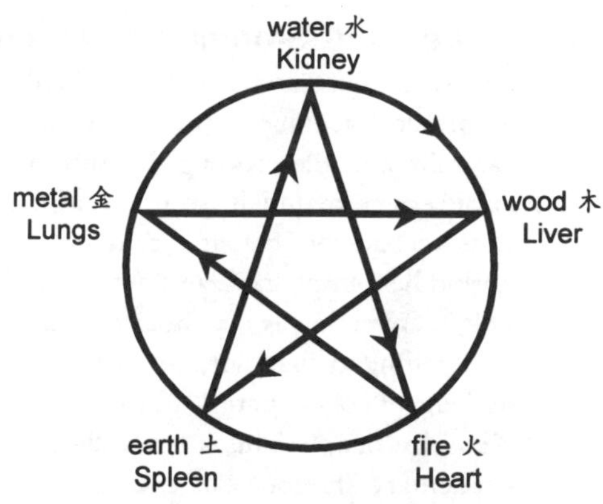

Figure 6.1. *The star represents the controlling cycle (ke 克), the circle the generative cycle (sheng 生)*

table, is a potent contributor to Liver and Spleen/Stomach disharmony.

Chronic Liver *qi* stagnation produces several commonly seen repercussions which complicate the basic *qi* stagnation pattern. The prolonged pressure in the system easily transforms into Heat, which, depending on duration and intensity of the aetiological conditions, can develop into stagnant Heat or the more severe Fire. If Heat is of sufficient intensity, it can cause Blood to move recklessly, contributing to diarrhoea with bleeding or *yin* damage. Long term *qi* stagnation can also lead to Blood stagnation and the development of masses or tumours in the Intestines. Liver *qi* invading the Spleen results in Spleen deficiency and the likely generation of Dampness. Dampness, once present, may then combine with any Heat in the system causing Damp Heat or Phlegm Heat. The mixture of Liver *qi* stagnation, Spleen deficiency and Damp Heat is referred to as the primary pathological triad (p.912).

In addition to the emotional factors that upset the Liver, worry, obsessive thinking and prolonged concentration in combination with a sedentary lifestyle and poor diet, will weaken Spleen *qi*, predisposing it to (or inviting) invasion by Liver *qi*, resulting in further damage.

Spleen and Stomach *qi* deficiency

Overwork, excessive worry or mental activity, irregular dietary habits, lack of physical activity or prolonged illness can weaken Spleen *qi*. Spleen *qi* naturally ascends creating the appropriate equilibrium for the descent of turbid waste materials, so it is said the Spleen governs 'the raising of the clear and descent of the turbid'. If this activity fails, the 'clear and turbid' (turbid here implying Dampness as well as waste materials) intermingle and sink, manifesting as diarrhoea or mucus in the stools.

Prolonged inactivity, or sitting for lengthy periods, especially while studying or concentrating the mind, can weaken the Spleen and deplete Spleen *qi* in some people. This is especially common in students, who often combine a sedentary, studious existence with poor dietary habits.

Chronic retention of Dampness following an unresolved external invasion, or from a damp environment or the diet, will eventually drain Spleen *qi* and cause deficiency. Damp Heat patterns that are treated too enthusiastically with bitter cold herbs or antibiotics can transform into Spleen deficiency or Cold Damp patterns.

Spleen and Kidney *yang* deficiency

Spleen (with or without Kidney *yang*) *yang* deficiency diarrhoea is usually a chronic condition, although it can, in some cases, be acute, following gastro-intestinal surgery or sudden excessive ingestion of cold substances.

Spleen *yang* is easily weakened by poor dietary habits (p.214).

Kidney *yang* deficiency may be an inherited condition, or may develop as a result of age, chronic illness, overexertion, overexposure to cold conditions and excessive lifting or standing. In men, Kidney *yang* can be depleted by excessive ejaculation; in women by having many pregnancies, or by insufficient recover between pregnancies.

Failure or disorder of the Spleen and Kidney *yang's* fluid transforming and metabolising action may lead to an accumulation of pathogenic fluids. Once fluid metabolism is compromised, these fluids can end up in different parts of the body, depending on the constitution of the patient and the aetiological conditions that gave rise to them. Most typically, pathological fluids end up as oedema or ascites. In the more unusual case of diarrhoea, they end up in the gastro-intestinal system, where the Large Intestine fails to reabsorb fluids from the solid waste matter.

Blood stagnation

Blood stagnation diarrhoea is most commonly the product of a chronic localised irritation of the Large Intestine by a focal stagnation. The initial stagnation that eventually gives rise to Blood stagnation may be prolonged Liver *qi* stagnation, or food stagnation which over time creates Heat and Dampness or Phlegm. By its very nature, *qi* stagnation will ultimately involve Blood stagnation, as '*qi* leads the Blood'. The Heat or Damp Heat produced by chronic food stagnation injures the Intestine by drying and scorching the Intestinal lining and its delicate *luo mai*. Phlegm, being a substantial pathogen and particularly cloying in nature, physically obstructs the circulation of *qi* and Blood at some point. Blood stagnation usually reflects a physical lesion of the Intestine.

Blood stagnation type diarrhoea may also follow abdominal trauma or abdominal surgery.

DIAGNOSIS

The first step is to clearly establish what the patient means by the term diarrhoea. Ask about the patient's normal pattern of bowel movements and how the presenting problem varies from normal. Other patterns not requiring specific treatment should be excluded, such as the loose stools that often occur during a course of treatment for another disorder, particularly in patients with Phlegm Damp patterns. Excess Phlegm Damp is discharged through the stools giving rise to diarrhoea. This type of diarrhoea generally doesn't last long, although in severe cases may persist for a month or two, and requires no specific change of treatment.

As always, the eight principles guide the diagnosis. The first thing to determine is whether the diarrhoea is acute or chronic. Acute disorders are generally less than a few weeks in duration. The diagnostic strategy is outlined

BOX 6.2 KEY DIAGNOSTIC POINTS

Aggravation
- with cold, raw food, or even just eating - Spleen deficiency
- with emotions and stress - Liver *qi* invading the Spleen

Amelioration
- pain that is eased with diarrhoea - Liver *qi* stagnation, food stagnation, Damp Heat, Cold Damp, Spleen and Kidney *yang* deficiency (an exception to the rule)

Nature of the diarrhoea
- explosive - external pathogens
- with mucus - Spleen *qi* deficiency, Liver *qi* stagnation
- preceded by cramping pain - Liver *qi* stagnation, Damp Heat, Summer Heat

Timing
- waking needing to go (often urgently) early in the morning - Spleen and Kidney *yang* deficiency
- soon after eating - Spleen *qi* deficiency

Accompanying symptoms
- with undigested food - Spleen and Kidney *yang* deficiency
- burning anus or tenesmus - Damp Heat
- severe distension, bad breath, belching - food stagnation
- alternating diarrhoea and constipation - Liver *qi* invading the Spleen
- fever - Summer Damp, Damp Heat
- with dark or purple stools or focal pain upon palpation - Blood stagnation

in Figure 6.2.

Take care to always palpate the abdomen, as impacted faeces with spurious diarrhoea is not uncommon, especially in elderly or bedridden patients. In addition, when analysing digestive disorders, abdominal palpation can provide valuable clues in complex or contradictory cases.

Abdominal palpation

In general, the state of the abdomen provides reliable information about the deficient or excess nature of a pattern. A typical example would be distinguishing between the diarrhoea of Cold Damp (excess) and Spleen deficiency. They can coexist, and in practice often look quite similar. In the absence of clear tongue and pulse evidence, how do we determine whether to focus on reducing the Cold Damp or supplementing the Spleen?. Simply supplementing the Spleen may aggravate Dampness; similarly, using

Dampness dispersing treatments may aggravate Spleen deficiency. The key is the abdomen. If the abdomen feels firm or resistant and the patient dislikes pressure, the balance of the pattern is tipped towards excess. If the abdomen is soft or yielding and either does not dislike pressure or welcomes it, the probability is deficiency. This appears to be a reliable sign, even in patients who appear quite the opposite to what the abdomen indicates.

Abdominal palpation can also give information about the Heat or Cold nature of a pathogen. This should be done in two stages at the beginning of the examination, before any actual palpation is done. Firstly, a hand is held just above the surface of the abdomen to detect any areas of radiant Heat or Cold, and then lightly touches the surface of the abdomen. If the practitioner's hand rests too long in one place or too firmly, it will alter the temperature at that locus. Certain temperature findings are common and quite consistent from patient to patient. For example, patients with Spleen *qi* or *yang* deficiency digestive problems often feel cooler in the upper abdomen and epigastrium; patients with Kidney *yang* deficiency often feel cooler in the lower abdomen, below a horizontal line drawn through the navel. Any locus of inflammation in the abdomen will be reflected in warmer tissues above, as any decrease in circulation, from Cold, Blood stagnation etc., will show in cooler areas above.

TCM DIFFERENTIAL DIAGNOSIS

- **Dysenteric disorder** (*li ji* 痢疾): Dysenteric disorder is an acute or chronic inflammation of the large intestine characterised by abdominal pain, tenesmus and diarrhoea mixed with blood, mucus and pus. The key feature is the presence of blood and/or mucus and/or pus.
- **Sudden Turmoil Disorder** (*huo luan* 霍乱): Sudden Turmoil Disorder is a group of transmissible disorders characterised by the acute and simultaneous onset of vomiting and diarrhoea. Biomedical disorders such as acute gastroenteritis, a variety of gastro-intestinal infections and food poisoning may be classified as *huo luan* when associated with sudden vomiting and diarrhoea.

TREATMENT

The patterns discussed here may appear separately or in combination, and patterns can change into one another over time. Complicated cases involving underlying deficiency with excess can be often be analysed and treated using the guidelines of the primary pathological triad (p.912). There are various cautions to observe with certain herbs when treating diarrhoea. Firstly, astringent and supplementing herbs are contraindicated in acute cases, where the principle of treatment is to expel pathogens. Secondly, bitter and cold Heat clearing herbs, if applied over-enthusiastically, can damage the Spleen and cause a deficient type of diarrhoea. Finally, the exclusive use of sweet warm herbs should be avoided when supplementing the Spleen as they can generate Dampness.

In general, both acute and chronic cases of diarrhoea respond well to TCM treatment, with persistence being the key in chronic patterns. The longer a patient has had a problem, the longer it will take to resolve. The more profound deficiency patterns and Blood stagnation may require months of treatment. In acute cases, it is wise to persist with treatment for a few days after the patient has recovered to ensure the complete expulsion of the pathogen.

The diet

In addition to the general dietary guidelines for each pathology, there are some foods that are specifically useful for diarrhoea, and some that should be avoided.

Foods specific for diarrhoea

Generally beneficial	plenty of non diuretic fluids (slightly sweetened, osmotic fluids such as lucozade, dilute juice or lemonade are best), well cooked porridge of rice, oats or barley, leek, eggplant, aduki beans, string beans, carrot, yam, button mushroom, olive, umeboshi plum
Damp Heat	millet or job's tears (yi ren) porridge, tofu, mung bean, pineapple, persimmon, peppermint
Qi and yang deficiency	black and cayenne pepper, dried ginger, nutmeg, chestnut, chicken egg
Restrict or avoid	moistening or laxative foods, honey, milk, apricots, plums and prunes (except umeboshi), sesame seeds, walnuts, pinenuts, oils, coffee, alcohol

Figure 6.2 *Diagnostic strategy for diarrhoea*

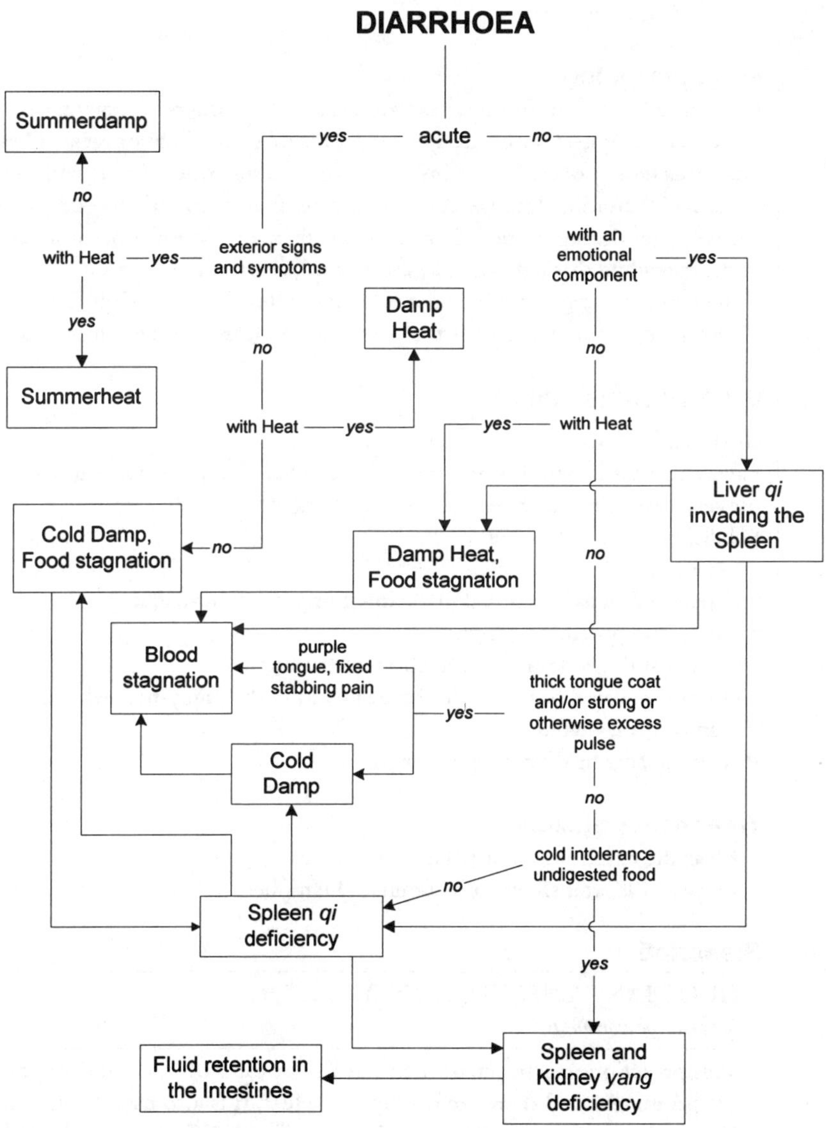

暑病

6.1 SUMMER (SEASONAL) DIARRHOEA

- Summerdamp
- Summerheat

Pathophysiology

- Summerdamp and Summerheat are seasonal disorders characterised by internal Dampness with exterior symptoms of either Cold or Heat. These patterns mostly occur during humid or wet weather, often during late Summer and Autumn, although they may occur at any time of the year. They also appear during sudden changes in weather, and typically occur in clusters, spreading through schools, the workplace or home.
- The main difference between the Summer patterns and the Cold Damp or Damp Heat acute patterns is the presence of clear external symptoms.

6.1.1 Summerdamp

Clinical features

- acute diarrhoea with borborygmus, abdominal cramping and pain; in severe cases the diarrhoea is watery and urgent
- chills, possible mild fever
- no sweating
- generalised muscle aches, dull occipital or general headache
- nausea and possibly vomiting
- fullness and discomfort in the chest and abdomen
- lethargy, malaise, heaviness in the head and body, foggy-headedness

T thin or greasy white coat
P floating, soft or slippery, possibly tight

Treatment principle

Clear the exterior and dispel Summerdamp
Dispel Cold, transform and eliminate Dampness

Prescription

HUO XIANG ZHENG QI SAN 藿香正气散
(*Agastache Formula*)

This prescription is selected when acute symptoms of internal Dampness are prominent and there are no signs of Heat. It is also used for internal Dampness patterns that are stirred up by Wind Cold invasion. This is an extremely effective and frequently used prescription. The diarrhoea may, in some cases, worsen initially as the Damp is discharged.

huo xiang (Herba Agastaches seu Pogostemi) 藿香 12-15g
fu ling (Sclerotium Poriae Cocos) 茯苓 12-15g

hou po (Cortex Magnoliae Officinalis) 厚朴 9-12g
zi su ye (Folium Perillae Frutescentis) 紫苏叶 9-12g
ban xia (Rhizoma Pinelliae Ternatae) 半夏 9-12g
da fu pi (Pericarpium Arecae Catechu) 大服皮 9-12g
bai zhu (Rhizoma Atractylodes Macrocephalae) 白术 9-12g
chen pi (Pericarpium Citri Reticulatae) 陈皮 9-12g
bai zhi (Radix Angelicae Dahuricae) 白芷 6-9g
jie geng (Radix Platycodi Grandiflori) 桔梗 6-9g
gan cao (Radix Glycyrrhizae Uralensis) 甘草 3-6g
sheng jiang (Rhizoma Zingiberis Officinalis Recens)
生姜 6-9g
da zao (Fructus Zizyphi Jujubae) 大枣 2pce

Method: Decoction. The herbs should be gently simmered for no longer than 20 minutes in a pot with a close fitting lid. If nausea is a problem, the decoction can be taken through a straw and sipped slowly, with the straw right at the back of the tongue. **Huo xiang** fragrantly disperses Damp turbidity and harmonises the Stomach; **zi su ye** and **bai zhi** dispel Wind Cold and transform Dampness; **hou po** and **chen pi** regulate and direct *qi* downwards and out, transform Phlegm Damp and alleviate fullness; **ban xia** transforms Phlegm Damp and stops vomiting; **da fu pi** directs *qi* and Damp downwards and out, and alleviates fullness; **bai zhu** and **fu ling** strengthen the Spleen, dry Damp and promote urination to clear Damp; **jie geng** assists the dispersing function of the Lungs; **gan cao**, **sheng jiang** and **da zao** harmonise the other herbs and regulate the Stomach. (Source: *Shi Yong Zhong Yi Nei Ke Xue*)

Modifications

- With severe exterior symptoms (chills, floating, tight pulse, occipital headache and stiff neck), increase the dose of **zi su ye** to 15g, and add **jing jie** (Herba seu Flos Schizonepetae Tenuifolia) 荆芥 12g and **fang feng** (Radix Ledebouriellae Divaricatae) 防风 12g.
- With severe Damp (severe vomiting, thick greasy tongue coat), delete **bai zhu**, and add **cang zhu** (Rhizoma Atractylodis) 苍术 12-15g and **pei lan** (Herba Eupatorii Fortuneii) 佩兰 9-12g.
- Some patients experience frequent severe waves of abdominal cramping preceding diarrhoea when the Cold component is strong. When this occurs, add **gan jiang** (Rhizoma Zingiberis Officinalis) 干姜 9-12g and **chuan jiao** (Pericarpium Zanthoxyli Bungeani) 川椒 3-6g.
- With spasms and cramps in the calf muscle, add **mu gua** (Fructus Chaenomelis) 木瓜 9-12g and **wu zhu yu** (Fructus Evodiae Rutaecarpae) 吴茱萸 3-6g, and increase isotonic fluid or salt intake.
- With scanty urine, add **mu tong** (Caulis Mutong) 木通 6-9g and **ze xie** (Rhizoma Alismatis Orientalis) 泽泻 9-12g.

Patent medicines

Xing Jun San 行军散 (Marching Powder, Five Pagodas Brand)

- This is one of the most effective patents for acute diarrhoea of a Summerdamp and Cold Damp type. An extremely fragrant green powder, it can be taken in small doses (¼ - ½ teaspoon) every 30-60 minutes.

Huo Xiang Zheng Qi Pian 藿香正气片 (Huo Xiang Zheng Qi Pian, Huo Hsiang Cheng Chi Pien)
Zhui Feng Su He Wan 追风苏合丸 (So Hup Yuen Medical Pills)
Shen Qu Cha 神曲茶 (Shen Chu Cha)

Acupuncture

See Summerheat.

6.1.2 Summerheat

Clinical features

- acute, frequent, urgent, foul, explosive diarrhoea
- relatively high fever which is unrelieved by sweating, possibly mild chills
- may or may not be sweating
- thirst, dry mouth
- concentrated urine
- irritability and restlessness
- heaviness in the body, foggy-headedness, headache
- nausea and vomiting
- fatigue and lethargy
- may be sore throat
- in general all symptoms are worse around mid afternoon

T greasy white or yellow coat
P floating, rapid, soggy, soft

Treatment principle

Clear the exterior and dispel Summerheat
Clear Heat, transform and eliminate Dampness

Prescription

XIN JIA XIANG RU YIN 新加香薷饮
(*Newly Augmented Elsholtzia Decoction*)

xiang ru (Herba Elsholtzia seu Moslae) 香薷 9-15g
jin yin hua (Flos Lonicerae Japonicae) 金银花 12-18g
lian qiao (Fructus Forsythia Suspensae) 连翘 6-9g
bian dou (Semen Dolichos Lablab) 扁豆 9-15g
hou po (Cortex Magnoliae Officinalis) 厚朴 6-9g

Method: Decoction. The herbs should be gently simmered for no longer than 20 minutes in a pot with a tight fitting lid. This formula should be taken cool as **xiang**

ru can cause vomiting when taken hot. **Xiang ru** promotes sweating and clears the exterior, expels Summerheat and transforms Dampness; **jin yin hua** and **lian qiao** clear Summerheat and Toxic Heat from the *qi* level and upper *jiao*; **bian dou** strengthens the Spleen and leaches out Dampness; **hou po** directs *qi* downwards and alleviates fullness. (Source: *Zhong Yi Nei Ke Lin Chuang Shou Ce*)

NB: The diarrhoea may initially worsen as the Dampness is discharged.

Patent medicines

Bao Ji Wan 保济丸 (Po Chai Pills)
Shen Qu Cha 神曲茶 (Shen Chu Cha)

Acupuncture (select from)

LI.11 (*qu chi* -) .... *he* sea point of the Large Intestine, clears Dampness and Damp Heat from *yang ming*
LI.4 (*he gu* -) .... *yuan* point of the Large Intestine, opens the pores and expels pathogens from the surface
zhi xie (N-CA-3) .... extra point for diarrhoea, located halfway between Ren.8 (*shen que*) and the pubic bone; add moxa if Cold
St.25 (*tian shu* -) .... *mu* point of the Large Intestine, regulates the Intestines, clears Dampness and Damp Heat and stops diarrhoea; add moxa if Cold
St.37 (*shan ju xu* -) .... lower *he* point of the Large Intestine, regulates and eliminates stagnation and accumulation from the Stomach and Intestines
Sp.9 (*yin ling quan*) .... *he* sea point of the Spleen, promotes urination to drains Dampness and Damp Heat
Bl.25 (*da chang shu* -) .... *shu* point of the Large Intestine, clears Dampness and Damp Heat and stops diarrhoea

- with high fever, add Du.14 (*da zhui* -) and SJ.5 (*wai guan* -)
- with chills and occipital headache, add Du.14 (*da zhui* Ω), Bl.13 (*fei shu* Ω) and LI.4 (*he gu* -)
- with nausea, add PC.6 (*nei guan*)
- with myalgia, add Sp.21 (*da bao*)
- with foggy-headedness, add *yin tang* (M-HN-3) and Du.20 (*bai hui*)
- with sudden severe diarrhoea, vomiting and fever, bleed PC.3 (*qu ze* ↓) and Bl.40 (*wei zhong* ↓) with a lancet and extract a few drops of blood. *See also* Chapter 24.2 Sudden Turmoil Disorder.
- with severe Cold causing strong griping pain that occurs in waves and precedes the diarrhoea, moxa can be applied with a moxa box over the umbilicus, or with moxa cones over slices of ginger. Select 2-3 abdominal points close to the pain.
- *Ear points*: lungs, large intestine, small intestine, spleen, abdomen, sympathetic

Clinical notes

- Summerdamp and Summerheat type diarrhoea may be diagnosed biomedically as acute gastroenteritis, food poisoning, gastric flu, influenza or acute colitis.
- The acute Summerdamp or Summerheat patterns respond well to early treatment, but have a tendency to drag on or become recurrent if neglected. This frequently occurs in patients who return to work or activity before they are fully recovered and the Dampness completely cleared. They may continue to have relapses for several weeks or longer. For patients prone to this pattern or those at risk (for example, those living in humid climates or who are run down), a small dose of the patent medicine *Xing Jun San* 行军散 (Marching Powder) at the first hint of gastro-intestinal distress can nip potential episodes in the bud.
- Fluid and electrolyte replacement is important, especially in infants and young children, who can become dangerously dehydrated quite quickly. Oral isotonic fluid replacement solution should be administered in small amounts frequently. Isotonic solution can be made by adding 3.5 grams of household salt ($NaCl$), 2.5 grams of sodium bicarbonate, 1.5 grams of potassium chloride (KCl) and 20 grams of sugar to one litre of water. Isotonic drinks are commercially available. Alternatively use lemonade with a teaspoon of salt.

Table 6.2. *Comparison of common causes of acute diarrhoea*

Pathogen	Location	Common features	Specific features	Prescription
Cold Damp	external (Summerdamp)	watery urgent diarrhoea with borborygmus, abdominal cramping and pain, thick tongue coat	chills and fever, myalgia, headache, floating pulse	HUO XIANG ZHENG QI TANG
	internal		slippery pulse, abdominal distension	PING WEI SAN WEI LING TANG
Damp Heat	external (Summerheat)	frequent, urgent, explosive, burning, foul smelling diarrhoea	fever and chills unrelieved by sweating, thirst, scanty urine, irritability, floating rapid pulse	XIN JIA XIANG RU YIN
	internal		slippery pulse, afternoon fever, tenesmus	GE GEN HUANG QIN HUANG LIAN TANG

大肠湿热

6.2 DAMP HEAT

Pathophysiology

- This pattern is usually due to invasion by pathogenic Damp Heat which prevails in Summer, late Summer and Autumn, but may occur at any time. It may also be associated with inappropriate use of purgative herbs during an external (*tai yang*) disorder that weakens the Spleen and Stomach, facilitating invasion by the pathogen into *yang ming*.
- Damp Heat diarrhoea can also be the result of internally generated Damp Heat, in which case it may present as either an acute episode of diarrhoea, or more chronic or recurrent diarrhoea. In either case, the diarrhoea is clearly related to ingestion of Damp Heat engendering foods and alcohol.
- In contrast to the Summer Dampness pattern, the Damp Heat symptoms in this pattern is more concentrated in the Intestines.

Clinical features

- acute or recurrent, frequent, urgent, foul smelling, hot diarrhoea, with a burning anus and/or tenesmus
- fever or afternoon fever which is unrelieved with sweating
- sweating that tends to come in waves and is worse in the afternoon
- restlessness and irritability
- cramping abdominal pain
- concentrated scanty urine
- thirst

T greasy yellow coat; may be red tongue body

P slippery and rapid

Treatment principle

Clear Damp Heat from the Intestines
Stop diarrhoea

Prescription

GE GEN HUANG GEN HUANG LIAN TANG 葛根黄芩黄连汤
(*Kudzu, Coptis and Scute Combination*)

wei ge gen (roasted Radix Puerariae) 煨葛根 12-15g
huang qin (Radix Scutellariae Baicalensis) 黄芩 9-12g
huang lian (Rhizoma Coptidis) 黄连 6-9g
gan cao (Radix Glycyrrhizae Uralensis) 甘草 3-6g

Method: Decoction. **Wei ge gen** dispels Heat and alleviates diarrhoea; **huang qin** and **huang lian** clear Damp Heat from the Intestines, **gan cao** protects the Stomach. (Source: *Shi Yong Zhong Yi Nei Ke Xue*)

Modifications

- With prominent Dampness (thick, greasy tongue coat and slippery pulse), add **cang zhu** (Rhizoma Atractylodis) 苍术 12-15g, **fu ling** (Sclerotium Poriae Cocos) 茯苓 12-15g and **yi ren** (Semen Coicis Lachryma-jobi) 苡仁 15-30g.
- With prominent Heat (strong fever, burning anus, yellow tongue coat, rapid pulse), add **jin yin hua** (Flos Lonicerae Japonicae) 金银花 15-30g, **lian qiao** (Fructus Forsythia Suspensae) 连翘 9-12g and **shan zhi zi** (Fructus Gardeniae Jasminoides) 山栀子 9-12g.
- With severe diarrhoea, add **ma chi xian** (Herba Portulacae Oleraceae) 马齿苋 15-18g.
- With cramping abdominal pain, add **mu xiang** (Radix Aucklandiae Lappae) 木香 6-9g and **bai shao** (Radix Paeoniae Lactiflorae) 白芍 9-12g.
- With bleeding, add **di yu** (Radix Sanguisorbae Officinalis) 地榆 9-12g and **huai hua mi** (Flos Sophorae Japonicae Immaturus) 槐花米 9-12g.
- With nausea or vomiting, add **ban xia** (Rhizoma Pinelliae Ternatae) 半夏 9-12g and **zhu ru** (Caulis Bambusae in Taeniis) 竹茹 12-15g.
- With abdominal distension, add **hou po** (Cortex Magnoliae Officinalis) 厚朴 9-12g and **zhi ke** (Fructus Citri Aurantii) 枳壳 9-12g.
- With difficult or scanty urination, add **hua shi** (Talcum) 滑石 12-18g.
- With food stagnation or diarrhoea associated with overindulgence, add **jiao shen qu** (baked Massa Fermentata) 焦神曲 15g, **chao mai ya** (dry fried Fructus Hordei Vulgaris Germinantus) 炒麦芽 15-30g, **jiao shan zha** (baked Fructus Crataegi) 焦山楂 15g.
- With signs of residual Wind Heat, or Damp Heat in the Intestines that is stirred up by a Wind Heat attack, add **jin yin hua** (Flos Lonicerae Japonicae) 金银花 15-30g, **lian qiao** (Fructus Forsythia Suspensae) 连翘 9-12g and **bo he** (Herba Mentha Haplocalycis) 薄荷 6g.
- With evidence of infection by the parasite *Giardia lamblia*, add **qing hao** (Herba Artemisiae Annuae) 青蒿 15g and **da suan** (Bulbus Alli Sativi) 大蒜 6-9g. These herbs can also be decocted separately and given as an enema.

Variations and additional prescriptions

Spurious diarrhoea

- Damp Heat diarrhoea should be distinguished from the false diarrhoea known as 'spurious', in which green, watery, foul, diarrhoea-like fluids are forced around an impacted stool in the descending or sigmoid colon. It occurs most commonly in the elderly or bedridden. The key finding is the mass that will be palpated in the left iliac fossa. *See* **HUANG LONG TANG** (*Yellow Dragon Decoction* 黄龙汤, p.176).

Patent medicines

Huang Lian Jie Du Wan 黄连解毒丸 (Huang Lian Jie Du Wan)
Chuan Xin Lian Kang Yan Pian 穿心莲抗炎片 (Chuan Xin Lian Antiphlogistic Tablets)
Bao Ji Wan 保济丸 (Po Chai Pills)
Huang Lian Su Pian 黄连素片 (Huang Lien Su Tablets)

Acupuncture (select from)

LI.11 (*qu chi* -) .... *he* sea point of the Large Intestine, clears Damp Heat from *yang ming*
zhi xie - (N-CA-3) .... extra point for diarrhoea, located halfway between Ren.8 (*shen que*) and the pubic bone
St.25 (*tian shu* -) .... *mu* point of the Large Intestine, regulates the Intestines, clears Damp Heat and stops diarrhoea
St.44 (*nei ting* -) .... *rong* spring and Water point of the Stomach, clears Heat from *yang ming*
Sp.9 (*yin ling quan* -) .... *he* sea point of the Spleen, promotes urination and drains Damp Heat
St.37 (*shang ju xu* -) .... lower *he* point of the Large Intestine, eliminates stagnation from the Stomach and Intestines and clears Damp Heat

- with high fever, add Du.14 (*da zhui* -) and LI.4 (*he gu* -)
- with nausea, add PC.6 (*nei guan*)
- with sudden severe diarrhoea, vomiting and fever, bleed PC.3 (*qu ze* ↓) and Bl.40 (*wei zhong* ↓) with a lancet and extract a few drops of blood. May also be needled with a reducing method.
- *Ear points*: large intestine, small intestine, spleen, abdomen, distal segment rectum, sympathetic

Clinical notes

- Damp Heat type diarrhoea may be diagnosed biomedically as acute or chronic gastroenteritis, acute or chronic enteritis, acute or chronic colitis, food poisoning, giardiasis or bacillary dysentery.
- Damp Heat patterns can linger, sometimes at a subclinical level, for long periods, and the classic signs of Damp Heat may be minimal or confused. This can occur because the patient's diet continually feeds the Damp Heat, or because the initial pathogen was never properly cleared and became latent. The latter is quite common in patients who contract an exotic gastro-intestinal bug while travelling in tropical countries. Erroneous attempts to supplement the Spleen on the assumption of some deficiency will clarify the diagnosis. The patient usually gets worse, or at least gets no better. *See also* p.245.

大肠寒湿

6.3 COLD DAMP

Pathophysiology

- Cold Damp in the gastro-intestinal system is due to overindulgence in cold and raw food, fruit, juices or tea, or exposure to external cold and damp. It also may occur following a course of antibiotics or other cooling drugs.
- Cold Damp in the Intestines can be acute, or intermittent and recurrent. When recurrent and chronic, it can be the result of an acute episode that was never resolved properly, or of a diet that consists largely of cold or Dampening foods.
- The presence of Cold Damp in the gastro-intestinal system will eventually weaken Spleen *yang*, so a mixed deficiency excess pattern may develop. There may, of course, have been pre-existing Spleen deficiency that allowed the Cold Damp to enter.
- In contrast to the Summerdamp pattern, which the Cold Damp pattern resembles, there are no exterior symptoms.

Clinical features

- Acute, or chronic and recurrent diarrhoea, which can range from simply loose to watery and urgent. The patient may double up in an attempt to warm the abdomen, and dislike abdominal palpation as it may increase any discomfort.
- cramping or colicky abdominal pain
- borborygmus
- fullness and distension in the epigastrium and abdomen
- loss of appetite, reduced sense of taste
- nausea
- increased desire to sleep
- heavy sensation in the body
- clear urine

T thick, greasy white coat
P moderate and slippery or soft

Treatment principle

Warm and dry Cold Damp (or drain Dampness with bland herbs)
Strengthen the Spleen and stop diarrhoea

Prescription

PING WEI SAN 平胃散
(*Magnolia and Ginger Formula*)

This prescription is selected in milder cases with loose stools.

cang zhu (Rhizoma Atractylodis) 苍术 12-15g

hou po (Cortex Magnoliae Officinalis) 厚朴 9-12g
chen pi (Pericarpium Citri Reticulatae) 陈皮 9-12g
zhi gan cao (honey fried Radix Glycyrrhizae Uralensis)
炙甘草 3-6g

Method: Grind the herbs to a powder and take 6-9 grams twice daily with warm water. May also be decocted with the quantities as shown. **Cang zhu** powerfully warms and dries Dampness; **hou po** regulates *qi* and transforms Dampness; **chen pi** regulates *qi*; **zhi gan cao** strengthens the Spleen and supplements *qi*. (Source: *Shi Yong Zhong Yi Nei Ke Xue*)

WEI LING TANG 胃苓汤
(*Magnolia and Hoelen Combination*)

This prescription is selected for urgent watery diarrhoea. It contains bland diuretic herbs to assist in the elimination of Dampness through urination.

cang zhu (Rhizoma Atractylodis) 苍术 12-15g
fu ling (Sclerotium Poriae Cocos) 茯苓 12-15g
zhu ling (Sclerotium Polypori Umbellati) 猪苓 12-15g
bai zhu (Rhizoma Atractylodes Macrocephalae) 白术 12-15g
hou po (Cortex Magnoliae Officinalis) 厚朴 9-12g
chen pi (Pericarpium Citri Reticulatae) 陈皮 9-12g
gui zhi (Ramulus Cinnamomi Cassiae) 桂枝 6-9g
ze xie (Rhizoma Alismatis Orientalis) 泽泻 9-12g
gan cao (Radix Glycyrrhizae Uralensis) 甘草 3-6g

Method: Grind the herbs to a powder and take 6-9 grams 2-3 times daily with warm water. May also be decocted with the quantities as shown. This prescription combines **PING WEI SAN** above with **WU LING SAN** (*Hoelen Five Formula* 五苓散) to increase the diuretic effect so as to lead Dampness away from the bowel to be eliminated through the urine. (Source: *Shi Yong Zhong Yi Nei Ke Xue*)

Modifications

- With severe Cold causing spasmodic abdominal pain that improves with warmth, add **gan jiang** (Rhizoma Zingiberis Officinalis) 干姜 6-9g and **gao liang jiang** (Rhizoma Alpiniae Officinari) 高良姜 9-12g.
- With nausea, add **ban xia** (Rhizoma Pinelliae Ternatae) 半夏 9-12g.
- With food stagnation, distension and indigestion, add **shen qu** (Massa Fermentata) 神曲 15g, **shan zha** (Fructus Crataegi) 山楂 15g and **chao lai fu zi** (dry fried Semen Raphani Sativi) 炒莱服子 15g.
- With acid reflux or sour regurgitation, add **huang lian** (Rhizoma Coptidis) 黄连 6g and **wu zhu yu** (Fructus Evodiae Rutaecarpae) 吴茱萸 2g.
- With a component of *qi* stagnation, add **xiang fu** (Rhizoma Cyperi Rotundi) 香附 9-12g, **mu xiang** (Radix Aucklandiae Lappae) 木香 6-9g and **fo shou** (Fructus Citri Sarcodactylis) 佛手 9-12g.

- With tenesmus, add **mu xiang** (Radix Aucklandiae Lappae) 木香 6-9g and **sha ren** (Fructus Amomi) 砂仁 6-9g.

Variations and additional prescriptions

With Spleen yang deficiency

- If there is underlying Spleen *yang* deficiency, or if retention of Cold damages Spleen *yang*, **LI ZHONG WAN** (*Ginseng and Ginger Formula* 理中丸, p.150) should be used following the resolution of the Dampness.

In difficult cases

- In recalcitrant or recurrent cases, consider the possibility of intestinal or systemic parasites (*see* Chapter 2.7, p.92), deeply rooted Dampness (p.245), or the primary pathological triad (p.912).

Patent medicines

Ping Wei San 平胃散 (Ping Wei San, Tabellae Pingwei)
Xiang Sha Liu Jun Zi Wan 香砂六君子丸 (Xiang Sha Liu Jun Wan, Aplotaxis-Ammomum Pills, Six Gentlemen Tea Pills)
- with Spleen *qi* deficiency

Fu Zi Li Zhong Wan 附子理中丸 (Fu Tzu Li Chung Wan, Carmichaeli Tea Pills, Li Chung Yuen Medical Pills)
- for *yang* deficiency with Cold

Xing Jun San 行军散 (Marching Powder, Five Pagodas Brand)
- For this pattern, this patent medicine is one of the backup formulae used in those cases that do not progress as expected. Sometimes a few days of this powder can powerfully root out deeply lodged Damp and help shift a difficult condition.

Acupuncture (select from)

St.25 (*tian shu* -▲) .... *mu* point of the Large Intestine, warms the Intestines, dispels Cold Damp and stops diarrhoea

zhi xie (N-CA-3 ▲) .... extra point for diarrhoea, located halfway between Ren.8 (*shen que*) and the pubic bone

St.36 (*zu san li* -▲) .... *he* sea point of the Stomach, powerfully warms and strengthens the Spleen and Stomach and supplements *qi* to overcome Cold Damp

St.37 (*shan ju xu* -) .... lower *he* point of the Large Intestine, eliminates Cold Damp from the Intestines

Sp.9 (*yin ling quan* -) .... *he* sea point of the Spleen, promotes urination and drains Dampness

Sp.6 (*san yin jiao* -) .... strengthens the Spleen to transform Dampness

Sp.3 (*tai bai* -) .... *yuan*, *shu* stream and Earth point of the Spleen, strengthens the Spleen to transforms Dampness

Bl.25 (*da chang shu* -) .... *shu* point of the Large Intestine, clears Dampness from the Large Intestine and stops diarrhoea

- with nausea, add PC.6 (*nei guan*)
- with cramping abdominal pain, moxa can be applied with a moxa box over the umbilicus, or with moxa cones over slices of ginger.
- *Ear points*: large intestine, small intestine, spleen, abdomen, distal segment rectum, sympathetic

Clinical notes

- Cold Damp diarrhoea may be diagnosed biomedically as gastroenteritis, food poisoning, cholera, stomach flu, functional weakness of the stomach, hypochlorhydria, chronic gastritis and colitis.
- This pattern usually responds well and quickly to correct treatment, however Cold Damp can sometimes persist and become latent. This sometimes follows inappropriate antibiotic treatment or a cold raw diet. Difficult cases which linger at a low level and never properly resolve, or which recur with the least provocation, may be due to deeply rooted Dampness that is never completely dried and expelled. *See* p.245.
- For dietary recommendations, see pp. 873, 880.

饮食积滞

6.4 FOOD STAGNATION

Pathophysiology

- Food stagnation is generally related to overindulgence or irregular eating habits. In the Western world, where people are generally sedentary and habitually eat too much, or eat hard to digest food, eat too quickly, at odd hours, or while working and stressed, the pattern can develops insidiously (*see* p.3). The Spleen and Stomach are regularly overtaxed by new food being ingested on top of partially digested food from the last meal. The digestion fails to cope with the consistent demands placed upon it and food putrefies before it can be processed. Most frequently, food stagnation gives rise to upper gastro-intestinal symptoms such as nausea, acid reflux or abdominal bloating. When complicated by Damp Heat, food stagnation is more likely to cause diarrhoea.
- Because chronic food stagnation is usually associated with a degree of Spleen weakness, there will usually be elements of Dampness. Similarly, chronic stagnation frequently generates Heat. Over time, the Dampness is congealed by the Heat into Damp Heat, Phlegm or Phlegm Heat.
- Clinically, food stagnation can be pure excess, or a mixture of excess and Spleen deficiency. As the pattern progresses, the deficiency elements may become more and more prominent.

Clinical features

- acute or chronic diarrhoea with foul smelling stools and possibly undigested food
- abdominal and epigastric distension and/or pain and/or and borborygmus, all of which are relieved following diarrhoea or belching; abdominal pain is worse for pressure
- foul belching, halitosis
- acid reflux, nausea
- foul flatulence

T thick white or yellow greasy coat

P wiry and slippery or slippery and rapid

Treatment principle

Alleviate food stagnation and harmonise the Stomach

Clear Damp Heat, transform Phlegm or Phlegm Heat, warm the Stomach, strengthen the Spleen (as necessary)

Prescription

BAO HE WAN 保和丸
(*Citrus and Crategus Formula*)

chao shan zha (dry fried Fructus Crataegi) 炒山楂 18-24g
chao shen qu (dry fried Massa Fermentata) 炒神曲 12-15g
fu ling (Sclerotium Poriae Cocos) 茯苓 12-15g
ban xia (Rhizoma Pinelliae Ternatae) 半夏 9-12g
chen pi (Pericarpium Citri Reticulatae) 陈皮 9-12g
chao lai fu zi (dry fried Semen Raphani Sativi)
炒莱服子 9-12g
lian qiao (Fructus Forsythia Suspensae) 连翘 6-9g

Method: Grind herbs to a powder and form into 9-gram pills with water. The dose is one pill 2-3 times daily. May also be decocted with the quantities as shown. **Chao shan zha**, **chao shen qu** and **chao lai fu zi** improve digestion and alleviate food stagnation; **chao lai fu zi** transforms Phlegm Damp; **ban xia** and **chen pi** harmonise the Stomach, resolve Phlegm and promote the movement of *qi*; **fu ling** strengthens the Spleen and leaches out Damp; **lian qiao** dissipates accumulations and clears Heat. (Source: *Shi Yong Zhong Yi Nei Ke Xue*)

Modifications

- With severe bloating, add **zhi shi** (Fructus Immaturus Citri Aurantii) 枳实 9-12g and **hou po** (Cortex Magnoliae Officinalis) 厚朴 9-12g.
- With nausea, add **sheng jiang** (Rhizoma Zingiberis Officinalis Recens) 生姜 9-12g.
- With Heat (irritability, red tongue tip and sides), add **shan zhi zi** (Fructus Gardeniae Jasminoides) 山栀子 9-12g and **huang lian** (Rhizoma Coptidis) 黄连 6-9g.
- With Phlegm Heat, add **zhu ru** (Caulis Bambusae in Taeniis) 竹茹 12-15g.
- With Cold in the Stomach, delete **lian qiao**, and add **gan jiang** (Rhizoma Zingiberis Officinalis) 干姜 6-9g and **sha ren** (Fructus Amomi) 砂仁 6-9g.
- With Spleen deficiency, delete **lian qiao** and add **bai zhu** (Rhizoma Atractylodes Macrocephalae) 白术 12-15g.

Variations and additional prescriptions

Chronic food stagnation with Damp Heat

- For more chronic cases, with significant digestive disruption and the generation of Damp Heat or Phlegm Heat, the aim of treatment is to guide stagnation downward and clear Damp Heat or Phlegm Heat with **ZHI SHI DAO ZHI WAN** (*Immature Bitter Orange Pill to Guide out Stagnation* 枳实导滞丸, p.181). This prescription uses **da huang**, normally contraindicated in diarrhoea, according to the principle of 'increasing movement to treat disorders characterised by too much movement'. Removal of the congested Damp Heat and food will alleviate the diarrhoea. For diarrhoea, this prescription is generally not used for more than a week or two.

With Spleen deficiency

- When there is significant Spleen and Stomach deficiency, either preceding, or as a result of, chronic food stagnation, the treatment is to strengthen the Spleen and Stomach while resolving food stagnation, with a prescription such as **JIAN PI WAN** (*Strengthen the Spleen Pill*) 健脾丸.

  dang shen (Radix Codonopsis Pilosulae) 党参 60g
  chao bai zhu (dry fried Rhizoma Atractylodes Macrocephalae) 炒白术 60g
  chao mai ya (dry fried Fructus Hordei Vulgaris Germinantus) 炒麦芽 30g
  chen pi (Pericarpium Citri Reticulatae) 陈皮 30g
  chao shan zha (dry fried Fructus Crataegi) 炒山楂 30g
  chao shen qu (dry fried Massa Fermentata) 炒神曲 30g
  zhi shi (Fructus Immaturus Citri Aurantii) 枳实 90g

  Method: Grind the herbs to a fine powder and form into 6-gram pills with water or ginger juice. The dose is 2-3 pills daily. May also be decocted with a 60-90% reduction in quantities. **Dang shen** and **chao bai zhu** strengthen the Spleen; **chao mai ya**, **chao shan zha** and **chao shen qu** alleviate food stagnation and improve digestion; **chen pi** regulates *qi*; **zhi shi** regulates *qi* and directs *qi* downwards. (Source: *Shi Yong Fang Ji Xue*)

Patent medicines

Bao He Wan 保和丸 (Bao He Wan)
Shen Qu Cha 神曲茶 (Shen Chu Cha)
Liu He Bao He Wan 六合保和丸 (Bo Wo Yuen Medical Pills)
Jian Pi Wan 健脾丸 (Jian Pi Wan)
 - with Spleen deficiency

Acupuncture (select from)

Ren.12 (*zhong wan* -) .... *mu* point of the Stomach, clears stagnation of food and Heat from the Stomach
St.25 (*tian shu* -) .... *mu* point of the Large Intestine, clears food stagnation and Heat from the Intestines and stops diarrhoea
St.40 (*feng long* -) .... *luo* point of the Stomach, clears stagnant food, Heat and Phlegm from the Stomach and Intestines
St.36 (*zu san li* -) .... *he* sea point of the Stomach, regulates and

strengthens the Spleen and Stomach and stops diarrhoea

St.37 (*shan ju xu* -) .... lower *he* point of the Large Intestine, regulates and eliminates stagnation from the Stomach and Intestines

St.44 (*nei ting* -) .... *rong* spring and Water point of the Stomach, clears Heat from the Stomach and alleviates food stagnation

LI.10 (*shou san li* -) .... benefits digestion and regulates gastro-intestinal function

- with nausea, add PC.6 (*nei guan* -)
- with abdominal bloating, add Sp.4 (*gong sun* -) or Sp.5 (*shang qiu* -)
- with Spleen deficiency, add Sp.6 (*san yin jiao*)
- with abdominal pain, add Sp.8 (*di ji* -) and Liv.5 (*li gou* -)
- *Ear points*: stomach, spleen, abdomen, large intestine, small intestine, sympathetic

Clinical notes

- This is a disorder of gluttony and dietary irregularity. In isolation it needs no treatment other than a sensible approach to diet and exercise, however if bad habits persist it can become a more serious problem.
- The Chinese have long known the benefits of sipping small amounts of certain teas while eating. The action of such teas helps assist digestion, especially of fats, and reduces the risk of food stagnation. European cultures use table wine in much the same way, hence 'a little wine for thy stomach's sake'. Similarly, 'bitters', combinations of bitter herbs and alcohol, are a common accompaniment to food, either as a digestive aid following a meal, or as an aperitive. The bitterness of the herbs assists the descent of Stomach *qi* and dries Damp.

肝气犯脾

6.5 LIVER QI INVADING THE SPLEEN

Pathophysiology

- The mechanism of the diarrhoea here is one of hypertonicity of the biomedical intestine, coupled with a gradual weakening of digestive function. The constant tension in the Intestinal wall leads to a reduction in circulation of *qi* and Blood and reduced harvesting of *qi* across the Intestinal wall. In addition, the weakened Spleen produced Dampness that sinks downwards.
- In the early stages of this pattern it tends to be intermittent and correspond with an escalation of stress; as it progresses the Spleen is progressively weakened, the Liver more readily invades, and the diarrhoea becomes more frequent.
- There are several complications that may occur as a result of the chronic *qi* stagnation. Stagnant Heat can be generated. The Heat may combine with any Dampness to create Damp Heat. Heat may damage Intestinal *yin*. Heat may cause Blood to move recklessly or damage the *luo mai* of the Intestine, causing bleeding. Chronic *qi* stagnation will eventually cause Blood to stagnate.

Clinical features

- Recurrent diarrhoea which may be urgent and preceded by cramping abdominal pain; the pain is relieved following defecation The diarrhoea may alternate with constipation. The diarrhoea may be frequent and explosive and initiated or aggravated by emotional stress and tension or by eating. There may be mucus in the stools or occasional bleeding.
- abdominal distension
- poor appetite, nausea
- heartburn, indigestion
- borborygmus
- flatulence and belching, which relieve abdominal discomfort
- hypochondriac discomfort, ache or tightness, generally worse on the right side
- irritability, depression, moodiness
- shoulder and neck tension, temporal or tension headaches
- cold fingers and toes
- premenstrual syndrome and breast tenderness

T normal or darkish body, or pale, or with slightly red edges; greasy coat, especially over to root (depending on the degree of Heat, deficiency and Dampness)

P wiry

Treatment principle

Harmonise the Liver and Spleen, regulate Liver *qi*
Support and strengthen the Spleen
Alleviate spasm and pain, and stop diarrhoea

Prescription

TONG XIE YAO FANG 痛泻要方
(*Important Formula for Painful Diarrhoea*)

This is the basic prescription to treat chronic abdominal pain and diarrhoea from Liver *qi* stagnation. It can be taken, modified appropriately, for months, and will gradually relax and restore the damaged Intestine.

chao bai shao (dry fried Radix Paeoniae Lactiflorae) 炒白芍 15-24g
chao bai zhu (dry fried Rhizoma Atractylodes Macrocephalae) 炒白术 12-15g
chen pi (Pericarpium Citri Reticulatae) 陈皮 9-12g
fang feng (Radix Ledebouriellae Divaricatae) 防风 9-12g

Method: Decoction. **Chao bai shao** softens the Liver and alleviates spasm and pain in the Intestine; **chao bai zhu** strengthens the Spleen to bolster it against invasion by the Liver; **chen pi** regulates *qi*; **fang feng** assists **chao bai shao** in alleviating cramping and calming the Intestines. (Source: *Zhong Yi Nei Ke Lin Chuang Shou Ce*)

Modifications

- To enhance the Liver *qi* moving action of the prescription, add **chai hu** (Radix Bupleuri) 柴胡 9-12g, **qing pi** (Pericarpium Citri Reticulatae Viridae) 青皮 9-12g and **xiang fu** (Rhizoma Cyperi Rotundi) 香附 9-12g.
- With watery diarrhoea, add **fu ling** (Sclerotium Poriae Cocos) 茯苓 12-15g and **che qian zi** (Semen Plantaginis) 车前子 9-12g.
- With severe abdominal pain, increase the dose of **bai shao** (Radix Paeoniae Lactiflorae) 白芍 to 30g, and add **gan cao** (Radix Glycyrrhizae Uralensis) 甘草 6-9g and **yan hu suo** (Rhizoma Corydalis Yanhusuo) 延胡索 9-12g.
- With flatulence, add **chao shan zha** (dry fried Fructus Crataegi) 炒山楂 15g and **chao shen qu** (dry fried Massa Fermentata) 炒神曲 15g.
- With tenesmus, add **mu xiang** (Radix Aucklandiae Lappae) 木香 6-9g and **bing lang** (Semen Arecae Catechu) 槟榔 9-12g.
- With bleeding, add **di yu** (Radix Sanguisorbae Officinalis) 地榆 9-12g and **san qi fen** (powdered Radix Notoginseng) 三七粉 3-6g.
- With mucus in the stools, add **cang zhu** (Rhizoma Atractylodis) 苍术 12-15g.
- With food stagnation (epigastric and abdominal fullness, foul belching, a thick tongue coat), add **chao mai ya** (dry fried Fructus Hordei Vulgaris Germinantus) 炒麦芽 15-30g, **chao shan zha** (dry fried Fructus Crataegi)

炒山楂 15g and **chao shen qu** (dry fried Massa Fermentata) 炒神曲 15g.

- With mild signs of stagnant Blood, add **dan shen** (Radix Salviae Miltiorrhizae) 丹参 12-15g, **yu jin** (Tuber Curcumae) 郁金 9-12g and **yan hu suo** (Rhizoma Corydalis Yanhusuo) 延胡索 9-12g.
- For patients who are nervous or anxious, add **he huan pi** (Cortex Albizziae Julibrissin) 合欢皮 15g, **wu wei zi** (Fructus Schizandrae Chinensis) 五味子 6g and **fu xiao mai** (Semen Tritici Aestivi Levis) 浮小麦 30g.
- With depression, add **yu jin** (Tuber Curcumae) 郁金 9-12g, **he huan pi** (Cortex Albizziae Julibrissin) 合欢皮 15g and **xiang fu** (Rhizoma Cyperi Rotundi) 香附 9-12g.
- In severe or resistant cases, select one two appropriate astringent herbs from Table 7.2 (p.301).

Variations and additional prescriptions

With Spleen qi deficiency

- If the Spleen is predominantly weak, 'inviting' the invasion of Liver *qi*, the resulting diarrhoea or loose stools are aggravated or initiated with stress, and are accompanied by dull hypochondriac pain, fatigue, poor appetite, shortness of breath, weak voice, abdominal distension, tightness in the epigastrium but a soft yeilding abdomen, a pale swollen tongue and a weak pulse. The aim of treatment is to focus firstly on strengthening the Spleen and secondly on regulating Liver *qi* with **SI JUN ZI TANG** (*Four Major Herbs Combination* 四君子汤) modified.

  dang shen (Radix Codonopsis Pilosulae) 党参 15-24g
  chao bai zhu (dry fried Rhizoma Atractylodes Macrocephalae) 炒白术 12-15g
  fu ling (Sclerotium Poria Cocos) 茯苓 12-15g
  zhi gan cao (honey fried Radix Glycyrrhizae Uralensis) 炙甘草 3-6g
  chao bai shao (dry fried Radix Paeoniae Lactiflorae) 炒白芍 12-24g
  chai hu (Radix Bupleuri) 柴胡 9-12g

  Method: Decoction. **Dang shen**, **chao bai zhu**, **fu ling** and **zhi gan cao** strengthen the Spleen and supplement *qi*; **chao bai shao** and **chai hu** soften the Liver, ease spasms and regulate Liver *qi*.

With stagnant Heat

- *See* Dysenteric disorder, p.283.

With Damp Heat

- *See* Dysenteric disorder, p.285.

With yin deficiency
- *See* Dysenteric disorder, p.285.

Patent medicines

Chai Hu Shu Gan Wan 柴胡疏肝丸 (Chai Hu Shu Gan Wan)
- Liver invading the Spleen and Stomach

Xiao Yao Wan 逍遥丸 (Xiao Yao Wan, Hsiao Yao Wan, Bupleurum Sedative Pills)
- with Spleen and Blood deficiency

Mu Xiang Shun Qi Wan 木香顺气丸 (Mu Xiang Shun Qi Wan)
- with food stagnation

Shu Gan Wan 舒肝丸 (Shu Gan Wan, Shu Kan Wan)
- with abdominal pain

Jia Wei Xiao Yao Wan 加味逍遥丸 (Jia Wei Xiao Yao Wan, Dan Zhi Xiao Yao Wan) - with stagnant Heat

Xiang Sha Yang Wei Wan 香砂养胃丸 (Xiang Sha Yang Wei Wan, Hsiang Sha Yang Wei Wan) - with Phlegm Damp

Acupuncture (select from)

Ren.12 (*zhong wan*) .... these points regulate *qi* in the abdomen by
Liv.13 (*zhang men*) strengthening the Spleen and Stomach,
St.25 (*tian shu*) harmonising the Liver and Spleen and regulating the Intestines

PC.6 (*nei guan* -) .... spreads Liver *qi* and regulates the middle *jiao*, especially good combined with Liv.3

St.36 (*zu san li*) .... *he* sea point of the Stomach, regulates and strengthens the Stomach and Intestines to prevent overcontrolling damage by Liver

Sp.6 (*san yin jiao*) .... strengthens the Spleen, regulates Liver *qi*, supplements *qi* and drains Dampness

LI.4 (*he gu*) .... the 'four gates', both *yuan* points, invigorate *qi*
Liv.3 (*tai chong* -) and Blood, exert powerful sedative and calming action, ease muscle spasm and calm the Intestines

Bl.18 (*gan shu* -) .... *shu* point of the Liver, regulates Liver *qi* and softens the Liver

Bl.25 (*da chang shu* -) .... *shu* point of the Large Intestine, regulates Intestinal *qi*

yin tang (M-HN-3) .... calms the *shen* and alleviates agitation

- Add *a shi* points along the Stomach channel as appropriate. Tender points will usually be found around St.37 (*shang ju xu*) or St.39 (*xia ju xu*).
- with significant Spleen deficiency, add Bl.20 (*pi shu* +) and Bl.21 (*wei shu* +)
- with signs of Heat add Liv.2 (*xing jian* -)
- with insomnia, lateral headaches or extreme nervousness, use SJ.5 (*wai guan*), GB.39 (*xuan zhong*) and Du.24 (*shen ting*) to soothe the Liver, regulate *qi* and calm the *shen.*
- *Ear points*: *shen men*, liver, stomach, spleen, large intestine, subcortex, sympathetic

Clinical notes

- Liver *qi* invading the Spleen type diarrhoea may be diagnosed biomedically as chronic gastritis, irritable bowel syndrome, colitis, ulcerative colitis, coeliac disease or nervous stomach.
- Liver *qi* stagnation type diarrhoea usually has a good prognosis, particularly if the source of external stress can be resolved. Acupuncture and herbs are certainly among the best and most reliable treatments for this distressing condition. Treatment often needs to be prolonged (3 months+) and must be combined with appropriate relaxation and stress management techniques, or other forms of *qi* mobilising activity. Particularly useful is walking, swimming, yoga or *tai ji chuan*, although all exercise is beneficial. Gentle and regular massage, particularly of the abdomen, neck and mid thoracic region is also useful.
- Diarrhoea of this type is frequently complicated by Spleen deficiency stagnant Heat or Damp Heat (the primary pathological triad, p.912).
- For dietary recommendations see p.878.

脾胃气虚

6.6 SPLEEN AND STOMACH QI DEFICIENCY

Pathophysiology

- Spleen *qi* deficiency is a common pattern of diarrhoea, especially in children. It is common in patients with a rigid or inappropriate dietary regime, and in those who consume an excess (for their constitution) of uncooked or cold natured foods, or sweet foods. It may also occur following antibiotic therapy, high doses of vitamin C, or ingestion of other cold natured drugs.
- Spleen *qi* deficiency diarrhoea is the product of weakness of digestive power. The Spleen is unable to process and extract all the goodness from ingested substances, leaving a residue of unprocessed food and Dampness which sinks into the Intestines and appears as diarrhoea.

Clinical features

- Frequent loose stools or diarrhoea, possibly with mucus. The diarrhoea is constant or intermittent and aggravated by fatigue, overexertion and certain foods. The bowels move soon after eating. In some patients diarrhoea and constipation alternate.
- abdominal distension or dull ache, improved by warmth
- poor appetite, early satiety, decreased sense of taste, nausea
- weakness and fatigue; tiredness may increase after eating
- weak, tired limbs
- pale, sallow complexion and lips
- puffiness around the eyes and in the fingers
- weight loss

T pale, with toothmarks and a white coat
P weak, thready, deficient, moderate

Treatment principle

Strengthen the Spleen and supplement *qi*
Dry Dampness and stop diarrhoea

Prescription

SHEN LING BAI ZHU SAN 参苓白术散
(*Ginseng and Atractylodes Formula*)

chao dang shen (dry fried Radix Codonopsis Pilosulae) 炒党参 15-30g
chao bai zhu (dry fried Rhizoma Atractylodes Macrocephalae) 炒白术 12-15g
chao yi ren (dry fried Semen Coicis Lachryma-jobi) 炒苡仁 15-30g
fu ling (Sclerotium Poriae Cocos) 茯苓 12-15g

chao bian dou (dry fried Semen Dolichos Lablab)
炒扁豆 12-15g
chao shan yao (dry fried Radix Dioscoreae Oppositae)
炒山药 15-18g
lian zi (Semen Nelumbinis Nuciferae) 莲子 12-15g
jie geng (Radix Platycodi Grandiflori) 桔梗 6-9g
sha ren (Fructus Amomi) 砂仁 6-9g
zhi gan cao (honey fried Radix Glycyrrhizae Uralensis)
炙甘草 3-6g

Method: Grind the herbs to a powder and take 9-grams, 2-3 times daily with warm water. May be decocted with quantities as shown. **Dang shen, chao bai zhu, chao yi ren, fu ling, chao bian dou, chao shan yao** and **zhi gan cao** strengthen the Spleen and supplement *qi*; **chao bai zhu** dries Dampness; **yi ren, fu ling** and **chao bian dou** leach out Dampness by promoting urination; **lian zi** astringes the Intestines and stops diarrhoea; **jie geng** directs *qi* upwards thus alleviating the diarrhoea; **sha ren** transforms Dampness and regulates *qi*. (Source: *Zhong Yi Nei Ke Lin Chuang Shou Ce*)

Modifications

- With severe Dampness, or Phlegm accumulation, (thick, greasy tongue coat, heaviness, distension etc.), add **cang zhu** (Rhizoma Atractylodis) 苍术 12-15g and **hou po** (Cortex Magnoliae Officinalis) 厚朴 9-12g, or consider **XIANG SHA LIU JUN ZI TANG** (*Saussurea and Cardamon Combination* 香砂六君子汤, p.149) as guiding prescription.
- With fluid retention, puffy eyes or oedema, increase the dose of **fu ling** (Sclerotium Poriae Cocos) 茯苓 to 18g, and add **ze xie** (Rhizoma Alismatis Orientalis) 泽泻 9-12g and **che qian zi** (Semen Plantaginis) 车前子 9-12g.
- With signs of Spleen *yang* deficiency (cold extremities, undigested food in the stools, abdominal pain which is better for warmth and a tight, slow or weak pulse, add **zhi fu zi** (Radix Aconiti Carmichaeli Praeparata) 制附子 6-12g (decocted for 30 minutes before the other herbs) and **pao jiang** (quick fried Rhizoma Zingiberis Officinalis) 炮姜 6-9g, or consider **FU ZI LI ZHONG WAN** (*Aconite, Ginseng and Ginger Formula* 附子理中丸, p.373) as guiding prescription.
- When Spleen deficiency is complicated by Liver *qi* stagnation, add **chai hu** (Radix Bupleuri) 柴胡 9-12g and **bai shao** (Radix Paeoniae Lactiflorae) 白芍 12-15g, or consider **SI JUN ZI TANG** (*Four Major Herbs Combination* 四君子汤, p.240) modified, as guiding prescription.
- With *wei qi* deficiency (spontaneous sweating, shortness of breath, frequent colds) add **zhi huang qi** (honey fried Radix Astragali Membranacei) 炙黄芪 15-30g and **wu wei zi** (Fructus Schizandrae Chinensis) 五味子 6-9g.
- With chronic and recalcitrant diarrhoea that is slow to improve, add some

astringent herbs such as **qian shi** (Semen Euryales Ferocis) 芡实 9-12g and **wei he zi** (roasted Fructus Terminaliae Chebulae) 煨诃子 6-9g. *See also* Table 7.2, p.301.

- With food stagnation, add **shan zha** (Fructus Crataegi) 山楂 15g, **chao mai ya** (dry fried Fructus Hordei Vulgaris Germinantus) 炒麦芽 15-30g and **chao shen qu** (dry fried Massa Fermentata) 炒神曲 15g.
- With frequent diarrhoea, rectal prolapse or haemorrhoids, add **zhi huang qi** (honey fried Radix Astragali Membranacei) 炙黄芪 30g, **chai hu** (Radix Bupleuri) 柴胡 9-12g and **sheng ma** (Rhizoma Cimicifugae) 升麻 6-9g, or consider **BU ZHONG YI QI TANG** (*Ginseng and Astragalus Combination* 补中益气汤, p.502) as guiding prescription, or in addition to the primary prescription.
- With intestinal candidiasis (or suspected *gu* parasites), add **bai zhi** (Radix Angelicae Dahuricae) 白芷 6-9g, **zi su ye** (Folium Perillae Frutescentis) 紫苏叶 9-12g and **bo he** (Herba Mentha Haplocalycis) 薄荷 6g.
- With evidence of infection by the parasite *Giardia lamblia*, add **qing hao** (Herba Artemisiae Annuae) 青蒿 15g and **da suan** (Bulbus Alli Sativi) 大蒜 6-9g. Because **qing hao** is cold natured, it may aggravate the deficiency in some patients. In these cases the **qing hao** and **da suan** can be decocted separately and given as an enema.

Variations and additional prescriptions

Unresponsive or resistant patients

- If the patient gets worse with the standard therapy and the diagnosis has been reconsidered and is reasonable, consider the following. Deeply lodged Dampness may be surfacing and is being eliminated. This can cause the diarrhoea to initially get worse, but the patient should feel better in themselves. Persisting with the therapy will bring about improvement. If, however, the patient feels worse, more lethargic and has persisting diarrhoea, then deeply lodged Dampness may be impeding the treatment. Short bursts (3-7 days) of a powerful, dispersing and fragrant Dampness resolving patent medicine, such as *Xing Jun San* 行军散 (Marching Powder) can often be sufficient to vaporise and start to move the Dampness and unfetter the Spleen. This formula can be used for up to a week in between courses of supplementing herbs. A small dose, ¼-½ teaspoon, 4-5 times daily is usually enough.

Patent medicines

Shen Ling Bai Zhu Wan 参苓白术丸 (Shen Ling Bai Zhu Wan)
 - for Spleen *qi* deficiency, excellent for children

Xiang Sha Liu Jun Zi Wan 香砂六君子丸 (Xiang Sha Liu Jun Wan, Aplotaxis-Ammomum Pills, Six Gentlemen Tea Pills)

- Spleen deficiency with Phlegm Damp

Jian Pi Wan 健脾丸 (Jian Pi Wan)

- Spleen deficiency with food stagnation

Fu Zi Li Zhong Wan 附子理中丸 (Fu Tzu Li Chung Wan, Carmichaeli Tea Pills, Li Chung Yuen Medical Pills)

- Spleen *yang* deficiency

Xing Jun San 行军散 (Marching Powder, Five Pagodas Brand)

Huo Xiang Zheng Qi Pian 藿香正气片 (Huo Xiang Zheng Qi Pian, Huo Hsiang Cheng Chi Pien)

- use one of the previous two medicines as a test for deep lying Dampness when patients do not respond as expected, or to use for a few days in between courses of supplementing prescriptions to enhance the clearance of any residual Dampness

Acupuncture (select from)

Ren.12 (*zhong wan* +▲) .. *mu* point of the Stomach, warms and strengthens the Spleen and Stomach and supplements *qi*

St.25 (*tian shu* +▲) .... *mu* point of the Large Intestine, warms and regulates the Intestines, improves Intestinal function and stops diarrhoea

zhi xie (N-CA-3 +▲) ..... extra point for diarrhoea, located halfway between Ren.8 (*shen que*) and the pubic bone

St.36 (*zu san li* +▲) .... *he* sea point of the Stomach, powerfully warms and strengthens the Spleen and Stomach, supplements *qi* and transforms Dampness

Sp.9 (*yin ling quan* -) .... together these points strengthen the Spleen
Sp.6 (*san yin jiao* +) and leach out and transform Dampness

Sp.5 (*shang qiu*) ....*jing* river point of the Spleen, strengthens the Spleen and transforms Dampness

Bl.20 (*pi shu* +▲) .... *shu* points of the Spleen and Stomach, warm
Bl.21 (*wei shu* +▲) and strengthen middle *jiao qi*

Bl.25 (*da chang shu* +▲) .. *shu* point of Large Intestine, warms, strengthens and regulates Intestinal *qi* and stops diarrhoea

- with abdominal pain, add Sp.4 (*gong sun*)
- with severe diarrhoea, strong moxa can be applied with a moxa stick to Du.20 (*bai hui*)

- with severe abdominal distension, add Sp.3 (*tai bai*) and Sp.15 (*da heng*)
- *Ear points*: spleen, stomach, large intestine, small intestine, abdomen, sympathetic

Clinical notes

- Spleen deficiency diarrhoea may be diagnosed biomedically as chronic gastritis, malabsorption syndrome, irritable bowel syndrome, coeliac disease, food intolerance or allergy, or functional weakness of the stomach.
- Spleen *qi* deficiency diarrhoea usually responds predictably and fairly quickly to correct treatment. In most cases, the patient should expect to see some improvement within a couple of weeks, then gradual resolution over several months.
- For dietary recommendations, see p.870.

脾肾阳虚

6.7 SPLEEN AND KIDNEY YANG DEFICIENCY

Pathophysiology

- The mechanism of Spleen and Kidney *yang* deficiency diarrhoea is similar to that of Spleen *qi* deficiency diarrhoea, albeit at a more severe level, with a serious lack of digestive power. The weakness of Kidney *yang* compounds the Spleen weakness by not supporting the Spleen with sufficient physiological Heat to process food and fluids, and by failing to regulate and control the 'lower *yin*' (the anus).
- There are two variations, depending on the state of fluid metabolism and the distribution of any unprocessed fluids; simple diarrhoea and accumulated pathological fluids in the Intestine (6.8).

Clinical features

- Diarrhoea which first occurs at dawn, or the patient wakes early needing to defecate. This often occurs between 5-7am, (thus 'cockcrow' or 'fifth watch' diarrhoea), but may be earlier. The diarrhoea is often watery, with undigested food residues; borborygmus and/or periumbilical pain may precede the diarrhoea, and ease after the defecation, although the patient may be exhausted. In severe cases there may be faecal incontinence.
- abdominal coldness and pain, better for warmth and pressure
- cold intolerance, cold extremities, especially legs
- copious clear urine, nocturia
- lower back and knee soreness or weakness
- poor appetite or anorexia, poor digestion, abdominal distension
- fatigue, exhaustion, depression and general disinterest
- increased desire to sleep

T pale and swollen with toothmarks and a white coat
P deep, thready and weak

Treatment principle

Warm, strengthen and supplement Spleen and Kidney *yang*
Astringe the Intestines and stop diarrhoea

Prescription

SI SHEN WAN 四神丸
(*Four Miracle Pill*) plus
LI ZHONG WAN 理中丸
(*Ginseng and Ginger Formula*)

bu gu zhi (Fructus Psoraleae Corylifoliae) 补骨脂 12-15g
rou dou kou (Semen Myristicae Fragrantis) 肉豆蔻 6-9g
wu wei zi (Fructus Schizandrae Chinensis) 五味子 6-9g

wu zhu yu (Fructus Evodiae Rutaecarpae) 吴茱萸 3-6g
dang shen (Radix Codonopsis Pilosulae) 党参 15-24g
chao bai zhu (dry fried Rhizoma Atractylodes Macrocephalae) 炒白术 12-15g
gan jiang (Rhizoma Zingiberis Officinalis) 干姜 9-12g
zhi gan cao (honey fried Radix Glycyrrhizae Uralensis) 炙甘草 6-9g

Method: Grind herbs into a fine powder and form into 9-gram pills with water. The dose is one pill 2-3 times daily. May also be decocted with the quantities shown. **Bu gu zhi** supplements Kidney *yang* and stops diarrhoea; **rou dou kou, wu zhu yu** and **gan jiang** warm middle *jiao yang* and dispel Cold; **wu wei zi** astringes the Intestines and stops diarrhoea; **dang shen**, **chao bai zhu** and **zhi gan cao** strengthen the Spleen and supplement *qi*. (Source: *Shi Yong Zhong Yi Nei Ke Xue*)

Modifications

- With significant abdominal pain, add **chao xiao hui xiang** (dry fried Fructus Foeniculi Vulgaris) 炒小茴香 15g and **gao liang jiang** (Rhizoma Alpiniae Officinari) 高良姜 9-12g.
- For elderly or severely ill patients with incessant diarrhoea, and possibly haemorrhoids or rectal prolapse, add lifting and astringing herbs like **zhi huang qi** (honey fried Radix Astragali Membranacei) 炙黄芪 30-60g, **he zi** (Fructus Terminaliae Chebulae) 诃子 12g and **chi shi zhi** (Halloysitum Rubrum) 赤石脂 30g. **Chi shi zhi** is divided into two doses, one of which is decocted, the other taken as powder with the strained decoction (*chong fu* 冲服). Note: Astringent herbs can only be used when there is no pathogen present. See also Table 7.2 (p.301) for more astringing possibilities.
- With severe Cold, add **zhi fu zi** (Radix Aconiti Carmichaeli Praeparata) 制附子 6-12g (decocted for 30 minutes before the other herbs).
- With *jing* and Blood deficiency, add **lu rong** (Cornu Cervi Parvum) 鹿茸 2-3g daily (taken separately in capsules).
- In chronic cases of *yang* deficiency, and frequently following gastro-intestinal surgery, the deficiency can be complicated by Blood stagnation (firm lower abdomen with pressure pain, spider vessels on the medial knee and ankle, pale purple tongue). It is best to experiment with mild Blood regulating herbs at relatively small doses first to avoid further dispersal of *yang qi* and aggravation of the diarrhoea. Suitable herbs include **gui zhi** (Ramulus Cinnamomi Cassiae) 桂枝, **lu lu tong** (Fructus Liquidambaris Taiwanianae) 路路通, **hong hua** (Flos Carthami Tinctorii) 红花, **jiang huang** (Rhizoma Curcumae Longae) 姜黄, **chuan xiong** (Radix Ligustici Chuanxiong) 川芎, **dan shen** (Radix Salviae Miltiorrhizae) 丹参, **sheng pu huang** (Pollen Typhae) 生蒲黄 and **ji xue teng** (Radix et Caulis Jixueteng) 鸡血藤.

Variations and additional prescriptions

- In severe or unresponsive cases, with chronic and unremitting diarrhoea to the point of incontinence, rectal prolapse and other deficient Cold signs and symptoms, the treatment can focus first on astringing leakage from the intestines, and second on warming *yang*. The guiding formula is **ZHEN REN YANG ZANG TANG** (*True Man's Decoction to Nourish the Organs* 真人养脏汤).

  zhi ying su ke (honey fried Pericarpium Papaveris Somniferi) 炙罂粟壳 6-15g
  wei he zi (roasted Fructus Terminaliae Chebulae) 煨诃子 9-12g
  chao bai shao (dry fried Radix Paeoniae Lactiflorae) 炒白芍 9-15g
  ren shen (Radix Ginseng) 人参 6-9g
  chao bai zhu (dry fried Rhizoma Atractylodes Macrocephalae) 炒白术 12-15g
  rou dou kou (Semen Myristicae Fragrantis) 肉豆蔻 6-9g
  mu xiang (Radix Aucklandiae Lappae) 木香 6-9g
  dang gui (Radix Angelicae Sinensis) 当归 6-9g
  zhi gan cao (honey fried Radix Glycyrrhizae Uralensis) 炙甘草 3-9g
  rou gui (Cortex Cinnamomi Cassiae) 肉桂 3-6g

  Method: Decoction. **Rou gui** is added towards the end of cooking (*hou xia* 后下). **Zhi ying su ke** and **wei he zi** astringe the Intestines and stop diarrhoea; **ren shen** (or **dang shen**), **chao bai zhu** and **zhi gan cao** strengthen the Spleen and supplement *qi*; **chao bai shao** and **dang gui** harmonise the Blood and stop pain; **rou gui** and **rou dou kou** warm the middle *jiao* and Kidney *yang* and disperse Cold; **mu xiang** regulates *qi* and alleviates tenesmus. Unfortunately **ying su ke** is rarely available, so may be substituted with **shi liu pi** (Pericarpium Punicae Granati) 石榴皮 9-15g. (Source: *Shi Yong Fang Ji Xue*)

Patent medicines

Fu Zi Li Zhong Wan 附子理中丸 (Fu Tzu Li Chung Wan, Carmichaeli Tea Pills, Li Chung Yuen Medical Pills)
- this pill can be used alone or combined with the one of the following patent medicines

Li Zhong Wan 理中丸 (Li Zhong Wan)

Ba Ji Yin Yang Wan 巴戟阴阳丸 (Ba Ji Yin Yang Wan)
- Spleen and Kidney *yang* deficiency

Jin Kui Shen Qi Wan 金匮肾气丸 (Fu Gui Ba Wei Wan, Sexoton Pills, Golden Book Tea)
- this pill is excellent for warming Kidney *yang*, however, as it contains **shu di**, which is 'greasy' and hard to digest, it can aggravate diarrhoea in some people. Best to start with a small

dose, in addition to the previous formula, increasing the dose gradually if the patient tolerates it.

Acupuncture (select from)

St.25 (*tian shu* +▲) .... *mu* point of the Large Intestine, warms and regulates the Intestines, improves Intestinal function and stops diarrhoea

Ren.8 (*shen que* ▲) .... Strong moxa on salt; place a piece of thin cloth over the navel and fill it with salt; burn large cones of moxa on the salt. The cloth enables quick removal of the salt and prevents excessive burning. Powerfully warms *yang* and stops diarrhoea

Ren.4 (*guan yuan* +▲) ..... warms and supplements *yuan qi* and Kidney *yang*

St.36 (*zu san li* +▲) .... *he* sea point of the Stomach, powerfully warms and strengthens the Spleen and Stomach, supplements *qi* and transforms Dampness

Sp.6 (*san yin jiao* +) .... strengthens the Spleen and Kidney and drains Dampness

Kid.3 (*tai xi* +) .... *yuan* point of the Kidney, supplements *yang*

Du.4 (*ming men* +▲) .... warms Kidney *yang*

Bl.20 (*pi shu* +▲) .... *shu* point of the Spleen, warms and strengthens the Spleen and supplements *qi*

Bl.23 (*shen shu* +▲) .... *shu* point of the Kidney, warms and stimulates Kidney *yang*

Bl.25 (*da chang shu* +▲) .. *shu* point of Large Intestine, warms, strengthens and astringes the Intestines

Du.20 (*bai hui* ▲) .... raises *yang* and astringes the Intestines

- *Ear points*: kidney, spleen, stomach, large intestine, prolapse, anus, *san jiao*, *shen men*, adrenal

Clinical notes

- Spleen and Kidney *yang* deficiency type diarrhoea may be diagnosed biomedically as chronic colitis, chronic dysentery, malabsorption syndrome, coeliac disease, ulcerative colitis, Crohn's disease, post intestinal surgery, A.I.D.S related diarrhoea or diarrhoea associated with the side effects of certain medications.
- Treatment will be need to be lengthy and regular to achieve a satisfactory result in this pattern; in many cases 6-12 months may be required for a sustained result.
- For dietary recommendations see p.873.

6.8 FLUID RETENTION IN THE INTESTINES

水饮留肠

Pathophysiology

- This pattern is a variation of *tan yin* in the Stomach and Intestines with Spleen and Kidney *yang* deficiency, a type of Fluid Accumulation Disorder, and as such, is related to the previous pattern (6.7). The difference between this and *yang* deficiency is the dominance of the pathological fluids in this case. Essentially a disorder of fluid metabolism from *yang* deficiency, fluids accumulate in the bowel instead of being reabsorbed and eliminated through the urine in the normal fashion. The mechanism of this pattern is similar to that which gives rise to collection of fluid in subcutaneous tissues, i.e. oedema.
- The location of the pathological fluids can vary from upper to lower digestive tract. In the upper digestive tract, the accumulated fluids tend to cause nausea and vomiting. In this case, however, fluids have accumulated in the lower Intestine and appear as watery diarrhoea.

Clinical features

- clear, watery, frothy diarrhoea; more water than diarrhoea
- borborygmus, with the sound of water sloshing in the abdomen when palpated
- emaciation
- nausea and/or vomiting of clear fluids
- abdominal distension
- scanty urination
- dry mouth
- dizziness

T pale with a greasy white coat
P slippery or soggy

Treatment principle

Warm and strengthen the Spleen and fluid metabolism
Drain Damp by promoting diuresis (or expulsion through the bowel)

Prescription

LING GUI ZHU GAN TANG 苓桂术甘汤
(*Atractylodes and Hoelen Combination*) plus
JI JIAO LI HUANG WAN 己椒苈黄丸
(*Stephania, Zanthoxylum, Descurainia and Rhubarb Pill*)

This is a relatively strong and somewhat cathartic prescription, designed to quickly expel the accumulated fluid through the bladder and bowel. It is selected in severe cases. The purgative and cathartic elements (**ting li zi** and **da huang**) should be deleted once fluids are moving.

fu ling (Sclerotium Poriae Cocos) 茯苓 12-15g
gui zhi (Ramulus Cinnamomi Cassiae) 桂枝 9-12g
chao bai zhu (dry fried Rhizoma Atractylodes Macrocephalae) 炒白术 12-15g
gan cao (Radix Glycyrrhizae Uralensis) 甘草 3-6g
han fang ji (Radix Stephaniae Tetrandrae) 汉防己 9-12g
jiao mu (Semen Zanthoxyli Bungeani) 椒目 3-6g
ting li zi (Semen Descurainiae seu Lepidii) 葶苈子 6-9g
da huang (Radix et Rhizoma Rhei) 大黄 6-9g

Method: Decoction. **Fu ling** strengthens the Spleen and promotes urination to drain pathological fluids; **bai zhu** strengthens the Spleen and dries Dampness; **gui zhi** opens up the flow of *yang qi* and assists fluid metabolism; **han fang ji** and **jiao mu** promote urination; **ting li zi** powerfully drives out fluids and assists **da huang** in clearing fluid accumulation in the Intestines by cathartically purging; **gan cao** protects the Stomach. (Source: *Shi Yong Zhong Yi Nei Ke Xue*)

Modifications

- With abdominal pain, add **chao bai shao** (dry fried Radix Paeoniae Lactiflorae) 炒白芍 12-18g, **chao xiao hui xiang** (dry fried Fructus Foeniculi Vulgaris) 炒小茴香 12-15g and **gao liang jiang** (Rhizoma Alpiniae Officinari) 高良姜 6-9g.

Variations and additional prescriptions

Spleen yang deficiency

- In cases with relatively severe digestive weakness and generalised pitting oedema, the aim of treatment is to warm *yang*, strengthen the Spleen and promote urination with **SHI PI YIN** (*Magnolia and Atractylodes Combination* 实脾饮).

zhi fu zi (Radix Aconiti Carmichaeli Praeparata) 制附子 6-12g
gan jiang (Rhizoma Zingiberis Officinalis) 干姜 6-9g
fu ling (Sclerotium Poria Cocos) 茯苓 12-15g
chao bai zhu (dry fried Rhizoma Atractylodes Macrocephalae) 炒白术 12-15g
mu gua (Fructus Chaenomelis) 木瓜 9-12g
hou po (Cortex Magnoliae Officinalis) 厚朴 6-9g
mu xiang (Radix Aucklandiae Lappae) 木香 6-9g
da fu pi (Pericarpium Arecae Catechu) 大腹皮 6-9g
cao guo (Fructus Amomi Tsao-ko) 草果 6-9g
sheng jiang (Rhizoma Zingiberis Officinalis Recens) 生姜 6-9g
gan cao (Radix Glycyrrhizae Uralensis) 甘草 3-6g

da zao (Fructus Zizyphi Jujubae) 大枣 3pce

Method: Decoction. **Zhi fu zi** is cooked for 30 minutes prior to the other herbs (*xian jian* 先煎). **Zhi fu zi** and **gan jiang** warm *yang* and promote transformation and mobilisation of pathological fluids; **fu ling** and **chao bai zhu** strengthen the Spleen and leach and dry Damp respectively; **mu gua** revives the Spleen, transforms Dampness and promotes urination; **hou po**, **mu xiang**, **da fu pi** and **cao guo** direct *qi* downwards and transform Dampness; **da fu pi** promotes urination; **sheng jiang**, **gan cao** and **da zao** protect the Stomach.

This prescription can be used until fluid metabolism is corrected, then replaced by a standard Spleen *yang* supplementing prescription such as **FU ZI LI ZHONG WAN** (*Aconite, Ginseng and Ginger Formula* 附子理中丸, p.373). (Source: *Shi Yong Zhong Yi Nei Ke Xue*)

Patent medicines

Fu Zi Li Zhong Wan 附子理中丸 (Fu Tzu Li Chung Wan, Carmichaeli Tea Pills, Li Chung Yuen Medical Pills)
- Spleen *yang* deficiency

Jin Kui Shen Qi Wan 金匮肾气丸 (Fu Gui Ba Wei Wan, Sexoton Pills, Golden Book Tea)
- Kidney *yang* deficiency

Acupuncture (select from)

Ren.9 (*shui fen* ▲) .... these points promote urination and
St.28 (*shui dao* ▲) transformation of fluids

Ren.4 (*guan yuan* +▲) ..... these points warm Kidney *yang* to promote
Ren.6 (*qi hai* +▲) transformation and metabolism of fluids

Sp.9 (*yin ling quan* -) .... these points stimulate the Spleen and fluid
Sp.6 (*san yin jiao* -) metabolism to promote urination and drain Dampness and fluids

Bl.39 (*wei yang* -) .... lower *he* point of the *san jiao*, regulates fluid metabolism and promotes urination

Kid.7 (*fu liu* -) .... *jing* river and Metal point of the Kidneys, regulates Kidney *qi* and strengthens fluid metabolism

St.36 (*zu san li* +▲) .... *he* sea point of the Stomach, powerfully warms and strengthens the Spleen and Stomach, supplements *qi* and transforms Dampness

Bl.20 (*pi shu* +▲) .... *shu* points of the Spleen, Kidney and Urinary
Bl.23 (*shen shu* +▲) Bladder respectively, warm *yang* and promote
Bl.28 (*pang guang shu* ▲) fluid metabolism

- *Ear points*: kidney, spleen, lung, stomach, large intestine, *san jiao*, *shen men*, adrenal

Clinical notes

- Fluid retention in the Intestine type diarrhoea may be diagnosed biomedically as ascites or cirrhosis of the liver.
- For dietary recommendations, see p.873.

瘀阻肠络

6.9 BLOOD STAGNATION

Pathophysiology

- Blood stagnation diarrhoea is usually a chronic problem. It mostly follows many years of pathology which disrupts the circulation of *qi* and Blood in the Intestinal vessels and *luo mai*. The common precursors are prolonged Liver *qi* stagnation, food stagnation and Damp Heat. Occasionally this type of diarrhoea may follow an acute abdominal trauma or abdominal surgery. There will usually be some overlap with this pattern and varieties of the TCM disease categories 'Intestinal abscess', 'Abdominal mass' and 'Abdominal pain'.

Clinical features

- Chronic diarrhoea with a feeling of incomplete evacuation or tenesmus. The stools may be purple or black, sticky or tarry. The diarrhoea may alternate with constipation.
- fixed and localised, sharp or stabbing abdominal pain (usually in the lower left quadrant) which is worse for pressure
- dark complexion, dark rings around the eyes, purple nails
- spider naevi or vascular abnormalities over the abdomen, face and legs (particularly around the inner knee and ankle)

T purple or with brown or purple stasis spots; sublingual veins dark and distended

P wiry, choppy or thready

Treatment principle

Transform and eliminate stagnant Blood from the Intestines

Prescription

SHAO FU ZHU YU TANG 少腹逐瘀汤
(*Drive Out Blood Stasis in the Lower Abdomen Decoction*)

This formula is designed for Blood stagnation with Cold.

dang gui (Radix Angelicae Sinensis) 当归 9-15g
chi shao (Radix Paeoniae Rubrae) 赤芍 9-12g
sheng pu huang (Pollen Typhae) 生蒲黄 9-12g
chao wu ling zhi (dry fried Excrementum Trogopteri seu Pteromi) 炒五灵脂 9-12g
yan hu suo (Rhizoma Corydalis Yanhusuo) 延胡索 9-12g
chuan xiong (Radix Ligustici Chuanxiong) 川芎 6-9g
chao xiao hui xiang (dry fried Fructus Foeniculi Vulgaris) 炒小茴香 9-15g
mo yao (Myrrha) 没药 6-9g

rou gui (Cortex Cinnamomi Cassiae) 肉桂 3g
pao jiang (quick fried Rhizoma Zingiberis Officinalis)
炮姜 3-6g

Method: Decoction. **Rou gui** is added towards the end of cooking (*hou xia* 后下). **Dang gui, chi shao, sheng pu huang, wu ling zhi, chuan xiong** and **mo yao** invigorate Blood and disperse stagnant Blood; **chuan xiong, chao xiao hui xiang** and **yan hu suo** regulate *qi* and stop pain; **rou gui** and **pao jiang** warm *yang* and invigorate the circulation of *qi* and Blood; **pao jiang** warms the Spleen and stops diarrhoea; **rou gui** promotes generation of new Blood. (Source: *Shi Yong Zhong Yi Nei Ke Xue*)

Modifications

- With a history of Liver *qi* stagnation, add **bai shao** (Radix Paeoniae Lactiflorae) 白芍 12-18g, **chen pi** (Pericarpium Citri Reticulatae) 陈皮 9-12g and **fang feng** (Radix Ledebouriellae Divaricatae) 防风 9-12g.
- With hypochondriac pain, add **yu jin** (Tuber Curcumae) 郁金 9-12g and **chuan lian zi** (Fructus Meliae Toosendan) 川楝子 9-12g.
- With abdominal distension, add **zhi shi** (Fructus Immaturus Citri Aurantii) 枳实 9-12g and **hou po** (Cortex Magnoliae Officinalis) 厚朴 9-12g.
- With an abdominal mass (or masses), add **zao jiao ci** (Spina Gelditsiae Sinensis) 皂角刺 6-9g, **dan shen** (Radix Salviae Miltiorrhizae) 丹参 12-15g, **e zhu** (Rhizoma Curcumae Ezhu) 莪术 9-12g, **san leng** (Rhizoma Sparganii Stoloniferi) 三棱 9-12g.
- With bleeding, add **san qi fen** (powdered Radix Notoginseng) 三七粉 3g, or the patent medicine *Yun Nan Bai Yao* 云南白药 (Yunnan Paiyao).
- With Heat, add **di yu** (Radix Sanguisorbae Officinalis) 地榆 9-12g and **sheng di** (Radix Rehmanniae Glutinosae) 生地 12-15g.
- With *qi* deficiency, add **huang qi** (Radix Astragali Membranacei) 黄芪 18-30g.

Variations and additional prescriptions

- If a patient with a pre-existing Blood stagnation pattern develops Heat, with fever, increased diarrhoea possibly with blood or pus, increasing abdominal pain and rigidity, tenesmus and burning around the anus, and a greasy yellow tongue coat, the likely diagnosis is Blood stagnation with Damp Heat lodged in the Intestine. The treatment is to move and regulate *qi* and Blood, clear Damp Heat and eliminate Toxin with a prescription such as **SHAO YAO TANG** (*Peony Decoction* 芍药汤, p.270).

Patent medicines

Xue Fu Zhu Yu Wan 血府逐瘀丸 (Xue Fu Zhu Yu Wan)
- *qi* and Blood stagnation

Fu Ke Wu Jin Wan 妇科乌金丸 (Woo Garm Yuen Medical Pills)
- with Cold and deficiency

Sheng Tian Qi Pian 生田七片 (Raw Tian Qi Ginseng Pills)
- this patent can be used in addition to one of the above medicines, especially if there is bleeding

Acupuncture (select from)

St.25 (*tian shu* -) .... *mu* point of the Large Intestine, regulates Intestinal function, eliminates stagnation and stops diarrhoea
Ren.6 (*qi hai* -) .... regulates *qi* and Blood in the lower *jiao*
a shi points .... over sites of pain in the abdomen
a shi points .... along the Stomach channel between St.36 (*zu san li*) and St.39 (*xia ju xu*)
Bl.17 (*ge shu* -) .... *hui* point for Blood, eliminates stagnant Blood

Bl.25 (*da chang shu* -) .... these points invigorate Blood circulation and eliminate Blood stagnation from the Intestine
Sp.10 (*xue hai* -)
Sp.8 (*di ji* -)
Sp.6 (*san yin jiao*)

LI.4 (*he gu* -) .... the 'four gates', both *yuan* points, invigorate *qi* and Blood, powerful sedative and calming action, stops pain
Liv.3 (*tai chong*)

- Bleeding the *ah shi* points of the *ba liao* (points over the sacral foramina), followed by strong cupping, can powerfully activate Blood in the lower *jiao*.
- with Cold, add moxa
- *Ear points*: large intestine, distal segment rectum, abdomen, *san jiao*, *shen men*, adrenal

Clinical notes

- Blood stagnation type diarrhoea may be diagnosed biomedically as diverticulitis, diverticulosis, Crohn's disease, intestinal polyps, ulcerative colitis or bowel cancer.
- Treatment of Blood stagnation diarrhoea generally takes a long time, and the result depends on the type of bowel pathology present. Ulcerative colitis often responds reasonably well to TCM treatment but takes a long time for good results (6-12 months). Crohn's disease also responds to prolonged treatment, although not as well as ulcerative colitis. Treatment is more difficult and results are not so good, however, when patients are dependent on steroids or have a long history of steroid use. Diverticular disease responds well, again to lengthy treatment. Bowel cancer is best treated with a combination of Western medicine and TCM as support.

SUMMARY OF GUIDING FORMULAE FOR DIARRHOEA

Acute patterns

Summer (seasonal) disorders

- Summerdamp - *Huo Xiang Zheng Qi Tang* 霍香正气汤
- Summerheat - *Xin Jia Xiang Ru Yin* 新加香薷饮

Damp Heat - *Ge Gen Huang Qin Huang Lian Tang* 葛根黄芩黄连汤

- with spurious diarrhoea - *Huang Long Tang* 黄龙汤

Cold Damp - *Ping Wei San* 平胃散

- watery diarrhoea - *Wei Ling Tang* 胃苓汤
- with *yang* deficiency - *Li Zhong Wan* 理中丸

Food stagnation - *Bao He Wan* 保和丸

- with Damp Heat - *Zhi Shi Dao Zhi Wan* 枳实导滞丸
- with Spleen deficiency - *Jian Pi Wan* 健脾丸

Chronic patterns

Liver *qi* invading the Spleen - *Tong Xie Yao Fang* 痛泻要方

- with Spleen deficiency - *Si Jun Zi Tang* 四君子汤

Spleen *qi* deficiency - *Shen Ling Bai Zhu San* 参苓白术散

Spleen and Kidney *yang* deficiency - *Si Shen Wan* 四神丸 plus *Li Zhong Wan* 理中丸

- severe cases or incontinence - *Zhen Ren Yang Zang Tang* 真人养脏汤

Fluid accumulation in the Intestines

- Severe cases - *Ling Gui Zhu Gan Tang* 苓桂术甘汤 plus *Ji Jiao Li Huang Wan* 己椒苈黄丸
- with scanty urination - *Shi Pi Yin* 实脾饮

Stagnant Blood - *Shao Fu Zhu Yu Tang* 少腹逐瘀汤

- with Damp Heat - *Shao Yao Tang* 芍药汤

Table 6.3 *Differential diagnosis of diarrhoea*

Pattern	Duration	Aggravated by	Ameliorated by	Nature of diarrhoea	Nature of patient	Pulse and tongue
Summerdamp Summerheat	acute	humid weather, changes of weather		watery, explosive, urgent, with cramping pain	all ages	T: greasy, white or yellow coat P: floating, soft, slippery
Damp Heat	mostly acute, may be chronic	humid weather spicy or greasy food, alcohol		frequent, burning, explosive, foul, with pain	all ages	T: greasy, yellow coat P: slippery, rapid
Cold Damp	often acute, but may become chronic	cold or raw food, sugar, dairy		watery, explosive, or mucoid, with pain	all ages	T: thick, greasy, white coat P: slippery
Food stagnation	acute or chronic	overindulgence	eating less, eating slowly, defecation	foul smelling, explosive	often overweight	T: thick, greasy, white or yellow coat P: slippery, full
Liver *qi* invading the Spleen	chronic with acute exacerbations	emotional upset and stress, eating while upset	when relaxed, asleep, happy pain better for defecation, exercise	urgent, preceded by griping or colicky pain; may alternate with constipation; often frequent, may be mucus	nervy, tense, most common 20-50 yrs, F>M	T: normal or dark P: wiry

Spleen *qi* deficiency	mostly chronic, but may be acute following high doses of antibiotics or abdominal surgery	Cold or Damp natured substances like dairy foods, uncooked food, juices, antibiotics, sugar; worry, fatigue, overexertion	avoidance of aggravating factors, warm, easily digested food	loose stools or diarrhoea, may be frequent	pale, run down, puffy around eyes and fingers	T: pale P: weak
Spleen and Kidney *yang* deficiency			avoidance of aggravating factors; pressure and warmth applied to abdomen	patient woken early in the morning with urgent need to defecate, undigested food in the stool, watery stool, with dull abdominal pain	pale, run down, possibly overweight or tends to oedema, cold intolerance	T: pale and swollen P: deep, slow, weak
Fluid retention in the Intestines	chronic, similar to Spleen and Kidney *yang* deficiency	excessive ingestion of fluids, cold substances		watery or frothy with borborygmus or watery splash in the abdomen		T: pale with a greasy coat P: soggy, slippery
Blood stagnation	chronic	pressure on the abdomen, overeating	defecation	dark or tarry stool with a feeling of incomplete evacuation, and fixed, stabbing abdominal pain	dark complexion, possibly emaciated, broken vessels or naevii	T: purple or with brown or purple spots, distended sublinguals P: wiry or choppy

7. Dysenteric Disorder

Damp Heat
Fulminating
Liver *qi* invading the Spleen
(with stagnant Heat, Damp Heat or Fire)
Cold Damp
Anorectic
Chronic relapsing
Spleen and Kidney *yang* deficiency
Yin deficiency (with residual Damp Heat)
Blood stagnation

7 DYSENTERIC DISORDER

li ji 痢疾

Dysenteric disorder is an acute or chronic inflammation of the large intestine characterised by diarrhoea mixed with blood, mucus and pus.

There are two broad types of biomedical disorder that may be classified under the TCM heading of dysenteric disorder. The first is true dysentery, that is, infection of the large intestine by bacteria such as *Shigella sonnei*, *S. flexneri*, *S. boydii* and *S. dysenteriae*, or protozoans including *Entamoeba histolytica*. Other organisms, such as *Salmonella* can sometime produce the typical symptoms of dysenteric disorder. In their severe acute forms, these infections are not common in the western clinic. However, we often see patients presenting with the after effects and various complications of an acute episode of infectious dysentery upon return from Asia, Africa or South America. Acute infections frequently follow a seasonal pattern, occurring more frequently in the warm humid months. They may become chronic and recurrent if not treated promptly.

The second type is associated with chronic inflammatory bowel disease. From a TCM perspective, disorders of this type are usually associated with internal organ dysfunction, and typically run a chronic course with occasional flare ups and systemic complications. From a practical point of view, the patterns of the infectious and non infectious types of dysenteric disorder are often indistinguishable, and the treatments, in general, are quite similar. The only difference in treatment is that there are certain herbs that have a specific action against the bacteria or protozoans that cause true dysentery. These herbs can be added to the appropriate primary prescription.

Knowledge of the biomedical basis of the disease is essential for prognosis. Infectious dysentery will generally clear up relatively quickly, while chronic inflammatory bowel disease usually takes lengthy treatment for satisfactory results.

AETIOLOGY

Pathogens

External Damp Heat (Toxic Heat)

The main external pathogens which cause acute dysenteric disorder are Damp Heat, epidemic Toxic Heat, and to a lesser extent, Summerheat. Damp Heat is the most common acute presentation of dysenteric disorder. Damp Heat and Toxic Heat can be a product of the season, most commonly occurring during hot or humid weather, and is more frequent in tropical climates. Damp Heat pathogens can also invade the Intestines directly with spoiled food, or by sudden overindulgence in Damp Hot substances, such as alcohol, fats, spices or chilli.

There are different degrees of Damp Heat, from quite mild, causing infrequent diarrhoea with relatively small amounts of mucus and blood, through to severe with massive bleeding and disturbances of consciousness. At the severe end of the scale, the pathogen is reclassified as Toxic Heat or fulminating dysenteric disorder. Acute Damp Heat and Toxic Heat pathogens tend to occur in epidemic waves, affecting individuals regardless of their constitution.

BOX 7.1 SOME BIOMEDICAL CAUSES OF DYSENTERIC DISORDER

Infectious
- bacterial or amoebic dysentery
- haemorrhagic colitis

Inflammatory
- ulcerative colitis
- Crohn's disease
- chronic colitis

Mental emotional
- irritable bowel syndrome

Other
- malabsorption syndrome
- bowel cancer

Internal Damp Heat

Internally generated Damp Heat can produce dysenteric disorder, or more commonly, can contribute to ongoing or recurrent dysenteric disorder, following an unresolved or incompletely resolved acute episode. This is usually associated with a diet rich in heating, Damp producing or greasy foods, or the continued production of Stagnant Heat from *qi* stagnation (*see* Emotion, below).

External Cold Damp

External Cold Damp is a less common variant of acute dysenteric disorder. It may represent a type of dysenteric disorder that is more frequent during cold weather, or that occurs in individuals with a Cold or *yang* deficient constitution. An invasion of external Cold Damp may stir up a pre-existing condition of Damp.

Internal Cold Damp

Internally generated Cold Damp can produce a type of dysenteric disorder characterised by profuse mucus streaked stools. This is usually associated with a cold, raw or otherwise *yang* weakening diet. Chronic Cold Damp eventually drains Spleen *yang*.

Diet

Various dietary factors can contribute to dysenteric disorder. Eating spoiled or contaminated food produces acute dysenteric disorder, which in TCM terms may resemble an attack of Damp or Toxic Heat, or Cold Damp. Overeating, eating irregularly, or at odd hours, especially late at night, weakens

Spleen and Stomach *qi* and leads to food stagnation (*see* p.3), which can then generate Dampness and Heat. Overconsumption in general and excessive consumption of rich and hot natured foods in particular can lead to the accumulation of food and Damp Heat in the Intestines. Starvation, obsessive dieting or fasting, and a diet heavy with cold or raw foods will contribute to Cold Damp accumulation and *yang* deficiency.

Drugs, such as Heat clearing herbs and antibiotics, that may be used for an acute episode of Damp Heat or Toxic Heat dysenteric disorder, can weaken the Spleen *qi* and *yang* or create Dampness when used to excess or used inappropriately. Similarly, the use of antidiarrhoeal agents, such as Lomotil or Imodium, in an acute episode, can lock a pathogen into the Intestine and contribute to chronic or relapsing dysenteric disorder.

Emotion

Prolonged or extreme emotional stress is an important contributing factor in the development of some types of recurrent dysenteric disorder. Frustration, anger, resentment, repressed emotions and stress disrupt the circulation of Liver *qi*, which over time, or suddenly in extreme cases, can both disrupt the Spleen and create stagnant Heat. In the case of dysenteric disorder, the Heat is a critical factor in the development of bleeding, the Heat scorching the *luo mai* of the Large Intestine and causing reckless movement of Blood. The mucus component is the product of the damage to the Spleen, such that Dampness is continually produced and sinks through the bowel to be expelled with the stool. Stagnant Heat and Dampness also combine to form Damp Heat. This combination of pathologies, Liver and Spleen disharmony, generation of Dampness and stagnant Heat, and the creation of Damp Heat, is frequently seen in patients with chronic dysenteric disorder (and other chronic gastro-intestinal complaints), presenting in the Western clinic. *See* the primary pathological triad, p.912 for more.

While the Liver is usually the main culprit in damaging the Spleen, other organ systems may contribute as well. Anxiety, prolonged fearfulness or a severe shock can disrupt the Heart and Small Intestine axis. Similarly the Large Intestine is easily affected via its relationship with the Lungs, by sadness, grief and acute separation and loss. Regardless of the initial cause, the Intestines in general are a common site for storage of unexpressed or inexpressible emotion, leading to damage from chronic low grade hypertonicity and consequent reduced and compromised circulation, oxygenation and nutrition.

Disruption to the regular distribution of Liver *qi* also occurs in patients who do variable shift work, especially a frequently rotating eight hour shift (for example, 6am-2pm, 2pm-10pm, 10pm-6am in 2 weekly cycles).

BOX 7.2 KEY DIAGNOSTIC POINTS

Onset
- acute - Damp Heat, Toxic Heat, Cold Damp, Summerheat
- chronic or recurrent - Liver *qi* invading the Spleen, lingering Damp Heat with *qi* deficiency, *yin* deficiency, *yang* deficiency

Nature of stools
- more blood than mucus - Damp Heat (Heat>Damp)
- more mucus than blood - Damp Heat (Damp>Heat)
- pure Blood - Toxic Heat (fulminating)
- mostly or all mucus - Cold Damp

Fever
- lingering afternoon - residual Damp Heat
- afternoon or evening - *yin* deficiency
- high and unrelenting - Toxic Heat

Aggravation of recurrent disorder
- with spicy foods or alcohol - Liver *qi* invading the Spleen with residual Damp Heat, or lingering Damp Heat
- cold or raw foods, beer - lingering Cold Damp, *yang* deficiency
- stress, emotional turmoil - Liver *qi* invading the Spleen

Yang deficiency

Yang deficiency dysenteric disorder is a chronic condition, following an unresolved or poorly treated acute episode of dysentery. Patients may be prone to develop *yang* deficiency patterns because they are constitutionally *yang* deficient to begin with, are elderly, have a cold or *yang* weakening diet or are taking cold natured medications. Additional factors are prolonged starvation or digestive insult, as occurs in patients with a history of anorexia nervosa or bulimia. Chronic Cold Damp dysenteric disorder will eventually weaken *yang*.

Yang deficiency patterns can also be iatrogenically produced by over-enthusiastic use of bitter cold herbs, or substances such as antibiotics, in the treatment of an acute episode.

There are a various degrees of *yang* deficiency, from unremitting watery diarrhoea with mucus and bleeding, to severe rectal prolapse and collapse of *yang*. The Kidney will often be involved, aggravating the loss of tone in the rectum and anus (the 'lower *yin*') leading to more severe prolapse.

Yin deficiency

Yin deficiency dysenteric disorder is a fairly common complication of long term Damp Heat retention in the Intestines. Smouldering Heat gradually consumes the *yin*. In addition, excessive or prolonged and inappropriate use of bitter cold Heat clearing herbs will damage not only the Spleen and Stomach, but also the *yin*, particularly in susceptible patients or those with a pre-existing tendency to *yin* deficiency. Similarly, incorrect or premature use of astringent herbs or antidiarrhoeal agents, may cause Damp Heat to get locked into the Intestine, which then gradually plunders *yin*.

Yin deficiency dysenteric disorder can also be a relatively acute disorder, following quickly after an episode of dysenteric disorder with severe Toxic Heat and high fever.

TCM DIFFERENTIAL DIAGNOSIS

- **Diarrhoea (*xie xie* 泄泻)**: Diarrhoea is the passage of unformed or watery stools, generally without blood or pus. Generally not as urgent as dysenteric disorder. There is usually no tenesmus. There may be mucus in some cases.
- **Intestinal Wind (*chang feng* 肠风)**: A disorder characterised by the passage of fresh red blood per rectum, usually preceding a bowel movement. There is no diarrhoea, pain or tenesmus. In between bowel movements the patient feels normal.

TREATMENT

In dysenteric disorder, regardless of whether deficiency or excess predominates, the Intestine has been damaged and the circulation of *qi* and Blood compromised.

In acute cases, the treatment principle is to first eliminate pathogens, then do any restoration work that may be required depending on the damage done to the Intestines and Spleen. Therapy should be continued for at least 4-7 days after the resolution of the symptoms to ensure the complete expulsion of the pathogen.

In chronic or recurrent cases, different treatment principles and treatments are applied depending on whether the dysenteric disorder is active or not. During the active phase or during an aggravation, treatment for acute patterns may apply, even though the overall duration of the disorder is chronic. In between episodes, strengthening, *qi* regulating and harmonising treatment should proceed. In many chronic cases, a mixture of pathogen elimination and *zheng qi* strengthening will be required, prescriptions being altered frequently to stay in tune with the flux of pathogenic and normal *qi*. In most chronic cases, a minimum of several months therapy is usually required.

Retention enemas enhance and speed the results in chronic dysenteric disorder. Enemas are especially useful when there is physical damage to the Intestinal wall.

Figure 7.1 *Diagnostic strategy for dysenteric disorder*

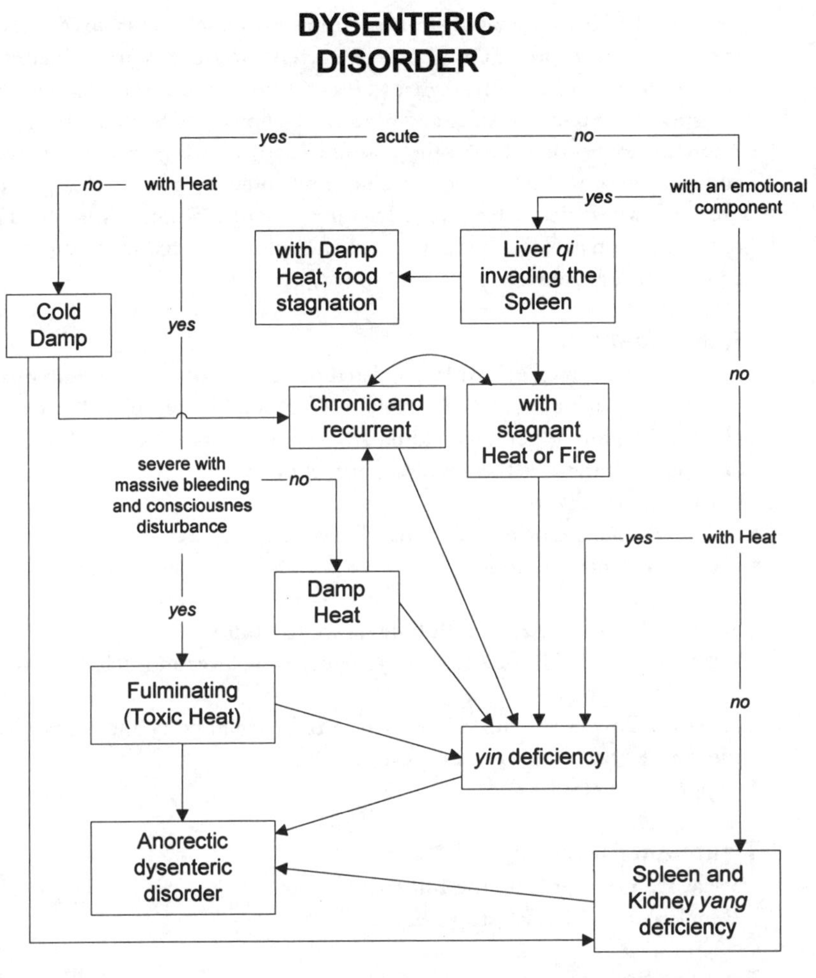

湿热痢疾

7.1 DAMP HEAT

Pathophysiology

- Acute Damp Heat dysenteric disorder is most commonly a seasonal disorder. It may, however, present as an acute exacerbation of a chronic pattern, such as *qi* stagnation with stagnant Heat. Once Damp Heat lodges in the Intestine, the circulation of *qi* and Blood is disrupted and becomes stagnant. The Heat forces Blood from the vessels causing bleeding from the bowel, and concentrates at certain points to generate intense, or Toxic, Heat, which breaks down tissues to form pus. The presence of Dampness manifests as mucus and can damage the function of the Spleen which then continues to produce more Damp.

Clinical features

- Frequent, foul smelling, explosive diarrhoea with blood, mucus and pus; the mixture of mucus and blood will vary depending on the balance of Heat and Damp. When Heat dominates there will be more blood, when Dampness dominates there will be more mucus.
- burning anus, tenesmus
- colicky abdominal pain, abdominal distension
- scanty concentrated urine
- red complexion, red eyes
- dry mouth, thirst (maybe with little desire to drink)
- in the early stages (the first few days) there may be fever and chills, headache and a floating pulse

T greasy yellow coat; with more Heat, a red tongue body and a dry coat; with more Dampness, a thick greasy tongue coat

P slippery and rapid

Treatment principle

Clear Damp Heat from the Intestine
Regulate *qi* and Blood, stop pain

Prescription

SHAO YAO TANG 芍药汤
(*Peony Decoction*)

This formula is selected when pus and blood are roughly equal in amount, and abdominal pain is a major feature.

bai shao (Radix Paeoniae Lactiflorae) 白芍 15-30g
huang qin (Radix Scutellariae Baicalensis) 黄芩 9-12g
dang gui (Radix Angelicae Sinensis) 当归 6-9g
bing lang (Semen Arecae Catechu) 槟榔 9-12g

huang lian (Rhizoma Coptidis) 黄连 6-9g
da huang (Radix et Rhizoma Rhei) 大黄 3-6g
mu xiang (Radix Aucklandiae Lappae) 木香 6-9g
gan cao (Radix Glycyrrhizae Uralensis) 甘草 3-6g
rou gui (Cortex Cinnamomi Cassiae) 肉桂 1-3g

Method: Decoction. **Bai shao** and **dang gui** harmonise and regulate Blood; **bai shao** and **gan cao** moderate spasms and stop pain; **mu xiang** and **bing lang** regulate *qi*, alleviate stagnation and tenesmus; **huang lian** and **huang qin** clear Damp Heat; **da huang** assists the previous two herbs in draining Heat by purging according to the principle of 'promoting flow to treat excessive flow'; **rou gui** and **gan cao** prevent the bitter cold herbs from damaging *yang qi*. (Source: *Shi Yong Zhong Yi Nei Ke Xue*)

Modifications

- In the early stages of acute Damp Heat dysenteric disorder, or if the Heat is intense, the **rou gui** is often replaced with **jin yin hua** (Flos Lonicerae Japonicae) 金银花 18-30g.
- In cases of bacillary dysentery (*Shigella* sp.), add **ma chi xian** (Herba Portulacae Oleraceae) 马齿苋 30g and **ban lan gen** (Radix Isatidis seu Baphicacanthi) 板蓝根 20g.
- In cases of amoebic dysentery (*Entamoeba histolytica*), add **bai tou weng** (Radix Pulsatillae Chinensis) 白头翁 15g.
- If Dampness is predominant (more mucus and pus than blood, abdominal fullness and distension), add **yi ren** (Semen Coicis Lachryma-jobi) 苡仁 15-30g, **fu ling** (Sclerotium Poriae Cocos) 茯苓 12-15g, **ze xie** (Rhizoma Alismatis Orientalis) 泽泻 9-12g, **cang zhu** (Rhizoma Atractylodis) 苍术 6-9g and **hou po** (Cortex Magnoliae Officinalis) 厚朴 9-12g.
- With Heat predominant (difficult stools, bleeding, thirst, dryness, red dry tongue, rapid pulse), delete **rou gui**, and add **jin yin hua** (Flos Lonicerae Japonicae) 金银花 18-30g, **chi shao** (Radix Paeoniae Rubrae) 赤芍 9-12g and **mu dan pi** (Cortex Moutan Radicis) 牡丹皮 9-12g. *See also* Variations and additional prescriptions.
- With significant bleeding, add **di yu** (Radix Sanguisorbae Officinalis) 地榆 12-15g and **zi zhu cao** (Folium Callicarpae) 紫珠草 12-15g.
- With severe abdominal pain, add **wu yao** (Radix Linderae Strychnifoliae) 乌药 9-12g and **zhi shi** (Fructus Immaturus Citri Aurantii) 枳实 12-15g.
- With exterior signs and symptoms (fever and chills and floating pulse), add **ge gen** (Radix Puerariae) 葛根 12g, **jing jie** (Herba seu Flos Schizonepetae Tenuifolia) 荆芥 12g, **lian qiao** (Fructus Forsythia Suspensae) 连翘 9-12g and **jin yin hua** (Flos Lonicerae Japonicae) 金银花 30g.
- With mild food stagnation, add two or three of the following herbs: **shen qu** (Massa Fermentata) 神曲 15g, **chao mai ya** (dry fried Fructus Hordei

Vulgaris Germinantus) 炒麦芽 15-30g, **shan zha** (Fructus Crataegi) 山楂 15g and **chao lai fu zi** (dry fried Semen Raphani Sativi) 炒莱服子 15g.

- Damp Heat can bottle up *yang* in the interior, obstructing its expression and leading to a situation of 'true Heat, false Cold' (a type of *jue* 厥 syndrome). The paradoxical signs of cold extremities and a minute pulse with the previously mentioned Damp Heat signs and symptoms are an indication for combining the primary prescription with **SI NI SAN** (*Bupleurum and Zhi Shi Formula* 四逆散, p.763).

Variations and additional prescriptions

Summerdamp or Summerheat dysenteric disorder

- In cases where Summerdamp or Summerheat symptoms are obvious (mild diarrhoea with small amounts of mucus and blood, chills and fever which are unrelieved by sweating, nausea and vomiting, heaviness in the body, foggy-headedness), the correct treatment is to expel Summerheat, clear Damp Heat and stop diarrhoea with **HUO XIANG ZHENG QI SAN** (*Agastache Formula* 藿香正气散) modified.

huo xiang (Herba Agastaches seu Pogostemi) 藿香 12-15g
fu ling (Sclerotium Poriae Cocos) 茯苓 12-15g
hou po (Cortex Magnoliae Officinalis) 厚朴 9-12g
zi su ye (Folium Perillae Frutescentis) 紫苏叶 9-12g
ban xia (Rhizoma Pinelliae Ternatae) 半夏 9-12g
da fu pi (Pericarpium Arecae Catechu) 大服皮 9-12g
bai zhu (Rhizoma Atractylodes Macrocephalae) 白术 9-12g
chen pi (Pericarpium Citri Reticulatae) 陈皮 9-12g
bai zhi (Radix Angelicae Dahuricae) 白芷 6-9g
jie geng (Radix Platycodi Grandiflori) 桔梗 6-9g
gan cao (Radix Glycyrrhizae Uralensis) 甘草 3-6g
huang lian (Rhizoma Coptidis) 黄连 6-9g
mu xiang (Radix Aucklandiae Lappae) 木香 9-12g

Method: Decoction. The herbs should be gently simmered for no longer than 20 minutes in a pot with a close fitting lid. If nausea is a problem, the decoction can be taken through a straw and sipped slowly, with the straw right at the back of the tongue. **Huo xiang** fragrantly disperses Dampness and harmonises the Stomach; **zi su ye** and **bai zhi** dispel Wind Cold and transform Dampness; **hou po** and **chen pi** regulate and direct *qi* downwards, transform Dampness and alleviate fullness; **ban xia** transforms Dampness and stops vomiting; **da fu pi** directs *qi* and Dampness downwards and alleviates fullness; **bai zhu** and **fu ling** strengthen the Spleen, dry Dampness and promote urination to clear Dampness; **jie geng** assists the dispersing function of the Lungs; **gan cao** harmonises the other herbs and regulates the Stomach; **huang lian** and **mu xiang** clear Heat from the Intestines and alleviate tenesmus respectively. (Source: *Shi Yong Zhong Yi Nei Ke Xue*)

With food stagnation

- When food stagnation is severe (diarrhoea with pus and blood alternating with constipation, severe abdominal fullness and pain which is worse for pressure, a thick greasy tongue coat and a slippery strong pulse), the aim of treatment is to move *qi*, guide out stagnation, and drain Heat with **MU XIANG BING LANG WAN** (*Aucklandia and Betel Nut Pill* 木香槟榔丸). The Damp Heat invasion may precede and contribute to food stagnation, causing an acute pattern. Alternatively prolonged food stagnation can generate Damp Heat, a more chronic pattern.

  mu xiang (Radix Aucklandiae Lappae) 木香 60g
  bing lang (Semen Arecae Catechu) 槟榔 60g
  qing pi (Pericarpium Citri Reticulatae Viridae) 青皮 60g
  huang lian (Rhizoma Coptidis) 黄连 60g
  huang bai (Cortex Phellodendri) 黄柏 60g
  da huang (Radix et Rhizoma Rhei) 大黄 60g
  xiang fu (Rhizoma Cyperi Rotundi) 香附 90g
  bai tou weng (Radix Pulsatillae Chinensis) 白头翁 90g
  bai shao (Radix Paeoniae Lactiflorae) 白芍 90g

  Method: Grind herbs to a fine powder and form into 3 gram pills with water. The dose is 1-3 pills two or three times daily. May also be decocted with an 80% reduction in quantities. **Mu xiang** and **bing lang** promote the movement of *qi*, alleviate stagnation and relieve tenesmus; **qing pi** and **xiang fu** regulate and break up stagnant *qi* and harmonise the Liver and Spleen; **huang lian** and **huang bai** clear Damp Heat; **da huang** clears Heat and purges accumulation through the Intestines; **bai tou weng** clears Toxic Heat from the Intestines and alleviates dysenteric disorder; **bai shao** softens the Liver, eases spasms and stops pain. (Source: Formulas and Strategies)

With Heat greater than Dampness

- If Heat predominates, with violent diarrhoea, more blood than pus, or passing pure blood, fever and thirst, the aim of treatment is to clear Toxic Heat with **BAI TOU WENG TANG** (*Pulsatilla Decoction* 白头翁汤, p.278).

With Intestinal dryness and yin damage

- Another variation can occur when excessive parching herbs or the existing Heat dry out the Intestine and damage *yin* fluids. The clinical features are diarrhoea with pus and thick blood, difficult evacuation, abdominal pain, burning anus, scanty urine, dryness of the mouth and tongue, fever, irritability and a flooding, rapid or thready and rapid pulse. The aim of treatment is to moisten Dryness, clear Heat and guide out and eliminate stagnation with **HE JIAN SHAO YAO HUANG LIAN TANG** (*Peony and Coptis Decoction to Bolster the River* 河间芍药黄连汤) modified. *See also yin* deficiency, p.306.

dang gui (Radix Angelicae Sinensis) 当归 9-12g
chi shao (Radix Paeoniae Rubrae) 赤芍 9-12g
da huang (Radix et Rhizoma Rhei) 大黄 6-9g
gan cao (Radix Glycyrrhizae Uralensis) 甘草 3-6g
huang lian (Rhizoma Coptidis) 黄连 6-9g
sheng di (Radix Rehmanniae Glutinosae) 生地 12-18g
shi hu (Herba Dendrobii) 石斛 12-15g

Method: Decoction. **Dang gui** and **chi shao** regulate Blood and eliminate stagnant Blood; **huang lian** and **da huang** clear Heat from the Intestines; **sheng di** and **shi hu** moisten dryness, protect *yin* and clear Heat; **gan cao** protects the Stomach and clears Heat. (Source: *Shi Yong Zhong Yi Nei Ke Xue*)

Patent medicines

Qing Fei Yi Huo Pian 清肺抑火片 (Ching Fei Yi Huo Pien)

Lian Qiao Bai Du Pian 连翘败毒片 (Lien Chiao Pai Tu Pien)

- Although neither of these patents is specific for dysenteric disorder, they both clear Damp Heat and Toxic Heat. They both contain rhubarb root (**da huang**), which here can aid the expulsion of the pathogen through the bowel. The standard dose should be increased 2-3 times. Combine either with one of the following general anti-Toxic patent medicines.

Huang Lian Jie Du Wan 黄连解毒丸 (Huang Lian Jie Du Wan)

- Damp Heat

Huang Lian Su Pian 黄连素片 (Huang Lien Su Tablets)

Chuan Xin Lian Kang Yan Pian 穿心连抗炎片 (Chuan Xin Lian Antiphlogistic Pills)

Fu Fang Nan Ban Lan Gen Pian 复方南板蓝根 (Fu Fang Nan Ban Lan Gen) - this medicine and the one above, can be added to one of the first four patent formulae to enhance the Toxic Heat clearing action

Acupuncture (select from)

St.25 (*tian shu* -) .... *mu* point of the Large Intestine, clears Damp Heat and stops diarrhoea

zhi xie - (N-CA-3) .... extra point for diarrhoea, located halfway between Ren.8 (*shen que*) and the pubic bone

St.37 (*shang ju xu* -) .... lower *he* point of the Large Intestine, eliminates stagnation and accumulation from the Stomach and Intestines and clears Damp Heat

ah shi points .... between St.36 (*zu san li*) and St.39 (*xia ju xu*), clear Heat and stagnation from the Intestines

LI.11 (*qu chi* -) .... *he* sea point of the Large Intestine, clears Damp Heat from *yang ming*

St.44 (*nei ting* -) .... together these points powerfully clear Heat
LI.4 (*he gu* -) from *yang ming*

- Acupuncture must be given frequently for a good result. One or two treatments daily is appropriate in severe cases.
- with high fever add Du.14 (*da zhui* -)
- with prominent Dampness, add Sp.9 (*yin ling quan* -)
- with nausea add PC.6 (*nei guan*) and Ren.12 (*zhong wan*)
- with tenesmus add Du.1 (*chang qiang* -), Bl.30 (*bai huan shu* -) and Ren.4 (*guan yuan*)
- *Ear points*: large intestine, small intestine, subcortex, sympathetic, lower portion of rectum

Retention enema

Retention enema is a useful additional treatment for chronic or recurrent Damp Heat patterns, with ulceration of, or damage to, the bowel wall. This may occur in biomedical diseases such as ulcerative colitis and Crohn's disease, or persistent infection. The herbs are brewed as for a normal decoction, strained and cooled to body temperature before 60-150 mls is inserted with a commercial enema device. The enema is given once daily for 7-14 days, and can be retained, with the patient lying down, for 30 minutes to 2 hours, or better, overnight, with the patients hips elevated in bed.

1. For cases with ulceration of the bowel wall

The main principle of treatment is to promote healing and to clear Damp Heat locally.

shi gao (Gypsum) 石膏 30g
dang gui (Radix Angelicae Sinensis) 当归 15g
bai zhi (Radix Angelicae Dahuricae) 白芷 12g
bai ji (Radix Bletillae Striatae) 白芨 12g
xue jie (Sanguis Draconis) 血竭 12g
ru xiang (Gummi Olibanum) 乳香 10g
mo yao (Myrrha) 没药 10g
gan cao (Radix Glycyrrhizae Uralensis) 甘草 10g
bing pian (Borneol) 冰片 3g

Method: Decoction for use as an enema. **Bing pian** is added as a powder to the strained decoction. **Shi gao**, **bing pian** and **gan cao** promote healing; **dang gui** nourishes Blood, **bai zhi** promotes discharge of pus; **bai ji** protects the lining of the Intestine and stops bleeding; **xue jie**, **ru xiang** and **mo yao** regulate Blood and promote healing.

2. With dominant Damp Heat

The main principle of treatment is to clear the accumulated Damp Heat from the bowel. This enema is also useful for cases with chronic infection.

ming fan (Alumen) 明矾 15g
bai ji (Radix Bletillae Striatae) 白芨 15g
ku shen (Radix Sophorae Flavescentis) 苦参 15g
huai hua (Flos Sophora Japonicae Immaturus) 槐花 15g
huang lian (Rhizoma Coptidis) 黄连 10g
da huang (Radix et Rhizoma Rhei) 大黄 10g

Method: Decoction for use as an enema. **Ming fan** stops bleeding and diarrhoea; **bai ji** protects the Intestinal wall and stops bleeding; **ku shen** and **huang lian** clear Damp Heat; **huai hua** clears Damp Heat and stops bleeding; **da huang** clears Heat.

In chronic or recurrent amoebic dysentery, add **bai tou weng** (Radix Pulsatillae Chinensis) 白头翁 30g, **da suan** (Bulbus Alli Sativi) 大蒜 10g and **shi liu pi** (Pericarpium Punicae Granati) 石榴皮 10g. For chronic bacterial dysentery, add **ma chi xian** (Herba Portulacae Oleraceae) 马齿苋 30g and **da suan** (Bulbus Alli Sativi) 大蒜 10g.

3. With persistent bleeding

Make an enema of a decoction of **shi gao** (Gypsum) 30g, **bai ji** (Radix Bletillae Striatae) 白芨 12g, and add the patent medicine *Yun Nan Bai Yao* 云南白药 (Yunnan Paiyao) or **san qi fen** (powdered Radix Notoginseng) 三七粉 3-6g.

Clinical notes

- Damp Heat dysenteric disorder may be diagnosed biomedically as bacillary dysentery, amoebic dysentery, food poisoning, acute gastroenteritis, acute exacerbation of ulcerative colitis or Crohn's disease.
- When due to an acute infection, Damp Heat dysenteric disorder responds quickly to correct treatment. Raw herbs are most effective.
- When associated with a chronic systemic disorder, such as a flare-up of ulcerative colitis or Crohn's, treatment is often quite effective but needs to be prolonged. The frequency and dose of herbs may also need to be increased until symptoms are under control. In severe cases, raw herbs, rather than powdered extracts, are often required to bring about quick alleviation of symptoms. One or two packets of raw herbs per day, using the upper end of the dosage range, may be necessary.
- Fluid replacement is an essential feature of treatment. In severe cases dehydration may be an important factor. Oral isotonic fluid replacement solution should be administered in small amounts frequently. Isotonic solution can be made by adding 3.5 grams of household salt (NaCl), 2.5 grams of sodium bicarbonate, 1.5 grams of potassium chloride (KCl) and 20 grams of sugar to one litre of water. Isotonic drinks are commercially available.
- In the early stages, a bland semiliquid diet is recommended. Solid foods may be added as the dysentery decreases in frequency. Avoid fats, oils,

fried foods, raw foods and fruit, dried foods, high density proteins like meat and fish. Rice porridge, **yi ren** (Semen Coicis Lachryma-jobi) 苡仁 porridge etc., are appropriate. *See also* p.220 and dietary recommendations p.884.

- Iatrogenic complications easily occur in this disorder. Over-enthusiastic use of cold herbs can aid transformation of Damp Heat into Cold Damp. Excessive use of parching herbs can dry the Intestine and cause a Dryness Heat pattern. Inappropriate or premature use of supplementing or astringent herbs, can lead to retention of Damp Heat and recurrent dysentery. Use of antidiarrhoeal agents such as Imodium or Lomotil can lock a pathogen into the bowel. Chronic Damp Heat frequently damages *yin*.
- Untreated Damp Heat dysentery will often damage *yin* or occasionally *yang* and transform into a deficient pattern. When chronic, Damp Heat dysenteric disorder is frequently associated with Spleen deficiency and Liver *qi* stagnation with stagnant Heat (the primary pathological triad, *see* p.912).
- Prevention may be enhanced in areas where true dysentery is endemic by ingesting two or three cloves of raw garlic daily, and plenty of the locally made yogurt.

Table 7.1 *Comparison of Damp Heat dysenteric disorder pattern variations*

Variation	Features	Prescription
Heat = Dampness	diarrhoea with approximately equal amounts of mucus and/or pus and blood, tenesmus, abdominal pain, burning anus, scanty urination, greasy yellow tongue coat, slippery, rapid pulse	SHAO YAO TANG
Heat > Dampness	diarrhoea with more blood than mucus or pus, or passing pure blood, high fever, thirst, tenesmus, abdominal pain, burning anus, red tongue with a greasy yellow tongue coat, rapid, flooding, wiry, slippery pulse	BAI TOU WENG TANG
Dampness > Heat	diarrhoea with more mucus than blood, abdominal fullness and distension, greasy yellow tongue coat,slippery, soft or soggy pulse	SHAO YAO TANG modified
Food stagnation	diarrhoea with mucus and blood alternating with constipation, severe abdominal fullness which is worse for pressure, flatulence, belching, a thick, greasy tongue coat and an slippery, strong pulse	MU XIANG BING LANG WAN

疫毒痢疾

7.2 FULMINATING DYSENTERIC DISORDER

Pathophysiology

• Fulminating dysenteric disorder is a severe variation of Damp Heat dysenteric disorder, with the intensity and focal nature of the Damp Heat creating Toxic Heat. The Heat is so intense that it easily affects the Blood causing massive bleeding and potential disturbances of consciousness. It tends to appear in epidemics, affecting both weak and strong individuals. This type of dysenteric disorder can be a dangerous and life threatening, the pathogen threatening to rapidly overwhelm the body's defences. A number of serious events can swiftly occur, including delirium, coma, shock and death. Severe patterns such as this will usually cause considerable damage to the patient's *yin* and *yang*, and frequently lead to chronic complications.

Clinical features

- Sudden onset of frequent, explosive diarrhoea with copious fresh red, dark red or purple blood, and possibly mucus and pus. Rarely, there may be diarrhoea like bloody water.
- abrupt onset of high fever
- severe abdominal pain and tenesmus
- thirst, dryness, dehydration
- pounding headache, malaise
- nausea, vomiting
- irritability, restlessness
- in severe cases there may be delirium or confusion, muscular spasms and cramps or convulsions, cold limbs, skin rashes and respiratory difficulties

T red or scarlet with a dry yellow coat
P slippery and rapid

Treatment principle

Clear Toxic Heat and Damp Heat
Cool the Blood, stop dysentery

Prescription

BAI TOU WENG TANG 白头翁汤
(*Pulsatilla Decoction*) modified

bai tou weng (Radix Pulsatillae Chinensis) 白头翁 30g
huang lian (Rhizoma Coptidis) 黄连 9-15g
huang bai (Cortex Phellodendri) 黄柏 9-12g
qin pi (Cortex Fraxini) 秦皮 12-15g
jin yin hua (Flos Lonicerae Japonicae) 金银花 30g

bai jiang cao (Herba cum Radice Patriniae) 败酱草 30g
sheng di (Radix Rehmanniae Glutinosae) 生地 18-30g
chi shao (Radix Paeoniae Rubrae) 赤芍 12-15g
mu dan pi (Cortex Moutan Radicis) 牡丹皮 9-12g
huai hua (Flos Sophora Japonicae Immaturus) 槐花 12-15g
gan cao (Radix Glycyrrhizae Uralensis) 甘草 3-6g

Method: Decoction. **Bai tou weng** clears Toxic Heat and stops dysentery; **huang lian, huang bai** and **qin pi** clear Damp Heat from the Intestines; **jin yin hua** and **bai jiang cao** clear Toxic Heat; **sheng di, chi shao** and **mu dan pi** cool the Blood; **huai hua** clears Damp Heat and stops bleeding; **gan cao** protects the Stomach. (Source: *Zhong Yi Nei Ke Lin Chuang Shou Ce*)

Modifications

- With muscle spasms, cramps or convulsions add **gou teng** (Ramulus Uncariae cum Uncis) 钩藤 12g and **shi jue ming** (Concha Haliotidis) 石决明 15g.
- With severe abdominal pain and cramping, delete **chi shao** and add **mu xiang** (Radix Aucklandiae Lappae) 木香 6-9g, **bing lang** (Semen Arecae Catechu) 槟榔 9-12g and **bai shao** (Radix Paeoniae Lactiflorae) 白芍 15-18g.
- With watery, bloody diarrhoea, double the dose of **huai hua** (Flos Sophora Japonicae Immaturus) 槐花 and add **wu mei** (Fructus Pruni Mume) 乌梅 15g, **huang qin tan** (charred Radix Scutellariae Baicalensis) 黄芩炭 15g and **di yu** (Radix Sanguisorbae Officinalis) 地榆 30g.
- With exterior signs (fever and chills and floating pulse, usually only the first day or two), delete **sheng di** and **mu dan pi**, and add **ge gen** (Radix Puerariae) 葛根 15g, **jing jie** (Herba seu Flos Schizonepetae Tenuifolia) 荆芥 12g and **lian qiao** (Fructus Forsythia Suspensae) 连翘 15g.

Variations and additional prescriptions

With disturbances of consciousness

- If Heat enters the *ying* or Blood, with severe high fever, confusion or delirium, the aim of treatment is to first cool the Blood and restore consciousness with the patent medicines *Zi Xue Dan* (Tze Hsueh Tan 紫雪丹) or *Zhi Bao Dan* (Zhi Bao Dan 至宝丹). There are versions of these famous medicines that claim to contain endangered species, and some that do not. Be sure to check the label before purchase. The pill is forced into the mouth or nose or given via a nasogastric tube until consciousness is restored. Once the patient is able to take herbs orally, combine the primary prescription with **SHUI NIU JIAO DI HUANG TANG** (*Water Buffalo Horn and Rehmannia Decoction* 水牛角地黄汤, p.454) to continue cooling the Blood.

Yang transforming into yin–collapse of yang

- In extreme cases, when the '*yangness*' of the pattern reaches a peak, it can suddenly transform into a critical *yin* pattern as *zheng qi* collapses. This is similar to shock, and is characterised by with cold limbs, profuse sweating, dyspnoea, grey pallid complexion, confusion, disorientation and an imperceptible pulse. The aim of treatment is to rescue *yang* with swift administration of **SHEN FU TANG** (*Ginseng and Prepared Aconite Decoction* 参附汤, p.458). In China this prescription is available in ampoules for injection.

A quick purge to eliminate locked in Toxic Heat

- In some cases, Toxic Heat can get 'locked in' to the interior of the body, with severe systemic symptoms but relatively mild dysentery. The aim of treatment is to purge the Toxic Heat and guide out accumulation with a combination of the primary prescription and **DA CHENG QI TANG** (*Major Rhubarb Combination* 大承气汤, p.69).

Rectal prolapse

- In severe cases, rectal prolapse may result from the severe diarrhoea and tenesmus. Once the Heat and pathogens have been cleared, a formula to elevate *yang* may be selected, such as **BU ZHONG YI QI TANG** (*Ginseng and Astragalus Combination* 补中益气汤, p.502) suitably modified. *See also* Rectal Prolapse, p.787.

Retention enema

Retention enema is impractical in cases of severe acute dysenteric disorder when the patient is suffering frequent diarrhoea. However, fulminant dysenteric disorder can become chronic or recurrent. If so, the same enemas as for Damp Heat apply.

Patent medicines

Qing Fei Yi Huo Pian 清肺抑火片 (Ching Fei Yi Huo Pien)
Lian Qiao Bai Du Pian 连翘败毒片 (Lien Chiao Pai Tu Pien)

- Although neither of these patents is specific for dysenteric disorder, they both clear Damp Heat and Toxic Heat. They both contain rhubarb root (**da huang**), which here can aid the expulsion of the pathogen through the bowel. The standard dose should be increased 2-3 times. Whichever one is selected should be combined with one of the following general anti-Toxic patent medicines.

Huang Lian Su Pian 黄连素片 (Huang Lien Su Tablets)
Jia Wei Xiang Lian Pian 加味香连片 (Chiawei Hsianglienpian)

Chuan Xin Lian Kang Yan Pian 穿心连抗炎片 (Chuan Xin Lian Antiphlogistic Pills)

Fu Fang Nan Ban Lan Gen Pian 复方南板蓝根 (Fu Fang Nan Ban Lan Gen) - this medicine and the one above, can be added to one of the first four patent formulae to enhance the Toxic Heat clearing action

One of the following emergency patent medicines may be used when delirium, confusion or loss of consciousness occurs (forced into the mouth or blown into the nose):

Zi Xue Dan 紫雪丹 (Tze Hsueh Tan)

Zhi Bao Dan 至宝丹 (Zhi Bao Dan)

Acupuncture (select from)

St.25 (*tian shu* -) .... *mu* point of the Large Intestine, clears Damp Heat and Toxic Heat

St.37 (*shang ju xu* -) .... lower *he* point of the Large Intestine, eliminates stagnation and accumulation from the Stomach and Intestines and clears Damp and Toxic Heat

LI.11 (*qu chi* -) .... *he* sea point of the Large Intestine, clears Damp Heat from *yang ming*

St.44 (*nei ting* -) .... together these points powerfully clear Heat
LI.4 (*he gu* -) from *yang ming*

PC.3 (*qu ze* ↓) .... *he* sea point of the Pericardium and Urinary
Bl.40 (*wei zhong* ↓) Bladder respectively, these points cool the Blood and clear Toxic Heat

- treatment can be given every 6-8 hours
- with high fever add Du.14 (*da zhui* -) and *shi xuan* (M-UE-1) ↓
- with confusion or delirium add *shi xuan* ↓ (M-UE-1) and Du.26 (*ren zhong*)
- with convulsions, add *yin tang* (M-HN-3), Sp.15 (*da heng*)
- with headache, add *tai yang* (M-HN-9), St.44 (*nei ting*)

With collapsing *yang* (shock)

- For collapsing *yang* (i.e. shock), apply strong moxa to Ren.8 (*shen que*). Place a piece of thin cloth over the navel and fill it with salt. Burn large cones of moxa on the salt. The cloth enables quick removal of the salt and prevents excessive burning. In addition, apply strong reinforcing needling on Ren.4 (*guan yuan* +) and St.36 (*zu san li* +).
- A modern method for shock is strong needling on Du.25 (*su liao* -), Kid.1 (*yong quan* -) and PC.6 (*nei guan* -). Du.25 (*su liao*) is needled to a

depth of 0.2-0.5 cun and manipulated continuously for 30 minutes. If these points are insufficient to elevate blood pressure, add LI.4 (*he gu* -), Du.26 (*ren zhong* -), and St.36 (*zu san li*).

- *Ear points*: *shen men*, subcortex, large intestine, small intestine, sympathetic, distal segment rectum

Clinical notes

- Fulminating dysenteric disorder may be diagnosed biomedically as fulminant bacillary dysentery or cholera.
- Fluids replacement is an essential feature of treatment. In severe cases dehydration may be an important factor. Oral isotonic fluid replacement solution should be administered in small amounts frequently. Isotonic solution can be made by adding 3.5 grams of household salt (NaCl), 2.5 grams of sodium bicarbonate, 1.5 grams of potassium chloride (KCl) and 20 grams of sugar to one litre of water. Isotonic drinks are commercially available.
- This pattern can be life threatening and should be managed in hospital.

肝气犯脾

7.3 LIVER QI INVADING THE SPLEEN (WITH STAGNANT HEAT, DAMP HEAT OR FIRE)

Pathophysiology

- Liver *qi* stagnation with stagnant Heat or Damp Heat is a common cause of chronic or recurrent dysenteric disorder. Years of stress and consequent punishment by the Liver of the Spleen, often combined with an irregular diet and poor quality food lead to chronic tension and Heat accumulation in the Large Intestine. The Heat gives rise to the reckless movement of Blood and bleeding. In addition, many patients will have elements of Spleen deficiency, and thus exhibit the primary pathological triad (*see* p.912).
- There are several approaches to this problem, depending on whether the patient has active bleeding, is between episodes of diarrhoea, or has other complicating pathology. The treatment strategy will vary accordingly. For example, during acute episodes or flare-ups, the focus of pathology may shift to being predominantly Damp Heat in nature, in which case prescriptions from that section are used.

Clinical features

- Chronic or recurrent diarrhoea with blood and/or mucus; the diarrhoea usually occurs in cycles which can vary from weeks to months, and has a clear emotional component. The diarrhoea may alternate with constipation.
- abdominal distension with cramping and pain typically preceding the diarrhoea
- irritability, easy anger, mood swings, depression
- temporal or tension headaches
- red, dry, sore eyes
- facial flushing
- nightsweats, the patient tends to feel hot generally
- bitter or metallic taste in the mouth, dry mouth
- poor appetite, acid reflux, nausea

T red, or with red edges or red spots on the edges of the tongue, and a yellow coat

P strong, wiry and rapid

Treatment principle

Regulate Liver *qi* and harmonise the Liver and Spleen
Clear stagnant Heat or Damp Heat from the Liver and Intestines
Cool the Blood and stop bleeding

Prescription

DAN ZHI XIAO YAO SAN 丹栀逍遥散
(*Bupleurum and Paeonia Formula*) modified

chai hu (Radix Bupleuri) 柴胡 9-12g
bai shao (Radix Paeoniae Lactiflora) 白芍 15-24g
dang gui (Radix Angelicae Sinensis) 当归 9-12g
bai zhu (Rhizoma Atractylodis Macrocephalae) 白术 9-12g
fu ling (Sclerotium Poriae Cocos) 茯苓 9-15g
zhi gan cao (honey fried Radix Glycyrrhizae Uralensis) 炙甘草 3-6g
shan zhi zi (Fructus Gardeniae Jasminoidis) 山栀子 9-12g
mu dan pi (Cortex Moutan Radicis) 牡丹皮 9-12g
bo he (Herba Mentha Haplocalycis) 薄荷 6g
fang feng (Radix Ledebouriellae Divaricatae) 防风 9-12g
sheng di (Radix Rehmanniae Glutinosae) 生地 12-15g
huai hua (Flos Sophora Japonicae Immaturus) 槐花 9-12g
qian cao gen (Radix Rubiae Cordifoliae) 茜草根 12-15g

Method: Decoction. **Bo he** is added towards the end of cooking (*hou xia* 后下). **Chai hu** and **bai shao** regulate and move Liver *qi*; **bai shao** softens the Liver and with **zhi gan cao** eases spasms and stops pain; **fu ling, bai zhu** and **zhi gan cao** strengthen the Spleen; **fu ling** leaches out Damp and promotes urination; **bai zhu** dries Damp; **dang gui** and **bai shao** nourish Blood and soften the Liver; **shan zhi zi** and **mu dan pi** cool the Liver and clear stagnant Heat; **bo he** clears Heat and assists **chai hu** in regulating *qi*; **fang feng** eases spasms in the Intestines; **sheng di** cools the Blood and protects *yin*; **huai hua** and **qian cao gen** clear Heat and stop bleeding.

Modifications

- With severe Heat (or Fire) add **long dan cao** (Radix Gentianae Longdancao) 龙胆草 6g and **huang qin** (Radix Scutellariae Baicalensis) 黄芩 9-12g.
- With severe abdominal pain, increase the dose of **bai shao** (Radix Paeoniae Lactiflorae) 白芍 to 30g, and add **yan hu suo** (Rhizoma Corydalis Yanhusuo) 延胡索 9-12g.
- With severe bleeding, add **di yu** (Radix Sanguisorbae Officinalis) 地榆 9-12g and **san qi fen** (powdered Radix Notoginseng) 三七粉 3g, the latter taken separately or added to the strained decoction.
- With mucus, add **cang zhu** (Rhizoma Atractylodis) 苍术 9-12g.
- With tenesmus, add **mu xiang** (Radix Aucklandiae Lappae) 木香 6-9g and **bing lang** (Semen Arecae Catechu) 槟榔 9-12g.
- With constipation, add **bing lang** (Semen Arecae Catechu) 槟榔 9-12g and **zhi shi** (Fructus Immaturus Citri Aurantii) 枳实 6-9g.
- With sore, red eyes, add **xia ku cao** (Spica Prunellae Vulgaris) 15g.

- With food stagnation (epigastric and abdominal fullness, foul belching, a thick tongue coat), add **chao mai ya** (dry fried Fructus Hordei Vulgaris Germinantus) 炒麦芽 15-30g, **jiao shan zha** (baked Fructus Crataegi) 焦山楂 15g and **jiao shen qu** (baked Massa Fermentata) 焦神曲 15g. In cases with severe food stagnation, consider a prescription that focuses on relieving the food stagnation as the primary strategy, with regulating *qi* secondary, such as **MU XIANG BING LANG WAN** (*Aucklandia and Betel Nut Pill* 木香槟榔丸, p.273).
- For tense or stressed patients, add **he huan pi** (Cortex Albizziae Julibrissin) 合欢皮 15g.
- With acid reflux, add **hai piao xiao** (Os Sepiae seu Sepiellae) 海螵蛸 15g and **mu li** (Concha Ostrea) 牡蛎 15-30g, or **huang lian** (Rhizoma Coptidis) 黄连 6g and **wu zhu yu** (Fructus Evodiae Rutaecarpae) 吴茱萸 2g, the latter pair especially when there is also nausea or vomiting.

Variations and additional prescriptions

With Damp Heat

- During a severe flare-up or aggravation of the condition, as may occur in response to periods of increased stress, heavy drinking or overeating, the main influence in the pattern may be the accumulated Damp Heat. The diarrhoea becomes more frequent, with severe cramping pain copious blood and mucus. The treatment during this time should focus on the branch (that is, the Damp Heat), until the symptoms settle and constitutional work can recommence. If pain is a main feature **SHAO YAO TANG** (*Peony Decoction* 芍药汤, p.270) may be selected; if abdominal distension is a main feature, select **ZHONG MAN FEN XIAO WAN** (*Separate and Reduce Fullness in the Middle Pill* 中满分消丸, p.27).

To regulate qi between episodes

- In between episodes of active dysenteric disorder, a general *qi* regulating formula should be given. A typical example in a young or otherwise relatively healthy individual might be a mixture (in patent medicine form) of **TONG XIE YAO FANG** (*Important Formula for Painful Diarrhoea* 痛泻要方, p.239), with either **XIAO YAO SAN** (*Bupleurum and Dang Gui Formula* 逍遥散, p.159), **DAN ZHI XIAO YAO SAN** (*Bupleurum and Paeonia Formula* 丹栀逍遥散, p.284) or **CHAI HU SHU GAN SAN** (*Bupleurum and Cyperus Formula* 柴胡疏肝丸, p.76). *See also* Liver *qi* invading the Spleen diarrhoea, p.238.

With yin deficiency

- In chronic cases with residual Heat, there will generally be a degree of *yin* deficiency. In between episodes of diarrhoea, a *yin* supplementing prescription may be selected if appropriate. Suitable formulae include **YI GUAN JIAN** (*Linking Decoction* 一贯煎, p.78) for Liver *yin* deficiency with *qi* stagnation, **QI JU DI HUANG WAN** (*Lycium, Chrysanthemum and Rehmannia Formula* 杞菊地黄丸, p.909) for Liver and Kidney *yin* deficiency, **ZHI BAI BA WEI WAN** (*Anemarrhena, Phellodendron and Rehmannia Formula* 知柏八味丸, p.718) for *yin* deficiency with deficient Heat. *See also yin* deficiency dysenteric disorder, p.306.

Patent medicines

During the active phase to clear Heat and cool the Liver

Jia Wei Xiao Yao Wan 加味逍遥丸 (Jia Wei Xiao Yao Wan, Dan Zhi Xiao Yao Wan) plus
Lian Qiao Bai Du Pian 连翘败毒片 (Lien Chiao Pai Tu Pien) or
Long Dan Xie Gan Wan 龙胆泻肝丸 (Long Dan Xie Gan Wan, Lung Tan Xie Gan Wan)

During the non-active phase to soothe the Liver

Shu Gan Wan 舒肝丸 (Shu Gan Wan, Shu Kan Wan)
Mu Xiang Shun Qi Wan 木香顺气丸 (Mu Xiang Shun Qi Wan, Aplotaxis Carminative Pills)
Xiao Yao Wan 逍遥丸 (Xiao Yao Wan, Hsiao Yao Wan, Bupleurum Sedative Pills)
Chai Hu Shu Gan Wan 柴胡疏肝丸 (Chai Hu Shu Gan Wan)

Acupuncture (select from)

Ren.12 (*zhong wan*)
Liv.13 (*zhang men*)
St.25 (*tian shu* -) .... these points regulate *qi* in the abdomen by strengthening the Spleen and Stomach, harmonising the Liver and Spleen and regulating the Intestines

St.37 (*shang ju xu* -) .... lower *he* point of the Large Intestine, clears Heat and stagnation from the Stomach and Intestines

St.36 (*zu san li*) .... *he* sea point of the Stomach, regulates and strengthens the Stomach and Intestines to prevent overcontrolling damage by the Liver

Liv.2 (*xing jian* -) .... *rong* spring and Fire point of the Liver, clears Heat from the Liver, regulates and moves stagnant *qi* and clears Heat from the lower *jiao*

Sp.6 (*san yin jiao*) .... strengthens the Spleen, regulates Liver *qi*, supplements *qi* and drains Dampness
a shi points .... along the Stomach channel, usually found between St.36 (*zu san li*) and St.39 (*xia ju xu*), and along the Urinary Bladder channel between Bl.18 (*gan shu*) and Bl.28 (*pang guang shu*)

LI.4 (*he gu*) .... the 'four gates', both *yuan* points, invigorate *qi*
Liv.3 (*tai chong* -) and Blood, have a powerful sedative and calming action, ease muscle spasm and calm the Intestines
yin tang (M-HN-3) .... calms the *shen* and alleviates agitation

- with severe bleeding, add Sp.10 (*xue hai* -) and Liv.1 (*da dun*)
- with nausea, add PC.6 (*nei guan*)
- with mucus, add St.40 (*feng long* -) and Sp.3 (*tai bai*)
- with hypochondriac pain, add Liv.14 (*qi men* -)
- If the patient is tense and stressed, and suffers insomnia and temporal headaches, use SJ.5 (*wai guan*), GB.39 (*xuan zhong*), and Du.24 (*shen ting*) to soothe the Liver, regulate *qi* and calm the *shen*.
- with grief or sadness (Lung involvement), add Lu.7 (*lie que*) and Lu.1 (*zhong fu*)
- with Spleen deficiency, add Bl.20 (*pi shu*)
- *Ear points*: liver, large intestine, distal segment rectum, *shen men*, subcortex, sympathetic

Retention enema

Retention enema is a useful additional treatment for Liver *qi* stagnation with ulceration or damage to the bowel wall. The main principle of treatment is to promote healing and relax the bowel. If Damp Heat is a significant feature, see p.276.

fang feng (Radix Ledebouriellae Divaricatae) 防风 10g
bai zhu (Rhizoma Atractylodes Macrocephalae) 白术 10g
bai shao (Radix Paeoniae Lactiflorae) 白芍 15g
chen pi (Pericarpium Citri Reticulatae) 陈皮 10g
ru xiang (Gummi Olibanum) 乳香 10g
mo yao (Myrrha) 没药 10g

Method: The herbs are brewed as for a normal decoction, strained and cooled to body temperature before 100-200 mls is inserted with a commercial enema device. The enema can be retained (with the patient lying down) for 30 minutes to 2 hours. **Fang feng**, **bai shao**, **bai zhu** and **chen pi** regulate Intestinal *qi* and ease spasm; **ru xiang** and **mo yao** promote healing.

Clinical notes

- Liver *qi* stagnation with stagnant Heat type dysenteric disorder may be diagnosed biomedically as ulcerative colitis, Crohn's disease or irritable bowel syndrome.
- This pattern appears to be particularly common in those who do variable shift work, especially a frequently rotating eight hour shift (for example 6am-2pm, 2pm-10pm, 10pm-6am in 2 weekly cycles). The cycles of the body which are regulated by the Liver, are thrown out of balance. Complete resolution of the dysenteric disorder is difficult unless the body's internal clock can be reset to a more balanced rhythm, with a more regular daily schedule. Due to the nature of shift work, many patients will have the complicating factor of an irregular diet and overconsumption of heating and irritant substances such as alcohol, coffee and fast or junk foods.
- Dysenteric disorder of a *qi* stagnation with stagnant Heat type can respond well to correct treatment, particularly if the source of external stress can be resolved. Treatment will usually need to persist for at least six months for a good result and must be combined with appropriate relaxation and stress management techniques, or other forms of *qi* mobilising activity. Particularly useful is walking, swimming, yoga or *tai ji chuan*, although all exercise is beneficial. Gentle and regular massage, particularly of the abdomen, neck and mid thoracic region is also useful.
- For dietary recommendations, see p.878.

寒湿痢疾

7.4 COLD DAMP

Pathophysiology

- Cold Damp represents a type of dysenteric disorder that may occur in a patient with a pre-existing Spleen *yang* deficiency, or dysenteric disorders during the winter. This pattern superficially resembles the Spleen deficiency chronic patterns which appear in the three following patterns. The key feature here is the predominance of the excess Cold Damp, relative to any deficiency.
- Cold Damp invades the Spleen and Intestines, disrupting the *qi* mechanism and transformation of food and fluids into useable *qi*. The resulting accumulated Damp sinks into the Intestines and appears as mucus in the stool, while the constricting Cold restrains *qi* and causes spasm and pain.
- Over time the pathogenic Cold Damp will drain Spleen *yang* further, and the pattern, if untreated or poorly treated, is likely to become predominantly deficient and chronic or recurrent.

Clinical features

- diarrhoea with more mucus than blood, or passing of pure mucus
- dull abdominal pain which is better for warmth, but dislikes pressure
- tenesmus
- epigastric and abdominal distension and fullness
- no thirst, decreased sense of taste, loss of appetite
- heaviness in the head and body, foggy-headedness
- clear urine
- lethargy and listlessness
- may be chills, mild fever, muscle aches, no sweating and a floating pulse (with the remnants of an external pathogen)

T normal or pale with a greasy white coat
P soft, soggy, moderate or slippery

Treatment principle

Warm the middle *jiao*, transform Cold Damp, regulate *qi*

Prescription

WEI LING TANG 胃苓汤
(*Magnolia and Hoelen Combination*) modified

cang zhu (Rhizoma Atractylodis) 苍术 12-15g
chao bai zhu (dry fried Rhizoma Atractylodes Macrocephalae) 炒白术 12-15g
hou po (Cortex Magnoliae Officinalis) 厚朴 9-12g
fu ling (Sclerotium Poriae Cocos) 茯苓 12-15g

zhu ling (Sclerotium Polypori Umbellati) 猪苓 9-12g
ze xie (Rhizoma Alismatis Orientalis) 泽泻 9-12g
rou gui (Cortex Cinnamomi Cassiae) 肉桂 3g
chen pi (Pericarpium Citri Reticulatae) 陈皮 6-9g
dang gui (Radix Angelicae Sinensis) 当归 6-9g
mu xiang (Radix Aucklandiae Lappae) 木香 6-9g
zhi shi (Fructus Immaturus Citri Aurantii) 枳实 6-9g
pao jiang (quick fried Rhizoma Zingiberis Officinalis) 炮姜 6-9g

Method: Decoction. **Cang zhu** and **hou po** powerfully warm and dry Dampness and alleviate fullness; **chao bai zhu** strengthens the Spleen and dries Dampness; **fu ling** strengthens the Spleen; **fu ling**, **zhu ling** and **ze xie** promote urination to drain Dampness; **rou gui** and **pao jiang** assist in the transformation of *qi* and promotion of fluid metabolism, and dispel Cold; **chen pi**, **zhi shi** and **mu xiang** regulate *qi*; **mu xiang** relieves tenesmus; **dang gui** harmonises Blood. (Source: *Shi Yong Zhong Yi Nei Ke Xue*)

Modifications

- With severe tenesmus, add **bing lang** (Semen Arecae Catechu) 槟榔 6-9g.
- With food stagnation and abdominal distension, add **lai fu zi** (Semen Raphani Sativi) 莱服子 12-15g and **da fu pi** (Pericarpium Arecae Catechu) 大服皮 9-12g.
- With severe Cold causing spasmodic abdominal pain that improves with warmth, add **gao liang jiang** (Rhizoma Alpiniae Officinari) 高良姜 9-12g.
- With nausea, add **ban xia** (Rhizoma Pinelliae Ternatae) 半夏 9-12g.
- With acid reflux or sour regurgitation, add **huang lian** (Rhizoma Coptidis) 黄连 3g and **wu zhu yu** (Fructus Evodiae Rutaecarpae) 吴茱萸 2g.
- With a component of *qi* stagnation, add **xiang fu** (Rhizoma Cyperi Rotundi) 香附 9-12g and **fo shou** (Fructus Citri Sarcodactylis) 佛手 9-12g.

Variations and additional prescriptions

With exterior signs and symptoms

- If the condition is acute and there are clear exterior signs, combine the primary prescription with several doses of another appropriate formula. For Wind Cold (chills greater than fever, no sweating, occipital headache, floating tight pulse) combine with **JING FANG BAI DU SAN** (*Schizonepeta and Ledebouriella Powder to Overcome Pathogenic Influences* 荆防败毒散, p.909). For Summerdamp (heaviness, muscle aches, more chills and fever, floating and soggy pulse), combine with **HUO XIANG ZHENG QI SAN** (*Agastache Formula* 霍香正气散, p.222).

Patent medicines

Ping Wei San 平胃散 (Ping Wei San, Tabellae Pingwei)

Xiang Sha Liu Jun Zi Wan 香砂六君子丸 (Xiang Sha Liu Jun Wan, Aplotaxis-Ammomum Pills, Six Gentlemen Tea Pills)
Fu Zi Li Zhong Wan 附子理中丸 (Fu Tzu Li Chung Wan, Carmichaeli Tea Pills, Li Chung Yuen Medical Pills)
- for *yang* deficiency with Cold

Xing Jun San 行军散 (Marching Powder, Five Pagodas Brand)
- A powerful Damp drying powder, good in acute cases with external symptoms.

Acupuncture (select from)

St.25 (*tian shu* -▲) .... *mu* point of the Large Intestine, warms the Intestines and eliminates Cold Damp
zhi xie (N-CA-3 ▲) .... extra point for diarrhoea, located halfway between Ren.8 (*shen que*) and the pubic bone
St.36 (*zu san li* -▲) .... *he* sea point of the Stomach, powerfully warms and strengthens the Spleen and Stomach and supplements *qi* to transform Cold Damp
St.37 (*shan ju xu* -) .... lower *he* point of the Large Intestine, eliminates Cold Damp from the Intestines
Sp.9 (*yin ling quan* -) .... *he* sea point of the Spleen, promotes urination and drains Dampness
Sp.6 (*san yin jiao* -) .... strengthens the Spleen, regulates Liver *qi*, supplements *qi* and drains Dampness

Sp.3 (*tai bai* -) .... *yuan luo* pair, strengthen the Spleen and
St.40 (*feng long* -) transform Dampness and Phlegm

Bl.25 (*da chang shu* -▲) ... *shu* points of the Large and Small Intestine
Bl.27 (*xiao chang shu* -▲) respectively, eliminate Cold Damp

- with nausea, add PC.6 (*nei guan*)
- with abdominal pain, moxa can be applied with a moxa box over the umbilicus, or use moxa cones over slices of ginger on the indicated points above.
- *Ear points*: spleen, large intestine, small intestine, sympathetic, distal segment rectum

Clinical notes

- Cold Damp dysenteric disorder may be diagnosed biomedically as dysentery, ulcerative colitis or irritable bowel syndrome.
- Chronic Cold Damp can occasionally generate Heat, resulting in occasional, usually mild, episodes of Damp Heat dysenteric disorder.
- For dietary recommendations, see p.873, 880.

噤口痢疾

7.5 ANORECTIC DYSENTERIC DISORDER

Pathophysiology

- Anorectic dysenteric disorder[1] follows unresolved or poorly treated Damp Heat, Cold Damp or fulminant dysenteric disorder. In most cases the pattern will not have a long history; most likely the patient will have had an acute illness for 1-2 weeks, then lapse into this state. Because patients are unable to eat, they deteriorate quickly, and the condition can be dangerous. The priority treatment principle is to get patients eating again, so they can recover their *qi*.
- The basic mechanism is a combination of residual Heat in the Intestines with serious underlying deficiency, leading to obstruction of the *qi* mechanism. This causes the pathogen to rebel upwards, disabling Stomach *qi*.
- The main feature, the *jin kou*, (literally 'silent or closed mouth'), is the inability to take any food or fluid without vomiting. There are two variants of the pattern, depending on the balance of deficiency and excess.

Clinical features

- small and decreasing amounts of diarrhoea with mucus; there may or may not be small amounts of blood.
- nausea and vomiting with anything taken through the mouth
- severe anorexia, inability or refusal to eat
- **when the residual Heat excess is prominent**: the above symptoms are accompanied by signs of Heat and excess, red complexion, thirst and dryness, fullness in the chest, foul taste in the mouth and restlessness

T greasy yellow tongue coat
P with Heat: slippery, rapid pulse

- **when the deficiency is prominent**: the patient is emaciated and continually nauseous, vomits upon eating and lacks thirst

T pale with little coat
P thready and weak

Treatment principle

Excess: Clear residual Heat, harmonise the Stomach and stop vomiting
Open the Stomach and encourage decent of *qi* with bitter pungent herbs

Deficiency: Strengthen the Spleen, harmonise the Stomach
Direct Stomach *qi* downwards and stop vomiting

---

[1]Wiseman's 'Food denying dysentery'

Prescription

KAI JIN SAN 开噤散
(*Powder for Treating Anorectic Dysentery*)

This prescription (literally 'open the closed powder') is suitable for excess patterns.

dong gua ren (Semen Benincasae Hispidae) 冬瓜仁 15g
dang shen (Radix Codonopsis Pilosulae) 党参 12g
shi lian zi (Semen Caesalpinae Minacis) 石莲子 9g
dan shen (Radix Salviae Miltiorrhizae) 丹参 9g
fu ling (Sclerotium Poriae Cocos) 茯苓 9g
chen cang mi (Fructus Oryzae Sativae) 陈仓米 9g
he ye di (Petiolus Nelumbinis Nuciferae) 荷叶蒂 9g
shi chang pu (Rhizoma Acori Graminei) 石菖蒲 9g
chen pi (Pericarpium Citri Reticulatae) 陈皮 9g
huang lian (Rhizoma Coptidis) 黄连 4.5g

Method: Decoction as powder. The decoction should be taken in small amounts as frequently as possible without provoking vomiting, or small amounts of the powder may be placed under the tongue. **Dong gua ren** clears Damp Heat and promotes downwards movement of *qi*; **dang shen, fu ling** and **chen cang mi** support the Spleen; **shi lian zi** clears Damp Heat and, with **shi chang pu**, opens the Stomach to be able to receive food; **dan shen** clears Heat, invigorates Blood and calms the *shen*; **chen pi** regulates *qi*; **huang lian** clears Damp Heat and directs *qi* downwards. (Source: *Shi Yong Zhong Yi Nei Ke Xue*)

Modifications

- With severe nausea, add **ban xia** (Rhizoma Pinelliae Ternatae) 半夏 12g.
- If prolonged vomiting damages Stomach *yin*, with red, dry, or peeled tongue, delete **chen pi**, and add two or three of the following herbs: **xi yang shen** (Radix Panacis Quinquefolii) 西洋参 9g, **mai dong** (Tuber Ophiopogonis Japonici) 麦冬 9g, **shi hu** (Herba Dendrobii) 石斛 9g or **lu gen** (Rhizoma Phragmitis Communis) 芦根 15g.

XIANG SHA LIU JUN ZI TANG 香砂六君子汤
(*Saussurea and Cardamon Combination*) modified

This prescription is selected when the patient is seriously weakened. The focus of treatment is on reviving the Spleen. It can be taken in small doses to start with, ideally combined with a light rice soup (to harmonise the Stomach). The dose taken daily can gradually be increased to 2 cups per day.

dang shen (Radix Codonopsis Pilosulae) 党参 12-15g
chao bai zhu (dry fried Rhizoma Atractylodes Macrocephalae) 炒白术 12-15g

fu ling (Sclerotium Poriae Cocos) 茯苓 12-15g
ban xia (Rhizoma Pinelliae Ternatae) 半夏 9-12g
chen pi (Pericarpium Citri Reticulatae) 陈皮 9-12g
zhi gan cao (honey fried Radix Glycyrrhizae Uralensis)
炙甘草 3-6g
mu xiang (Radix Aucklandiae Lappae) 木香 6-9g
sha ren (Fructus Amomi) 砂仁 6-9g
gan jiang (Rhizoma Zingiberis Officinalis) 干姜 6-9g
rou gui (Cortex Cinnamomi Cassiae) 肉桂 3g
bu gu zhi (Fructus Psoraleae Corylifoliae) 补骨脂 9-12g
lian zi (Semen Nelumbinis Nuciferae) 莲子 9-12g
shi chang pu (Rhizoma Acori Graminei) 石菖蒲 6-9g

Method: Decoction. **Dang shen** supplements *qi* and strengthens the Spleen; **chao bai zhu** strengthens the Spleen and dries Dampness; **fu ling** strengthens the Spleen and leaches out Dampness through the urine; **ban xia** transforms Phlegm, dries Dampness, directs rising Stomach *qi* downwards and stops nausea and vomiting; **chen pi** transforms Phlegm and dries Dampness, regulates middle *jiao qi* and corrects the *qi* mechanism; **zhi gan cao** strengthens the Spleen and harmonises the Stomach; **mu xiang** and **sha ren** regulate *qi* and open the Stomach; **gan jiang**, **bu gu zhi** and **rou gui** warm *yang* and stop vomiting; **lian zi** and **shi chang pu** open the Stomach to pique the appetite. (Source: *Shi Yong Zhong Yi Nei Ke Xue*)

Variations and additional prescriptions

- SHEN LING BAI ZHU SAN (*Ginseng and Atractylodes Formula* 参苓白术散, p.243) is a suitable alternative for deficient cases, with the same modifications as directly above.
- If the patient is unable to take any medicine at all, 1 gram of **YU SHU DAN** (*Jade Pivot Special Pill* 玉枢丹, p.748) can be held in the mouth until the Stomach settles enough to enable the patient to sip the main prescription.

Acupuncture (select from)

Ren.12 (*zhong wan*) .... *mu* point of the Stomach, warms and regulates the Stomach and directs Stomach *qi* downwards; add moxa in deficient cases

St.25 (*tian shu* -) .... *mu* point of the Large Intestine, clears Dampness and Heat from the Intestines; add moxa in deficient cases

PC.6 (*nei guan*) .... *luo* point of the Pericardium, master point of *yin wei mai*, regulates the middle *jiao* and stops nausea and vomiting

LI.4 (*he gu* -) ....*yuan* point of the Large Intestine, clears Heat from, and regulates, *yang ming*

Sp.4 (*gong sun*) .... *luo* point of the Spleen, master point of *chong mai*, regulates the Spleen and Stomach
St.36 (*zu san li*) .... *he* sea point of the Stomach, powerfully warms and strengthens the Spleen and Stomach and supplements *qi*; add moxa in deficient cases
St.37 (*shang ju xu* -) .... lower *he* point of the Large Intestine, clears stagnation and accumulation from the Stomach and Intestines and clears Dampness and Heat
Sp.6 (*san yin jiao* +) .... strengthens the Spleen, regulates Liver *qi*, supplements *qi* and drains Dampness
Bl.20 (*pi shu*) .... *shu* point of the Spleen, warms and supplements Spleen *qi* and *yang*; add moxa in deficient cases

- *Ear points*: *shen men*, spleen, stomach, sympathetic

Retention enema

See Damp Heat, p.275.

Clinical notes

- This is a serious and potentially dangerous development in the progress of a dysenteric disorder. It should be managed in hospital.
- Dietary suggestions are a moot point in a condition such as this, but powdered buckwheat mixed with a little sugar and water is recommended.

休息痢疾

7.6 CHRONIC RELAPSING DYSENTERIC DISORDER

Pathophysiology

- If an acute episode of dysenteric disorder is untreated or poorly treated, it can become chronic and relapsing. Over-enthusiastic or premature use of astringent herbs in the treatment of a Damp Heat or Toxic Heat pattern can cause a pathogen to become lodged in the Intestines. *Zheng qi* is gradually weakened, and a complex state of deficiency, excess, Heat and Cold result. Depending on the longevity of the condition and the constitution of the patient, the manifestation of the dysenteric disorder may be Damp Heat, Cold Damp, Spleen deficiency, *yin* deficiency or a combination of these.
- Damp Heat or Cold Damp can get locked away in the Intestines, occasionally surfacing in response to an invasion of an exterior pathogen, the ingestion of certain foods, including supplementing and astringent herbs, or when the patient is stressed or fatigued. This is a type of latent (*fu* 伏) pathogen.
- Treatment depends on where the patient is in the cycle of exacerbation and remission, and the severity of the symptoms. During the quiescent phase, the main principle is primarily to strengthen the Spleen and Stomach, and secondarily to clear Damp Heat. During exacerbation however, the dysenteric disorder may be characterised by Damp Heat, Toxic Heat or Cold Damp, in which case the treatments outlined in those sections apply. The treatments described below are suitable when patients present with mixtures of deficiency and excess.

Clinical features

- Chronic intermittent diarrhoea with variable mixtures of mucus, pus and blood, triggered or aggravated by overexertion, colds, fatigue, stress, or with no obvious trigger. During active phases the diarrhoea may occur many times daily and be accompanied by the following:
- fatigue and tiredness
- tenesmus
- abdominal distension, mild abdominal pain that improves with warmth and possibly pressure
- loss of appetite and sense of taste
- in long standing cases there will usually be obvious deficiency - emaciation, sallow or pallid complexion, listlessness, lethargy, increased desire to sleep, cold intolerance and cold extremities

T normal, pale or red with a greasy coat
P thready and choppy or soft and weak

Treatment principle

Strengthen the Spleen, supplement *qi*
Regulate *qi*, clear Damp Heat, Cold Damp, Toxic Heat (as necessary)

Prescription

ZI SHENG WAN 资生丸
(*Aid Life Pill*) modified

This formula is selected when deficiency is predominant. It is suitable for prolonged cases with Spleen deficiency and some residual Damp and a tendency to food stagnation.

dang shen (Radix Codonopsis Pilosulae) 党参 100g
bai zhu (Rhizoma Atractylodes Macrocephalae) 白术 100g
fu ling (Sclerotium Poriae Cocos) 茯苓 45g
bian dou (Semen Dolichos Lablab) 扁豆 45g
yi ren (Semen Coicis Lachryma-jobi) 苡仁 45g
zhi shi (Fructus Immaturus Citri Aurantii) 枳实 45g
mu xiang (Radix Aucklandiae Lappae) 木香 45g
shan zha (Fructus Crataegi) 山楂 60g
shen qu (Massa Fermentata) 神曲 45g
mai ya (Fructus Hordei Vulgaris Germinantus) 麦芽 60g
zhi gan cao (honey fried Radix Glycyrrhizae Uralensis)
炙甘草 15g
huang lian (Rhizoma Coptidis) 黄连 10g

Method: Grind herbs to a fine powder and form into 9-gram pills with water. The dose is one pill 2-3 times daily. May also be decocted with an 80-90% reduction in quantities. **Dang shen**, **bai zhu**, **fu ling**, **yi ren**, **bian dou** and **zhi gan cao** strengthen the Spleen and supplement *qi*; **bai zhu** dries Dampness; **yi ren**, **fu ling** and **bian dou** leach out Dampness by promoting urination; **zhi shi**, **mu xiang**, **shan zha**, **shen qu** and **mai ya** move *qi*, improve digestion and alleviate food stagnation; **huang lian** clears Damp Heat. (Source: *Shi Yong Zhong Yi Nei Ke Xue*)

WU MEI WAN 乌梅丸
(*Mume Pill*) modified

This formula, with its mix of hot, cold, and astringent herbs, treats a variety of complex patterns characterised by a mixture of Heat, Cold and deficiency. The prescription warms the Intestines, expels pathogens and stops dysenteric disorder. The clinical features of the disorder are recurrent diarrhoea with mucus and blood, abdominal pain that is relieved by warmth and pressure, and a red tongue.

wu mei (Fructus Pruni Mume) 乌梅 .... 48(30)g
huang lian (Rhizoma Coptidis) 黄连 .... 48(9)g
gan jiang (Rhizoma Zingiberis Officinalis) 干姜 .... 30(6)g
huang bai (Cortex Phellodendri) 黄柏 .... 18(9)g
xi xin (Herba cum Radice Asari) 细辛 .... 18(3)g
zhi fu zi (Radix Aconiti Carmichaeli Praeparata)
制附子 .... 18(6)g

gui zhi (Ramulus Cinnamomi Cassiae) 桂枝 .... 18(6)g
dang shen (Radix Codonopsis Pilosulae) 党参 .... 18(9)g
chuan jiao (Pericarpium Zanthoxyli Bungeani) 川椒 .... 12(3)g
dang gui (Radix Angelicae Sinensis) 当归 .... 12(9)g
mu xiang (Radix Aucklandiae Lappae) 木香 .... 12(9)g

Method: Grind herbs to a fine powder and form into 9-gram pills with water. The dose is one pill 2-3 times daily. May also be decocted with quantities shown in brackets, in which case **zhi fu zi** is cooked for 30 minutes before adding the other herbs (*xian jian* 先煎). **Wu mei** astringes the Intestines and stops diarrhoea; **chuan jiao** and **xi xin** warm the interior and disperse Cold; **huang lian** and **huang bai** attack parasites by making the environment hostile, and drain parasites downwards with their bitter coldness; **gan jiang**, **zhi fu zi** and **gui zhi** warm *yang* and dispel Cold and balance the bitter coldness of the previous two herbs; **dang gui** and **dang shen** supplement and replenish *qi* and Blood; **mu xiang** regulates *qi* and relieves tenesmus.

Modifications

- Chronic amoebic dysentery (*Entamoeba histolytica*) typically follows this relapsing pattern. The stools are the consistency and colour of blackcurrant jam. In this case, the seeds of *Brucea javanica* (**ya dan zi** 鸦胆子) may be taken in addition to the appropriate decoction. The dose is 15 seeds three times daily after eating. One course is seven to ten days. Because **ya dan zi** are so bitter they are not decocted. Instead they are usually wrapped in a dried longan fruit (**long yan rou** 龙眼肉) or in gelatine capsules, and taken separately.

Variations and additional prescriptions

With Liver qi stagnation

- This pattern is frequently complicated by Liver *qi* stagnation with stagnant Heat or residual Damp Heat. *See* p.284.

Treatment in between episodes to strengthen and regulate

- In between episodes, a gentle formula to strengthen the Spleen, clear any residual Dampness and move *qi* may be used. There are numerous possibilities depending on the nature of the patient and the other symptoms they exhibit.
  - For patients with Spleen deficiency and residual Phlegm Damp (abdominal distension, indigestion, reflux, foggy-headedness, pale tongue with a thick white coat), **XIANG SHA LIU JUN ZI TANG** (*Saussurea and Cardamon Combination* 香砂六君子汤, p.149) may be selected as the guiding formula.
  - When there is a strong component of anxiety, phobias or panic attacks and sleep disturbance, and episodes of dysenteric disorder are provoked or aggravated by worry, anxiety or fatigue, combine the

primary prescription with **GUI PI TANG** (*Ginseng and Longan Combination* 归脾汤, p.728).

- Recurrent dysenteric disorder may also be associated with repeated battering of the Spleen and Intestines by an aggressive and overcontrolling Liver. Combine the principal prescription with an appropriate *qi* moving prescription, such as **TONG XIE YAO FANG** (*Important Formula for Painful Diarrhoea* 痛泻要方, p.239), **XIAO YAO SAN** (*Bupleurum and Dang Gui Formula* 逍遥散, p.159), **DAN ZHI XIAO YAO SAN** (*Bupleurum and Paeonia Formula* 丹栀逍遥散, p.284) or **CHAI HU SHU GAN SAN** (*Bupleurum and Cyperus Formula* 柴胡疏肝丸, p.76).
- With Spleen *yang* deficiency, combine with **WEN PI TANG** (*Warm the Spleen Decoction* 温脾汤, p.62).

Patent medicines

Zi Sheng Wan 资生丸 (Zi Sheng Wan, Zi Sheng Stomachic Pills)
Xiang Lian Wan 香连丸 (Xiang Lian Wan)
- add when there is clear residual Damp Heat and tenesmus

Acupuncture (select from)

Ren.12 (*zhong wan*) .... these points regulate *qi* in the abdomen by
Liv.13 (*zhang men*) strengthening the Spleen and Stomach,
St.25 (*tian shu* -) harmonising the Liver and Spleen and regulating the Intestines

St.36 (*zu san li* +) .... *he* sea point of the Stomach, regulates and strengthens the Stomach and Intestines to prevent overcontrolling damage by Liver, supplements *qi* and stops diarrhoea
St.37 (*shang ju xu* -) .... lower *he* point of the Large Intestine, eliminates stagnation from the Stomach and Intestines and regulates the Intestines
Sp.6 (*san yin jiao*) .... strengthens the Spleen, regulates Liver *qi*, supplements *qi* and drains Dampness

Bl.20 (*pi shu*) .... *shu* points of the Spleen, Stomach and Large
Bl.21 (*wei shu*) Intestine respectively, strengthen and regulate
Bl.25 (*da chang shu*) the gastro-intestinal system and supplement *qi*

- Add *a shi* points along the Stomach channel as appropriate. Tender points will often be found around St.37 (*shang ju xu*) or St.39 (*xia ju xu*).
- add moxa when there is little or no residual Heat

- with bleeding, add Sp.1 (*yin bai* ▲) and Liv.1 (*da dun*)
- with mucus, add St.40 (*feng long* -) and Sp.3 (*tai bai*)
- with *qi* stagnation, add Liv.3 (*tai chong* -) and GB.34 (*yang ling quan* -)
- with stagnant Heat, add Liv.2 (*xing jian* -)
- with hypochondriac pain, add Liv.14 (*qi men* -)
- If the patient is tense and stressed, and suffers insomnia and lateral headaches, use SJ.5 (*wai guan*), GB.39 (*xuan zhong*), and Du.24 (*shen ting*) to soothe the Liver, regulate *qi* and calm the *shen*.
- *Ear points*: spleen, large intestine, small intestine, subcortex, sympathetic, distal segment rectum

Retention enema

See p.275.

Clinical notes

- Relapsing dysenteric disorder may be diagnosed biomedically as persistent amoebic or bacterial dysentery, giardia, ulcerative colitis, Crohn's disease or irritable bowel syndrome.
- This pattern can be quite complicated and often involves several distinct pathologies. The most common mix is the primary pathological triad. Selection of the appropriate prescription depends on the balance of the pathologies. *See* p.912 for more detail.
- For dietary recommendations, see pp.870, 880, 884.

Table 7.2 *Astringent herbs for dysenteric disorder or chronic diarrhoea*

Chi Shi Zhi 赤石 脂 (Halloysium Rubrum)	Kaolin; sweet, sour, astringent, warm. An important substance for chronic diarrhoea and dysenteric disorders, particularly when severe to the point of incontinence, and accompanied by bleeding. Often combined with Yu Yu Liang.
Yu Yu Liang 禹余粮 (Limonite)	Mineral composed largely of iron oxide ($Fe_2O_3.nH_2O$); sweet, astringent, neutral. For severe or intractable diarrhoea or dysenteric disorder to the point of incontinence or with bleeding. Often combined with Chi Shi Zhi.
He Zi 诃子 (Fructus Terminaliae Chebulae)	Terminalia fruit; bitter, sour, astringent, neutral. For chronic diarrhoea and dysenteric disorder. Being neutral, it can be used for hot or cold patterns depending on the other herbs with which it is combined.
Wu Mei 乌梅 (Fructus Pruni Mume)	Umeboshi plum; sour, warm. For chronic diarrhoea and dysenteric disorder, especially with bleeding or parasites.
Shi Liu Pi 石 榴皮 (Pericarpium Punicae Granati)	Pomegranate husk; sour, astringent and warm. For chronic diarrhoea and dysenteric disorder with Cold; best when the diarrhoea has led to haemorrhoids or rectal prolapse.
Chun Gen Pi 椿根皮 (Cortex Ailanthi Altissimae)	Ailanthus bark; bitter, astringent, cold. Especially for chronic residual Damp Heat patterns causing recurrent diarrhoea, dysenteric disorder with bleeding or vaginal discharge.
Rou Dou Kou 肉豆蔻 (Semen Myristicae Fragrantis)	Nutmeg; acrid, warm. Particularly for *yang* deficiency type chronic, recurrent or intractable diarrhoea, particularly when the patient is woken from sleep in the early morning with an urge to defecate.
Lian Zi 莲子 (Semen Nelumbinis Nuciferae)	Lotus seed; sweet, astringent, neutral. Strengthens the Spleen to stop diarrhoea. Useful when Spleen deficiency diarrhoea is accompanied by *shen* disturbance causing anxiety and insomnia.
Qian Shi 芡实 (Semen Euryales Ferocis)	Fox nut; sweet, astringent, neutral. Strengthens the Spleen and drains Damp to stop diarrhoea. Especially useful for Spleen deficiency diarrhoea in children.

阳虚痢疾

7.7 SPLEEN AND KIDNEY YANG DEFICIENCY

Pathophysiology

- Spleen and Kidney *yang* deficiency dysenteric disorder follows improperly or incompletely treated fulminant or Damp Heat dysenteric disorder, and reflects the prominence of weakened *zheng qi* and *yang*. If severe enough this pattern can overlap with anorectic dysentery. The difference between this and relapsing dysenteric disorder is that, in this pattern, there is negligible pathogen remaining and treatment thus focuses simply on restoring Spleen function.

Clinical features

- Chronic and relentless dysenteric diarrhoea which is thin, watery and mucoid, and may contain pus and blood. In severe cases there may be incontinence of stools and rectal prolapse. The diarrhoea is worse for exposure to cold and cold foods.
- mild tenesmus, or a dragging sensation in the lower abdomen, not relieved by the diarrhoea
- mild, persistent abdominal pain, which is better for warmth and pressure
- loss of appetite, listlessness, fatigue, exhaustion, depression
- waxy pale or sallow complexion
- cold extremities, cold intolerance
- weakness and soreness of the lower back and legs

T pale and swollen with a thin, white coat
P deep, thready, weak, slow

Treatment principle

Warm and strengthen Spleen and Kidney *yang*
Disperse Cold, transform Dampness
Astringe diarrhoea and elevate *qi*

Prescription

FU ZI LI ZHONG WAN 附子理中丸
(*Aconite, Ginseng and Ginger Formula*) modified

This prescription is suitable for milder cases.

zhi fu zi (Radix Aconiti Carmichaeli Praeparata) 制附子 9-12g
gan jiang (Rhizoma Zingiberis Officinalis) 干姜 9-12g
dang shen (Radix Codonopsis Pilosulae) 党参 15-24g
chao bai zhu (dry fried Rhizoma Atractylodes Macrocephalae) 炒白术 12-15g

zhi gan cao (honey fried Radix Glycyrrhizae Uralensis) 炙甘草 6-9g
bu gu zhi (Fructus Psoraleae Corylifoliae) 补骨脂 9-12g
rou dou kou (Semen Myristicae Fragrantis) 肉豆蔻 6-9g
wu wei zi (Fructus Schizandrae Chinensis) 五味子 3-6g
wu zhu yu (Fructus Evodiae Rutaecarpae) 吴茱萸 3-6g

Method: Decoction. **Zhi fu zi** is cooked for 30 minutes before the other herbs (*xian jian* 先煎). **Zhi fu zi** and **gan jiang** warm Spleen *yang*; **dang shen**, **bai zhu** and **zhi gan cao** strengthen the Spleen and supplement *qi*; **bu gu zhi** supplements Kidney *yang* and stops diarrhoea; **rou dou kou** and **wu zhu yu** warm middle *jiao yang* and dispel Cold; **wu wei zi** astringes the Intestines and stops diarrhoea. (Source: *Shi Yong Zhong Yi Nei Ke Xue*)

ZHEN REN YANG ZANG TANG 真人养脏汤
(*True Man's Decoction to Nourish the Organs*) plus
TAO HUA TANG 桃花汤
(*Peach Blossom Decoction*)

This prescription is selected in severe cases with incessant diarrhoea and prolapsed rectum.

chi shi zhi (Halloysitum Rubrum) 赤石脂 30g
zhi ying su ke (honey fried Pericarpium Papaveris Somniferi) 炙罂粟壳 6-15g
wei he zi (roasted Fructus Terminaliae Chebulae) 煨诃子 .. 9-12g
chao bai zhu (dry fried Rhizoma Atractylodes Macrocephalae) 炒白术 12-15g
chao bai shao (dry fried Radix Paeoniae Lactiflorae) 炒白芍 9-15g
fu ling (Sclerotium Poriae Cocos) 茯苓 15g
ren shen (Radix Ginseng) 人参 6-9g
gan jiang (Rhizoma Zingiberis Officinalis) 干姜 9-12g
rou dou kou (Semen Myristicae Fragrantis) 肉豆蔻 6-9g
mu xiang (Radix Aucklandiae Lappae) 木香 6-9g
dang gui (Radix Angelicae Sinensis) 当归 6-9g
rou gui (Cortex Cinnamomi Cassiae) 肉桂 3-6g
zhi gan cao (honey fried Radix Glycyrrhizae Uralensis) 炙甘草 3-9g

Method: Decoction. **Rou gui** is added towards the end of cooking (*xian jian* 先煎). **Chi shi zhi** is usually given separately as a powder. **Chi shi zhi**, **zhi ying su ke** and **wei he zi** astringe the Intestines and stop diarrhoea; **ren shen** (or **dang shen**), **chao bai zhu** and **zhi gan cao** strengthen the Spleen and reinforce *qi*; **chao bai shao** and **dang gui** harmonise the Blood and stop pain; **rou gui** and **rou dou kou** warm the middle *jiao* and Kidney *yang* and disperse Cold; **mu xiang** regulates *qi* and alleviates tenesmus. Unfortunately **ying su ke** is rarely available, so may be substituted with **shi liu pi** (Pericarpium Punicae Granati) 石榴皮 9-15g. (Source: *Shi Yong Zhong Yi Nei Ke Xue*)

Modifications (to either prescription, where not already included)

- With severe cold, add **zhi fu zi** (Radix Aconiti Carmichaeli Praeparata) 制附子 9-15g (decocted for 30 minutes before the other herbs).
- With severe prolapse, add **yu liang shi** (Limonite) 禹粮石 12-18g, **huang qi** (Radix Astragali Membranacei) 黄芪 30-60g, **chai hu** (Radix Bupleuri) 柴胡 6-9g and **sheng ma** (Rhizoma Cimicifugae) 升麻 6-12g, or combine with **BU ZHONG YI QI TANG** (*Ginseng and Astragalus Combination* 补中益气汤, p.502).
- A small dose of a Kidney *yang* supplementing formula like **JIN KUI SHEN QI WAN** (*Rehmannia Eight Formula* 金匮肾气丸) in patent pill form can be added, as the patient's digestion improves. This pill is excellent for warming Kidney *yang*, however, as it contains **shu di**, which is 'greasy' and hard to digest, it can aggravate the diarrhoea in some people.

Patent medicines

Fu Zi Li Zhong Wan 附子理中丸 (Fu Tzu Li Chung Wan, Carmichaeli Tea Pills, Li Chung Yuen Medical Pills)
Bu Zhong Yi Qi Wan 补中益气丸 (Bu Zhong Yi Qi Wan, Central Qi Pills) - add with rectal prolapse
Jin Kui Shen Qi Wan 金匮肾气丸 (Fu Gui Ba Wei Wan, Sexoton Pills, Golden Book Tea)

Acupuncture (select from)

St.25 (*tian shu* +▲) .... *mu* point of the Large Intestine, warms and regulates the Intestines, improves Intestinal function and stops diarrhoea
Ren.8 (*shen que* ▲) .... Strong moxa on salt; place a piece of thin cloth over the navel and fill it with salt; burn large cones of moxa on the salt. The cloth enables quick removal of the salt and prevents excessive burning. Powerfully warms *yang* and stops diarrhoea.
Ren.4 (*guan yuan* +▲) ..... warms and supplements *yuan qi* and Kidney *yang*
St.36 (*zu san li* +▲) .... *he* sea point of the Stomach, powerfully warms and strengthens the Spleen and Stomach, supplements *qi* and transforms Dampness
Sp.6 (*san yin jiao* +) .... strengthens the Spleen and Kidney, drains Dampness to stop diarrhoea
Kid.3 (*tai xi* +) .... *yuan* point of the Kidney, supplements *yang*
Du.4 (*ming men* +▲) .... warms Kidney *yang*

Bl.20 (*pi shu* +▲) .... *shu* point of the Spleen, warms and strengthens the Spleen and supplements *qi*

Bl.23 (*shen shu* +▲) .... *shu* point of the Kidney, warms and stimulates Kidney *yang*

Bl.25 (*da chang shu* +▲) .. *shu* point of Large Intestine, warms, strengthens and astringes the Intestines to stop diarrhoea

Du.20 (*bai hui* ▲) .... strong moxa to help raise *yang* and astringe the Intestines

- a moxa box over the lower abdomen is useful
- *Ear points*: spleen, large intestine, small intestine, sympathetic, adrenal, distal segment rectum

Retention enema

The main principle of treatment is to warm and astringe the Intestines, promote healing and stop dysenteric disorder. May be used every few days until the main symptoms are managed and subsiding.

liu huang (Sulphur) 硫磺 5g
zhi fu zi (Radix Aconiti Carmichaeli Praeparata)
制附子 8g
xian ling pi (Herba Epimedii) 仙灵脾 10g
bai zhi (Radix Angelicae Dahuricae) 白芷 10g
gan cao (Radix Glycyrrhizae Uralensis) 甘草 10g
bu gu zhi (Fructus Psoraleae Corylifoliae) 补骨脂 10g
shi liu pi (Pericarpium Punicae Granati) 石榴皮 10g

Method: **Zhi fu zi** is cooked for 30 minutes before the other herbs (*xian jian* 先煎). The prescription is then brewed as for a normal decoction, strained and cooled to body temperature before 100-200 mls is inserted with a commercial enema device. The enema can be retained (with the patient lying down) for 30 minutes to 2 hours. **Liu huang** and **zhi fu zi** powerfully warm *yang* and dispel Cold; **xian ling pi** and **bu gu zhi** supplement Kidney *yang*; **bai zhi** and **gan cao** aid in discharge of pus and assist in healing; **shi liu pi** astringes the Intestines.

Clinical notes

- *Yang* deficiency dysenteric disorder may be diagnosed biomedically as persistent chronic colitis, chronic dysentery, ulcerative colitis, Crohn's disease and irritable bowel syndrome.
- Treatment will be need to be lengthy and regular to achieve a satisfactory result in this pattern; in many cases 6-12 months may be required for a sustained result and to rebuild *yang*.
- For dietary recommendations, see p.873.

阴虚痢疾

7.8 YIN DEFICIENCY (WITH RESIDUAL DAMP HEAT)

Pathophysiology

- *Yin* deficiency dysenteric disorder often follows unresolved Damp Heat or fulminant dysenteric disorder, where the intense or smouldering Heat damages and dries *yin*. It also occurs in patients who had a pre-existing *yin* deficiency condition before contracting dysenteric disorder.
- This pattern will often be accompanied by elements of residual Damp Heat, however the pattern is defined by the prominence of the deficiency.

Clinical features

- Chronic diarrhoea with small quantities of sticky mucus and blood. Frequent urge to defecate but often in vain.
- mild lower abdominal pain, tenesmus
- loss of appetite, nausea, dry mouth and lips, thirst worse at night
- afternoon or tidal fever, worse at night
- heat in the palms and soles, nightsweats, flushing
- emaciation, weight loss

T red or scarlet and dry, with a greasy or peeled coat
P thready and rapid

Treatment principle

Nourish and supplement *yin* and clear residual Damp Heat
Nourish and regulate Blood, and stop dysentery

Prescription

HUANG LIAN E JIAO TANG 黄连阿胶汤
(*Coptis and Ass-Hide Gelatin Decoction*) plus
ZHU JU WAN 驻车丸
(*Stop the Chariot Pill*) modified

This prescription assumes a degree of residual Damp Heat, common when an acute episode of dysenteric disorder quickly damages *yin*. This strategy has to be used with some caution however, as the bitter cold herbs can exacerbate the already damaged *yin* if no Damp Heat is present.

e jiao (Gelatinum Corii Asini) 阿胶 9-12g
dang gui (Radix Angelicae Sinensis) 当归 9-12g
huang qin (Radix Scutellariae Baicalensis) 黄芩 9-12g
huang lian (Rhizoma Coptidis) 黄连 3-6g
bai shao (Radix Paeoniae Lactiflorae) 白芍 9-12g
sheng di (Radix Rehmanniae Glutinosae) 生地 9-12g
shi hu (Herba Dendrobii) 石斛 9-12g
mai dong (Tuber Ophiopogonis Japonici) 麦冬 9-12g

mu dan pi (Cortex Moutan Radicis) 牡丹皮 9-12g
wu mei (Fructus Pruni Mume) 乌梅 9-12g

Method: Grind herbs to a fine powder and form into 9-gram pills with water. The dose is one pill 2-3 times daily. May also be decocted with dosages as shown. When decocted, **e jiao** is melted in the warm strained decoction (*yang hua* 烊化). **E jiao**, **dang gui**, and **bai shao** nourish *yin* and Blood and stop bleeding; **bai shao** and **wu mei** astringe *yin* and the Intestine; **huang lian** and **huang qin** clear residual Damp Heat from the Intestine; **sheng di** and **mu dan pi** cool the Blood; **mai dong** and **shi hu** nourish Stomach *yin*. (Source: *Zhong Yi Nei Ke Shou Ce*)

Modifications

- With significant bleeding, add **han lian cao** (Herba Ecliptae Prostratae) 旱莲草 9-12g and **di yu tan** (charred Radix Sanguisorbae Officinalis) 地榆炭 9-12g.
- With difficulty passing stools, add **gua lou** (Fructus Trichosanthis) 栝楼 12-18g and **xuan shen** (Radix Scrophulariae Ningpoensis) 玄参 18-24g.
- With significant residual Damp Heat (sticky Blood and mucus) add **bai hua she she cao** (Herbs Hedyotis Diffusae) 白花蛇舌草 30g and **qin pi** (Cortex Fraxini) 秦皮 12-15g.
- With insomnia, sleep disturbances or anxiety, add **zhen zhu mu** (Concha Margaritaferae) 珍珠母 15g and **long chi** (Dens Draconis) 龙齿 15g.
- With low grade or afternoon fevers, add **yin chai hu** (Radix Stellariae Dichotomae) 银柴胡 9-12g.

Patent medicines

Zhi Bai Ba Wei Wan 知柏八味丸 (Zhi Bai Ba Wei Wan, Chih Pai Pa Wei Wan)

Xiang Lian Wan 香连丸 (Xiang Lian Wan)
- add when there is residual Damp Heat and tenesmus

Acupuncture (select from)

Ren.12 (*zhong wan*) .... *mu* point of the Stomach, supplements *qi* and *yin* in combination with St.36

St.25 (*tian shu* +) .... *mu* point of the Large Intestine, regulates the Intestines, clears Damp Heat and stops diarrhoea

Ren.4 (*guan yuan* +) .... meeting point of the *yin*, regulates *qi* in the lower *jiao*, strengthens the Kidneys and supplements *yin*, especially with Sp.6

Sp.6 (*san yin jiao*) .... supplements and regulates *qi* and *yin* and strengthens the Kidneys

St.37 (*shan ju xu* -) .... lower *he* point of the Large Intestine, clears residual Damp Heat from the Intestines and

regulates the Intestines
St.36 (*zu san li* +) .... *he* sea point of the Stomach, powerfully strengthens the Spleen and Stomach and supplements *qi* and *yin*
Sp.9 (*yin ling quan* +)........ *he* sea point of the Spleen, promotes urination and drains Damp
Kid.3 (*tai xi* +)................*yuan* point of the Kidney, supplements *yin*

Bl.20 (*pi shu* +)................ *shu* points of the Spleen, Kidney and Large
Bl.23 (*shen shu* +) Intestine, benefit *yin*, clear residual pathogens
Bl.25 (*da chang shu* +) and regulate the Intestines

- patients with *yin* deficiency patterns are often hypersensitive to needles so a gentle approach with few points is recommended to begin with
- *Ear points*: spleen, stomach, kidney, large intestine, small intestine, sympathetic, distal segment rectum, *shen men*

Retention enema

The main principle of treatment is nourish and supplement *yin* and Blood, and repair the Intestinal wall. May be used every few days until the main symptoms are managed and subsiding.

dang gui (Radix Angelicae Sinensis) 当归 10g
e jiao (Gelatinum Corii Asini) 阿胶 10g
bai shao (Radix Paeoniae Lactiflorae) 白芍 10g
bai ji (Radix Bletillae Striatae) 白芨 10g
ru xiang (Gummi Olibanum) 乳香 5g
mo yao (Myrrha) 没药 5g
gan cao (Radix Glycyrrhizae Uralensis) 甘草 5g

Method: Decoction for use as an enema. **E jiao** is melted in the warm strained decoction (*yang hua* 烊化). **E jiao**, **dang gui**, and **bai shao** nourish *yin* and Blood and stop bleeding; **bai ji** protects the lining of the Intestine and stops bleeding; **ru xiang** and **mo yao** regulate Blood and promote healing; **gan cao** and **bai shao** combine sweet and sour flavours to ease spasms and generate *yin*.

Clinical notes

- *Yin* deficiency dysenteric disorder may be diagnosed biomedically as the convalescent stage of amoebic or bacterial dysentery, persistent chronic colitis, ulcerative colitis or Crohn's disease.
- This can be a difficult pattern to treat successfully, but may respond reasonably well to prolonged treatment. In long standing cases, 6-12 months of treatment may be necessary for a satisfactory result. More recent cases that follow a febrile illness will usually respond faster.
- For dietary recommendations, see p.876.

瘀阻肠络

7.9 BLOOD STAGNATION

Pathophysiology

- Blood stagnation type dysenteric disorder is a chronic pattern that complicates other long term disorders. It is usually associated with significant damage to the Intestinal wall.

Clinical features

- Chronic diarrhoea with a feeling of incomplete evacuation or tenesmus. The diarrhoea may be purple or black, sticky or tarry and contain mucus and clots of blood.
- fixed and localised, sharp or stabbing abdominal pain, usually in the lower left quadrant, which is worse for pressure; masses may be palpable
- dark complexion and lips, dark rings around the eyes
- spider naevi or vascular abnormalities over the abdomen, face and legs, particularly around the inner knee and ankle

T purplish or with purple or brown petechial spots with little or no coat; dark and distended sublingual veins

P wiry, choppy or thready

Treatment principle

Regulate *qi* and Blood and eliminate stagnant Blood from the Intestine

Prescription

SHAO FU ZHU YU TANG 少腹逐瘀汤
(*Drive Out Blood Stasis in the Lower Abdomen Decoction*) modified

This formula is designed for Blood stagnation with Cold.

dang gui (Radix Angelicae Sinensis) 当归 9-15g
chi shao (Radix Paeoniae Rubrae) 赤芍 9-12g
chao wu ling zhi (dry fried Excrementum Trogopteri seu Pteromi) 炒五灵脂 9-12g
sheng pu huang (Pollen Typhae) 生蒲黄 9-12g
yan hu suo (Rhizoma Corydalis Yanhusuo) 延胡索 9-12g
chuan xiong (Radix Ligustici Chuanxiong) 川芎 6-9g
chao xiao hui xiang (dry fried Fructus Foeniculi Vulgaris) 炒小茴香 6-9g
pao jiang (quick fried Rhizoma Zingiberis Officinalis) 炮姜 3-6g
di yu (Radix Sanguisorbae Officinalis) 地榆 12-15g

Method: Decoction. **Dang gui, chi shao, chuan xiong, chao wu ling zhi** and **sheng pu huang** regulate and invigorate Blood, and eliminate stagnant Blood; **yan hu suo** and **chao xiao hui xiang** regulate *qi* and Blood and stop pain; **pao jiang** warms the middle *jiao* and stops diarrhoea; **di yu** cools the Blood and stops bleeding. (Source: *Zhong Yi Zhi Liao Yi Nan Za Bing Mi Yao*)

Modifications

- With abdominal distension, add **zhi shi** (Fructus Immaturus Citri Aurantii) 枳实 9-12g and **hou po** (Cortex Magnoliae Officinalis) 厚朴 9-12g.
- With tenesmus, add **mu xiang** (Radix Aucklandiae Lappae) 木香 6-9g and **bing lang** (Semen Arecae Catechu) 槟榔 9-12g.
- With severe pain, add **bai shao** (Radix Paeoniae Lactiflorae) 白芍 18-24g, **ru xiang** (Gummi Olibanum) 乳香 6-9g and **mo yao** (Myrrha) 没药 6-9g.
- With abdominal masses, add **san leng** (Rhizoma Sparganii Stoloniferi) 三棱 9-12g and **e zhu** (Rhizoma Curcumae Ezhu) 莪术 9-12g.
- With severe bleeding, add **san qi fen** (powdered Radix Notoginseng) 三七粉 3-6g, or the patent *Yun Nan Bai Yao* 云南白药 (Yunnan Paiyao).
- With residual Damp Heat (sticky Blood and mucus) add **bai hua she she cao** (Herbs Hedyotis Diffusae) 白花蛇舌草 30g.
- With Cold, add **rou gui** (Cortex Cinnamomi Cassiae) 肉桂 3g.
- With Heat, add **sheng di** (Radix Rehmanniae Glutinosae) 生地 12-15g and **mu dan pi** (Cortex Moutan Radicis) 牡丹皮 9-12g.
- With Phlegm or Dampness, add **cang zhu** (Rhizoma Atractylodis) 苍术 9-12g, **yi ren** (Semen Coicis Lachryma-jobi) 苡仁 15-24g and **fu ling** (Sclerotium Poriae Cocos) 茯苓 12-15g.
- With *qi* deficiency, add **huang qi** (Radix Astragali Membranacei) 黄芪 15-30g, **dang shen** (Radix Codonopsis Pilosulae) 党参 15-30g and **bai zhu** (Rhizoma Atractylodes Macrocephalae) 白术 9-12g.
- With Liver *qi* stagnation, add **bai shao** (Radix Paeoniae Lactiflorae) 白芍 12-24g, **chen pi** (Pericarpium Citri Reticulatae) 陈皮 9-12g and **fang feng** (Radix Ledebouriellae Divaricatae) 防风 9-12g.
- With hypochondriac pain, add **yu jin** (Tuber Curcumae) 郁金 9-12g and **chuan lian zi** (Fructus Meliae Toosendan) 川楝子 9-12g.

Patent medicines

Xue Fu Zhu Yu Wan 血府逐瘀丸 (Xue Fu Zhu Yu Wan)
- *qi* and Blood stagnation

Fu Ke Wu Jin Wan 妇科乌金丸 (Woo Garm Yuen Medical Pills)
- with a degree of deficiency and Cold

Sheng Tian Qi Pian 生田七片 (Raw Tian Qi Ginseng Tablets)
- this patent can be combined with another, especially with bleeding

Tong Jing Wan 痛经丸 (Tong Jing Wan)
- for severe Blood stagnation with pain

Acupuncture (select from)

St.25 (*tian shu* -) .... *mu* point of the Large Intestine, regulates Intestinal function and eliminates stagnation

Ren.6 (*qi hai* -) .... regulates *qi* and Blood in the lower *jiao*

St.29 (*gui lai* -)	eliminates stagnant Blood from the lower *jiao*
a shi points	over sites of pain in the abdomen
a shi points	along the Stomach channel between St.36 (*zu san li*) and St.39 (*xia ju xu*), and on the Urinary Bladder channel between Bl.18 (*gan shu*) and Bl.28 (*pang guang shu*)
St.37 (*shang ju xu* -)	lower *he* point of the Large Intestine, eliminates stagnation from the Intestines and regulates Intestinal *qi* and Blood
Bl.17 (*ge shu* -)	*hui* point for Blood, eliminates stagnant Blood
Bl.25 (*da chang shu* -) Sp.10 (*xue hai* -) Sp.8 (*di ji* -) Sp.6 (*san yin jiao*)	these points invigorate Blood circulation and eliminate Blood stagnation from the Intestine
LI.4 (*he gu* -) Liv.3 (*tai chong*)	the 'four gates', both *yuan* points, invigorate *qi* and Blood, powerful sedative and calming action, stop pain

- Bleeding the *ah shi* points of the *ba liao* (points over the sacral foramina) followed by strong cupping, can powerfully activate Blood in the lower *jiao*.
- with Cold, add moxa
- *Ear points*: distal segment rectum, large intestine, small intestine, appendix, sympathetic

Retention enema

The main principle is to regulate Blood and promote healing.

dang gui (Radix Angelicae Sinensis) 当归 12g
chi shao (Radix Paeoniae Rubrae) 赤芍 12g
xue jie (Sanguis Draconis) 血竭 12g
ru xiang (Gummi Olibanum) 乳香 10g
mo yao (Myrrha) 没药 10g

Method: Decoction for use as an enema. **Dang gui** and **chi shao** regulate and nourish Blood; **xue jie**, **ru xiang** and **mo yao** regulate Blood and promote healing.

Clinical notes

- Blood stagnation type dysenteric disorder may be diagnosed biomedically as ulcerative colitis, bowel cancer, diverticulosis, intestinal polyps or Crohn's disease.
- This is obviously a serious and most likely sinister development of dysenteric disorder, and the patient should be thoroughly evaluated by specialists. In cases of cancer, TCM can assist, but a combination of TCM and biomedicine should be employed. Long term therapy (12 months+), will be necessary for any satisfactory result. *See also* Clinical notes, p.258.

SUMMARY OF GUIDING FORMULAE FOR DYSENTERIC DISORDER

Damp Heat - *Shao Yao Tang* 芍药汤
- with Summerheat or Summerdamp - *Huo Xiang Zheng Qi San* 藿香正气散
- with food stagnation - *Mu Xiang Bing Lang Wan* 木香槟榔丸
- with Heat greater than Dampness - *Bai Tou Weng Tang* 白头翁汤
- with *yin* damage and dryness - *He Jian Shao Yao Huang Lian Tang* 河间芍药黄连汤

Fulminating (Toxic Heat) - *Bai Tou Weng Tang* 白头翁汤
- with disturbance of consciousness - *Shui Niu Jiao Di Huang Tang* 水牛角地黄汤
- with collapsing *yang* - *Shen Fu Tang* 参附汤
- with locked in Toxic Heat - *Da Cheng Qi Tang* 大承气汤

Liver *qi* invading the Spleen with stagnant Heat - *Dan Zhi Xiao Yao San* 丹栀逍遥散
- with Damp Heat - *Shao Yao Tang* 芍药汤, *Zhong Man Fen Xiao Wan* 中满分消丸

Cold Damp - *Wei Ling Tang* 胃苓汤
- with Wind Cold - *Jing Fang Bai Du San* 荆防败毒散
- with Summerdamp - *Huo Xiang Zheng Qi San* 藿香正气散

Anorectic dysenteric disorder - *Kai JinTang* 开噤汤
- with deficiency - *Xiang Sha Liu Jun Zi Tang* 香砂六君子汤

Chronic relapsing - *Zi Sheng Tang* 资生汤
- with Heat, Cold and deficiency - *Wu Mei Wan* 乌梅丸

Spleen and Kidney *yang* deficiency - *Fu Zi Li Zhong Wan* 附子理中丸
- severe cases - *Zhen Ren Yang Zang Tang* 真人养脏汤 plus *Tao Hua Tang* 桃花汤

Yin deficiency - *Huang Lian E Jiao Tang* 黄连阿胶汤 plus *Zhu Ju Tang* 驻车丸

Stagnant Blood - *Shao Fu Zhu Yu Tang* 少腹逐瘀汤

8. Dysphagia

Phlegm and *qi* accumulation
Heat drying Fluids and *yin*
Phlegm and Blood stagnation
Qi and *yang* deficiency

8 DYSPHAGIA

yi ge 壹膈

Dysphagia describes a sensation of difficulty swallowing, with or without pain. It is often described by the patient as a 'feeling of food getting stuck on the way down'. Dysphagia can be related to disorders of the mouth, pharynx and oesophagus. Oral and pharyngeal causes of dysphagia are usually related to painful infection, inflammation or ulceration, and will be differentiated according to the TCM defined disease symptoms of mouth ulcers or sore throat (Volume 1).

Oesophageal causes of dysphagia may be obstructive or motor. Obstructive dysphagia is associated with narrowing of the lumen of the oesophagus by a lesion such as a stricture or tumour. Patients with obstructive dysphagia usually have difficulty with food but can swallow liquids without difficulty. Motor dysphagia is associated with dysfunction of the smooth muscle of the oesophagus, and is characterised by difficulty swallowing both solids and liquids.

Disorders of the pharynx can cause ingested food or drink to pass into the trachea, causing coughing or spasm of the larynx.

The elderly are most frequently affected, with as many as 40% of people over the age of 75 affected to some degree. Ageing leads to weakness of the jaw muscles, loss of teeth and reduced salivation. The elderly are also more likely to suffer conditions that produce dysphagia as a secondary effect, such as stroke, Parkinson's disease, motor neurone disease and cancer.

Accident related head and neck injuries and cancers of the throat and mouth are the most common causes in younger patients. Regardless of age or health status, it is essential for all patients presenting with dysphagia to be thoroughly investigated.

In TCM, the oesophagus is influenced by dysfunction of the Spleen and Stomach, and Liver organ systems and channel pathways. It is part of the Spleen and Stomach organ system, and as such can be directly damaged by any pathology affecting these organs. The Liver organ system affects the oesophagus through the Liver channel, which passes along the oesophagus, throat, mouth and eyes to the vertex. Liver *qi* stagnation and Liver Heat easily disrupt Spleen and Stomach function.

There are four basic pathological elements that can give rise to dysphagia either singly, or more commonly, in combination. These are stagnant *qi*, Phlegm, stagnant Blood and *yin* deficiency.

In the early stages of the disorder, an excess pattern is most likely, typically *qi* stagnation, with or without Phlegm due to dysfunction of the Liver and Spleen. If *qi* stagnation persists, deficiency of the Spleen and Kidneys becomes more and more dominant. In the later stages, as deficiency and stagnation intensify, Blood and Phlegm stagnation masses develop, and, with the continued difficulty in getting adequate nutrition, *zheng qi* starts to decline.

Complications of dysphagia

Swallowing difficulty can lead to significant morbidity and further complication, as *zheng qi* and *yang* are depleted through malnutrition and dehydration. Patients with significant dysphagia can deteriorate quite quickly.

In addition, dysphagia may result in aspiration of food or liquids into the airways. Aspiration is, in turn, associated with the development of chest infections and pneumonia, an especially dangerous complication in patients already weakened from some other pathology, such as Wind stroke.

On an emotional level, frequent coughing, choking and spluttering during eating can contribute to significant embarrassment, anxiety and depression in some patients, who may choose to isolate themselves at meal times or miss meals altogether.

BOX 8.1 BIOMEDICAL CAUSES OF DYSPHAGIA

Most Common

- tonsillitis, oral ulceration
- stricture (from reflux oesophagitis or corrosive ingestion)
- oesophageal motility disorders
- candidiasis
- herpes simplex
- globus
- motility disorders (achalasia, oesophageal spasm)
- masses in the neck and mediastinum (swollen lymph nodes, goitre, bronchogenic carcinoma, etc.)
- tumours, carcinoma

Other

- scleroderma, dermatomyositis
- systemic lupus erythematosus
- multiple sclerosis
- myasthenia gravis
- motor neurone disease
- post cerebrovascular accident
- Chagas' disease
- anorexia nervosa
- anaphylaxis
- pharyngeal diverticulum
- hiatus hernia
- syringobulbia
- Plummer-Vinson syndrome
- cervical spondylosis
- Parkinson's disease
- foreign body
- radiation or operative injury following tumour treatment

AETIOLOGY

Emotion

Dysphagia often begins as a relatively mild and benign disorder associated with Liver *qi* stagnation. Numerous emotional patterns can give rise to Liver *qi* stagnation, affecting the structures associated with the Liver organ system (here the throat). Internalised and repressed emotion, in particular anger, resentment, frustration, bitterness, hatred and anxiety may all play a part in generating stagnant *qi*. Inability to express or vocalise these feelings especially affects the area of the larynx and throat. Similarly, difficulty in accepting (or swallowing) change or a new situation can create *qi* stagnation in the throat. Patients may be stressed and under pressure; they may be fed up with various elements of their lives–'I can't swallow any more!'. Once *qi* becomes stagnant, a number of other pathological mechanisms may be set in motion, complicating the initial pattern. Liver *qi* stagnation can interfere with the function of the Spleen and Stomach. If the Liver invades the Spleen, the Spleen is weakened and may produce Dampness as a by-product of inefficient digestion. If the Liver invades the Stomach, Stomach *qi* can ascend carrying the acid contents up through the oesophagus. Prolonged *qi* stagnation often generates Heat, which intensifies the rising tendency of the already disordered Stomach *qi*. The Heat plus the increased acid reflux damages Stomach *yin*, drying and tightening the oesophagus and associated structures.

In addition, stagnant *qi* slows and retards fluids which may congeal into Phlegm. Any Heat that has developed may combine with pre-existing Dampness forming Phlegm or Phlegm Heat. Because Phlegm tends to follow *qi* and sticks where the *qi* is stagnant, the Phlegm lodges with the stagnant *qi* in the throat. Once Phlegm or Phlegm Heat is formed, the nature of the obstruction is more substantial, and physical changes take place in the tissues of the throat and oesophagus.

Prolonged accumulation of *qi* and Phlegm, and perhaps Heat and *yin* deficiency, will gradually slow and obstruct the circulation of Blood, and more sinister lesions may develop.

Liver *qi* stagnation type dysphagia is characterised by the variable nature of the swallowing difficulty. It tends to be intermittent, and varies with the emotional state of the patient. The addition of Phlegm tends to create a more substantial obstruction, but, in the early stages, the Phlegm can congeal and dissipate according to the state of the *qi*. As the pathology develops however, the Phlegm component becomes more and more prominent and the dysphagia becomes more or less constant.

Emotions that influence the Lungs can have a bearing on pathology of the throat. Sadness, grief, loss and unshed tears can cause Lung *qi* to accumulate at the level of the throat, often experienced as a sensation of a lump. In TCM this is usually described as 'plum stone throat'.

Diet

Foods that generate Heat and/or Dampness and Phlegm are implicated in the development of dysphagia. The introduction of Heat into the Stomach can cause Stomach *qi* to rise, and with it gastric acids which directly damage, dry and tighten the oesophagus. Foods cooked with chillies and spices, or rich oily foods or alcohol can create Heat and Dampness in the Stomach.

Tobacco can also contribute to the generation of Stomach Heat. Phlegm and Dampness producing foods can cause stagnation in the Spleen and Stomach, block *qi* movement and the *qi* mechanism, and generate Heat.

Phlegm producing and Heat inducing foods can also contribute indirectly to dysphagia. What this means is that rather than damaging the throat and oesophagus directly, they can induce damage to other organ systems that influence these structures, thus disrupting their function. Examples of this are the dysphagia that may follow Wind Stroke, or occur as part of a *wei* syndrome.

Habitual overeating will generate food stagnation, disrupting the *qi* mechanism and generating Dampness and/or Heat in the Stomach.

TCM DIFFERENTIAL DIAGNOSIS

- **Plum stone throat** (*mei he qi* 梅核气): Plum stone throat is a functional disorder of the upper oesophagus associated with Liver and/or Lung *qi* stagnation and Phlegm. The sensation is of something lodged in the throat, but in fact, swallowing is normal. The sensation is intermittent and visual investigations of the throat and larynx are negative. Because there are similarities in aetiology and pathology between plum stone throat and mild dysphagia, some of the treatments recommended for dysphagia can be applied to plum stone throat.
- **Regurgitation** (*fan wei* 反胃): Regurgitation of the contents of the previous meal, largely or completely undigested, some hours later. There is, however, no difficulty in ingesting food.
- **Vomiting** (*ou tu* 呕吐): Ejection of gastric contents associated with rebellious Stomach *qi*. There is no difficulty in swallowing.

TREATMENT

The treatment of dysphagia can be complicated, not least by the fact that the patient may have difficulty ingesting medicine. By the time a patient has real difficulty swallowing, the pathology is quite advanced and treatment is difficult. When the cause of the dysphagia is functional, TCM treatment is effective and can often resolve the problem. Where there is a structural lesion of some description, the prognosis with TCM treatment alone is not so favourable, and will depend on the nature of the lesion. When a neoplasm is the culprit, TCM treatment usually takes second place to biomedical or surgical therapy, and provides more of a supportive role.

痰气交阻

8.1 PHLEGM AND QI ACCUMULATION

Pathophysiology

- Phlegm and *qi* accumulation most commonly represents a functional motility disorder of the oesophagus, oesophageal spasm or decrease in lumen circumference, associated with benign nodule formation in the oesophagus or pharynx. This patterns occurs during the early stage of dysphagia.
- Prolonged stagnation of *qi* leads to accumulation of *qi* at the level of the chest and throat; the sluggish *qi* leads to a retardation in the movement of fluids which congeal into Phlegm. Prolonged stagnation of *qi* and/or Phlegm can easily generate Heat, damaging *yin* and drying the mouth and throat, compounding the difficulty and contributing to thick Phlegm formation. Over time the basic pattern may be complicated by *yin* deficiency or Blood stagnation.
- When *qi* stagnation is dominant, this pattern usually has a clear emotional component, and may represent plum stone throat rather than dysphagia.

Clinical features

- Difficulty swallowing, often with an emotional component–the difficulty is alleviated when the patient is relaxed and aggravated when upset or stressed. The difficulty may be constant, in which case the Phlegm component is likely to be dominant, or occur only when stressed, pointing to dominance of Liver *qi* stagnation.
- fullness and/or discomfort in the chest, or dull chest pain, sensation of tightness or constriction in the throat
- hiccoughs, belching, acid reflux
- vomiting, sometimes a mucus like material or food streaked with mucus
- dry mouth and throat
- sluggish or difficult stools
- gradual weight loss

T unremarkable or red or with red edges and a thin or thick greasy white or yellow coat

P wiry and slippery, possibly rapid or thready

Treatment principle

Regulate *qi*, soothe and soften the Liver
Transform Phlegm
Moisten dryness, clear Heat (as necessary)

Prescription

BAN XIA HOU PO TANG 半夏厚朴汤
(*Pinellia and Magnolia Combination*)

This prescription is used for 'plum stone throat', and is useful for early stage functional dysphagia. The tongue coat is usually greasy and the pulse slippery.

ban xia (Rhizoma Pinelliae Ternatae) 半夏 9-12g
hou po (Cortex Magnoliae Officinalis) 厚朴 6-9g
fu ling (Sclerotium Poriae Cocos) 茯苓 12-15g
sheng jiang (Rhizoma Zingiberis Officinalis Recens) 生姜 9-15g
zi su ye (Folium Perillae Frutescentis) 紫苏叶 6-9g

Method: Decoction. **Ban xia** transforms Phlegm, directs *qi* downwards and harmonises the Stomach; **hou po** directs *qi* downwards, transforms Phlegm and alleviates sensations of fullness and distension; **fu ling** leaches out Dampness and assists the previous herbs in transforming Phlegm; **sheng jiang** harmonises the Stomach; **zi su ye** promotes movement of *qi* in the chest. (Source: *Shi Yong Fang Ji Xue*)

QI GE SAN 启隔散
(*Open the Diaphragm Powder*)

This is the primary prescription when there is true dysphagia and Phlegm is the dominant feature. Swallowing is more or less constantly impaired.

dan shen (Radix Salviae Miltiorrhizae) 丹参 30g
sha shen (Radix Adenophorae seu Glehniae) 沙参 30g
fu ling (Sclerotium Poria Cocos) 茯苓 30g
chuan bei mu (Bulbus Fritillariae Cirrhosae) 川贝母 9-12g
yu jin (Tuber Curcumae) 郁金 9-12g
sha ren (Fructus Amomi) 砂仁 9-12g
he ye di (Stipa Folium Nelumbinis Nuciferae) 荷叶蒂 9-12g

Method: Decoction. **Dan shen, yu jin** and **sha ren** regulate *qi* and Blood, relieve constraint, transform Phlegm and harmonise the Stomach; **sha shen** nourishes *yin*, moistens the throat and loosens dry Phlegm; **fu ling** and **chuan bei mu** improve metabolism of fluids, transform Phlegm and dissipate accumulation; **he ye di** directs *qi* downwards and harmonises the Stomach. (Source: *Shi Yong Zhong Yi Nei Ke Xue*)

XIAO YAO SAN 逍遥散
(*Bupleurum and Dang Gui Formula*) modified

This prescription is selected when Liver *qi* stagnation is the dominant pathology (an obvious emotional component, intermittent dysphagia, tightness and constriction in the throat, irritability, menstrual disorders, wiry pulse). The primary aim of treatment is to spread Liver *qi*, direct *qi* downward and ease the throat, secondarily to transform Phlegm and dissipate masses.

chai hu (Radix Bupleuri) 柴胡 9-12g
dang gui (Radix Angelicae Sinensis) 当归 9-12g
bai shao (Radix Paeoniae Lactiflorae) 白芍 12-15g
bai zhu (Rhizoma Atractylodes Macrocephalae) 白术 12-15g
fu ling (Sclerotium Poria Cocos) 茯苓 12-15g
ji xing zi (Semen Impatiens Balsamina) 急性子 12-15g
xuan fu hua (Flos Inulae) 旋复花 12-15g
dai zhe shi (Haematitum) 代赭石 18-30g
zhu ru (Caulis Bambusae in Taeniis) 竹茹 9-12g
ba yue zha (Fructus Akebiae) 八月扎 9-12g
wei ling xian (Radix Clematidis) 威灵仙 12-18g

Method: Decoction. **Xuan fu hua** is decocted in a cloth bag (*bao jian* 包煎). **Chai hu** moves Liver *qi* and relieves constraint; **dang gui** and **bai shao** nourish the Blood and soften the Liver; **fu ling** and **bai zhu** strengthen the Spleen and clear Dampn;ess **ji xing zi** softens hardness and disperses accumulation; **xuan fu hua** directs *qi* downwards and transforms Phlegm; **dai zhe shi** heavily weighs down *qi*; **zhu ru** clears Heat from the Stomach; **ba yue zha** regulates *qi*, disperses accumulation and stops pain; **wei ling xian** promotes movement through the channels, softens hardness and disperses Phlegm. (Source: *Zhong Yi Zhi Liao Yi Nan Za Bing Mi Yao*)

Modifications (apply to all prescriptions)

- If the patient has signs of dryness (parched mouth and throat), reduce or delete **fu ling** and add **mai dong** (Tuber Ophiopogonis Japonici) 麦冬 9-12g, **xuan shen** (Radix Scrophulariae) 玄参 18-24g, **tian hua fen** (Radix Trichosanthis Kirilowii) 天花粉 9-12g and a spoon of honey.
- With fullness and discomfort in the chest, add **quan gua lou** (Fructus Trichosanthis) 全栝楼 18-24g and **chen pi** (Pericarpium Citri Reticulatae) 陈皮 9-12g.
- With Phlegm nodules encroaching on the oesophagus, add **xuan shen** (Radix Scrophulariae) 玄参 18-24g, **mu li** (Concha Ostreae) 牡蛎 24-30g and **huang yao zi** (Bulbus Dioscorea Bulbifera) 黄药子 9-12g, and substitute **zhe bei mu** (Bulbus Fritillariae Thunbergii) 浙贝母 for **chuan bei mu**.
- With a degree of Blood stagnation, add **tao ren** (Semen Persicae) 桃仁 9-12g, **hong hua** (Flos Carthami Tinctorii) 红花 9-12g and **chuan xiong** (Radix Ligustici Chuanxiong) 川芎 6-9g.
- With frequent belching, add **chen pi** (Pericarpium Citri Reticulatae) 陈皮 9-12g and **chen xiang** (Lignum Aquilariae) 沉香 3-6g.

Variations and additional prescriptions

With rebellious Stomach qi

- A prescription that has the action of heavily weighting and driving down *qi*, is **XUAN FU DAI ZHE TANG** (*Inula and Haematite Decoction* 旋复代赭汤) modified. This prescription can be used when there is a sensation of constriction behind the sternum, with strong signs of rebellious Stomach *qi* such as belching, heartburn, regurgitation or vomiting. The patient may be clearing his or her throat or spitting mucus frequently.

  dai zhe shi (Haematitum) 代赭石 18-30g
  xuan fu hua (Flos Inulae) 旋复花 12-15g
  ban xia (Rhizoma Pinelliae Ternatae) 半夏 9-12g
  dan nan xing (Pulvis Arisaemae cum Felle Bovis) 胆南星 6-9g
  ji xing zi (Semen Impatiens Balsamina) 急性子 12-15g
  quan gua lou (Fructus Trichosanthis) 全栝楼 19-24g
  tai zi shen (Radix Pseudostellariae Heterophyllae) 太子参 12-15g

  Method: Decoction. **Xuan fu hua** is decocted in a cloth bag (*bao jian* 包煎). **Dai zhe shi** and **xuan fu hua** regulate *qi* and powerfully direct *qi* downwards; **ban xia, dan nan xing, ji xing zi** and **quan gua lou** direct *qi* downwards, transform and dispel Phlegm; **tai zi shen** supports the Stomach. (Source: *Shi Yong Zhong Yi Nei Ke Xue*).

Phlegm Heat

- Stagnation of Phlegm and *qi* will often generate Heat. The features of the resulting Phlegm Heat in the Stomach and oesophagus include difficulty swallowing, a feeling of obstruction in the upper chest, fullness and discomfort in the epigastrium and chest, burning epigastric and retrosternal discomfort, heartburn, a greasy yellow tongue coat and slippery pulse. The aim of treatment is to clear and transform Phlegm Heat and open the chest with **XIAO XIAN XIONG TANG** (*Minor Sinking Into the Chest Decoction* 小陷胸汤) modified.

  quan gua lou (Fructus Trichosanthis) 全栝楼 18-24g
  ban xia (Rhizoma Pinelliae Ternatae) 半夏 9-12g
  huang lian (Rhizoma Coptidis) 黄连 3-6g
  chuan bei mu (Bulbus Fritillariae Cirrhosae) 川贝母 6-9g
  yu jin (Tuber Curcumae) 郁金 9-12g
  zhi ke (Fructus Citri Aurantii) 枳壳 9-12g
  shan zhi zi (Fructus Gardeniae Jasminoidis) 山栀子 9-12g

  Method: Decoction. **Quan gua lou, ban xia** and **chuan bei mu** transform and clear Phlegm Heat; **huang lian** and **shan zhi zi** clear Heat and Fire from the upper *jiao*; **yu jin** and **zhi ke** regulate *qi* and relieve constraint of *qi*. (Source: *Zhong Yi Zhi Liao Yi Nan Za Bing Mi Yao*)

Patent medicines

Xiao Yao Wan 逍遥丸 (Xiao Yao Wan, Hsiao Yao Wan, Bupleurum Sedative Pills)

Jia Wei Xiao Yao Wan 加味逍遥丸 (Jia Wei Xiao Yao Wan, Dan Zhi Xiao Yao Wan) - *qi* stagnation with stagnant Heat

Hai Zao Wan 海藻丸 (Hai Zao Wan)
- specific for Phlegm masses, combine with one of the above patent medicines

Nei Xiao Luo Li Wan 内消瘰疬丸 (Nei Xiao Luo Li Wan)
- specific for Phlegm and Blood stagnation masses, combine with one of the first two patent medicines

Acupuncture (select from)

Ren.22 (*tian tu*) .... these points regulate *qi* and Blood in the chest
Ren.17 (*shan zhong*) and oesophagus, direct *qi* downwards, correct
Ren.14 (*ju que*) the *qi* mechanism in the chest, resolve Phlegm and relax the diaphragm

LI.18 (*fu tu* -) .... local point for the throat, transforms Phlegm

Kid.27 (*shu fu* -) .... local point for oesophageal spasm, select if tender

PC.5 (*jian shi* -) .... specific for plum stone throat, regulates Liver *qi* and transforms Phlegm

Kid.4 (*da zhong* -) .... *luo* point of the Kidney, a special point for stricture in the oesophagus

PC.6 (*nei guan* -) .... *luo* point of the Pericardium, master point of *yin wei mai*, opens the chest, eases spasms, regulates Liver *qi* and regulates the middle *jiao*

St.40 (*feng long* -) .... *luo* point of the Stomach, transforms Phlegm

- with Lung involvement associated with prolonged sadness or grief, add Lu.3 (*tian fu*) and Lu.7 (*lie que*)
- *Ear points*: liver, stomach, oesophagus, throat, *shen men*

Clinical notes

- Phlegm and *qi* accumulation type dysphagia may be diagnosed biomedically as oesophageal spasm, a functional or motor disorder of the oesophagus, reflux oesophagitis, or oesophageal stricture or spasm related to stress or grief.
- This pattern responds well to correct treatment, and long term results will be enhanced by appropriate measures to combat the effects of stress–avoidance, exercise, meditation, yoga and active relaxation are all valuable parts of a treatment strategy. *See also* Clinical Notes, p.808.
- For dietary recommendations, see p.878 and 880.

津亏热结

8.2 HEAT DRYING FLUIDS AND YIN (OF THE THROAT AND OESOPHAGUS)

Pathophysiology

- The Heat in this pattern can be either excess Heat (less common), deficient Heat, or a mixture of both (common). The pathology follows prolonged Heat in the Stomach and Liver, and is analogous to Stomach Heat with *yin* deficiency. There will typically be a history of indigestion or heartburn.
- The treatment will vary according to the relative degree of *yin* deficiency and excess Heat.

Clinical features

- Difficulty swallowing, possibly accompanied by a burning or painful sensation; food is difficult to swallow but fluids can be ingested. After eating, the bulk of the ingested food may be vomited up again, possibly mixed with mucus.
- gradual weight loss
- dryness of the mouth and throat, thirst, dry skin
- pain in the chest and upper back
- uncomfortable burning sensation in the epigastrium
- hoarse or croaky voice
- sensation of heat in the palms and soles
- low grade or afternoon fever
- nightsweats, facial flushing
- tendency to constipation

T red and dry with multiple surface cracks, maybe a yellow coat
P wiry, thready and rapid

Treatment principle

Nourish and moisten *yin* and fluids
Clear Heat and disperse accumulations

Prescription

WU ZHI AN ZHONG YIN 五汁安中饮
(*Five Juices Drink to Calm the Middle*)

This prescription is appropriate when the dryness and dysphagia are relatively severe. The juices lubricate the oesophagus and throat and redirect *qi* downwards.

jiu cai zhi (chinese chive juice) 韭菜汁 20ml
niu ru (cows milk) 牛乳 .... 2 cup
sheng jiang zhi (ginger juice) 生姜汁 6ml
li zhi (pear juice) 李汁 20ml

ou zhi (lotus juice) 藕汁 20ml

Method: Extract the juice from the fresh materials with a juice extractor and add to the milk. Sip the juice mixture frequently. The doses given are suitable for a day. **Jiu cai zhi** harmonises the Stomach, eliminates stagnant Blood, relaxes the oesophagus and directs *qi* downwards; **niu ru**, **li zhi** and **ou zhi** generate fluids, moisten dryness and benefit the Stomach; **sheng jiang zhi** harmonises the Stomach, stops vomiting, transforms Phlegm and eases the diaphragm. (Source: *Zhong Yi Nei Ke Shou Ce*)

Modifications

- To augment the *yin* nourishing and lubricating, Heat clearing action of the juice mix, decoct **sheng di** (Radix Rehmanniae Glutinosae) 生地 15-18g, **sha shen** (Radix Adenophorae seu Glehniae) 沙参 12-15g, and **shi hu** (Herba Dendrobi) 石斛 12-15g and sip frequently.
- With significant Stomach Heat, add **huang lian** (Rhizoma Coptidis) 黄连 3-6g, **huang qin** (Radix Scutellariae Baicalensis) 黄芩 9-12g, **huang bai** (Cortex Phellodendri) 黄柏 9-12g, **shan zhi zi** (Fructus Gardeniae Jasminoidis) 山栀子 9-12g.
- The juices above can also be used in combination with one of the prescriptions listed below.

Variations and additional prescriptions

With severe dryness, lack of saliva and constipation

- When Heat has significantly damaged gastro-intestinal *yin*, the tissues of the upper digestive tract can become tight and hard. The clinical features are persistent dysphagia with dryness of the mouth, lips and throat, lack of saliva, sore tight throat, sense of constriction or mass in the throat and upper oesophagus, food getting stuck in the upper oesophagus, the need to sip fluid to get food down, hoarse voice, upper chest and back pain, afternoon fever, nightsweats, constipation, a red dry tongue and thready pulse. The aim of treatment is to nourish *yin*, generate fluids, and clear Toxic Heat with **ZENG YE TANG** (*Increase the Fluids Decoction* 增液汤) modified.

xuan shen (Radix Scrophulariae) 玄参 18-24g
mai dong (Tuber Ophiopogonis Japonici) 麦冬 12-15g
sheng di (Radix Rehmanniae Glutinosae) 生地 15-18g
tian hua fen (Radix Trichosanthis Kirilowii) 天花粉 12-15g
zhi mu (Rhizoma Anemarrhenae Asphodeloides) 知母 9-12g
yu zhu (Rhizoma Polygonati Odorati) 玉竹 9-12g
shi hu (Herba Dendrobi) 石斛 9-12g
shan dou gen (Radix Sophorae Tonkinensis) 山豆根 9-12g
lou lu (Radix Rhapontici seu Echinops) 漏芦 15-30g
bai hua she she cao (Herba Hedyotidis Diffusae)
白花蛇舌草 30-60g

Method: Decoction. **Xuan shen**, **mai dong**, **sheng di**, **yu zhu** and **shi hu** moisten dryness and nourish *yin*; **tian hua fen** and **zhi mu** clear Heat and generate fluids; **shan dou gen**, **lou lu** and **bai hua she she cao** clear Toxins and dissipate accumulations. (Source: *Zhong Yi Zhi Liao Yi Nan Za Bing Mi Yao*)

Lung and Stomach yin deficiency

- Lung and Stomach *yin* are closely related, and damage to Stomach *yin* can easily affect Lung *yin*. When this occurs, the tissues of throat are affected by the *yin* deficiency. The features are constant dysphagia of solids and a sense of a mass in the throat or upper oesophagus, pain with swallowing, frequent dry cough, sore dry throat, dry stools, heat in the palms and soles and nightsweats. The aim of treatment is to nourish Lung and Stomach *yin* and dissipate masses with **SHA SHEN MAI MEN DONG TANG** (*Adenophora and Ophiopogon Combination* 沙参麦门冬汤) modified.

sha shen (Radix Adenophorae seu Glehniae) 沙参 18-30g
mai dong (Tuber Ophiopogonis Japonici) 麦冬 12-15g
yu zhu (Rhizoma Polygonati Odorati) 玉竹 12-15g
tian hua fen (Radix Trichosanthis Kirilowii) 天花粉 12-15g
sheng di (Radix Rehmanniae Glutinosae) 生地 12-15g
xuan shen (Radix Scrophulariae) 玄参 18-24g
jin yin hua (Flos Lonicerae Japonicae) 金银花 15-18g
zhi mu (Rhizoma Anemarrhenae Asphodeloides) 知母 9-12g
yin chai hu (Radix Stellariae Dichotomae) 银柴胡 9-12g
shan dou gen (Radix Sophorae Tonkinensis) 山豆根 9-12g
xu chang qing (Herba cum Radice Cynanchum Paniculatum) 徐长卿 12-15g

Method: Decoction. **Sha shen**, **mai dong** and **yu zhu** nourish Lung and Stomach *yin*; **sheng di** and **xuan shen** cool the Blood and nourish *yin*; **tian hua fen** and **zhi mu** clear Heat and generate fluids; **jin yin hua** clears Toxic Heat; **yin chai hu** clears deficient Heat; **shan dou gen** and **xu chang qing** clear Toxic Heat and disperse accumulations. (Source: *Shi Yong Zhong Yi Nei Ke Xue*)

Yin damage following radiotherapy

- Dysphagia that occurs following radiotherapy for a neoplasm of the breast or lung is usually associated with *yin* damage and residual Heat. The features are a feeling of obstruction and burning in the throat or oesophagus, vomiting, and a pink or red, dry tongue. The aim of treatment is to cool the oesophagus and throat, redirect *qi* downwards and harmonise the Stomach with **LIANG GE SAN** (*Cool the Diaphragm Powder* 凉膈散) modified.

da huang (Radix et Rhizoma Rhei) 大黄 6-9g
mang xiao (Mirabilitum) 芒硝 6-9g
huang qin (Radix Scutellariae Baicalensis) 黄芩 9-12g

shan zhi zi (Fructus Gardeniae Jasminoidis) 山栀子 9-12g
lian qiao (Fructus Forsythia Suspensae) 连翘 9-12g
gan cao (Radix Glycyrrhizae Uralensis) 甘草 6-9g
chen pi (Pericarpium Citri Reticulatae) 陈皮 6-9g
huang lian (Rhizoma Coptidis) 黄连 3-6g
wu zhu yu (Fructus Evodiae Rutaecarpae) 吴茱萸 2-3g
yu xing cao (Herba Houttuyniae) 鱼腥草 30g

Method: Decoction. **Mang xiao** is dissolved in the strained decoction (*chong fu* 冲服). **Da huang** and **mang xiao** clear Heat through the bowels; **huang qin**, **huang lian** and **shan zhi zi** clear Damp Heat from the upper *jiao*; **chen pi** regulates *qi*; **lian qiao** and **yu xing cao** clear Toxic Heat and disperse accumulations; **wu zhu yu** combined with **huang lian** clears Liver and Stomach Heat and alleviates heartburn and rising Stomach *qi*. (Source: *Zhong Liu Ke Zhuan Bing*)

Modifications (apply to all prescriptions, where not already included)

- With tumours of the oesophagus, specific Toxic Heat and hardness softening herbs may be added. Select two or three of the following herbs: **gui zhen cao** (Herba Bidens Bipinnata) 鬼针草 30g, **ji xing zi** (Semen Impatiens Balsamina) 急性子 30g, **shu yang quan** (Herba Solanum Lyratum) 蜀羊泉 30g, **shan ci gu** (Pseudobulbus Shancigu) 山慈菇 0.6-0.9g (as powder added to the strained decoction), **bai hua she she cao** (Herba Hedyotidis Diffusae) 白花蛇舌草 60-120g, **ban zhi lian** (Herba Scutellariae Barbatae) 半枝连 30g, or **huang yao zi** (Bulbus Dioscorea Bulbifera) 黄药子 9-12g.

Patent medicines

Luo Han Guo Chong Ji 罗汉冲剂 (Luo Han Kuo Beverage)
Liu Wei Di Huang Wan 六味地黄丸 (Liu Wei Di Huang Wan, Six Flavour Tea)
- Kidney *yin* deficiency

Mai Wei Di Huang Wan 麦味地黄丸 (Mai Wei Di Huang Wan, Ba Xian Chang Shou Wan)
- Lung, Stomach and Kidney *yin* deficiency

Gu Ben Wan 固本丸 (Gu Ben Wan, Ren Shen Ku Pen Wan)
- Stomach *yin* and *qi* deficiency

Acupuncture

Ren.22 (*tian tu*) .... these points regulate *qi* and Blood in the chest
Ren.17 (*shan zhong*) and oesophagus, direct *qi* downwards, correct
Ren.14 (*ju que*) the *qi* mechanism in the chest, resolve Phlegm and relax the diaphragm
LI.18 (*fu tu* -) .... local point for the throat, transforms Phlegm
Kid.27 (*shu fu* -) .... local point for oesophageal spasm

Lu.7 (*lie que*) .... master and couple point of *ren mai* and *yin qiao*
Kid.6 (*zhao hai*) *mai* respectively, used together they can ease spasm in the midline, correct movement of *qi* through the midline and moisten the throat

St.36 (*zu san li* +) .... *he* sea point of the Stomach, powerfully strengthens the Spleen and Stomach system and supplements *qi* and *yin*

Sp.6 (*san yin jiao* +) .... strengthens the Spleen, regulates Liver *qi*, supplements *yin* and strengthens the Kidneys, invigorates *qi* and Blood and removes obstruction from the channels

- with Stomach Heat, add PC.8 (*lao gong* -) and St.44 (*nei ting* -)
- *Ear points*: stomach, oesophagus, diaphragm, throat, kidney, lung, *shen men*

Clinical notes

- Dysphagia associated with Heat, dryness and *yin* deficiency may be diagnosed biomedically as cancer of the oesophagus, reflux oesophagitis or oesophageal stricture.
- Dysphagia of this type will often show tissue changes consistent with neoplasm, or precursor stages to neoplasm. Thorough investigation is essential, and if neoplasm is confirmed, TCM is useful as support for any biomedical treatment.
- For dietary recommendations, see pp.876, 887.

痰瘀内结

8.3 PHLEGM AND BLOOD STAGNATION

Pathophysiology

- Phlegm and Blood stagnation is always a chronic pattern, and usually the result of long term Liver *qi* stagnation or a complication of *yin* deficiency. It most likely represents some type of physical lesion in the lumen of the oesophagus and should be viewed with suspicion. If the pattern tends towards Blood stagnation, the likely lesion is a carcinoma or similar; if towards Phlegm a benign growth is more likely.

Clinical features

- Difficulty swallowing, in severe cases to the point of not being able to eat solid food at all; even fluids may be difficult.
- vomiting may follow attempts to eat; the vomitus may be watery and tinged red or brown
- localised, possibly sharp or piercing central chest pain
- tendency to constipation with hard dry stools; possibly black tarry stools
- weight loss, emaciation
- dry scaly skin, brittle pitted nails
- spider naevi on the face and chest, dark distended vessels on the legs and abdomen
- dull, sallow or darkish complexion; dark or purplish lips and conjunctiva
- dark rings around the eyes

T purplish or with purple or brown petechial spots, with little or no coat; sublingual vessels are distended and dark

P thready and choppy

Treatment principle

Invigorate Blood, break up Blood stagnation, disperse masses
Nourish and supplement *yin* and Blood

Prescription

TONG YOU TANG 通幽汤
(*Open the Pyloric Sphincter Decoction*)

sheng di (Radix Rehmanniae Glutinosae) 生地 15-18g
shu di (Radix Rehmanniae Glutinosae Conquitae) 熟地 15-18g
dang gui (Radix Angelicae Sinensis) 当归 12-15g
tao ren (Semen Persicae) 桃仁 9-12g
hong hua (Flos Carthami Tinctorii) 红花 9-12g
sheng ma (Rhizoma Cimicifugae) 升麻 9-12g
gan cao (Radix Glycyrrhizae Uralensis) 甘草 6-9g

Method: Decoction. **Sheng di**, **shu di** and **dang gui** nourish *yin* and Blood; **tao ren** and **hong hua** invigorate Blood and eliminate stagnant Blood; **sheng ma** elevates *qi* to stimulate the *qi* mechanism and thus facilitate the natural descent of *qi*, **gan cao** strengthens the Spleen and harmonises the Stomach. (Source: *Shi Yong Zhong Yi Nei Ke Xue*)

Modifications

- In general, if the dominant pathology is Blood stagnation, herbs to enhance the Blood moving action of the prescription may be added. Select two or three of the following herbs: **san qi fen** (powdered Radix Notoginseng) 三七粉 3-6g, **dan shen** (Radix Salviae Miltiorrhizae) 丹参 12-18g, **chi shao** (Radix Paeoniae Rubrae) 赤芍 9-12g, **liu ji nu** (Herba Artemesiae Anomalae) 刘寄奴 9-12g or **wu ling zhi** (Excrementum Trogopteri seu Pteromi) 五灵脂 9-12g.
- With severe Blood stagnation, add one or two or the following substances: **shui zhi** (Hirudo seu Whitmania) 水蛭 3-6g, **meng chong** (Tabanus) 虻虫 1.5-3g, **di bie chong** (Eupolyphaga seu Opisthoplatia) 地鳖虫 6-12g or **jiu cai zhi** (chinese chive juice) 韭菜汁 20ml.
- With Phlegm and Phlegm nodules dominant, add two or three of the following herbs: **hai zao** (Herba Sargassii) 海藻 12-15g, **kun bu** (Thallus Algae) 昆布 12-15g, **wa leng zi** (Concha Arcae) 瓦楞子 15-30g, **zhe bei mu** (Bulbus Fritillariae Thunbergii) 浙贝母 12-15g, **quan gua lou** (Fructus Trichosanthis) 全栝楼 18-24g, **mu li** (Concha Ostreae) 牡蛎 15-30g or **huang yao zi** (Bulbus Dioscorea Bulbifera) 黄药子 9-12g.
- With mucus like vomiting, add **lai fu zi** (Semen Raphani Sativi) 莱服子 9-12g and **sheng jiang** (Rhizoma Zingiberis Officinalis Recens) 生姜 9-12g.
- With copious mucus (cough, constant throat clearing), add **zhu li** (Succus Bambusae) 竹沥 12-15g, **hai fu shi** (Pumice) 海浮石 9-12g, **mu li** (Concha Ostreae) 牡蛎 15-30g or **wa leng zi** (Concha Arcae) 瓦楞子 15-30g; or combine with the patent medicine *She Dan Chuan Bei Ye* (Snake Bile and Fritillary Liquid 蛇胆川贝液, 3-4 vials daily).
- With *qi* deficiency, add **dang shen** (Radix Codonopsis Pilosulae) 党参 15-24g and **huang qi** (Radix Astragali Membranacei) 黄芪 18-30g.
- If vomiting prevents ingestion, a small dose of **YU SHU DAN** (*Jade Pivot Special Pill* 玉枢丹, p.748) under the tongue may settle the stomach enough for the patient to take the herbs.
- With tumours of the oesophagus, specific Toxic Heat and hardness softening herbs may be added. Select two or three of the following herbs: **gui zhen cao** (Herba Bidens Bipinnata) 鬼针草 30g, **ji xing zi** (Semen Impatiens Balsamina) 急性子 30g, **shu yang quan** (Herba Solanum Lyratum) 蜀羊泉 30g, **shan ci gu** (Pseudobulbus Shancigu) 山慈菇 0.6-0.9g (as powder added to the strained decoction), **bai hua she she cao** (Herba Hedyotidis Diffusae) 白花蛇舌草 60-120g, **ban**

zhi lian (Herba Scutellariae Barbatae) 半枝连 30g, or **huang yao zi** (Bulbus Dioscorea Bulbifera) 黄药子 9-12g.

Patent medicines

The pills can be crushed and steeped in hot water (drink the water) to facilitate their ingestion

Xue Fu Zhu Yu Wan 血府逐瘀丸 (Xue Fu Zhu Yu Wan)
- general *qi* and Blood moving medicine

Nei Xiao Luo Li Wan 内消瘰疬丸 (Nei Xiao Luo Li Wan)
- Phlegm and Blood stagnation masses

Hai Zao Wan 海藻丸 (Hai Zao Wan)
- Phlegm masses

She Dan Chuan Bei Ye 蛇胆川贝液 (Snake Bile and Fritillary Liquid)

Acupuncture (select from)

Ren.22 (*tian tu*) .... these points regulate *qi* and Blood in the chest
Ren.17 (*shan zhong*) and oesophagus, direct *qi* downwards, correct
Ren.14 (*ju que*) the *qi* mechanism in the chest, resolve Phlegm and relax the diaphragm

Kid.27 (*shu fu* -) .... local point for oesophageal spasm, select if tender

LI.18 (*fu tu* -) .... local point for the throat, transforms Phlegm

Bl.17 (*ge shu* -) .... *hui* point for Blood, transforms stagnant Blood, regulates diaphragm function

Bl.46 (*ge guan* -) .... reinforces the effect of Bl.17

PC.5 (*jian shi* -) .... specific for constriction in the throat

PC.6 (*nei guan* -) .... *luo* point of the Pericardium, master point of *yin wei mai*, opens the chest, eases spasms, spreads Liver *qi*, regulates the middle *jiao*

St.36 (*zu san li* -) .... *he* sea point of the Stomach, powerfully regulates the Spleen and Stomach, supplements *qi*

- *Ear points*: stomach, oesophagus, liver, throat, diaphragm, *shen men*

Clinical notes

- Phlegm and Blood stagnation type dysphagia will most likely be diagnosed biomedically as an organic lesion obstructing the oesophagus such as tumour, carcinoma, nodules, stricture, or scleroderma.
- Blood stagnation type dysphagia is a difficult condition to treat successfully with TCM alone and is a potentially dangerous condition. Patients presenting without prior investigation should be referred for biomedical diagnosis. TCM may be more useful in a supporting role if the patient requires surgery or chemotherapy. Phlegm nodules, however, often respond quite well, but relatively lengthy treatment is usually required.

气虚阳微

8.4 QI AND YANG DEFICIENCY

Pathophysiology

- *Qi* and *yang* deficiency represents a late stage of dysphagia where the patient's *zheng qi* is becoming weaker. The focus of treatment at this stage shifts from attacking and expelling the pathogen to supporting the *qi*. The Spleen and Kidneys are the main organ systems affected and keeping them functioning is the main priority.

Clinical features

- difficulty swallowing, may only be able to ingest liquids
- weight loss, emaciation
- severe fatigue, exhaustion and weakness
- pale, sallow complexion
- cold intolerance and cold extremities
- hypersalivation, drooling; spitting or vomiting frothy sputum
- shortness of breath
- oedema of the face and ankles or generalised oedema
- abdominal distension

T pale and swollen

P thready, weak, imperceptible

Treatment principle

Warm and supplement the Spleen and Kidneys

Strengthen *qi* and support *yang*

Prescription

BU QI YUN PI TANG 补气运脾汤
(*Decoction to Supplement* Qi *and Invigorate the Spleen*)

ren shen (Radix Ginseng) 人参 12-15g
zhi huang qi (honey fried Radix Astragali Membranacei) 炙黄芪 18-30g
fu ling (Sclerotium Poriae Cocos) 茯苓 12-15g
chao bai zhu (dry fried Rhizoma Atractylodes Macrocephalae) 炒白术 12-15g
chen pi (Pericarpium Citri Reticulatae) 陈皮 9-12g
ban xia (Rhizoma Pinelliae Ternatae) 半夏 9-12g
da zao (Fructus Zizyphi Jujubae) 大枣 4pce
sheng jiang (Rhizoma Zingiberis Officinalis Recens) 生姜 6-9g
sha ren (Fructus Amomi) 砂仁 6-9g
gan cao (Radix Glycyrrhizae Uralensis) 甘草 3-6g

Method: Decoction. **Ren shen, huang qi, fu ling, bai zhu** and **gan cao** strengthen the Spleen and supplement *qi*; **chen pi** and **ban xia** regulate *qi* and direct *qi* downwards, and transform Phlegm; **da zao, sheng jiang** and **sha ren** harmonise the Stomach. (Source: *Zhong Yi Nei Ke Shou Ce*)

Modifications

- In most cases, herbs such as **xuan fu hua** (Flos Inulae) 旋复花 12-15g and **dai zhe shi** (Haematitum) 代赭石 15-30g can be added to assist the descent of *qi*.
- With severe vomiting, delete **zhi huang qi**, and add **xuan fu hua** (Flos Inulae) 旋复花 12-15g, **dai zhe shi** (Haematitum) 代赭石 15-30g and **jiu cai zhi** (chinese chive juice) 韭菜汁 10ml.
- With loose stools or diarrhoea, substitute **gan jiang** (Rhizoma Zingiberis Officinalis) 干姜 for **sheng jiang**, and add **rou dou kou** (Semen Myristicae Fragrantis) 肉豆蔻 6g.
- With constipation, add **dang gui** (Radix Angelicae Sinensis) 当归 9-12g and **rou cong rong** (Herba Cistanches Deserticolae) 肉苁蓉 24-30g.
- With severe Cold, cold intolerance and cold extremities add **zhi fu zi** (Radix Aconiti Carmichaeli Praeparata) 制附子 6-12g (decocted for 30 minutes before the other herbs) and **rou gui** (Cortex Cinnamomi Cassiae) 肉桂 3g.
- With Kidney *yang* deficiency, add **bu gu zhi** (Fructus Psoraleae Corylifoliae) 补骨脂 12-15g and **zhi fu zi** (Radix Aconiti Carmichaeli Praeparata) 制附子 6-12g (decocted for 30 minutes before the other herbs).
- With nausea and vomiting of thin fluids, (Cold in the Stomach) add **wu zhu yu** (Fructus Evodiae Rutaecarpae) 吴茱萸 3-6g.

Variations and additional prescriptions

Spleen yang deficiency with Phlegm accumulation

- With Spleen *yang* deficiency and Phlegm accumulation, Spleen *yang* must be restored sufficiently before even simple foods can be processed and strength regained. The aim of treatment is to warm Spleen *yang* and promote movement of *yang* and fluids with **FU ZI LI ZHONG WAN** (*Aconite, Ginseng and Ginger Formula* 附子理中丸) modified.

  zhi fu zi (Radix Aconiti Carmichaeli Praeparata) 制附子 6-12g
  gan jiang (Rhizoma Zingiberis Officinalis) 干姜 9-12g
  ren shen (Radix Ginseng) 人参 9-12g
  chao bai zhu (dry fried Rhizoma Atractylodes Macrocephalae) 炒白术 12-15g
  zhi gan cao (honey fried Radix Glycyrrhizae Uralensis) 炙甘草 6-9g
  rou gui (Cortex Cinnamomi Cassiae) 肉桂 3g

sheng jiang zhi (ginger juice) 生姜汁 10ml
jiu cai zhi (chinese chive juice) 韭菜汁 10ml

Method: Decoction. **Zhi fu zi** is decocted for 30 minutes before the other herbs (*xian jian* 先煎). **Zhi fu zi**, **gan jiang** and **rou gui** warm *yang* and stimulate movement of *qi*; **ren shen** (or **dang shen**), **bai zhu** and **zhi gan cao** strengthen the Spleen and supplement *qi*; **sheng jiang zhi** harmonises the Stomach, stops vomiting, transforms Phlegm and eases the diaphragm; **jiu cai zhi** harmonises the Stomach, eliminates stagnant Blood, relaxes the oesophagus and directs *qi* downwards.

Qi and Blood deficiency

- With *qi* and Blood deficiency (sallow dull complexion, dizziness, emaciation), the aim of treatment is to supplement *zheng qi* and Blood with **BA ZHEN TANG** (*Ginseng and Dang Gui Eight Combination*) modified.

dang shen (Radix Codonopsis Pilosulae) 党参 15-24g
chao bai zhu (dry fried Rhizoma Atractylodes Macrocephalae) 炒白术 12-15g
dang gui (Radix Angelicae Sinensis) 当归 9-12g
bai shao (Radix Paeoniae Lactiflorae) 白芍 12-18g
shu di (Radix Rehmanniae Glutinosae Conquitae) 熟地 12-18g
chi shao (Radix Paeoniae Rubrae) 赤芍 9-12g
zhi huang qi (honey fried Radix Astragali Membranacei) 炙黄芪 18-30g
yu jin (Tuber Curcumae) 郁金 9-12g
bai hua she she cao (Herba Hedyotidis Diffusae) 白花蛇舌草 30-60g
xia ku cao (Spica Prunellae Vulgaris) 夏枯草 15-18g

Method: Decoction. **Dang shen**, **huang qi** and **chao bai zhu** strengthen the Spleen and supplement *qi*; **dang gui** and **shu di** nourish Blood; **chi shao** and **yu jin** regulate Blood and eliminate stagnant Blood; **bai hua she she cao** and **xia ku cao** dissipate masses. (Source: *Zhong Yi Zhi Liao Yi Nan Za Bing Mi Yao*)

Kidney yang deficiency

- If the patient exhibits Kidney *yang* deficiency, a decoction of **YOU GUI WAN** (*Eucommia and Rehmannia Formula* 右归丸) may be useful to support the Spleen and Kidneys, and warm *yang*.

shu di (Radix Rehmanniae Glutinosae Conquitae) 熟地 18-24g
shan zhu yu (Fructus Corni Officinalis) 山茱萸 12-15g
shan yao (Radix Dioscoreae Oppositae) 山药 15-18g
gou qi zi (Fructus Lycii) 枸杞子 12-15g
tu si zi (Semen Cuscutae Chinensis) 菟丝子 12-15g
du zhong (Cortex Eucommiae Ulmoidis) 杜仲 9-12g
zhi fu zi (Radix Aconiti Carmichaeli Praeparata) 制附子 6-12g

rou gui (Cortex Cinnamomi Cassiae) 肉桂 3-6g
dang gui (Radix Angelicae Sinensis) 当归 9-12g
lu jiao jiao (Cornu Cervi Gelatinum) 鹿角胶 9-12g

Method: Decoction. **Zhi fu zi** is cooked for 30 minutes before the other herbs (*xian jian* 先煎); **lu jiao jiao** is melted in the strained decoction (*yang hua* 烊化). Sip slowly as often as possible. **Shu di**, **gou qi zi** and **dang gui** nourish Kidney *yin* and Blood; **shan zhu yu** supplements the Liver; **shan yao** strengthens the Spleen and Kidneys; **tu si zi** and **du zhong** supplement Kidney *yang*; **zhi fu zi** and **rou gui** warm *yang*; **lu jiao jiao** benefits *yang* and *jing*.

Patent medicines

The pills can be crushed and steeped in hot water (drink the water) to facilitate their ingestion

Jin Kui Shen Qi Wan 金匮肾气丸 (Fu Gui Ba Wei Wan, Sexoton Pills, Golden Book Tea)
- Kidney *yang* deficiency

Fu Zi Li Zhong Wan 附子理中丸 (Fu Tzu Li Chung Wan, Carmichaeli Tea Pills, Li Chung Yuen Medical Pills)
- Spleen *yang* deficiency

Acupuncture (select from)

Ren.22 (*tian tu*) .... these points regulate *qi* and Blood in the chest
Ren.17 (*shan zhong*) and oesophagus, direct *qi* downwards, correct
Ren.14 (*ju que*) the *qi* mechanism in the chest, resolve Phlegm and relax the diaphragm

Ren.12 (*zhong wan* +▲) .. *mu* point of the Stomach, warms and regulates the Stomach and Spleen, directs Stomach *qi* downwards

Ren.4 (*guan yuan* ▲) .... these points warm Kidney *yang* and *yuan*
Ren.6 (*qi hai* ▲) *qi*, and aid the Kidneys in anchoring the dissipating *yang*

PC.6 (*nei guan*) .... *luo* point of the Pericardium, master point of *yin wei mai*, regulates the middle *jiao*

Lu.9 (*tai yuan*) ....*yuan* and *shu* stream point of the Lungs, *hui* point for the vessels, strengthens the Lungs and supplements *qi*

St.36 (*zu san li* +▲) .... *he* sea point of the Stomach, powerfully warms and strengthens the Spleen and Stomach and supplements *qi*

Kid.4 (*da zhong* ▲) .... *luo* point of the Kidneys, a special point for stricture in the oesophagus

Bl.17 (*ge shu* ▲) .... *shu* point for the diaphragm, regulates diaphragm function and Blood

Bl.20 (*pi shu* +▲) .... *shu* point of the Spleen, warms and supplements Spleen *qi* and *yang*

- a moxa box over the abdomen is useful
- with severe Kidney *yang* deficiency, add Bl.23 (*shen shu* +▲) and Du.4 (*ming men* +▲)
- *Ear points*: spleen, stomach, kidney, lungs, oesophagus, *shen men*

Clinical notes

- The general prognosis of patients with this pattern and degree of dysphagia is not good, but strength and well being can be improved.
- Thin Chinese rice porridge (*zhou* 粥) made with nutritive substances like chicken stock, ginger and dates may be useful.
- For other dietary recommendations, see pp.870-873.

SUMMARY OF GUIDING FORMULAE FOR DYSPHAGIA

Qi and Phlegm accumulation - *Ban Xia Hou Po Tang* 半夏厚朴汤
- with dominant Phlegm - *Qi Ge San* 启隔散
- with dominant *qi* stagnation - *Xiao Yao San* 逍遥散
- with rebellious Stomach *qi* - *Xuan Fu Dai Zhe Tang* 旋复代赭汤
- with Phlegm Heat - *Xiao Xian Xiong Tang* 小陷胸汤

Heat drying fluids and *yin* - *Wu Zhi An Zhong Yin* 五汁安中饮
- with severe dryness - *Zeng Ye Tang* 增液汤
- with Lung and Stomach *yin* deficiency - *Sha Shen Mai Men Dong Tang* 沙参麦门冬汤
- following radiotherapy - *Liang Ge San* 凉隔散

Phlegm and Blood stagnation - *Tong You Tang* 通幽汤

Qi and *yang* deficiency - *Bu Qi Yun Pi Tang* 补气运脾汤
- with Spleen *yang* deficiency - *Fu Zi Li Zhong Wan* 附子理中丸
- with *qi* and Blood deficiency - *Ba Zhen Tang* 八珍汤
- with Kidney *yang* deficiency - *You Gui Wan* 右归丸

9. Epigastric pain

Excess patterns

Cold congealing Stomach *qi*
Food stagnation
Liver *qi* stagnation
Stomach Heat
Blood stagnation

Deficient patterns

Spleen and Stomach *qi* (*yang*) deficiency
Spleen and Stomach *yin* deficiency

9 EPIGASTRIC PAIN

wei wan tong 胃脘痛

Epigastric pain[1] is pain in the area defined as the epigastrium. The epigastric region is the area medial to the nipples, above the umbilicus and beneath the ribs (Fig.9.1). Most commonly, epigastric pain is experienced in a fist sized area beneath the notch of the ribs. The pain may radiate to the hypochondriac region or back, and may be associated with symptoms such as indigestion, flatulence, nausea, vomiting, acid reflux, indeterminate gnawing hunger, coldness in the body, black sticky stools or constipation and diarrhoea.

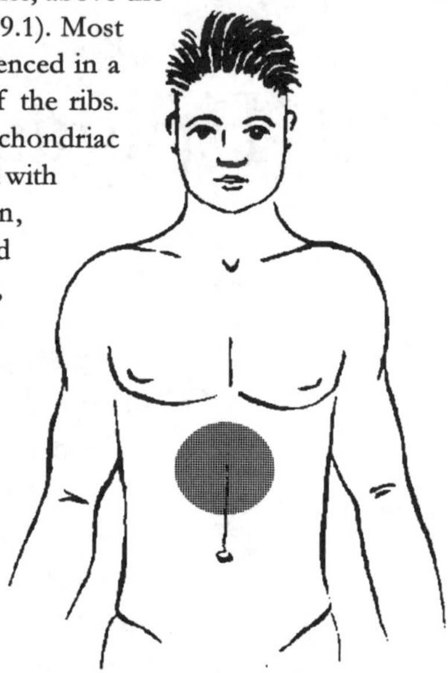

Figure 9.1 *The epigastric region*

The epigastric region is under the control of the Stomach, Spleen and Liver, and *ren* and *chong mai*. Most epigastric pain is associated with Stomach and/or Liver pathology. The most common patterns clinically are Liver and Stomach disharmony, Stomach *qi* or *yang* deficiency, and Stomach Heat and *yin* deficiency.

Epigastric pain can be acute or chronic, or chronic with acute exacerbations. When acute and severe, possible surgical emergencies, such as perforated peptic ulcer, should be kept in mind and the patient appropriately referred. In general, it is chronic or recurrent epigastric pain that brings patients to seek TCM treatment, and for which TCM is usually quite successful.

Epigastric pain should be differentiated from abdominal pain (p.46) and hypochondriac pain (*see* Volume 1). Abdominal pain, for the purposes of TCM disease diagnosis, is pain in the area bounded superiorly by a line running horizontal a couple of centimetres above the navel and inferiorly by the inguinal ligaments. Hypochondriac pain is pain in the area lateral to the epigastric area, just beneath the ribs.

[1]Wiseman's 'Stomach Duct Pain'

AETIOLOGY

Cold

External Cold

External Cold can be introduced into the body in association with Wind, or directly, by ingestion of large quantities of cold natured or physically cold foods, drinks or medications. Environmental Cold can invade the gastro-intestinal system directly through the mouth, bypassing the surface altogether. Invasion of external Cold is facilitated by a pre-existing weakness of Spleen and Stomach *qi* and/or *yang*. Cold invasion usually causes acute epigastric pain.

BOX 9.1 SOME BIOMEDICAL CAUSES OF EPIGASTRIC PAIN

Gastro-intestinal
- acute and chronic gastritis
- peptic ulcers
- acute and chronic pancreatitis
- oesophagitis/reflux
- cholecystitis
- cholelithiasis
- gastrospasm
- carcinoma - stomach, oesophagus, pancreas
- 'nervous' stomach
- irritable bowel syndrome
- dyspepsia

Cardiac
- referred myocardial infarction

Respiratory
- referred lower lobe pneumonia

Medications
- aspirin/NSAIDS
- cortisone
- alcohol abuse

Other
- poisoning

Internal Cold

Internal Cold is the product of a deficiency of Spleen and/or Kidney *yang*, whereby *yin* Cold becomes predominant relative to warming active *yang*. Depending on the degree of deficiency and the degree of Cold, the pain produced can vary. When the deficiency elements are primary, the pain tends to be mild and dull, relieved by both warmth and pressure. When *yin* Cold excess is predominant, the pain tends to be fairly severe and cramping, relieved by warmth but made worse by pressure.

Heat

External Heat

External Heat can invade the gastro-intestinal system directly, or follow a virulent, or unresolved, acute exterior disorder. Heat, or Cold which transforms into Heat as it penetrates deeper into the body, pushes through the surface, the *shao yang* level, and lodges in the *yang ming* level, the Stomach and Intestines. Occasionally, febrile illnesses can leave a residue of Phlegm Heat in the Stomach, causing pain and discomfort. External Heat type epigastric pain is mostly acute.

Internal Heat
Consumption of heating foods introduces Heat directly into the Stomach (*see* Diet, below). Internally generated Heat that affects the Stomach may also be the product of chronic Liver *qi* stagnation that generates stagnant Heat or Fire. Once stagnant Heat is present in the Liver system, it can be introduced into the Stomach via the controlling (*ke* 克) cycle, *see* p.214. Similarly, but less commonly, prolonged worry, anxiety and depression, or a sudden shock can retard the movement of Heart *qi*. The resulting accumulation of *qi* creates a focus of pressure in the chest, which can result is Heart Fire. Heart Fire can be transmitted via the generating cycle (*sheng* 生) to influence and heat the Stomach.

Internal Heat can also be created by *yin* deficiency. The Stomach needs a degree of moisture for efficient operation, and is thus easily dried out and heated up by a systemic increase in Heat from *yin* deficiency.

Diet

The type of food consumed and the way it is consumed are important factors in the genesis of epigastric pain. Eating spoiled or contaminated food can produce acute pain, which in TCM terms may resemble an attack of Cold or Damp Heat.

Too much cold natured or raw food can introduce Cold and weaken Spleen and Stomach *qi* and *yang*. Some drugs weaken the middle *jiao* and deplete Spleen and Stomach *qi* and *yang* (*see* below). Reduced food intake as a result of strict dieting, or prolonged starvation or digestive insult, such as occurs in patients with a history of anorexia nervosa, bulimia or during famine, serious damages Spleen *yang*.

Overconsumption in general, and excessive consumption of rich, heating or supplementing foods in particular, can lead to the accumulation of stagnant food and Heat or Damp Heat in the Stomach. Food stagnation is a common precursor to a host of pathologies that may give rise to epigastric pain (*see* p.3). Eating large quantities of foods that heat the Stomach and Liver, specifically substances like chilli and spices, alcohol, coffee and chocolate, causes Heat to accumulate. Once Heat is resident in the Stomach it easily damages Stomach *yin*. The natural tendency of Heat to rise can contribute to acid reflux which may damage the lining of the oesophagus and cause pain. Some specific foods are notorious for being indigestible to some people, and easily cause acid and pain. These include acid foods like the citrus family, tomatoes, uncooked peppers and capsicums, radishes, onions and garlic.

Sugar and dairy products create Dampness and Phlegm.

Drugs

Numerous therapeutic agents, both herbal and pharmaceutical, legal or illicit

BOX 9.2 KEY DIAGNOSTIC POINTS

Pain
- severe, acute, colicky pain - usually Cold
- intermittent pain, fullness or distension that is directly related to the patient's emotional state and stress level - Liver *qi* stagnation
- vague, difficult to localise pain/discomfort - *qi* stagnation
- fixed, sharp or stabbing pain which the patient can point to with a finger - Blood stagnation
- burning pain with acid reflux and belching - excess or deficient Heat
- mild, dull, continuous pain that is relieved by eating, pressure and warmth - deficiency of *qi* or *yang*
- mild, dull, distending pain with nausea - Phlegm or Dampness
- sudden violent pain is usually associated with a pathogen, typically Cold or overeating (food stagnation)

Aggravation
- with eating - excess
- with emotion and stress - Liver *qi* stagnation
- with not eating - deficiency
- with pressure - excess

Amelioration
- with eating - deficiency
- with warmth and pressure - Cold and deficiency
- with vomiting, defecation or belching - excess, *qi* stagnation
- rest - deficiency
- activity, exercise - *qi* stagnation

Timing
- waking around 2-3am with pain - Liver *qi* stagnation
- worse at night in general - Blood stagnation, *yin* deficiency
- worse upon waking - Phlegm Damp

Associated symptoms
- acid reflux - Liver *qi* invading the Stomach, Heat, Phlegm Damp, food stagnation
- flatulence, belching - Liver *qi* stagnation, food stagnation, Phlegm Damp
- morning nausea - Phlegm Damp

can cause epigastric pain. Probably the most common are those that are cold in nature, such as non steroidal anti-inflammatory agents (NSAIDs) purgative laxatives and occasionally antibiotics. Non steroidal anti-inflammatory agents are well known for physically damaging the lining of the stomach. Drugs that are heating can also damage the Stomach, consume *yin* and cause pain. These include corticosteroids, alcohol, inappropriate *yang* supplementing medicines, and stimulants such as cocaine and speed.

Emotion

Emotional factors, particularly those that contribute to stagnant Liver *qi*, are a major factor in the development of epigastric pain. Liver *qi* stagnation is most commonly produced by repression of emotion, the buried frustrations of everyday life, the suppressed anger and resentments. It also arises from exposure to ongoing stress or emotional tension, whether at work, at home or school. A particular cause of *qi* stagnation related epigastric pain is tension or fighting around the dinner table.

Prolonged *qi* stagnation can contribute to several complications which also cause pain, such as Blood stagnation, stagnant Heat and Spleen deficiency with the eventual generation of internal Cold or Dampness. In addition, *qi* stagnation leads to a generalised hypertonicity of both skeletal and smooth muscle, further restricting the circulation of *qi* and Blood to the tissues.

Less commonly, prolonged worry, anxiety, or a sudden shock can retard the movement of Heart *qi*. The resulting accumulation of *qi* creates a focus of pressure in the chest, which can create Heart Fire. Heart Fire is transmitted to the Stomach via the generating cycle.

In addition to the emotional factors that upset the Liver, worry, obsessive thinking and prolonged concentration in combination with a sedentary or studious lifestyle and poor diet, will weaken Spleen and Stomach *qi*. When weak, the Stomach is predisposed to invasion by Liver *qi* resulting in further damage.

Spleen and Stomach deficiency

Spleen *yang* deficiency pain may be associated with the diet (*see* above) or medication. Excessive mental strain or prolonged concentration may deplete Spleen *qi*. The damage is aggravated when an irregular diet is combined with sustained mental activity and too much sitting. The Spleen and Stomach can also be weakened following an acute invasion of Cold and/or Dampness. Gastric surgery can also deplete Spleen *yang*, and cause Blood stagnation.

Stomach *yin* deficiency may follow a febrile disease, long term consumption of spicy heating foods, or excessive consumption of drugs such as steroids, illicit stimulants and *yang* supplementing substances. It also may result from prolonged or excessive vomiting or another chronic Stomach pathology, especially one characterised by Heat or dryness.

Spleen and Stomach deficiency may also be constitutional, and in patients with a component of inherited weakness, there will often be a history of 'tummy aches' since childhood.

Blood stagnation

Blood stagnation type epigastric pain may be acute or, more commonly, chronic. Acute pain may follow gastric trauma or surgery. Chronic pain follows long term Stomach pathology, typically Liver *qi* stagnation or *yin* deficiency. Any pathology, however, regardless of whether it is excess or deficient, may lead to Blood stasis or involve elements of Blood stasis if long lasting enough. Some pathologies are particularly good at causing Blood stagnation. Cold pathologies (Cold and *yang* deficiency) can cause Blood stagnation by 'freezing and constricting' the vessels and slowing circulation. Hot pathologies (Heat, Damp Heat, Phlegm Heat and *yin* deficiency) can cause stagnation by 'evaporating' Blood and increasing the viscosity and stickiness of Blood. Blood stagnation frequently complicates *yang* deficiency, *yin* deficiency, Phlegm accumulation and prolonged Liver *qi* stagnation.

PHYSIOLOGY OF EPIGASTRIC PAIN

As with all pain, epigastric pain can be subdivided into two general types, excess and deficiency. All varieties of epigastric pain are ultimately due to obstruction to the circulation of *qi* and Blood in the Stomach.

Pain associated with excess

Excess pain is due to the presence of a pathogen which may be of external or internal origin, or due to stagnation of some kind, typically *qi* or Blood stagnation. Typical external pathogens are Heat and Cold which can directly invade the Stomach, and stagnated food. Internal pathogens include Liver *qi* invasion of the Stomach, Phlegm Damp, Damp Heat and Blood stagnation.

Excess pathology usually causes strong, spasmodic pain. The intensity of the pain is usually related to the degree of accumulation, or the strength of the pathogen. The spasmodic nature of the pain reflects the buildup and discharge of *qi* and Blood behind the obstruction, or the periodic release of the pathogenic accumulation. This is especially evident with *qi* stagnation. Excess pain can be constant as well, as is often the case in Blood stagnation patterns. The pathogen in excess pain patterns tends to be located in the Stomach, in contrast to the deficiency patterns which tend to be more systemic.

Excess pain patterns can be acute or chronic and recurrent. When prolonged, they will often transform into, or overlap with, another pattern or patterns. Eventually, excess pain patterns will develop a degree of deficiency, or become entirely deficient. In clinical practice, patients will often manifest more than one pattern. A patient may experience different types of pain. For example, a patient may have elements of *qi* stagnation, Blood stagnation and Heat, all of which cause different types of pain, at different times.

Pain associated with deficiency

The deficiency patterns are characterised by the lack of an essential physiological entity, *qi*, *yang* or *yin*, and can be further subdivided into functional or structural disorders. *Qi* or *yang* deficiency patterns are associated with a functional weakness of one or more of the organ systems of the epigastric region, usually the Stomach and Spleen. Pain is produced by the weak circulation, and subsequent pooling and stagnation, of *qi* and Blood.

In contrast, *yin* deficiency patterns are often associated with atrophy or deterioration of organ structure. For example, in Stomach *yin* deficiency patterns, the lining of the stomach organ may be found to have lost some of its rugae or folds and the gastric mucosa atrophic to some degree.

The epigastric pain of a deficient pattern tends to be mild yet constant, and the pathology, while focused in the epigastrium, is usually systemic, and may involve systems not directly related to the epigastrium. For example, Spleen *yang* deficiency will often drain, and be complicated by, Kidney *yang* deficiency; Spleen *qi* deficiency may be complicated by Heart and Lung *qi* deficiency.

Deficiency patterns will often involve a degree of excess. If *qi* or *yang* are unable to sufficiently move and process Blood, fluids and food, the latter will accumulate or begin to slow or congeal. Thus we find the pain of a deficiency pattern occasionally replaced by excess type pain as the relative balance between the excess and deficiency aspects shifts and changes in response to varying stimuli.

DIAGNOSIS

The first thing to ascertain in the exact location of the pain. Many patients complain of 'stomach pain' or 'stomach ache', but on further questioning the area referred to can range from the upper to lower abdomen and may be analysed differently (*see* Ch.2 Abdominal pain, p.46 and Hypochondriac pain in Volume.1 of this series). A current and recent history of medications taken is essential.

Epigastric pain often involves several overlapping patterns, and can be quite complex.

Typical pattern combinations

The following are examples of transformation from one excess pattern to another excess or deficient pattern, illustrating possible combination of patterns:

- Liver *qi* invading the Stomach which eventually begins to show signs of Blood stagnation.
- Liver *qi* stagnation which generates Heat that gradually damages Stomach *yin*.

- Spleen *qi* deficiency which promotes accumulation of Phlegm Damp, which obstructs the Blood, eventually causing Blood stagnation, or transforms into Phlegm Heat.
- Acute invasion of external Heat into the Stomach and damage to Stomach *yin*.
- External Cold invasion into *tai yin*, collapse of Spleen *yang* and accumulation of Cold Damp
- Food stagnation that weakens the Spleen, generates Phlegm Heat and obstructs *qi* movement and the *qi* mechanism.

A note on abdominal palpation

Abdominal palpation is an important diagnostic tool in deciding the nature of epigastric pain. Pain that is worse, and stays worse, when pressure is applied is excess, regardless of the deficient or otherwise weak state of the patient. Pain that is relieved, or at least not made worse with pressure is deficient, regardless of the robust nature or excess appearance of the patient. Pain that is worse initially and then eases off with continued pressure is associated with *qi* stagnation. When a pattern appears contradictory, the epigastric and abdominal palpation findings should be regarded as the primary diagnostic finding. For example, a thin pale patient with obvious signs of *qi* deficiency complains of epigastric pain which is definitely worse with palpation. Even though the patient is weak, the primary aim of therapy should be to clear the excess in the epigastrium, with secondary support for *zheng qi*.

TREATMENT

Treatment of epigastric pain is generally quite successful with TCM, especially when combined with dietary and life habit modifications. In fact, because of the prevalence of diet as an aetiological feature, changes to the diet and eating habits alone will often make significant improvements.

Acupuncture is effective for relieving acute pain and for the gradual removal of the stagnation which contributes to chronic epigastric pain. Herbs are usually required to replenish Blood and *yin*.

Figure 9.2 *Diagnostic strategy for acute epigastric pain*

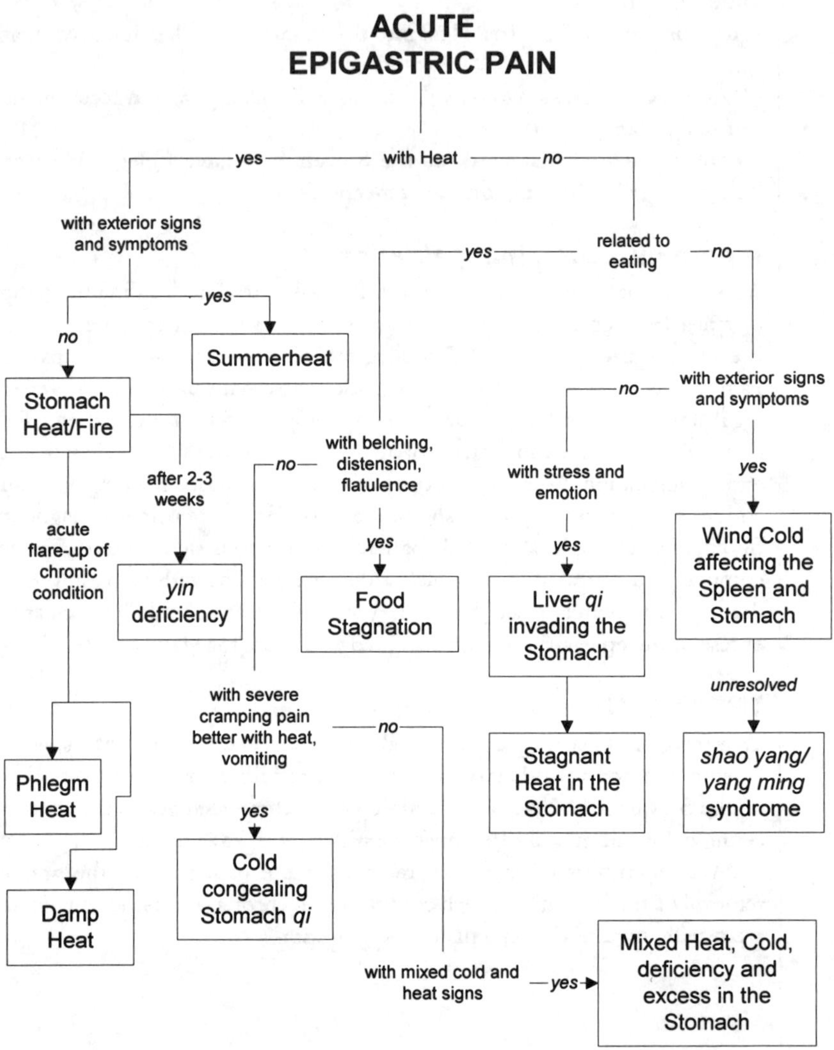

Figure 9.3 *Diagnostic strategy for chronic epigastric pain*

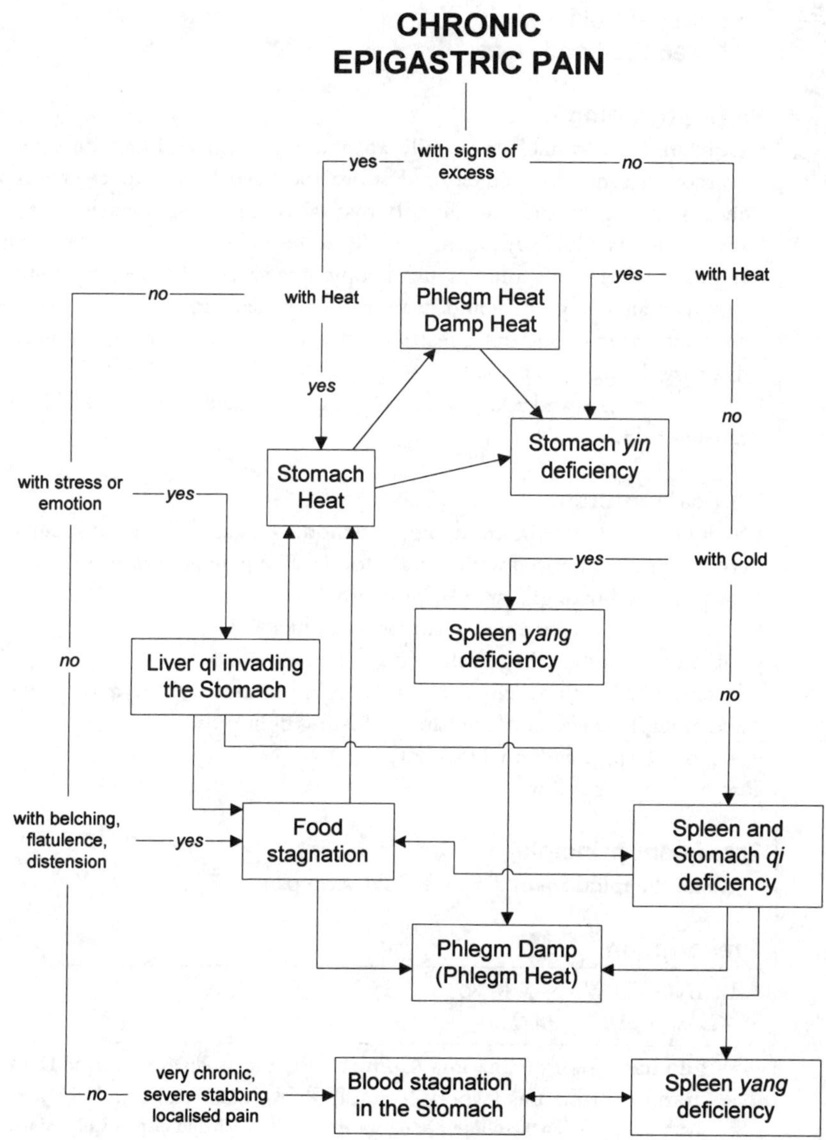

寒凝气滞

9.1 COLD INVADING THE STOMACH

- Internal Cold
- External Cold
- Mixed Cold and Heat

Pathophysiology

- Cold in the Stomach is usually an acute pattern and can be due to overconsumption of cold natured or raw foods, such as fruit, ice cream or beer, particularly on hot days. It may also follow an invasion of an environmental Cold pathogen, typically at the end of Summer or Autumn, as the weather cools and catches people unawares. The development of Cold can also be gradual and protracted, especially in those with cooling diets such as raw food diets, restricted weight loss diets and vegan diets. In this case the pain is episodic.
- The cold 'freezes and congeals', obstructing the circulation of *qi* and Blood causing pain.

Clinical features

- Sudden, often violent, cramping, spasmodic epigastric pain, or recurrent colicky pain associated with certain foods. The pain is significantly better for warmth, but aggravated by pressure.
- absence of thirst, or a desire for warm drinks
- nausea or vomiting, hypersalivation
- if associated with an environmental Cold pathogen, there may be fever and chills, myalgia, headache and a floating tight pulse

T normal or pale with a white coat
P wiry or tight or slow

Treatment principle

Warm the middle *jiao*, disperse Cold, stop pain

Prescription

LIANG FU WAN 良附丸
(*Galangal and Cyperus Pill*)

gao liang jiang (Rhizoma Alpiniae Officinari) 高良姜 9-12g
xiang fu (Rhizoma Cyperi Rotundi) 香附 9-12g

Method: Decoction. **Gao liang jiang** warms the Stomach and dispels Cold; **xiang fu** regulates *qi* and stops pain. (Source: *Shi Yong Zhong Yi Nei Ke Xue*)

Modifications

- With severe Cold, add **gan jiang** (Rhizoma Zingiberis Officinalis) 干姜

6-9g and **wu zhu yu** (Fructus Evodiae Rutaecarpae) 吴茱萸 3-6g.

- With *qi* stagnation (epigastric distension and belching), add **mu xiang** (Radix Aucklandiae Lappae) 木香 6-9g and **chen pi** (Pericarpium Citri Reticulatae) 陈皮 9-12g.
- With food stagnation, add **zhi shi** (Fructus Immaturus Citri Aurantii) 枳实 9-12g, **shen qu** (Massa Fermentata) 神曲 15g and **ji nei jin** (Endothelium Corneum Gigeriae Galli) 鸡内金 15g.
- With nausea, add **sheng jiang** (Rhizoma Zingiberis Officinalis Recens) 生姜 6-9g and **ban xia** (Rhizoma Pinelliae Ternatae) 半夏 9-12g.

Variations and additional prescriptions

External Wind Cold Damp

- With fever and chills, myalgia, heaviness, lethargy and other exterior symptoms, add **zi su ye** (Folium Perillae Frutescentis) 紫苏叶 9-12g and **sheng jiang** (Rhizoma Zingiberis Officinalis Recens) 生姜 6-9g, or use **HUO XIANG ZHENG QI SAN** (*Agastache Formula* 藿香正气散, p.744).

Cold transforming into Heat

- If the Cold lingers and stagnates, it can transform into Heat, giving rise to a common pattern of chronic epigastric discomfort. Along with a mixture of Heat and Cold signs and symptoms, the key feature is a sensation of blockage, distension and discomfort in the epigastrium. In addition, there is loss of appetite, nausea and vomiting or dry retching, borborygmus and diarrhoea, a thin, yellow, greasy tongue coat and a soft, and/or rapid pulse. The aim of treatment is to harmonise the Stomach, correct the *qi* mechanism and redirect *qi* downwards with **BAN XIA XIE XIN TANG** (*Pinellia Combination* 半夏泻心汤, p.32).

Patent medicines

Li Zhong Wan 理中丸 (Li Zhong Wan)

Fu Zi Li Zhong Wan 附子理中丸 (Carmichaeli Tea Pills, Fu Tzu Li Chung Wan, Li Chung Yuen Medical Pills)

- for severe Cold and severe pain

Xing Jun San 行军散 (Marching Powder, Five Pagodas Brand)

- for pain associated with an external Wind Cold or Damp invasion

Huo Xiang Zheng Qi Pian 藿香正气片 (Huo Xiang Zheng Qi Pian, Huo Hsiang Cheng Chi Pien)

Acupuncture (select from)

Ren.12 (*zhong wan* -▲) .... *mu* point of the Stomach, dispels Cold, regulates *qi* and stops pain

St.21 (*liang men* -▲) .... warms the Stomach and dispels Cold
St.36 (*zu san li* +▲) .... *he* sea point of the Stomach, powerfully warms and strengthens the Spleen and Stomach and supplements *qi*
St.34 (*liang qiu* -) .... *xi* cleft point of the Stomach, stops pain
Sp.4 (*gong sun*) .... *luo* point of the Spleen, master point of *chong mai*, regulates the Spleen and Stomach and stops pain
Bl.20 (*wei shu* +▲) .... *shu* point of the Stomach, warms the Stomach and disperses Cold

- a moxa box over the epigastrium is excellent, as are moxa cones burnt on slices of ginger over the main area of pain
- with nausea, add PC.6 (*nei guan*)
- with Dampness, add Sp.3 (*tai bai* -)
- with abdominal distension, add Sp.3 (*tai bai*) and Sp.15 (*da heng*)
- *Ear points*: stomach, spleen, abdomen, *shen men*, sympathetic

Clinical notes

- Cold type epigastric pain may be diagnosed biomedically as food poisoning, acute gastroenteritis, gastritis, irritable bowel syndrome, nervous stomach or peptic ulcer disease.
- In mild cases a strong decoction of raw ginger root may be sufficient to relieve the pain.
- For dietary recommendations, p.873.

饮食积滞

9.2 FOOD STAGNATION

Pathophysiology

- Food stagnation is directly related to overeating or irregular eating habits. In the developed world (and increasingly in the developing world) where many people consistently overeat and are generally sedentary, the pattern often combines with weakness of Spleen and Stomach *qi*, and pathological food stagnation develops gradually. Clinically, this pattern is mixed excess and deficiency. As the pattern progresses, the deficiency will become more and more prominent.
- Food stagnation is also frequently complicated by, or is the by-product of, other excess accumulations, such as Liver *qi* stagnation, Phlegm and Phlegm Heat.

Clinical features

- epigastric distension, fullness, discomfort and pain which is relieved by vomiting and belching, and is worse for pressure and eating
- sour, foul belching, indigestion
- acid reflux, heartburn
- halitosis, flatulence
- nausea and vomiting with undigested food
- constipation, sluggish, foul stools or diarrhoea that relieves the pain

T thick, greasy, white or yellow coat
P slippery and full

Treatment principle

Eliminate stagnant food, regulate digestion

Prescription

BAO HE WAN 保和丸
(*Citrus and Crategus Formula*) modified

chao shan zha (dry fried Fructus Crataegi) 炒山楂 18-24g
fu ling (Sclerotium Poriae Cocos) 茯苓 12-15g
chao shen qu (dry fried Massa Fermentata) 炒神曲 12-15g
ban xia (Rhizoma Pinelliae Ternatae) 半夏 9-12g
chen pi (Pericarpium Citri Reticulatae) 陈皮 9-12g
lai fu zi (Semen Raphani Sativi) 莱服子 9-12g
lian qiao (Fructus Forsythia Suspensae) 连翘 6-9g
qing pi (Pericarpium Citri Reticulatae Viridae) 青皮 9-12g
yan hu suo (Rhizoma Corydalis Yanhusuo) 延胡索 9-12g

Method: Grind herbs to a powder and form into 9-gram pills with water. The dose is 1 pill twice daily. May also be decocted with quantities as shown. **Chao**

shan zha, **chao shen qu** and **chao lai fu zi** improve digestion and alleviate food stagnation; **chao lai fu zi** also directs *qi* downwards; **ban xia** and **chen pi** harmonise the Stomach, resolve Phlegm and promote the movement of *qi*; **fu ling** strengthens the Spleen and leaches out Damp; **lian qiao** dissipates accumulations and clears Heat; **qing pi** breaks up *qi* accumulation; **yan hu suo** regulates *qi* and Blood and stops pain. (Source: *Shi Yong Zhong Yi Nei Ke Xue*)

Modifications

- With severe pain, add **san leng** (Rhizoma Sparganii Stoloniferi) 三棱 9-12g, **e zhu** (Rhizoma Curcumae Ezhu) 莪术 9-12g.
- With severe distension or reflux, add **zhi shi** (Fructus Immaturus Citri Aurantii) 枳实 9-12g and **bing lang** (Semen Arecae Catechu) 槟榔 9-12g.
- With constipation or sluggish stools, add **bing lang** (Semen Arecae Catechu) 槟榔 9-12g and **da huang** (Radix et Rhizoma Rhei) 大黄 6-9g.
- With Liver *qi* stagnation, add **fo shou** (Fructus Citri Sarcodactylis) 佛手 9-12g, and **mei gui hua** (Flos Rosae Rugosae) 玫瑰花 6-9g.
- With vomiting or diarrhoea, add **huo xiang** (Herba Agastaches seu Pogostemi) 藿香 12-15g and **pei lan** (Herba Eupatorii Fortunei) 佩兰 9-12g.
- With persistent vomiting, add **xuan fu hua** (Flos Inulae) 旋复花 12-15g.
- With Spleen deficiency, add **bai zhu** (Rhizoma Atractylodes Macrocephalae) 白术 9-12g.
- If the stagnation is associated with excessive meat consumption, increase the dose of **shan zha** (Fructus Crataegi) 山楂 to 24g.
- If the stagnation is associated with starchy foods and carbohydrates, increase the dose of **lai fu zi** to 15g.
- If there are signs of Heat (irritability, red tongue tip and sides, yellow tongue coat) add **shan zhi zi** (Fructus Gardeniae Jasminoides) 山栀子 9-12g and **huang lian** (Rhizoma Coptidis) 黄连 3-6g.

Variations and additional prescriptions

Severe pain and constipation (food stagnation with yang ming fu syndrome)

- In patients with severe pain, constipation and a dry, yellow tongue coat, a few doses of a mild purge, like **TIAO WEI CHENG QI TANG** (*Regulate the Stomach and Order the* Qi *Decoction* 调胃承气汤, p.468) may be useful at first to vigorously clear the stagnation through the bowel.

Chronic cases with Damp Heat

- In chronic cases, the stagnation and digestive disruption may transform into Damp Heat, which can have a systemic influence. The features are relentless epigastric discomfort and pain, heartburn, persistent belching, foul breath, diarrhoea or constipation, flatulence, scanty, concentrated urination, a red tongue with a greasy yellow coat and a deep strong pulse. The aim of treatment is to guide stagnation downward, clear Heat and dispel Damp with **ZHI SHI DAO ZHI WAN** (*Immature Bitter Orange Pill to Guide out Stagnation* 枳实导滞丸, p.181).

Patent medicines

Bao He Wan 保和丸 (Bao He Wan)
Mu Xiang Shun Qi Wan 木香顺气丸 (Mu Xiang Shun Qi Wan)
Jian Pi Wan 健脾丸 (Jian Pi Wan)
- with Spleen deficiency

Zi Sheng Wan 资生丸 (Zi Sheng Wan, Zi Sheng Stomachic Pills)
- with Spleen deficiency and diarrhoea

Shen Qu Cha 神曲茶 (Shen Chu Cha)
Chen Xiang Hua Qi Wan 沉香化气丸 (Chen Xiang Hua Qi Wan)
- with constipation

Acupuncture (select from)

Ren.12 (*zhong wan* -) .... these points regulate the Stomach and alleviate stagnation and pain
Ren. 13 (*shang wan* -)
St.21 (*liang men* -)

St.36 (*zu san li* -) .... *he* sea point of the Stomach, regulates and strengthens the Stomach and digestion and stops pain
St.40 (*feng long* -) .... *luo* point of the Stomach, transforms Phlegm and clears stagnant food, Phlegm and Phlegm Heat from the Stomach
St.34 (*liang qiu* -) .... *xi* cleft point of the Stomach, stops pain
LI.10 (*shou san li* -) .... benefits digestion and regulates gastro-intestinal function
St.44 (*nei ting* -) .... *rong* spring and Water point of the Stomach, clears Heat from the Stomach, alleviates food stagnation

- with severe pain, add Sp.4 (*gong sun* -)
- with nausea or vomiting, add PC.6 (*nei guan*)
- with constipation, add St.25 (*tian shu* -) and St.37 (*shang ju xu* -)
- with Heat, bleed St.45 (*li dui* ↓)
- with abdominal bloating, add St.25 (*tian shu* -), Ren.6 (*qi hai*) and Sp.5 (*shang qiu* -)
- with Spleen deficiency, add Sp.6 (*san yin jiao* +) and Bl.20 (*pi shu* +)

- with Liver *qi* stagnation, add GB.34 (*yang ling quan* -)
- *Ear points*: stomach, spleen, abdomen, small intestine, pancreas, *shen men*, sympathetic

Clinical notes

- A liquid, semiliquid diet or total fasting should be maintained for the first few days of the treatment, and small meals, perhaps more frequently, considered afterwards. Because this is largely a disorder of overindulgence and irregular dietary habits, the patient should be counselled accordingly, and, in uncomplicated cases, this is usually enough to cure the problem. Epigastric pain from food stagnation may be diagnosed biomedically as functional dyspepsia or indigestion.
- The Chinese and other Asian cultures have long known the benefits of sipping small amounts of certain teas while eating. The action of such teas helps assist digestion, especially of fats, and reduces the risk of food stagnation. European cultures use table wine in much the same way, hence 'a little wine for thy stomach's sake'. Similarly, 'bitters', combinations of bitter herbs and alcohol, are a common accompaniment to food, either as a digestive aid following a meal, or as an aperitive. The bitterness of the herbs assists the descent of Stomach *qi* and dries Damp.

肝气犯胃

9.3 LIVER QI INVADING THE STOMACH

- with Heat
- with *yin* deficiency

Pathophysiology

- Liver *qi* invading the Stomach is a common pattern that tends to occur in stressed, angry or tense people, and in those who work, have meetings or argue while eating. This is a form of rebellious *qi*, with wood (the Liver) 'over controlling' earth (the Stomach). Pain is caused by the obstruction to the circulation of *qi* and Blood and disruption to the *qi* mechanism, which here causes a chronic or recurrent spasm of the gastric musculature.
- In the early stages of this pattern, the epigastric pain may appear sporadically following some emotional event, with the patient feeling quite well before and after the episode. As this pattern progresses however, other pathologies can intervene and complicate the picture, and commonly Heat is generated. In addition, Spleen and Stomach *qi* and/or *yin* deficiency, food stagnation, Damp or Phlegm Heat, or Blood stagnation, may occur.

Clinical features

- Spasmodic epigastric pain, distension, fullness, and discomfort, which may radiate to the hypochondriac region. There is usually an emotional component. The patient may note a long history of a 'knot in the stomach' when tense or emotional. The pain and distension are worse with pressure, although prolonged pressure or massage may actually ease it, as the *qi* is moved. The pain is better for exercise and when the patient is relaxed.
- frequent sighing, belching and flatulence, which relieve the discomfort
- variable appetite, bloating, acid reflux, heartburn
- tension headaches, dizziness
- alternating constipation and diarrhoea
- fullness or tightness in the chest
- depression, moodiness, irritability
- irregular menstruation, premenstrual syndrome and breast tenderness, dysmenorrhoea
- poor circulation, cold fingers and toes
- **with Heat**: burning epigastric pain or indeterminate gnawing hunger, severe heartburn, severe restlessness and irritability, easy anger, bitter taste in the mouth, thirst, concentrated urine, constipation

T a normal or dark tongue with thin white coat; with Heat, red tongue or red edges on the tongue and a dry, yellow coat

P wiry (and rapid)

Treatment principle

Soothe the Liver and regulate *qi*
Harmonise the Liver and Stomach, stop pain
Clear Heat

Prescription

CHAI HU SHU GAN SAN 柴胡疏肝散
(*Bupleurum and Cyperus Formula*)

chai hu (Radix Bupleuri) 柴胡 9-12g
cu bai shao (vinegar fried Radix Paeoniae Lactiflorae) 醋白芍 15-24g
zhi ke (Fructus Citri Aurantii) 枳壳 9-12g
chuan xiong (Radix Ligustici Chuanxiong) 川芎 6-9g
chen pi (Pericarpium Citri Reticulatae) 陈皮 9-12g
xiang fu (Rhizoma Cyperi Rotundi) 香附 9-12g
zhi gan cao (honey fried Radix Glycyrrhizae Uralensis) 炙甘草 3-6g

Method: Decoction. **Chai hu** regulates and invigorates Liver *qi* and relieves constraint of *qi*; **cu bai shao** softens the Liver, nourishes *yin* and Blood, thus preventing excessive dispersal of, and damage to, *qi* and Liver *yin* by **chai hu**, and with **zhi gan cao** eases spasms and stops pain–the vinegar assists in stopping pain; **zhi shi** breaks up stagnant *qi*, directs *qi* downwards and alleviates distension, it's descending action neatly balances the ascending nature of **chai hu**, thus facilitating the correct functioning of the *qi* mechanism; **zhi gan cao** harmonises the Stomach and strengthens the Spleen, and, with **cu bai shao**, eases spasms, thereby alleviating cramping pain; **chuan xiong** and **xiang fu** regulate *qi* and Blood to stop pain; **chen pi** regulates *qi* and corrects the *qi* mechanism. (Source: *Zhong Yi Nei Ke Lin Chuang Shou Ce*)

Modifications (where not already included)

- With severe pain, add two or three of the following herbs: **chuan lian zi** (Fructus Meliae Toosendan) 川楝子 9-12g, **yu jin** (Tuber Curcumae) 郁金 9-12g, **mu xiang** (Radix Aucklandiae Lappae) 木香 6-9g and **yan hu suo** (Rhizoma Corydalis Yanhusuo) 延胡索 9-12g or **fo shou** (Fructus Citri Sarcodactylis) 佛手 9-12g.
- With epigastric distension, add **zhi shi** (Fructus Immaturus Citri Aurantii) 枳实 9-12g and **jie geng** (Radix Platycodi Grandiflori) 桔梗 6-9g.
- With nausea, add **ban xia** (Rhizoma Pinelliae Ternatae) 半夏 9-12g and **sheng jiang** (Rhizoma Zingiberis Officinalis Recens) 生姜 6-9g.
- Prolonged or severe *qi* stagnation will often generate Heat, especially when the diet includes heating foods. The features are increasing acid reflux and heartburn, burning epigastric pain, sour belching, bitter taste in the mouth, red sore eyes and a yellow tongue coat. Add **shan zhi zi**

(Fructus Gardeniae Jasminoidis) 山栀子 9-12g, **mu dan pi** (Cortex Moutan Radicis) 牡丹皮 9-12g, **wu zhu yu** (Fructus Evodiae Rutaecarpae) 吴茱萸 2-3g and **huang lian** (Rhizoma Coptidis) 黄连 3-6g. *See also* **DAN ZHI XIAO YAO SAN** (*Bupleurum and Paeonia Formula* 丹栀逍遥散, p.604).

- Note: Be careful when using strong bitter, pungent and/or dispersing herbs (**huang lian, wu zhu yu**), as excessive or prolonged use can damage Stomach *yin* and lead to complications. Monitor the patient carefully, and reduce or delete these elements as the patient's condition improves. When in doubt, or if there are elements of *yin* deficiency (centrally peeled tongue etc.), gentle herbs that move *qi* without damaging *yin* may be employed. These include **fo shou** (Fructus Citri Sarcodacylis) 佛手 9-12g, **ba yue zha** (Fructus Akebiae) 八月扎 9-12g, **mei gui hua** (Flos Rosae Rugosae) 玫瑰花 6-9g and **xiang yuan pi** (Pericarpium Citri Medica) 香橼皮 9-12g.
- With severe heartburn and hyperacidity, add **hai piao xiao** (Os Sepiae seu Sepiellae) 海螵蛸 15g and **duan wa leng zi** (calcined Concha Arcae) 煅瓦楞子 15g.
- With excessive belching or sighing, add two or three of the following herbs: **bai dou kou** (Fructus Amomi Kravanh) 白豆蔻 6-9g, **mei gui hua** (Flos Rosae Rugosae) 玫瑰花 6-9g, **chen xiang** (Lignum Aquilariae) 沉香 3-6g and **xuan fu hua** (Flos Inulae) 旋复花 12-15g.
- If the patient is tense and stressed, add **he huan pi** (Cortex Albizziae Julibrissin) 合欢皮 15g, **suan zao ren** (Semen Zizyphi Spinosae) 酸枣仁 15g and **mu li** (Concha Ostreae) 牡蛎 15-30g. In most cases it is valuable to add some *shen* calming herbs.
- With food stagnation, add **shan zha** (Fructus Crataegi) 山楂 15g.
- With *qi* deficiency, add **dang shen** (Radix Codonopsis Pilosulae) 党参 15-24g.
- With mild signs of *yin* deficiency, add **sheng di** (Radix Rehmanniae Glutinosae) 生地 12-15g and **mu dan pi** (Cortex Moutan Radicis) 牡丹皮 9-12g (see also Variations and additional prescriptions).
- With mild signs of Blood stagnation (occasional stabbing pain), add **dan shen** (Radix Salviae Miltiorrhizae) 丹参 12-15g and **san qi fen** (powdered Radix Notoginseng) 三七粉 3g.
- With *Helicobacter pylori* infection, add **pu gong ying** (Herba Taraxaci Mongolici) 蒲公英 18-30g and **huang qin** (Radix Scutellariae Baicalensis) 黄芩 9-12g.

Variations and additional prescriptions

Chronic stagnant Heat damaging Liver and Stomach yin

- Chronic stagnant *qi* can damage Stomach *yin*, either through the Heat that is generated or simply by the repeated insult to the Stomach lining. The features are nagging, and occasionally spasmodic, epigastric pain made worse by emotional upset, dry mouth and throat, acid reflux, a red, dry tongue and a thready, wiry pulse. The aim of treatment is to nourish *yin* and spread Liver *qi* with **YI GUAN JIAN** (*Linking Decoction* 一贯煎) modified.

sheng di (Radix Rehmanniae Glutinosae) 生地 18-30g
gou qi zi (Fructus Lycii) 枸杞子 12-18g
sha shen (Radix Adenophorae seu Glehniae) 沙参 9-12g
mai dong (Tuber Ophiopogonis Japonici) 麦冬 9-12g
dang gui (Radix Angelicae Sinensis) 当归 9-12g
chuan lian zi (Fructus Meliae Toosendan) 川楝子 6-9g
bai shao (Radix Paeoniae Lactiflora) 白芍 15-30g
gan cao (Radix Glycyrrhizae Uralensis) 甘草 6-12g

Method: Decoction. **Sheng di, gou qi zi, sha shen** and **mai dong** moisten and nourish Liver and Stomach *yin*; **dang gui, bai shao** and **gou qi zi** nourish Liver Blood, soften the Liver and preserve *yin*; **chuan lian zi** regulates *qi* and stops pain; **bai shao** and **gan cao** are especially effective in creating *yin* (combining sweet and sour flavours), and alleviating spasmodic pain.

Patent medicines

Shu Gan Wan 舒肝丸 (Shu Gan Wan, Shu Kan Wan)
- the main patent medicine for *qi* stagnation type epigastric pain

Mu Xiang Shun Qi Wan 木香顺气丸 (Aplotaxis Carminative Pills)
- especially good with sluggish bowel movements

Xiao Yao Wan 逍遥丸 (Xiao Yao Wan, Hsiao Yao Wan, Bupleurum Sedative Pills)
- *qi* stagnation with Blood and Spleen deficiency

Jia Wei Xiao Yao Wan 加味逍遥丸 (Jia Wei Xiao Yao Wan, Dan Zhi Xiao Yao Wan)
- Liver and Stomach stagnant Heat

Wei Te Ling 胃特灵 (Wei Te Ling Stomach Sedative)
- added to primary formula when there is significant heartburn

Acupuncture (select from)

Ren.12 (*zhong wan* -) .... these points harmonise the Liver and Stomach,
St.21 (*liang men* -) regulate *qi* and stop pain
Liv.13 (*zhang men* -)

PC.6 (*nei guan* -) .... these points calm and regulate Liver *qi*,
Liv.3 (*tai chong* -) harmonise the Stomach, nourish Liver Blood and settle the *shen*

St.34 (*liang qiu* -) .... *xi* cleft point of the Stomach, stops pain
GB.34 (*yang ling quan*) ...... *he* sea point of the Gallbladder, *hui* point for the tendons, pacifies the Liver, harmonises the Liver and Stomach and stops spasm
St.36 (*zu san li*) .... *he* sea point of the Stomach, strengthens the Spleen and Stomach to fortify them against invasion by the Liver

Bl.18 (*gan shu* -) .... *shu* points of the Liver, Spleen and Stomach,
Bl.20 (*pi shu*) harmonise the Liver and middle *jiao*
Bl.21 (*wei shu*)

- for severe pain, add Liv.5 (*li gou* -), Sp.8 (*di ji* -) and Sp.4 (*gong sun*)
- with hypochondriac pain (or when tender), add Liv.14 (*qi men* -)
- with Heat in the Liver and Stomach, add Liv.2 (*xing jian* -) and St.44 (*nei ting* -)
- in most cases, points to calm the *shen* should be added: select one or two points from *yin tang* (M-HN-3), Du.19 (*hou ding*), Du. 24 (*shen ting*)
- *Ear points*: *shen men*, liver, stomach, subcortex, endocrine, sympathetic

Clinical notes

- Liver invading the Stomach type epigastric pain may be diagnosed biomedically as nervous stomach, dyspepsia, irritable bowel syndrome, 'food allergies', chronic gastritis, peptic ulcer disease, chronic cholecystitis, and chronic hepatitis.
- Liver *qi* invading the Stomach responds well to correct treatment, with most patients feeling better quite quickly. For long term results, reduction of stress triggers, stress management and daily exercise are essential to keep the *qi* moving. Calm and tranquillity while eating is essential. Acupuncture is of particular benefit in this pattern as, over time, it appears to alter and improve the physiological response of the patient to stressors. To achieve this however, at least one and preferably more courses of acupuncture treatment (between 10-14 sessions each course), should be given over some months.
- Strong peppermint tea can provide temporary relief from acute *qi* stagnation pain. Mint preparations for epigastric and abdominal pain are also available in pharmacies and drug stores.
- For dietary recommendations, see p.878.

胃热炽盛

9.4 STOMACH HEAT (FIRE)

Pathophysiology

- Stomach Heat patterns can be due to invasion by external pathogens, or, more commonly, to internally generated Heat or heating foods and beverages. The external patterns are generally acute, while internal Heat patterns are usually chronic or recurrent. The external pattern usually associated with an a Damp Heat or Summerheat invasion, or follows an unresolved Wind Cold or Wind Heat attack.
- Internal Stomach Heat is usually related to a heating diet. It also develops after repeated encroachment on the Stomach by Liver *qi*. If there is some overlap between Liver *qi* invading the Stomach and Stomach Heat, the dominant pathology can be determined by the relationship of the symptoms to the emotional state. If there is a relationship to the emotional state, the Liver is dominant; if not, the Stomach is dominant.
- There are two common complications of Stomach Heat patterns. Firstly, the Heat can dry and damage Stomach *yin*, so mixtures of excess Heat and *yin* deficiency commonly occur. The Heat may also cook and congeal fluids to Damp Heat or Phlegm Heat, particularly if plenty of Damp natured foods are being ingested, in particular alcohol, dairy, sugar and fatty foods.
- The difference between Heat and Fire is in the intensity of the symptoms. Fire causes bleeding of the Stomach and gums.

Clinical features

- burning epigastric pain which is worse for pressure and heating foods
- epigastric distension
- thirst with desire for cold drinks
- excessive appetite, hungry again soon after eating
- sour belching, heartburn and acid reflux
- halitosis, sore or swollen gums
- mostly constipation, but may be diarrhoea
- restlessness and irritability

T red with a thick, dry, yellow coat; in chronic cases the centre of the tongue may be peeled, or there may be a wide shallow central crack.

P slippery, strong, rapid

- **with Fire**: swelling, pain, ulceration or bleeding of the gums, toothache or vomiting blood

Treatment principle

Clear Heat and Fire from the Stomach
Stop pain

Prescription

QING WEI SAN 清胃散
(*Clear the Stomach Powder*)

This prescription is suitable for prolonged smouldering Stomach Heat, generated by an overly heating diet. The pain is chronic or recurrent.

huang lian (Rhizoma Coptidis) 黄连 6-9g
sheng di (Radix Rehmanniae Glutinosae) 生地 12-18g
mu dan pi (Cortex Moutan Radicis) 牡丹皮 9-12g
dang gui (Radix Angelicae Sinensis) 当归 6-9g
sheng ma (Rhizoma Cimicifugae) 升麻 6-9g

Method: Decoction. The main herb, bitter and cold **huang lian** clears Heat from the Stomach and directs Stomach *qi* and turbid *qi* downward; pungent, sweet, cool and elevating **sheng ma** encourages the ascent of clear *qi*, clears Toxic Heat from the Stomach and balances the descending nature of **huang lian**; together this pair, one ascending, one descending, clear Heat without drying, and correct the *qi* mechanism; **mu dan pi** cools the Blood and disperses stagnant Blood; **sheng di** cools the Blood and nourishes *yin*; **dang gui** nourishes and regulates Blood, and protects it against the drying effects of the Heat. (Source: *Shi Yong Zhong Yao Xue*)

Modifications

- With severe pain, add **yu jin** (Tuber Curcumae) 郁金 9-12g, **chuan lian zi** (Fructus Meliae Toosendan) 川楝子 9g and **yan hu suo** (Rhizoma Corydalis Yanhusuo) 延胡索 9-12g.
- With strong Heat (severe thirst and dryness), add **shi gao** (Gypsum) 石膏 15-30g and **huang qin** (Radix Scutellariae Baicalensis) 黄芩 9-12g.
- With Fire (vomiting Blood, bleeding or ulcerated gums), add one or two of the following herbs: **huang qin** (Radix Scutellariae Baicalensis) 黄芩 9-12g, **ban lan gen** (Radix Isatidis seu Baphicacanthi) 板蓝根 12-18g, **zi hua di ding** (Herba cum Radice Violae Yedoensitis) 紫花地丁 9-12g, **pu gong ying** (Herba Taraxaci Mongolici) 蒲公英 15-30g, **lu gen** (Rhizoma Phragmitis Communis) 芦根 24-30g, **si gua luo** (Fasciculus Vascularis Luffae) 丝瓜络 9-12g and **lu dou** (Semen Phaseoli Radiati) 绿豆 9-12g.
- With persistent, focal, gnawing pain and bleeding (suggestive of gastric ulceration), powder equal amounts of **hai piao xiao** (Os Sepiae seu Sepiellae) 海螵蛸, **bai ji** (Rhizoma Bletillae Striatae) 白芨 and **gan cao** (Radix Glycyrrhizae Uralensis) 甘草 and take 3 grams three times daily.
- With constipation, add **da huang** (Radix et Rhizoma Rhei) 大黄 6-9g.
- With Liver *qi* stagnation, add **chai hu** (Radix Bupleuri) 柴胡 9-12g, **zhi shi** (Fructus Immaturus Citri Aurantii) 枳实 9-12g and **bai shao** (Radix Paeoniae Lactiflora) 白芍 12-18g.
- With hyperacidity and heartburn, add powdered **hai piao xiao** (Os Sepiae seu Sepiellae) 海螵蛸 15g and powdered **duan wa leng zi** (calcined Concha Arcae) 煅瓦楞子 15g.

- With hypoacidity, add **shan zha** (Fructus Crataegi) 山楂 15g and **wu mei** (Fructus Pruni Mume) 乌梅 9-12g.
- With excessive belching, or nausea and vomiting, add **xuan fu hua** (Flos Inulae) 旋复花 12-15g and **dai zhe shi** (Haematitum) 代赭石 15g.
- With mild *yin* deficiency, add **xuan shen** (Radix Scrophulariae) 玄参 18-24g (*See also* Variations and additional prescriptions).
- With ulcers on the gums or mouth, apply the patent powder *Xi Gua Shuang* 西瓜霜 (Watermelon Frost) topically.
- With *Helicobacter pylori*, add **pu gong ying** (Herba Taraxaci Mongolici) 蒲公英 15-30g and **huang qin** (Radix Scutellariae Baicalensis) 黄芩 9-12g.

Variations and additional prescriptions

Acute pain from Summerheat invasion

- Acute Heat type epigastric pain may be associated with an invasion of Summerheat into the Stomach. The features in addition to the pain, are relatively high fever unrelieved by sweating, heaviness in the head and body, muscle aches, thirst, irritability, vomiting, diarrhoea, a floating, rapid, soggy pulse and a greasy, yellow tongue coat. The aim of treatment is to promote sweating to clear the exterior and expel Summerheat with **XIN JIA XIANG RU YIN** (*Newly Augmented Elsholtzia Decoction* 新加香薷饮, p.224).

Shao yang / yang ming syndrome

- An unresolved or virulent external pathogen, either Heat or Cold, can penetrate through the *tai yang* level and lodge simultaneously at the *shao yang* and *yang ming* levels, causing acute epigastric pain. In addition, there are features of both *shao yang* and *yang ming* syndrome, such as alternating fever and chills, nausea and vomiting, constipation or burning diarrhoea, pounding temporal headaches, dizziness, a yellow, greasy tongue coat and a wiry, rapid pulse.

  This is mostly an acute pattern, and typically follows an unresolved Wind attack. It may also, however, occur as an acute episode of a chronic subacute Damp Heat accumulation. In this case, it may overlap with such biomedically defined conditions as acute cholecystitis, gallstones, or pancreatitis. The aim of treatment is to harmonise *shao yang* and purge *yang ming* with **DA CHAI HU TANG** (*Major Bupleurum Combination* 大柴胡汤).

  chai hu (Radix Bupleuri) 柴胡 9-12g
  huang qin (Radix Scutellariae Baicalensis) 黄芩 9-12g
  zhi shi (Fructus Immaturus Citri Aurantii) 枳实 9-12g
  da huang (Radix et Rhizoma Rhei) 大黄 6-9g
  bai shao (Radix Paeoniae Lactiflora) 白芍 12-18g

ban xia (Rhizoma Pinelliae Ternatae) 半夏 9-12g
sheng jiang (Rhizoma Zingiberis Officinalis Recens)
生姜 6-9g
da zao (Fructus Zizyphi Jujubae) 大枣 4pce

Method: Decoction. **Chai hu** and **huang qin** clear Heat and pathogens from *shao yang*; **zhi shi** regulates *qi* and promotes downward movement of *qi*; **da huang** clears Heat by purging the bowels; **bai shao** nourishes the Blood, softens the Liver and alleviates spasmodic pain; **sheng jiang** and **da zao** harmonise and protect the Stomach; **da zao** also increases the ability of **bai shao** to stop pain.

Phlegm Heat

◆ Phlegm Heat is a common complication of Stomach Heat, and tends to occur in stressed individuals who work and play hard, often smoke and drink, and exercise little or only sporadically. Such patients tend to be overweight, and appear robust. The features are prolonged nagging pain and distension, thirst with no desire to drink, nausea, vomiting (the vomit sometimes mucus-like or streaked with blood), alternating constipation and diarrhoea, variable appetite, heavy sensations in the body, lethargy, a greasy tongue coat and a wide, shallow central tongue crack with a thick, rough coat in the crack. The aim of treatment is to clear Phlegm Heat, soothe the Liver and harmonise the Stomach with **XIAO XIAN XIONG TANG** (*Minor Sinking Into the Chest Decoction* 小陷胸汤) modified.

gua lou (Fructus Trichosanthis) 栝楼 24-30g
ban xia (Rhizoma Pinelliae Ternatae) 半夏 9-12g
huang lian (Rhizoma Coptidis) 黄连 3-6g
chai hu (Radix Bupleuri) 柴胡 9-12g
huang qin (Radix Scutellariae Baicalensis) 黄芩 9-12g
zhi shi (Fructus Immaturus Citri Aurantii) 枳实 9-12g
bai shao (Radix Paeoniae Lactiflora) 白芍 12-18g
xiang fu (Rhizoma Cyperi Rotundi) 香附 9-12g
yu jin (Tuber Curcumae) 郁金 9-12g
yan hu suo (Rhizoma Corydalis Yanhusuo) 延胡索 9-12g

Method: Decoction. **Gua lou** and **ban xia** transform Phlegm and clear Heat; **huang lian** and **huang qin** clear Heat from the upper *jiao* and Heart; **chai hu** regulates and moves Liver *qi* and clears Heat; **zhi shi** regulates *qi* and promotes descent of *qi*; **bai shao** softens the Liver and stops spasmodic pain; **xiang fu**, **yu jin** and **yan hu suo** regulate *qi* and stop pain.

Damp Heat

• In patients with an overly rich, greasy or Damp Heat producing diet, Heat and Dampness combine to produce a chronic problem that manifests in a slightly different fashion than that caused by Heat alone. Damp Heat can also be a by-product of chronic food stagnation (*see* p.3, and 352-353). Patients will have clear signs of Heat such as burning epigastric pain and distension, halitosis, a yellow tongue coat and a rapid pulse. The Damp, however, will modify the picture causing thirst with little desire to drink, epigastric distension, tendency to sluggish malodorous stools. In addition, these patients may have acne problems or a tendency to boils and sores, greasy skin, and strong body odour. This pattern can also be acute, following a period of heavy alcohol consumption. The treatment is to modify the patient's diet, and to assist in clearing Damp Heat with **HUANG LIAN JIE DU TANG** (*Coptis and Scute Combination* 黄连解毒汤).

huang lian (Rhizoma Coptidis) 黄连 3-6g
huang qin (Radix Scutellariae Baicalensis) 黄芩 9-12g
huang bai (Cortex Phellodendri) 黄柏 9-12g
shan zhi zi (Fructus Gardeniae Jasminoidis) 山栀子 9-12g

Method: Decoction. **Huang lian**, **huang qin** and **huang bai** clear Damp Heat from the upper, middle and lower *jiao* respectively; **shan zhi zi** clears Heat from the *san jiao*, and alleviates irritability.

Da huang (Radix et Rhizoma Rhei) 大黄 3-6g may be added initially if there is constipation. This formula is generally not used for more than 6-8 weeks.

With yin deficiency

- If the pattern is recurrent or chronic, Stomach *yin* may be damaged, leading to a mixed excess (Heat) and deficiency condition (thick but rootless tongue coat, dry mouth and tongue, weak, thready pulse). The aim of treatment is to drain Heat from the Stomach and nourish *yin* with **YU NU JIAN** (*Jade Woman Decoction* 玉女煎). *See also* p.376.

shi gao (Gypsum) 石膏 18-30g
shu di (Radix Rehmanniae Glutinosae Conquitae) 熟地 18-30g
mai dong (Tuber Ophiopogonis Japonici) 麦冬 9-12g
zhi mu (Rhizoma Anemarrhenae Asphodeloides) 知母 9-12g
chuan niu xi (Radix Cyathulae Officinalis) 川牛膝 12-15g

Method: Decoction. **Shi gao** and **zhi mu** clear Heat from the Stomach; **shu di** nourishes *yin* and Blood and Kidney Water to restrain Fire; **mai dong** nourishes Stomach *yin*; **chuan niu xi** directs *qi* downwards.

Patent medicines

Niu Huang Jie Du Pian 牛黄解毒片 (Niu Huang Chieh Tu Pien)
- particularly with mouth ulcers

Niu Huang Qing Huo Wan 牛黄清火丸 (Niuhuang Qinghuo Wan)
- with constipation

Qing Fei Yi Huo Pian 清肺抑火片 (Ching Fei Yi Huo Pien)
- suitable for *shao yang* / *yang ming* syndrome

Qing Qi Hua Tan Wan 清气化痰丸 (Pinellia Expectorant Pills)
- although this patent is used primarily for Phlegm Heat cough, it may also be used for Phlegm Heat in the Stomach.

Wen Dan Wan 温胆丸 (Wen Dan Wan)
- Phlegm Heat

Acupuncture (select from)

Ren.12 (*zhong wan* -) .... these points harmonise the Liver and Stomach,
St.21 (*liang men* -) regulate *qi* and stop pain

St.44 (*nei ting* -) .... *rong* spring and Water point of the Stomach, clears Heat from *yang ming*, the Stomach and Stomach channel

St.34 (*liang qiu* -) .... *xi* cleft point of the Stomach, stops pain

St.36 (*zu san li* -) .... *he* sea point of the Stomach, strengthens the Spleen and Stomach to fortify them against invasion by the Liver

ah shi points .... along the course of the Stomach channel, between St.36 (*zu san li*) and St.39 (*xia ju xu*)

PC.7 (*da ling*) .... *yuan* and *shu* stream point of the Pericardium, calms the *shen*, harmonises the Stomach and clears Heat

PC.8 (*lao gong* -) .... *rong* spring and Fire point of the Pericardium, drains Heat from the Stomach channel and cools the Blood and Heart Fire

LI.4 (*he gu* -) .... *yuan* point of the Large Intestine, clears Heat from *yang ming*, (especially good with St.44), and stops pain

- with *yin* deficiency add Bl.21 (*wei shu* +) and Bl.23 (*shen shu* +)
- with vomiting or spitting of blood, add PC.4 (*xi men* -)
- with fever, add LI.11 (*qu chi* -)
- With Phlegm Heat, add St.40 (*feng long* -)
- For *shao yang* / *yang ming* syndrome, add SJ.5 (*wai guan* -), GB.39 (*xuan zhong* -) and St.25 (*tian shu* -)
- *Ear points*: stomach, duodenum, abdomen, *shen men*, sympathetic

Clinical notes

- Stomach Heat type epigastric pain may be diagnosed biomedically as acute infectious gastroenteritis, functional dyspepsia, peptic ulcer disease, acute or chronic gastritis, acute or chronic pancreatitis, or acute or chronic cholecystitis.
- This is a relatively common pattern of epigastric pain, and usually responds well to correct treatment. The more prolonged, however, and the greater the degree of *yin* deficiency, the more treatment is required.
- For dietary recommendations, see pp.882-885.

血瘀阻胃

9.5 BLOOD STAGNATION

Pathophysiology

- Blood stagnation epigastric pain is usually a chronic condition, and typically follows pre-existing Stomach pathology. It almost always appears in conjunction with, or following, prolonged *qi* stagnation, Heat, and *qi* and/or *yin* deficiency. It may be more acute, however, following gastric surgery or trauma.
- As a consequence of other pathology, Blood stagnation tends to develop slowly, the symptoms progressing from mild to severe as the stagnation intensifies. Initially, movement of Blood is simply sluggish, but over time the Blood stops and becomes focally stagnant. Blood stagnation in the Stomach may first manifest when long term epigastric pain changes from generalised and ill defined to more sharp or localised. When acute, the characteristic systemic signs and symptoms of Blood stagnation may be absent.
- Blood stagnation patterns may tend towards Heat, Cold or neither, and present with or without significant deficiency.

Clinical features

- Epigastric pain that is fixed, sharp, stabbing or boring, and worse for pressure, eating and at night. In the early stages, the pain may be intermittent, but as the pattern develops, it becomes more constant. The pain may refer through to the back.
- nausea, belching, acid reflux; in severe cases there may be vomiting of dark or purplish, coffee ground like material, and the stools may be black and tarry
- darkish or purplish or blotchy complexion, lips and conjunctivae with dark rings around the eyes; in cases with significant underlying deficiency from chronic blood loss, the complexion is sallow or pale, and there may be dizziness.
- spider naevi on the cheeks, over the epigastrium and trunk and around the inner ankle and knee
- poor appetite or anorexia
- weight loss

T dark or purplish body, with purple or brown stasis spots; dark, distended sublingual veins

P wiry, or thready and choppy

Treatment principle

Transform and eliminate stagnant Blood, stop pain
Nourish Blood, stop bleeding, soften the Liver (as necessary)

Prescription

9.5.1 Relatively mild stagnation and pain

SHI XIAO SAN 失笑散
(*Break Into a Smile Powder*) plus
DAN SHEN YIN 丹参饮
(*Salvia Decoction*) modified

pu huang (Pollen Typhae) 蒲黄 9-12g
wu ling zhi (Excrementum Trogopteri seu Pteromi)
五灵脂 9-12g
dan shen (Radix Salviae Miltiorrhizae) 丹参 18-30g
sha ren (Fructus Amomi) 砂仁 6-9g
tan xiang (Lignum Santali Albi) 檀香 9-12g
xiang fu (Rhizoma Cyperi Rotundi) 香附 9-12g
san qi fen (powdered Radix Notoginseng) 三七粉 3-6g

Method: Decoction. **San qi fen** is added to the strained decoction (*chong fu* 冲服). **Pu huang** and **wu ling zhi** are a specific combination for pain from stagnant Blood; **dan shen** and **san qi fen** invigorate Blood and eliminate stagnant Blood; **sha ren**, **tan xiang** and **xiang fu** regulate *qi* and stop pain.

Modifications

- With severe pain add **yan hu suo** (Rhizoma Corydalis Yanhusuo) 延胡索 9-12g, or **ru xiang** (Gummi Olibanum) 乳香 6-9g and **mo yao** (Myrrha) 没药 6-9g.
- With severe *qi* stagnation (distension, belching), add **zhi shi** (Fructus Immaturus Citri Aurantii) 枳实 9-12g and **qing pi** (Pericarpium Citri Reticulatae Viridae) 青皮 9-12g.
- With active bleeding of dark blood (tarry stools, coffee ground vomitus) increase the dose of **san qi** powder to 9g and add **bai ji** (Rhizoma Bletillae Striatae) 白芨 9-15g. Both these herbs can also be taken separately as powder.
- With vomiting of fresh red blood and mild signs of Heat, add **huang qin** (Radix Scutellariae Baicalensis) 黄芩 9-12g, **huang lian** (Rhizoma Coptidis) 黄连 6-9g, **bai mao gen** (Rhizoma Imperatae Cylindricae) 白茅根 30g and **mu dan pi** (Cortex Moutan Radicis) 牡丹皮 9-12g.
- With Cold, add **gan jiang** (Rhizoma Zingiberis Officinalis) 干姜 6-9g and **gui zhi** (Ramulus Cinnamomi Cassiae) 桂枝 6-9g.
- With *qi* deficiency add **huang qi** (Radix Astragali Membranacei) 黄芪 18-30g, **bai zhu** (Rhizoma Atractylodes Macrocephalae) 白术 12-15g and **huang jing** (Rhizoma Polygonati) 黄精 12-15g.
- With *yin* deficiency, add **sheng di** (Radix Rehmanniae Glutinosae) 生地 12-15g and **sha shen** (Radix Adenophorae seu Glehniae) 沙参 12-15g.
- When the biomedical diagnosis is stomach cancer, add two or three of

the following herbs to enhance the detoxifying, accumulation eliminating action: **bai hua she she cao** (Herba Hedyotidis Diffusae) 白花蛇舌草 30-60g, **ban zhi lian** (Herba Scutellariae Barbatae) 半枝连 15g, **shu yang quan** (Herba Solanum Lyratum) 蜀羊泉 30g, **teng li gen** (Radix Actinidia Arguta) 藤梨根 60-120g, **she mei** (Herba Duchesnea Indica) 蛇莓 30g, **zhong jie feng** (Herba Sarcandra Glabrae) 肿节风 15g or **gui zhen cao** (Herba Bidens Bipinnata) 鬼针草 24g.

- Most patients with Blood stagnation in the Stomach will have quite impaired digestion and may have difficulty processing some Blood moving herbs. In most cases it is useful to add some digestion improving herbs, such as **shan zha** (Fructus Crataegi) 山楂 15g and **shen qu** (Massa Fermentata) 神曲 15g.

9.5.2 Severe Blood stagnation, pain and palpable masses

GE XIA ZHU YU TANG 膈下逐瘀汤
(*Drive out Blood Stasis Below the Diaphragm Decoction*) p.821

9.5.3 *Qi* and Blood stagnation

XUE FU ZHU YU TANG 血府逐瘀汤
(*Achyranthes and Persica Combination*) p.83

This prescription is selected for Blood and *qi* stagnation type epigastric pain, typically pain that follows years of Liver *qi* invading the Stomach.

Variations and additional prescriptions

With significant Heat

- When stagnant Blood is complicated by significant Heat, causing sporadic gastro-intestinal bleeding of fresh red blood, a purplish red tongue with a yellow coat and a wiry, rapid pulse, the aim of treatment is to clear Heat, cool the Blood and stop bleeding with **DA HUANG HUANG QIN XIE XIN TANG** (*Rhubarb and Scute Decoction to Drain the Epigastrium* 大黄黄芩泻心汤, p.472) modified. This formula is used until the bleeding ceases, after which a more general Blood moving formula may be selected.

With Cold and deficiency

- When Blood stagnation is complicated by deficiency and Cold, with vomiting of dark blood, tarry stools, fatigue and weakness, a sallow complexion, cold intolerance and cold extremities, the aim of treatment is to warm *yang*, strengthen the Spleen and stop bleeding with **HUANG TU TANG** (*Yellow Earth Decoction* 黄土汤, p.438).

Patent medicines

Xue Fu Zhu Yu Wan 血府逐瘀丸 (Xue Fu Zhu Yu Wan)
- a general *qi* and Blood stagnation invigorating formula

Shi Xiao Wan 失笑丸 (Shi Xiao Wan)
- add to enhance analgesic action

Sheng Tian Qi Pian 生田七片 (Sheng Tien Qi Pien)
- excellent when there is mild bleeding.

Fu Ke Wu Jin Wan 妇科乌金丸 (Woo Garm Yuen Medical Pills)
- good for Blood stagnation with a degree of deficiency (mostly *yang* or *qi* deficiency).

Tong Jing Wan 痛经丸 (Tong Jing Wan)
- severe Blood stagnation with masses

Yun Nan Bai Yao 云南白药 (Yunnan Paiyao)
- this famous patent medicine can be used for Blood stagnation and bleeding from the Stomach

Acupuncture (select from)

ah shi points .... over the site of pain, move *qi* and Blood locally
Ren.12 (*zhong wan* -) .... *mu* point of the Stomach, regulates movement of *qi* and Blood in the Stomach
St.21 (*liang men* -) .... regulates Stomach *qi*
St.34 (*liang qiu* -) .... *xi* cleft point of the Stomach, encourages circulation of *qi* and Blood in the Stomach and stops pain
St.36 (*zu san li* -) .... *he* sea point of the Stomach, powerfully invigorates movement of *qi* and Blood and regulates the Stomach
Bl.17 (*ge shu* -) .... *hui* point for Blood, transforms stagnant Blood
Bl.18 (*gan shu* -) .... *shu* point of the Liver, invigorates Liver *qi* and Blood
Bl.21 (*wei shu* -) .... *shu* point of the Stomach, eliminates Stagnant Blood from the Stomach
Du.8 (*jin suo* -) .... special point for spasm and pain
Sp.10 (*xue hai* -) .... regulates and invigorates Blood
Sp.6 (*san yin jiao*) .... strengthens the Spleen, regulates Liver *qi* and invigorates *qi* and Blood circulation
Sp.4 (*gong sun*) .... *luo* point of the Spleen, master point of *chong mai*, regulates the Spleen and Stomach and stops pain

- with nausea and vomiting, add PC.6 (*nei guan*)
- with Liver *qi* invading the Stomach, add Liv.13 (*zhang men* -)

- with irritability or depression, add Liv.3 (*tai chong*) or Liv.1 (*da dun* ▲)
- for severe pain, add LI.4 (*he gu* -) and Liv.5 (*li gou* -)
- *Ear points*: *shen men*, stomach, duodenum, liver, sympathetic

Clinical notes

- Blood stagnation type epigastric pain may be diagnosed biomedically as stomach cancer, chronic gastritis, chronic pancreatitis, peptic ulcer disease, perforated peptic ulcer, bleeding peptic ulcer or oesophageal varices.
- It is not uncommon to see patients with relatively severe cases of Blood stasis in TCM clinics, and treatment needs to be prolonged for a satisfactory result. Mild or early cases of Blood stagnation are more common, and in general respond reasonably well to correct and prolonged treatment. If the Blood stagnation is associated with cancer, TCM treatment is best in a supporting role. Keep in mind that sudden acute exacerbations of Blood stagnation type epigastric pain may indicate a medical and surgical emergency, such as a perforation of a peptic ulcer. Such patients require hospital attention.
- Severe bleeding from the digestive tract is a medical emergency and should be treated in hospital.
- For dietary recommendations, see p.886.

脾胃虛寒

9.6 SPLEEN AND STOMACH QI (YANG) DEFICIENCY

Pathophysiology

- The mechanisms that can give rise to pain of a deficiency Cold type are as follows:
  1. When Spleen and Stomach *qi* is weak, food and fluids are poorly processed and can accumulate in the Stomach as food stagnation, pathological fluids, or Phlegm Damp. Mixed patterns of deficiency and excess are common, and the balance of deficiency and excess will tend to fluctuate from time to time, depending on what happens in the patient's life. Phlegm Damp is perhaps the most common complicating factor, and on occasion may become the predominant pathology.
  2. Insufficient *qi* can lead to sluggish movement of *qi* and Blood through the Stomach–*qi* and Blood slow and accumulate, causing obstruction to the *qi* mechanism and pain.
  3. When *yang* is weak, the resulting Cold further constricts the circulation of *qi* and Blood, causing more intense pain.

Clinical features

- chronic mild, dull, nagging, continuous epigastric pain, which is relieved by warmth, pressure and sometimes by eating warm cooked foods
- vomiting of thin watery fluids
- poor appetite or anorexia
- loose stools or diarrhoea
- abdominal distension, worse with eating
- borborygmus
- tiredness, heaviness and lethargy, worse after eating
- fluid retention, especially fingers, eyelids and abdomen
- waxy pale or sallow complexion
- cold extremities, cold intolerance
- weight loss

T pale and swollen with toothmarks; the coat will vary from thin (in simple deficiency) to thick and greasy (with accumulated Phlegm Damp)

P moderate and weak, or deep and slow

Treatment principle

Warm and strengthen the Spleen and Stomach
Harmonise the Stomach and stop pain
Transform Phlegm Damp

Prescription

HUANG QI JIAN ZHONG TANG 黄芪健中汤
(*Astragalus Decoction to Construct the Middle*)

zhi huang qi (honey fried Radix Astragali Membranacei) 黄芪 18-30g
gui zhi (Ramulus Cinnamomi Cassiae) 桂枝 9-12g
bai shao (Radix Paeoniae Lactiflorae) 白芍 12-15g
zhi gan cao (honey fried Radix Glycyrrhizae Uralensis) 炙甘草 6-9g
sheng jiang (Rhizoma Zingiberis Officinalis Recens) 生姜 9-12g
da zao (Fructus Zizyphi Jujubae) 大枣 4pce
yi tang (Saccharum Granorum) 饴糖 30g

Method: Decoction. **Yi tang** is dissolved in the strained decoction (*chong fu* 冲服). **Zhi huang qi** warms and strengthens the Spleen and Stomach and supplements *qi*; **gui zhi** warms the middle *jiao* and dispels Cold; **gui zhi** and **yi tang** combine pungent and sweet flavours to bolster *yang*; **bai shao**, **zhi gan cao** and **yi tang** moderate spasmodic pain; **sheng jiang** and **da zao** harmonise and warm the Stomach. (Source: *Shi Yong Zhong Yi Nei Ke Xue*)

Modifications

- With significant pain, add **gao liang jiang** (Rhizoma Alpiniae Officinari) 高良姜 9-12g and **xiang fu** (Rhizoma Cyperi Rotundi) 香附 9-12g.
- With Phlegm Damp or vomiting of thin watery fluids, add **chen pi** (Pericarpium Citri Reticulatae) 陈皮 9-12g, **ban xia** (Rhizoma Pinelliae Ternatae) 半夏 9-12g and **fu ling** (Sclerotium Poriae Cocos) 茯苓 12-15g.
- With acid reflux or heartburn, delete **yi tang**, and add **wu zhu yu** (Fructus Evodiae Rutaecarpae) 吴茱萸 3g and **hai piao xiao** (Os Sepiae seu Sepiellae) 海螵蛸 15g.
- With food stagnation, add **zhi shi** (Fructus Immaturus Citri Aurantii) 枳实 9-12g, **shen qu** (Massa Fermentata) 神曲 15g and **mai ya** (Fructus Hordei Vulgaris Germinantus) 麦芽 15-30g.
- With black tarry stools or occult blood in the stools, add **gan jiang tan** (charred Rhizoma Zingiberis Officinalis) 干姜炭 6-9g, **di yu tan** (charred Radix Sanguisorbae Officinalis) 地榆炭 9-12g and **bai ji** (Rhizoma Bletillae Striatae) 白芨 9-15g or consider **HUANG TU TANG** (*Yellow Earth Decoction* 黄土汤 see p.438).

Variations and additional prescriptions

Spleen yang deficiency

- If Spleen *qi* deficiency deteriorates, Spleen *yang* will be depleted and the patient will begin to exhibit signs of Cold (cold extremities, cold intolerance, undigested food in the stools, inability to keep food down, more intense colicky pain and a weak pulse). The aim of treatment is to warm Spleen *yang* with **FU ZI LI ZHONG WAN** (*Aconite, Ginseng and Ginger Formula* 附子理中丸).

zhi fu zi (Radix Aconiti Carmichaeli Praeparata) 制附子 6-12g
gan jiang (Rhizoma Zingiberis Officinalis) 干姜 9-12g
dang shen (Radix Codonopsis Pilosulae) 党参 15-24g
chao bai zhu (dry fried Rhizoma Atractylodes Macrocephalae) 炒白术 12-15g
zhi gan cao (honey fried Radix Glycyrrhizae Uralensis) 炙甘草 3-9g

Method: Decoction. **Zhi fu zi** is decocted for 30 minutes before the other herbs (*xian jian* 先煎). **Zhi fu zi** and **gan jiang** warm Spleen *yang* and dispel Cold; **dang shen**, **chao bai zhu** and **zhi gan cao** strengthen the Spleen and supplement *qi*.

With severe Cold

- If the Cold symptoms suddenly become severe, causing intense pain, short term use of **DA JIAN ZHONG TANG** (*Major Zanthoxylum Combination* 大建中汤) may be useful.

chuan jiao (Pericarpium Zanthoxyli Bungeani) 川椒 6-9g
gan jiang (Rhizoma Zingiberis Officinalis) 干姜 9-12g
dang shen (Radix Codonopsis Pilosulae) 党参 15-24g
yi tang (Saccharum Granorum) 饴糖 30g

Method: Decoction. **Yi tang** is added to the strained decoction (*chong fu* 冲服). **Chuan jiao** and **gan jiang** dispel Cold and stop pain; **dang shen** and **yi tang** strengthen the Spleen and Stomach and stop spasms. (Source: *Shi Yong Zhong Yi Nei Ke Xue*)

With Phlegm Damp (Phlegm Heat)

- Prolonged Spleen and Stomach *qi* deficiency will often be complicated by Phlegm Damp, or occasionally Damp Heat or Phlegm Heat, as chronic stagnation can easily transform into Heat. When the Phlegm Damp aspects become the primary pathology, the pattern will assume some distinctive features, and the primary focus of treatment should be to transform the Phlegm Damp. The important features of Phlegm Damp in the Stomach are epigastric pain that is worse in the morning and with pressure, severe distension, morning nausea, vomiting of mucus like substance, acid reflux, dizziness, heaviness in the body, foggy-headedness and a thick, greasy tongue coat. Once the Phlegm Damp has been resolved, the balance of treatment can change to strengthening the Spleen and supplementation of *qi*. Suitable base prescriptions to transform Phlegm Damp include **ER CHEN TANG** (*Citrus and Pinellia Combination* 二陈汤, p.756) and **PING WEI SAN**

(*Magnolia and Ginger Formula* 平胃散, p.153); **WEN DAN TANG** (*Bamboo and Hoelen Combination* 温胆汤, p.606) may be considered with Phlegm Heat.

Complex of Heat, Cold and deficiency

- Also useful when the pattern is complicated by a mix of excess and deficiency, Heat and Cold, such as, *qi* deficiency, Phlegm or Damp Heat accumulation in the Stomach and Cold in the Intestines, is **BAN XIA XIE XIN TANG** (*Pinellia Combination* 半夏泻心汤, p.32). The main features for the use of this prescription are epigastric discomfort and distension, nagging pain, acid reflux, indigestion, loss of appetite, morning nausea, tendency to loose stools, and greasy, yellowish tongue coat.

To improve gastro-intestinal function during recovery

- After the pain has abated, formulae that strengthen the Spleen and Stomach should be used for a lengthy period to consolidate the treatment and replenish *qi*. Prescription selection will depend on the patient, but prescriptions such as **LIU JUN ZI TANG** (*Six Major Herbs Combination* 六君子汤, p.769) and **XIANG SHA LIU JUN ZI TANG** (*Saussurea and Cardamon Combination* 香砂六君子汤, p.149) are usually excellent for long term Spleen and Stomach strengthening and *qi* supplementation.

Patent medicines

Li Zhong Wan 理中丸 (Li Zhong Wan)
- for Spleen *yang* deficiency

Fu Zi Li Zhong Wan 附子理中丸 (Carmichaeli Tea Pills, Fu Tzu Li Chung Wan, Li Chung Yuen Medical Pills)
- for Spleen *yang* deficiency and severe Cold

Xiang Sha Liu Jun Zi Wan 香砂六君子丸 (Xiang Sha Liu Jun Wan, Aplotaxis-Ammomum Pills, Six Gentlemen Tea Pills)
- Spleen and Stomach *qi* deficiency with Phlegm Damp

Xiang Sha Yang Wei Wan 香砂养胃丸 (Xiang Sha Yang Wei Wan, Hsiang Sha Yang Wei Wan)
- with *qi* stagnation

Zi Sheng Wan 资生丸 (Zi Sheng Wan, Zi Sheng Stomachic Pills)
- with food stagnation

Acupuncture (select from)

Ren.12 (*zhong wan* +▲) .. local points to warm, strengthen and regulate
Ren.13 (*shang wan* +▲) the Stomach and dispel Cold

St.36 (*zu san li* +▲) .... *he* sea point of the Stomach, powerfully warms and strengthens the Spleen and Stomach and supplements *qi*

Sp.6 (*san yin jiao* +▲)...... strengthens the Spleen and Kidney and invigorates *qi* and Blood

LI.11 (*qu chi* +▲) .... *he* sea point of the Large Intestine, warms *yang ming* and stimulates *yang qi* in general when moxaed

Lu.9 (*tai yuan*) .... *yuan* and *shu* stream point of the Lungs, *hui* point for the vessels, strengthens the Lungs, supplements *qi* and eases epigastric pain

Bl.20 (*pi shu* +▲) .... *shu* points of the Spleen and Stomach, warm,
Bl.21 (*wei shu* +▲) supplement and regulate middle *jiao qi*

- A moxa box over the epigastrium is excellent, especially for *yang* deficiency.
- With obvious bleeding or occult blood in the stools, apply rice grain moxa on Sp.1 (*yin bai*). It usually takes several cones before the patient feels the heat; once felt, a minimum of 7-10 cones should be applied.
- with loose stools or diarrhoea, add *zhi xie* +▲ (N-CA-3)
- with fluid retention and oedema, add Sp.9 (*yin ling quan* -) and Ren.9 (*shui fen* ▲)
- with heaviness, add St.40 (*feng long* -) and Sp.3 (*tai bai*)
- with nausea, add PC.6 (*nei guan*)
- with Phlegm Damp, add St.40 (*feng long* -), Sp.3 (*tai bai*) and PC.5 (*jian shi* -)
- *Ear points*: stomach, spleen, abdomen, large intestine, small intestine, *shen men*, sympathetic

Clinical notes

- Spleen *qi* or *yang* deficiency type epigastric pain may be diagnosed biomedically as chronic gastritis, indigestion, functional dyspepsia, peptic ulcer disease or chronic pancreatitis.
- Pain of this type responds reliably to correct TCM treatment, but the greater the deficiency, the longer the course or treatment required. Spleen *yang* deficiency may need 3-9 months of treatment.
- For dietary recommendations, see pp.870-873.

胃陰不足

9.7 STOMACH YIN DEFICIENCY

Pathophysiology

- The pain of Stomach *yin* deficiency is due to the Stomach being adversely affected by lack of physiological *yin* fluids. In addition, because Stomach function is affected, food and fluids are inefficiently processed and cause food stagnation.
- Stomach *yin* deficiency is usually a complication of some other long standing pathology, most commonly Liver *qi* invading the Stomach, or the chronic Heat patttterns. It can, however, be more acute, and follow sudden damage to Stomach *yin* following a febrile illness, such as *yang ming* syndrome.
- Stomach *yin* is a superficial form of *yin*, relative to the deeper Kidney *yin*. The main feature of Stomach *yin* deficiency, at least initially, will often be dryness rather than Heat. As the deficiency deepens, the signs of Heat appear. Depending on the degree of deficiency and the length of the problem, Kidney *yin* may eventually be drained leading to the onset of deeper deficiency Heat symptoms, such as night sweats and 'bone steaming'.

Clinical features

- Vague, dull, nagging or burning epigastric pain which is worse when the stomach is empty, and may improve with pressure. The pain tends to be worse at night, and the patient may wake with pain in the early hours of the morning.
- dryness of the mouth, throat, mucous membranes and skin
- thirst with desire for cool drinks
- mild nausea, tending to be worse in the morning and when hungry; in severe cases dry retching
- poor appetite, or indeterminate gnawing hunger with no real desire to eat, or the patient may desire cold and bland foods, or a liquid diet
- constipation or dry stools

T slightly red and peeled in the centre, or red and dry with little or no coat; in severe or long standing cases, the tongue may be so denuded of papillae as to resemble a piece of liver (mirror tongue) or have numerous surface cracks or a wide shallow central crack.

P thready and rapid or thready and wiry

Treatment principle

Nourish and supplement Stomach *yin*, generate fluids
Clear deficient Heat
Supplement *yin* in general

Prescription

YI WEI TANG 益胃汤
(*Benefit the Stomach Decoction*) modified

sha shen (Radix Adenophorae seu Glehniae) 沙参 12-18g
mai dong (Tuber Ophiopogonis Japonici) 麦冬 9-12g
yu zhu (Rhizoma Polygonati Odorati) 玉竹 12-15g
sheng di (Radix Rehmanniae Glutinosae) 生地 15-24g
tian dong (Tuber Asparagi Cochinchinensis) 天冬 9-12g
bai shao (Radix Paeoniae Lactiflora) 白芍 15-24g
gan cao (Radix Glycyrrhizae Uralensis) 甘草 6-9g
dan zhu ye (Herba Lophatheri Gracilis) 淡竹叶 6-9g

Method: Decoction. **Sha shen, mai dong, yu zhu, sheng di** and **tian dong** nourish Stomach *yin* and clear Heat; **bai shao** and **gan cao** combine sour and sweet to generate *yin* and alleviate pain; **dan zhu ye** clears residual Heat from the Stomach and Heart and alleviates irritability. (Source: *Zhong Yi Nei Ke Shou Ce*)

Modifications

- With significant or nagging pain, include herbs that gently move *qi* without damaging *yin*. These include **fo shou** (Fructus Citri Sarcodacylis) 佛手 9-12g, **ba yue zha** (Fructus Akebiae) 八月扎 9-12g, **mei gui hua** (Flos Rosae Rugosae) 玫瑰花 6-9g or **xiang yuan pi** (Pericarpium Citri Medica) 香橼皮 9-12g.
- With acid reflux, heartburn, burning pain and nausea, add **duan wa leng zi** (calcined Concha Arcae) 煅瓦楞子 15g, or if there is Heat **wu zhu yu** (Fructus Evodiae Rutaecarpae) 吴茱萸 1-3g and **huang lian** (Rhizoma Coptidis) 黄连 3-6g.
- With residual Stomach Fire, add **shi gao** (Gypsum) 石膏 15-30g.
- With residual Phlegm Heat, add **gua lou** (Fructus Trichosanthis) 栝楼 15-24g, **tian hua fen** (Radix Trichosanthis Kirilowii) 天花粉 9-12g and **chuan bei mu** (Bulbus Fritillariae Cirrhosae) 川贝母 9-12g.
- With significant deficiency Heat, add **zhi mu** (Rhizoma Anemarrhenae Asphodeloides) 知母 9-12g and **xuan shen** (Radix Scrophulariae) 玄参 18-24g.
- With loss of appetite, add **mai ya** (Fructus Hordei Vulgaris Germinantus) 麦芽 15-30g and **ji nei jin** (Endothelium Corneum Gigeriae Galli) 鸡内金 15g.
- With hypoacidity, add **wu mei** (Fructus Pruni Mume) 乌梅 9-12g, **shi hu** (Herba Dendrobi) 石斛 12-15g and **shan zha** (Fructus Crataegi) 山楂 15g.
- With *qi* deficiency (swollen tongue with many surface cracks), add **tai zi shen** (Radix Pseudostellariae Heterophyllae) 太子参 15-24g and **wu wei zi** (Fructus Schizandrae Chinensis) 五味子 6g.

- With stagnant *qi*, add **mei gui hua** (Flos Rosae Rugosae) 玫瑰花 6-9g and **fo shou** (Fructus Citri Sarcodacylis) 佛手 9-12g, or consider **YI GUAN JIAN** (*Linking Decoction* 一贯煎, p.78).
- With stagnant Blood (intermittent stabbing pain, or a focal area that is worse with pressure), add **dan shen** (Radix Salviae Miltiorrhizae) 丹参 12-18g and **tao ren** (Semen Persicae) 桃仁 9-12g.
- With constipation, add **sheng he shou wu** (unprocessed Radix Polygoni Multiflori) 生何首乌 12-15g and **huo ma ren** (Semen Cannabis Sativae) 火麻仁 9-12g.
- With *Helicobacter pylori*, add **pu gong ying** (Herba Taraxaci Mongolici) 蒲公英 15-30g.
- With obvious bleeding or occult blood in the stools, add **e jiao** (Gelatinum Corii Asini) 阿胶 9-12g (melted in the hot strained decoction) and **bai ji** (Rhizoma Bletillae Striatae) 白芨 9-15g, or **san qi fen** (powdered Radix Notoginseng) 三七粉 3g washed down with the decoction.
- For atrophy of the gastric mucosa, add **dan shen** (Radix Salviae Miltiorrhizae) 丹参 12-18g and **zhi huang qi** (honey fried Radix Astragali Membranacei) 炙黄芪 18-30g.
- If Kidney and/or Liver *yin* is also weakened (lower back ache, flushing, nightsweats and tinnitus) combine with **LIU WEI DI HUANG WAN** (*Rehmannia Six Formula* 六味地黄丸). Patent pills are sufficient.

Patent medicines

Gu Ben Wan 固本丸 (Gu Ben Wan, Ren Shen Ku Pen Wan)
- Stomach *qi* and *yin* deficiency

Liu Wei Di Huang Wan 六味地黄丸 (Liu Wei Dihuang Wan)
- combine with the principal formula when there is Kidney *yin* deficiency

Zhi Bai Ba Wei Wan 知柏八味丸 (Zhi Bai Ba Wei Wan, Chih Pai Pa Wei Wan) - *yin* deficiency with Heat

Luo Han Guo Chong Ji 罗汉冲剂 (Luo Han Kuo Beverage)

Shen Ling Bai Zhu Wan 参苓白术丸 (Shen Ling Bai Zhu Wan)
- Spleen and Stomach *qi* and *yin* deficiency

Sheng Mai San Wan 生脉散丸 (Sheng Mai San Wan)
- Lung and Stomach *qi* and *yin* deficiency

Acupuncture (select from)

Ren.12 (*zhong wan* +)....... *mu* point of the Stomach, nourishes Stomach *yin*, regulates the Stomach and directs Stomach *qi* downwards

Ren.4 (*guan yuan* +) .... meeting point of the *yin* channels, nourishes *yin* in combination with Sp.6

St.36 (*zu san li* +) .... *he* sea point of the Stomach, powerfully strengthens the Spleen and Stomach and supplements *qi* and *yin*
Sp.6 (*san yin jiao*) .... strengthens the Spleen, regulates *qi*, benefits the Kidneys and supplements *qi* and *yin*

Bl.20 (*pi shu* +) .... these points strengthen the source of all
Bl.21 (*wei shu* +) acquired *yin*, the Spleen and Stomach

Bl.23 (*shen shu* +) .... these points strengthen the source of all
Kid.6 (*zhao hai* +) inherited *yin*, the Kidney, releasing stored *yin*
Kid.3 (*tai xi* +) to support Stomach *yin*

- with deficient Heat, add St.43 (*xian gu* -) and Kid.2 (*ran gu*)
- with sharp pain, add Kid.2 (*ran gu*)
- with nausea, add PC.6 (*nei guan*)
- *Ear points*: stomach, spleen, abdomen, kidney, *shen men*, sympathetic

Clinical notes

- Stomach *yin* deficiency type epigastric pain may be diagnosed biomedically as chronic atrophic gastritis, reflux oesophagitis, gastro-oesophageal reflux disease, heartburn, peptic ulcer disease or stomach cancer.
- This is a relatively common pattern seen in TCM clinics, and responds reasonably well to prolonged treatment. Even though the pain may be alleviated within a relatively short period of weeks, treatment will need to continue so as to rebuild *yin*. In long standing cases, 6-9 months of treatment may be necessary for a satisfactory long term result.
- For dietary recommendations, see p.876.

SUMMARY OF GUIDING FORMULAE FOR EPIGASTRIC PAIN

Excess patterns

Cold congealing Stomach *qi* - *Liang Fu Wan* 良附丸
- from Wind Cold - *Huo Xiang Zheng Qi San* 藿香正气散
- mixed with Heat - *Ban Xia Xie Xin Tang* 半夏泻心汤

Food stagnation - *Bao He Wan* 保和丸
- with severe pain and constipation - *Tiao Wei Cheng Qi Tang* 调胃承气汤
- with Damp Heat - *Zhi Shi Dao Zhi Wan* 枳实导滞丸

Liver *qi* invading the Stomach - *Chai Hu Shu Gan Wan* 柴胡疏肝丸
- with *yin* deficiency - *Yi Guan Jian* 一贯煎

Stomach Heat - *Qing Wei San* 清胃散
- with Damp Heat - *Huang Lian Jie Du Tang* 黄连解毒汤
- with a *shao yang* and *yang ming* pathogen - *Da Chai Hu Tang* 大柴胡汤
- with Phlegm Heat - *Xiao Xian Xiong Tang* 小陷胸汤
- with *yin* deficiency - *Yu Nu Jian* 玉女煎

Blood stagnation - *Shi Xiao San* 失笑散 + *Dan Shen Yin* 丹参饮
- in severe cases with masses - *Ge Xia Zhu Yu Tang* 膈下逐瘀汤
- with *qi* stagnation - *Xue Fu Zhu Yu Tang* 血府逐瘀汤
- with Heat - *Da Huang Huang Qin Xie Xin Tang* 大黄黄芩泻心汤
- with Cold and bleeding - *Huang Tu Tang* - 黄土汤

Deficient patterns

Spleen and Stomach *qi* deficiency - *Huang Qi Jian Zhong Tang* 黄芪健中汤
- Spleen *yang* deficiency - *Fu Zi Li Zhong Wan* 附子理中丸
- severe pain - *Da Jian Zhong Tang* 大健中汤
- with Phlegm Damp - *Er Chen Tang* 二陈汤, *Ping Wei San* 平胃散
- mixed with Heat and excess - *Ban Xia Xie Xin Tang* 半夏泻心汤

Stomach *yin* deficiency - *Yi Wei Tang* 益胃汤

Table 9.1 *Differential diagnosis of epigastric pain*

Pattern	Duration	Aggravated by	Ameliorated by	Nature of pain	Nature of patient	Pulse and tongue
Cold invading the Stomach	mostly acute	ingesting cold substances, pressure on the epigastrium	warmth on the epigastrium	violent, cramping, colicky, may come in spasmodic waves	all ages	T: white coat P: wiry, tight
Food stagnation	chronic with acute exacerbations	eating	belching, vomiting, fasting	distending, full	may tend to be overweight	T:thick, greasy coat P: slippery, full
Liver qi invading the Stomach	mostly chronic with acute exacerbations	emotion and stress	relaxation, expulsion of gas	crampy, 'knot in the Stomach'	tense, uptight, nervy, most common 20-50 yrs F>M	T: normal, or dark, or with red edges P: wiry
Stomach Heat	acute or chronic	pressure on the epigastrium, heating foods and fluids	fasting	burning, nagging, distending	all ages (may be tense when associated with qi stagnation)	T: red with a yellow coat P: slippery, rapid
Blood stagnation	chronic but may be acute following trauma or surgery	pressure, eating, at night		severe, sharp, boring, fixed in location	mostly older, looks unwell, weight loss	T: dark, purple, or with purple spots P:wiry, choppy, thready

Spleen and Stomach qi deficiency	chronic	fatigue, cold natured, hard to digest or excessively sweet foods	warmth, pressure, eating warm foods	mild, dull, continuous, nagging	pale, fatigued, puffy eyes, low vitality	T: pale, with tooth marks P: weak, deficient
Spleen yang deficiency	chronic, although may be acute following surgery	fatigue, cold natured, hard to digest or excessively sweet foods	warmth, pressure, eating warm foods	dull and nagging, with occasional severe, colicky, cramping pain	pale, cold intolerant, emaciated	T:pale and swollen P: deep, slow
Stomach yin deficiency	chronic (but may follow an acute febrile disease)	with an empty stomach and at night	pressure, moistening foods	vague, dull, burning, indeterminate gnawing discomfort	older patients, thin, flushed, heat intolerant	T: peeled in the centre or red and peeled P: thready, rapid

10. Gingivitis, Periodontitis

Stomach Heat, Fire
Stomach *yin* deficiency with Heat
Qi and Blood deficiency
Blood stagnation

10 GINGIVITIS, PERIODONTITIS

feng chi 风齿, *ya xuan*[1] 牙宣

Gingivitis and periodontitis are disorders of the gums and associated structures. They are similar, and indeed the Chinese medical aetiology is the same for both.

Gingivitis is inflammation of the gums characterised by redness, swelling, suppuration and bleeding. Dental plaque accumulation at the gingival margin causes gingivitis and plaque removal usually resolves it. Plaque is a matrix of cellular elements, including bacteria, epithelial cells, erythrocytes and leucocytes. In well developed plaque, fungi, protozoans and mycoplasmas may be found.

Periodontitis is the inflammation of the supporting structures of the teeth. It is more serious than gingivitis and frequently leads to irreversible damage. Not all gingivitis evolves into periodontitis, but all periodontitis is preceded by gingivitis. While calculus[2] deposits of the gingival margin are frequently involved, plaque remains the effective causal agent. Whether acute or chronic in nature, attachment of the gums to the teeth is affected and supporting bone is lost. Untreated teeth become loose and may be lost.

Periodontitis is occasionally complicated by abscess formation (*see* Chapter 25. Tooth abscess).

Though the primary causative agent of periodontal disease is plaque, other risk factors will place individuals at a higher susceptibility to the disease process. These are summarised in Box 10.1.

Maintenance of healthy gums and teeth is an essential feature of overall health maintenance and well being into old age. The mouth is the beginning of the digestive process, and thorough chewing improves the ability of the Spleen and Stomach to extract the maximum nutrition from food. Facilitating digestion, however, is not the only function of healthy gums and teeth. From a biomedical perspective, periodontal disease is a significant contributor to both morbidity and mortality as a result of poor nutritional status and disseminated infection. The gums can act as a reservoir for pathogenic bacteria which can enter the blood stream. There appears to be an increased risk of cardiovascular disease and diabetic complications in those with periodontitis.

This chapter is primarily concerned with the systemic patterns that exacerbate the gum disease process. TCM treatment is secondary to appropriate dentistry and oral hygiene. Treatment with TCM usually proceeds when gum

---

[1] Wiseman gives *ya xuan* as gaping gums.

[2] Calculus is formed when accumulated plaque mineralises due to deposition of salts present in the saliva. Calculus acts as a plaque trap, exacerbating plaque buildup.

disease does not improve following appropriate dental work, or when it is clearly complicated by a contributing pathology.

BOX 10.1 SOME BIOMEDICAL CAUSES OF GINGIVITIS AND PERIODONTITIS

Most common
- poor oral hygiene and buildup of plaque on the teeth
- diabetes[1]
- smoking[2]
- HIV infection
- psychological stress
- genetics

Medications
- Dilantin
- Cyclosporin
- Calcium channel blockers
- any medication that decreases secretion of saliva

Other
- gingival lesion from fungal: bacterial and viral infection; candida, herpes, streptococcal
- malnutrition: scurvy, pellagra
- physiological: puberty, menstruation, pregnancy
- osteoporosis
- leukaemia
- trauma
- exposure to heavy metals

Physiology of the mouth

The mouth is governed by the Spleen, Stomach, Heart and Kidney organ systems.

Spleen

The buccal cavity as a whole is overseen by the Spleen (as the 'orifice' of the Spleen). In particular, the cheeks and lips reflect the health of the Spleen. The state of the Blood and Spleen *qi* are reflected in the lustre and colour of the lips, and the efficiency of fluid metabolism and distribution can be observed in the cheeks and tongue. In addition, the Spleen channel spreads out over the ventral surface of the tongue.

Stomach

The gums are governed by the Stomach, both through the channel pathway and directly via the organ system, and various pathology of the Stomach can be reflected in the gums. Because the Stomach requires a moist environment to function efficiently, pathological processes that heat and/or dry the Stomach are those most likely to directly damage the Stomach, and thence the gums. Stomach *yin* deficiency and Stomach Heat are the most frequently observed patterns of gum disease.

Heart

The tongue is considered to be the 'sprout of the Heart', and Heat or *yin* deficiency patterns frequently involve the tongue (*see also* Chapter 20. Mouth Ulcers).

[1] 2-3x increase risk of periodontitis.

[2] 2x increase with light smoking (<10/day), 7x increase with heavy smoking (>10/day).

BOX 10.2 KEY DIAGNOSTIC POINTS

These apply to the oral cavity in general (gums, tongue, buccal cavity and lips)

Pain

- better for application of cold (ice etc.) - excess or deficient Heat
- better for warm drinks - excess or deficient Cold
- variable intensity - mixed *zheng qi* deficiency and pathological excess (the variation reflects the changes in fortune of the pathogen and the *zheng qi*)
  - continuous pain - ascendant pathogen, primary excess pattern
  - occasional exacerbation of low grade or dull pain - primary deficiency pattern with intermittent excess pathogen
- chronic pain that is worse later in the day and in the evening - *yin* deficiency
- chronic pain that is worse earlier in the day and improves as the day progresses - *yang* deficiency

Swelling and redness

- redness, swelling and pain - excess Heat (Wind Heat/Fire, Stomach Heat/Fire, Damp Heat)
  - acute Wind Heat/Fire
  - chronic or acute flare-up of a chronic disorder - Stomach Heat/Fire, Damp Heat
- mild swelling with little or no redness or pain, or with dull pain that increases towards the end of the day - *yin* deficiency
- soft swelling with distension and no redness - Phlegm Damp
- atrophy - *yin* deficiency, *qi* and Blood deficiency, Blood stagnation

Ulceration

- acute, with raised red margins and yellow exudate - excess Heat
- chronic or recurrent ulceration with a pale or greyish base, margins not especially red or raised - *yin* deficiency
- vesicular eruptions that burst and ulcerate - Wind Heat with Dampness
- acute white, porridge like spots or plaques - Damp Heat
- chronic, recurrent and often extensive yet shallow ulcerations that are not particularly painful and are the same colour as the surrounding tissue - *yang* deficiency
- with dryness and cracking - *yin* and Blood deficiency

Bleeding and suppuration

- copious yellow malodorous exudate - Stomach Fire, Toxic Heat
- continuous inoffensive thin suppuration or exudate - Spleen and Kidney deficiency, *qi* and Blood deficiency
- frequent copious bleeding - excess Heat
- mild bleeding with contact (brushing, chewing) - *yin* deficiency
- dark or clotted blood - Blood stagnation

Kidneys

The teeth are considered an outgrowth of the bones and therefore the province of the Kidneys. In particular the Kidneys (through *jing*) maintain the integrity and solidity of the teeth in the jaw, and of the teeth themselves. Loose or easily chipped or broken teeth may reflect a weakness of Kidney function.

Liver

The Liver channel encircles the internal aspect of the lips. The Liver can have an indirect but major effect on the structures of the mouth, through *qi* stagnation and stagnant Heat, which then influence the Stomach, Spleen and Heart through the generative (*sheng* 生) or controlling (*ke* 克) cycle.

AETIOLOGY

Poor oral hygiene

The most common cause of gingivitis and periodontitis is poor oral hygiene, and regardless of the systemic aspects of the pattern, this is the crucial factor. Patients can have a variety of systemic patterns that affect the gums and mouth, but if they look after their mouths properly, the oral manifestations may never eventuate. Of course, even in the absence of systemic imbalance, oral pathology will occur when oral hygiene is not maintained.

Diet

The most important aspects of the diet that contribute to gingivitis and periodontitis are those that heat the Stomach and thence the gums. Simple overeating or overconsumption of heating foods, such as spicy hot foods, alcohol and inappropriate *yang* supplementing substances, can cause Stomach Heat directly. Sugar is also a major contributing factor to the buildup of plaque.

Emotion

The most common emotional pattern giving rise to gum disease is that which affects the Liver and then the Stomach. Liver *qi* stagnation is caused by repressed emotion, frustration, anger and resentment. These emotions, especially when chronically unexpressed, can gradually lead to the development of stagnant Heat as the pressure builds up behind the area of congestion. Once Heat has been generated, either primarily in the Liver and transmitted to the Stomach, or directly in the Stomach as a result of the repeated insult to the Stomach, it will rise to affect the superior structures of the Stomach system, the mouth and gums.

Liver *qi* stagnation can also disrupt Spleen function and digestive efficiency.

Spleen weakness and inefficient digestion will contribute to the pathological residue Dampness, which in turn may obstruct *qi* circulation and generate Heat.

Prolonged *qi* stagnation can lead to several complications which also contribute to chronic gum disease. These include Blood stagnation, stagnant Heat, damage to *yin* and the Spleen, with consequent weakness of *qi* and Blood.

TREATMENT

The single most important element of treatment is regular dentistry and good oral hygiene, regular brushing and flossing. Daily removal of plaque with dental floss and a toothbrush and regular biannual cleaning by dental specialists can help prevent gingival disease. If dental hygiene is not maintained, TCM treatment will not deliver its full benefit.

Cessation of smoking makes a big difference. Modification of the diet will be a major factor in most cases involving the Stomach and/or Liver.

胃火上蒸

10.1 STOMACH HEAT/FIRE

Pathophysiology

- Stomach Heat is usually associated with the diet. An excess of Stomach heating foods and drink, or overconsumption of hot supplementing herbs can create the conditions which cause focal accumulation of Heat in the gums. Stomach Heat may also occur as a secondary effect of Liver Fire invading via the controlling cycle.
- This is a chronic pattern of gingivitis, although there may be occasional flare-ups and aggravations, depending on the eating or drinking habits of the individual concerned.

Clinical features

- Redness, swelling and pain in the gums; the gums easily and frequently bleed and may be ulcerated. There may be occasional suppuration. The pain may radiate to the head, cheek or jaw and is eased by the application of cold.
- halitosis, dry mouth, thirst, bad taste in the mouth
- frontal headaches
- epigastric discomfort
- ravenous hunger, or indeterminate gnawing hunger
- red flushed face, red lips
- tendency to constipation or sluggish stools; rarely, diarrhoea
- concentrated urine

T red and dry with a yellow coat, thicker in the centre of the tongue
P slippery, strong and rapid

Treatment principle

Clear Heat and Fire from the Stomach
Reduce swelling and stop pain

Prescription

QING WEI SAN 清胃散
(Clear the Stomach Powder)

This prescription is suitable when there are clear signs of Stomach Heat without constipation.

huang lian (Rhizoma Coptidis) 黄连 6-9g
sheng di (Radix Rehmanniae Glutinosae) 生地 12-18g
mu dan pi (Cortex Moutan Radicis) 牡丹皮 9-12g
dang gui (Radix Angelicae Sinensis) 当归 6-9g
sheng ma (Rhizoma Cimicifugae) 升麻 6-9g

Method: Decoction. The main herb, bitter and cold **huang lian** clears Heat from the Stomach and directs Stomach *qi* and turbid *qi* downward; **mu dan pi** cools the Blood and disperses stagnant Blood; **sheng di** cools the Blood and nourishes *yin*; **dang gui** nourishes and regulates Blood and protects it against the drying effects of the Heat; pungent, sweet, cool and elevating **sheng ma** encourages the ascent of clear *qi*, clears Toxic Heat from the Stomach and balances the descending nature of **huang lian**; together this pair, one ascending, one descending, clear Heat without drying, and correct the *qi* mechanism. (Source: *Zhong Yi Er Bi Hou Ke Xue*)

Modifications

- With severe redness and swelling of the gums, add two or three of the following herbs: **ma bian cao** (Herba Verbenae Officinalis) 马鞭草 9-12g, **pu gong ying** (Herba Taraxaci Mongolici) 蒲公英 15-30g, **shui niu jiao** (Cornu Bubali) 水牛角 15-30g, **niu bang zi** (Fructus Arctii Lappae) 牛蒡子 9-12g, **niu xi** (Radix Achyranthis Bidentatae) 牛膝 9-12g and **shan zhi zi** (Fructus Gardeniae Jasminoidis) 山栀子 9-12g or **qian cao gen** (Radix Rubiae Cordifoliae) 茜草根 9-12g.
- With toothache, add **fang feng** (Radix Ledebouriellae Divaricatae) 防风 9-12g and **bo he** (Herba Mentha Haplocalycis) 薄荷 6-9g.
- With severe thirst and dryness from damage to Stomach fluids, delete **dang gui** and add **tian hua fen** (Radix Trichosanthes Kirilowii) 天花粉 12-15g, **shi hu** (Herba Dendrobii) 石斛 12-15g and **zhi mu** (Rhizoma Anemarrhenae Asphodeloides) 知母 9-12g.
- With Blood stagnation, add **dan shen** (Radix Salviae Miltiorrhizae) 丹参 12-18g, **chuan xiong** (Radix Ligustici Chuanxiong) 川芎 6-9g and **chi shao** (Radix Paeoniae Rubrae) 赤芍 9-12g.
- With suppuration, add **ma bo** (Fructificatio Lasiosphaerae seu Calvatiae) 马勃 3-6g, **tian hua fen** (Radix Trichosanthes Kirilowii) 天花粉 12-15g and **zao jiao ci** (Spina Gleditsiae Sinensis) 皂角刺 9-12g.
- With constipation, add **da huang** (Radix et Rhizoma Rhei) 大黄 6-9g and **mang xiao** (Mirabilitum) 芒硝 6-9g.
- With incessant bleeding, add **niu xi** (Radix Achyranthis Bidentatae) 牛膝 12-15g, **bai mao gen** (Rhizoma Imperatae Cylindricae) 白茅根 18-30g, **xian he cao** (Herba Agrimoniae Pilosae) 仙鹤草 12-15g and **ou jie** (Nodus Nelumbinis Nuciferae Rhizomatis) 藕节 9-12g.

Variations and additional prescriptions

Liver Fire invading the Stomach

- Liver Fire can invade the Stomach, heating the Stomach system and causing marked redness, swelling and bleeding of the gums. The key to this pattern is the aggravation or initiation of the symptoms by emotional stress. The development of Liver Fire is aided by overindulgence in heating foods and beverages, especially alcohol. The aim of treatment is to cool the

Liver and stop bleeding with **LONG DAN XIE GAN TANG** (*Gentiana Combination* 龙胆泻肝汤) modified.

long dan cao (Radix Gentianae Longdancao) 龙胆草 6-9g
sheng di (Radix Rehmanniae Glutinosae) 生地 12-18g
shan zhi zi (Fructus Gardeniae Jasminoidis) 山栀子 9-12g
huang qin (Radix Scutellariae Baicalensis) 黄芩 9-12g
chai hu (Radix Bupleuri) 柴胡 9-12g
ze xie (Rhizoma Alismatis Orientalis) 泽泻 9-12g
che qian zi (Semen Plantaginis) 车前子 9-12g
mu tong (Caulis Mutong) 木通 3-6g
dang gui (Radix Angelicae Sinensis) 当归 6-9g
gan cao (Radix Glycyrrhizae Uralensis) 甘草 3-6g
mai dong (Tuber Ophiopogonis Japonici) 麦冬 9-12g
zhi mu (Rhizoma Anemarrhenae Asphodeloides) 知母 9-12g
bai mao gen (Rhizoma Imperatae Cylindricae) 白茅根 18-30g
xian he cao (Herba Agrimoniae Pilosae) 仙鹤草 12-15g

Method: Decoction. **Che qian zi** is usually cooked in a cloth bag (*bao jian*). **Long dan cao** cools the Liver and clears Fire; **sheng di** cools the Blood; **shan zhi zi** and **huang qin** clear Heat from the Heart, Stomach and Liver; **chai hu** assists in clearing Heat and alleviating constraint; **ze xie**, **che qian zi** and **mu tong** promote urination to provide an escape route for the Heat; **dang gui** nourishes and protects Blood; **gan cao** protects the Stomach; **mai dong** and **zhi mu** nourish *yin* and clear Heat; **bai mao gen** and **xian he cao** stop bleeding. (Source: *Shi Yong Zhong Yi Nei Ke Xue*)

Toxic Heat

- Severe Heat, or an acute flare-up of a chronic disorder, may manifest as a Toxic Heat pattern. This can result from an external invasion that aggravates a pre-existing condition, or can follow invasion of the Stomach by a particularly intense and virulent pathogen. The features are suppuration, bleeding gums with copious fresh red blood (and probably other sites of bleeding, nose, sclera, skin etc.), fever and chills or high fever, malaise, irritability, restlessness, severe thirst, halitosis, muscle and bone aches, constipation or diarrhoea, concentrated urine, a red tongue with a yellow coat and a forceful and rapid, or hollow pulse. The treatment aims to clear Toxic Heat from the Stomach and cool the Blood with **HUANG LIAN JIE DU TANG** (*Coptis and Scute Combination* 黄连解毒汤) modified.

huang lian (Rhizoma Coptidis) 黄连 6-9g
huang qin (Radix Scutellariae Baicalensis) 黄芩 9-12g
huang bai (Cortex Phellodendri) 黄柏 9-12g
shan zhi zi (Fructus Gardeniae Jasminoidis) 山栀子 9-12g
sheng di (Radix Rehmanniae Glutinosae) 生地 12-15g
ce bai ye (Cacumen Biotae Orientalis) 侧柏叶 12-15g

ou jie (Nodus Nelumbinis Nuciferae Rhizomatis) 藕节 12-15g
qing dai (Indigo Pulverata Levis) 青黛 1-3g

Method: Decoction. **Qing dai** is added to the strained decoction (*chong fu* 冲服). **Huang lian, huang qin, huang bai** and **shan zhi zi** clear Heat, Damp Heat and Toxic Heat from all three *jiao*; **sheng di** cools the Blood and nourishes *yin*; **ce bai ye** and **ou jie** stop bleeding; **qing dai** cools the Liver and clears Toxic Heat. (Source: *Shi Yong Zhong Yi Nei Ke Xue*)

Topical treatment

- Boil 15 grams of **huang qin** (Radix Scutellariae Baicalensis) 黄芩 in one cup of water for 20 minutes and hold the liquid in the mouth for as long as possible.
- With dental caries and relatively severe pain, gargle with a decoction of **lu feng fang** (Nidus Vespae) 露蜂房 12g and **hai tong pi** (Cortex Erythrinae) 海桐皮 12g.
- **BING PENG SAN** (*Borneol and Borax Powder* 冰硼散) modified, may be applied topically to the affected area.

bing pian (Borneol) 冰片 1.5g
xuan ming fen (Mirabilitum Purum) 玄明粉 15g
peng sha (Borax) 硼砂 15g

Method: Grind substances to a fine powder. Blow a small amount onto affected area 2-3 times daily. **Bing pian, xuan ming fen** and **peng sha** clear Heat and promote healing. (Source: *Zhong Yi Er Bi Hou Ke Xue*)

Patent medicines

Huang Lian Jie Du Wan 黄连解毒丸 (Huang Lian Jie Du Wan)
- Stomach Heat, Damp Heat

Niu Huang Qing Huo Wan 牛黄清火丸 (Niu Huang Qing Huo Wan)
- with constipation

Bei Jing Niu Huang Jie Du Pian 牛黄解毒片 (Peking Niu Huang Chieh Tu Pien) - Heat in the upper body

Huang Lian Shang Qing Pian 黄连上清片 (Huang Lian Shang Ching Pien) - Heat in the upper body

Long Dan Xie Gan Wan 龙胆泻肝丸 (Long Dan Xie Gan Wan, Lung Tan Xie Gan Wan) - with Liver Fire

Shuang Liao Hou Feng San 双料喉风散 (Superior Sore Throat Powder)
- can be massaged into the affected area to relieve pain and swelling

Xi Gua Shuang 西瓜霜 (Watermelon Frost)
- topically to relieve pain and swelling

Acupuncture (select from)

Ren.12 (*zhong wan* -) .... *mu* point of the Stomach, reducing method clears Heat from the Stomach

St.44 (*nei ting* -) .... together these points clear Heat from *yang*
LI.4 (*he gu* -) *ming* when reduced; they also have a special effect on oral diseases

SJ.2 (*ye men* -) .... *rong* spring and Water point of the *san jiao*, clears Heat from the *san jiao*

PC.8 (*lao gong* -) .... *rong* spring and Fire point of the Pericardium, drains Heat from the Stomach channel and cools Heart Fire

LI.11 (*qu chi* -) .... *he* sea point of the Large Intestine, clears Heat and Dampness from *yang ming*

St.6 (*jia che* -) .... local points for disease of the gums and
St.7 (*xia guan* -) mouth

- with swelling, add SJ.20 (*jiao sun*) and SI.8 (*xiao hai* -)
- with severe pain, add LI.2 (*er jian* -) and SI.5 (*yang gu* -)
- with severe Heat, bleed St.45 (*li dui* ↓)
- with constipation, add SJ.6 (*zhi gou* -) and St.25 (*tian shu* -)
- with Liver Fire, add Liv.2 (*xing jian* -)
- *Ear points*: stomach, mouth, tragus apex, upper jaw, lower jaw, *shen men*

With Toxic Heat, add

PC.3 (*qu ze* ↓) .... *he* sea point of the Pericardium and Urinary
Bl.40 (*wei zhong* ↓) Bladder respectively, together these points cool the Blood and clear Toxic Heat

St.45 (*li dui* ↓) ....*jing* well point of the Stomach, powerfully clears Heat from the Stomach and Stomach channel

Clinical notes

- The constitutional aspects of Stomach and Liver Heat/Fire patterns generally respond well to treatment, as long as appropriate dietary and life habit changes are made. Several months of treatment may be necessary.
- For dietary recommendations, see pp.882-885.

陰虛火旺

10.2 STOMACH YIN DEFICIENCY WITH HEAT

Pathophysiology

- This pattern is usually a complication of Stomach Heat/Fire, as any Heat in the system will dry the affected tissues and ultimately consume *yin*. The Stomach is especially prone to dryness and *yin* deficiency, as it needs some moisture to function normally. In prolonged cases, Kidney *yin* will be drained, and the Kidney deficiency elements will tend to become more prominent as the pattern develops. As the Kidney governs the integrity of the bones (the teeth being outgrowths of bone), the teeth are progressively loosened and lost.

Clinical features

- atrophy and retraction of the gums; the roots of the teeth are revealed; there may be frequent bleeding
- may be ulceration of the gums, the margins of which are only slightly red; possible occasional suppuration
- possibly loose, chipped or broken teeth; may be pain with chewing
- general dryness of mucous membranes and skin, thirst, dry mouth and throat
- dizziness, tinnitus, blurred vision, poor memory
- malar or facial flushing, nightsweats
- sensation of heat in the palms and soles ('five hearts hot')
- lower back ache

T red and dry with little or no coat, especially in the centre
P thready and rapid or wiry and rapid

Treatment principle

Nourish and supplement Stomach and Kidney *yin*
Clear Heat and deficient Heat
Benefit *jing* and strengthen the teeth

Prescription

YU NU JIAN 玉女煎
(*Jade Woman Decoction*) modified

This prescription is selected when there is obvious Stomach Fire in addition to the underlying *yin* deficiency.

shi gao (Gypsum) 石膏 18-30g
shu di (Radix Rehmanniae Glutinosae Conquitae) 熟地 18-30g
zhi mu (Rhizoma Anemarrhenae Asphodeloides) 知母 9-12g
mai dong (Tuber Ophiopogonis Japonici) 麦冬 9-12g
chuan niu xi (Radix Cyathulae Officinalis) 川牛膝 9-15g

nu zhen zi (Fructus Ligustri Lucidi) 女贞子 9-12g

Method: Decoction. **Shi gao** is decocted for 30 minutes before the other herbs (*xian jian* 先煎). **Shi gao** and **zhi mu** clear Heat from the Stomach; **shu di** nourishes *yin* and Blood and Kidney water to restrain Fire; **mai dong** and **nu zhen zi** clear Heat and nourish *yin*; **chuan niu xi** directs *qi* downwards away from the head. (Source: *Zhong Yi Er Bi Hou Ke Xue*)

Modifications

- With frequently bleeding gums, substitute **sheng di** (Radix Rehmanniae Glutinosae) 生地 for **shu di**, and add **bai mao gen** (Rhizoma Imperatae Cylindricae) 白茅根 18-30g, **qian cao gen** (Radix Rubiae Cordifoliae) 茜草根 12-15g and **mu dan pi** (Cortex Moutan Radicis) 牡丹皮 9-12g.
- With severe thirst and dryness in the mouth, add **tian hua fen** (Radix Trichosanthes Kirilowii) 天花粉 12-15g and **shi hu** (Herba Dendrobii) 石斛 12-15g.
- With mild signs of Blood stagnation, add **tao ren** (Semen Persicae) 桃仁 9-12g and **hong hua** (Flos Carthami Tinctorii) 红花 9-12g.

Variations and additional prescriptions

With Kidney yin deficiency

- With prominent Kidney *yin* deficiency (loose or broken teeth), or gum disease in the elderly, the aim of treatment is to supplement Kidney *yin* and strengthen the teeth with **LIU WEI DI HUANG WAN** (*Rehmannia Six Formula* 六味地黄丸) modified.

shu di (Radix Rehmanniae Glutinosae Conquitae) 熟地 240g
shan yao (Radix Dioscoreae Oppositae) 山药 120g
shan zhu yu (Fructus Corni Officinalis) 山茱萸 120g
fu ling (Sclerotium Poria Cocos) 茯苓 90g
ze xie (Rhizoma Alismatis Orientalis) 泽泻 90g
mu dan pi (Cortex Moutan Radicis) 牡丹皮 90g
gou ji (Rhizoma Cibotii Barometz) 狗脊 90g
gu sui bu (Rhizoma Drynariae) 骨碎补 120g
gou qi zi (Fructus Lycii) 枸杞子 90g
tu si zi (Semen Cuscutae Chinensis) 菟丝子 90g

Method: Grind the herbs to powder and form into 9-gram pills with honey. The dose is 2-3 pills daily. May also be decocted with a 90% reduction in quantities. **Shu di** and **gou qi zi** supplement Blood, and Liver and Kidney *yin*; **shan yao** strengthens the Spleen; **shan zhu yu** supplements Liver *yin*; **fu ling**, **ze xie** and **mu dan pi** prevent the supplementing herbs from clogging up the digestive system; **mu dan pi** invigorates Blood and eliminates stagnant Blood; **gou ji** and **gu sui bu** supplement the Liver and Kidneys and strengthen the bones and teeth; **tu si zi** benefits *jing*.

With significant deficient Heat, add **zhi mu** (Rhizoma Anemarrhenae Asphodeloides) 知母 90g and **huang bai** (Cortex Phellodendri) 黄柏 90g. (Source: *Zhong Yi Er Bi Hou Ke Xue*)

Topical treatment

- Rinse the mouth with a decoction brewed from **han lian cao** (Herba Ecliptae Prostratae) 旱连草 60-120g.

Patent medicines

Liu Wei Di Huang Wan 六味地黄丸 (Liu Wei Di Huang Wan, Six Flavour Tea) - Kidney *yin* deficiency

Gu Ben Wan 固本丸 (Gu Ben Wan, Ren Shen Ku Pen Wan) - Stomach *qi* and *yin* deficiency

Zhi Bai Ba Wei Wan 知柏八味丸 (Zhi Bai Ba Wei Wan, Chih Pai Pa Wei Wan) - with deficient Heat

Tian Wang Bu Xin Dan 天王补心丹 (Emperors Tea, Tien Wang Pu Hsin Tan) - with ulceration, Heart and Kidney *yin* deficiency

Xi Gua Shuang 西瓜霜 (Watermelon Frost) - topical to relieve pain and swelling

Acupuncture (select from)

Ren.12 (*zhong wan*) .... *mu* point of the Stomach, nourishes Stomach *yin*, regulates the Stomach and clears Heat

Ren.4 (*guan yuan* +) .... meeting point of the *yin* channels, nourishes and supplements the *yin* of whole body, with Sp.6

St.36 (*zu san li* +) .... *he* sea point of the Stomach, powerfully strengthens the Spleen and Stomach and supplements *qi* and *yin*

Sp.6 (*san yin jiao* +) .... with Ren.4, nourishes *yin* of the whole body

Kid.6 (*zhao hai* +) .... together these points open *yin qiao mai* and *ren*
Lu.7 (*lie que* +) *mai*, supplement *yin* and benefit the mouth and throat

LI.4 (*he gu*) .... special point for all oral disorders

Kid.3 (*tai xi* +) ....*yuan* point to nourish Kidney *yin*

Bl.21 (*wei shu*) .... these points supplement Stomach and Spleen
Bl.20 (*pi shu* +) *yin*

- several points around the mouth can be added to reinforce the local circulation of *qi* and *yin* to the mouth–St.4 (*di cang*), Ren.24 (*cheng jiang*), Du.26 (*ren zhong* -), *ah shi* points
- *Ear points*: stomach, kidney, mouth, upper jaw, lower jaw, *shen men*

Clinical notes

- Stomach *yin* deficiency gingivitis and periodontitis is a chronic problem and will take a while to achieve satisfactory results. Treatment will need to be continuous so as to rebuild *yin*. In long standing cases, 6-9 months of treatment may be necessary for long term results.
- For dietary recommendations, see p.876.

气血不足

10.3 QI AND BLOOD DEFICIENCY

Pathophysiology

- *Qi* and Blood deficiency patterns of gum disease are associated with a lack of nutrition to the gum tissues and consequent loss of integrity of the tissues.

Clinical features

- atrophy of the gums revealing the roots of the teeth; the gums are pale and the teeth loose; the gums bleed easily with brushing and chewing
- there may be other sites of bleeding, for example easy bruising, epistaxis, heavy menstrual period or uterine bleeding
- waxy, pale complexion, pale lips and conjunctivae
- postural dizziness, blurring vision
- loss of appetite
- abdominal distension
- loose stools
- fatigue, weakness, shortness of breath, low voice
- insomnia, frequent vivid dreaming, restless sleep
- palpitations

T pale with thin white coat
P thready and weak, or hollow if there has been significant blood loss

Treatment principle

Supplement *qi* and Blood
Aid discharge of pus, promote healing

Prescription

BA ZHEN TANG 八珍汤
(*Ginseng and Dang Gui Eight Combination*)

shu di (Radix Rehmanniae Glutinosae Conquitae) 熟地 12-18g
dang shen (Radix Codonopsis Pilosulae) 党参 15-24g
dang gui (Radix Angelicae Sinensis) 当归 9-15g
bai shao (Radix Paeoniae Lactiflorae) 白芍 12-18g
chao bai zhu (dry fried Rhizoma Atractylodes Macrocephalae) 炒白术 12-15g
fu ling (Sclerotium Poriae Cocos) 茯苓 12-15g
chuan xiong (Radix Ligustici Chuanxiong) 川芎 6-9g
zhi gan cao (honey fried Radix Glycyrrhizae Uralensis) 炙甘草 3-6g

Method: Decoction. **Shu di, dang gui** and **bai shao** nourish Blood and *yin*; **chuan xiong** regulates *qi* and Blood; **dang shen, chao bai zhu, fu ling** and **zhi gan cao** strengthen the Spleen and supplement *qi*. (Source: *Zhong Yi Er Bi Hou Ke Xue*)

Modifications

- With bleeding, add **e jiao** (Gelatinum Corii Asini) 阿胶 9-12g (melted in the hot strained decoction), **xue yu tan** (Crinis Carbonisatus Hominis) 血余炭 6-9g and **ou jie** (Nodus Nelumbinis Nuciferae Rhizomatis) 藕节 9-12g.
- With signs of *yang* deficiency, cold and prominent Spleen deficiency, (loose stools, poor appetite, cold intolerance) add **zhi huang qi** (honey fried Radix Astragali Membranacei) 炙黄芪 18-30g and **rou gui** (Cortex Cinnamomi Cassiae) 肉桂 3-6g.

Variations and additional prescriptions

Heart Blood and Spleen qi deficiency

- With Heart Blood and Spleen *qi* deficiency (insomnia, palpitations, anxiety) the treatment aims to supplement *qi* and Blood, strengthen the Spleen and calm the *shen* with **GUI PI TANG** (*Ginseng and Longan Combination* 归脾汤) modified.

zhi huang qi (honey fried Radix Astragali Membranacei)
炙黄芪 18-30g
dang shen (Radix Codonopsis Pilosulae) 党参 15-24g
fu ling (Sclerotium Poriae Cocos) 茯苓 12-15g
suan zao ren (Semen Zizyphi Spinosae) 酸枣仁 12-15g
long yan rou (Arillus Euphoriae Longanae) 龙眼肉 12-15g
yuan zhi (Radix Polygalae Tenuifoliae) 远志 6-9g
mu xiang (Radix Aucklandiae Lappae) 木香 6-9g
gan cao (Radix Glycyrrhizae Uralensis) 甘草 6-9g
ce bai ye (Cacumen Biotae Orientalis) 侧柏叶 12-15g
e jiao (Gelatinum Corii Asini) 阿胶 9-12g

Method: Decoction. **E jiao** is melted before being added to the strained decoction (*yang hua* 烊化). **Huang qi**, **dang shen**, **fu ling** and **gan cao** strengthen the Spleen and supplement *qi*; **suan zao ren**, **long yan rou** and **e jiao** nourish Blood; **suan zao ren**, **long yan rou**, **fu ling** and **yuan zhi** calm the *shen*; **mu xiang** regulates *qi*; **ce bai ye** and **e jiao** stop bleeding. (Source: *Zhong Yi Er Bi Hou Ke Xue*)

Spleen and Kidney yang deficiency

- If Spleen and Kidney *yang* are deficient (loose teeth with pale, puffy gums, pale swollen tongue, cold intolerance and extremities, and nocturia), the aim of treatment is to warm and supplement Spleen and Kidney *yang* with a guiding prescription such as **YOU GUI WAN** (*Eucommia and Rehmannia Formula* 右归丸, p.333), or **JIN KUI SHEN QI WAN** (*Rehmannia Eight Formula* 金匮肾气丸, p.724), plus the addition of herbs such as **zhi huang qi** (honey fried Radix Astragali Membranacei) 炙黄芪 and **dang shen** (Radix Codonopsis Pilosulae) 党参 to supplement *qi*.

Patent medicines

Ba Zhen Wan 八珍丸 (Ba Zhen Wan, Women's Precious Pills)
Shi Quan Da Bu Wan 十全大补丸 (Shi Quan Da Bu Wan, Ten Flavour Tea) - *qi* and Blood deficiency with Cold
Gui Pi Wan 归脾丸 (Gui Pi Wan, Angelicae Longana Tea, Kwei Be Wan)
Jin Kui Shen Qi Wan 金匮肾气丸 (Fu Gui Ba Wei Wan, Sexoton Pills, Golden Book Tea) - Kidney *yang* deficiency

Acupuncture (select from)

Ren.12 (*zhong wan* +▲) .. *mu* point of the Stomach, strengthens the Stomach and Spleen and supplements *qi* and Blood
Ren.4 (*guan yuan* +▲) ..... warms the Kidneys and *yuan qi* to promote transformation of *qi*
LI.4 (*he gu*) .... special point for all oral disorders
LI.11 (*qu chi* +▲) .... *he* sea point of the Large Intestine, warms *yang ming* and stimulates *yang qi* in general when moxaed
St.36 (*zu san li* +▲) .... *he* sea point of the Stomach, powerfully warms and strengthens the Spleen and Stomach and supplements *qi* and Blood
Sp.6 (*san yin jiao* +▲) ...... strengthens the Spleen and Kidney and invigorates and supplements *qi* and Blood
Bl.20 (*pi shu* +▲) .... *shu* points of the Spleen and Stomach, warm,
Bl.21 (*wei shu* +▲) supplement and regulate middle *jiao qi*

- with Kidney *yang* deficiency, add Bl.23 (*shen shu* +▲), Du.4 (*ming men* +▲) and Kid.3 (*tai xi* +)
- with frequent bleeding add Sp.1 (*yin bai* ▲)
- several points around the mouth can be added to reinforce the local circulation of *qi* and Blood to the mouth–St.4 (*di cang*), Ren.24 (*cheng jiang*), Du.26 (*ren zhong* -)
- *Ear points*: stomach, spleen, mouth, upper jaw, lower jaw, *shen men*

Clinical notes

- *Qi* and Blood deficiency patterns tend to produce the more chronic and difficult periodontitis, where the inflammatory elements are muted and the atrophic aspects are prominent. This pattern takes a long time and persistent treatment to improve, although further deterioration may be prevented. Massaging the gums with an electric toothbrush is useful.
- For dietary recommendations, see pp.870-874.

血瘀牙宣

10.4 BLOOD STAGNATION

Pathophysiology

- Blood stagnation is a chronic pattern of gum disease, and one that usually follows years of some other pathology, frequently Liver *qi* stagnation or Stomach *yin* deficiency.

Clinical features

- Chronic gum disease with discoloured, purplish, patchy or dark red atrophic gums; loose teeth, painful receding gums, frequently bleeding gums.
- persistent insomnia with much dreaming and restlessness; low grade fever at night
- irritability, short temper, depression, mood swings
- dizziness and forgetfulness
- dry, scaly skin, hair loss on the head and body
- broken vessels or spider naevi on the face, trunk, inner knee and ankle
- purplish lips, sclera, conjunctivae and nails
- dark rings around the eyes

T dark or red purple, or with brown or purple stasis spots; sublingual veins are distended and dark

P deep and choppy or wiry

Treatment principle

Invigorate Blood, eliminate stagnant Blood
Regulate *qi*, promote healing

Prescription

XUE FU ZHU YU TANG 血府逐瘀汤
(*Achyranthes and Persica Combination*) modified

dang gui (Radix Angelicae Sinensis) 当归 9-12g
sheng di (Radix Rehmanniae Glutinosae) 生地 12-15g
chi shao (Radix Paeoniae Rubrae) 赤芍 9-12g
chuan xiong (Radix Ligustici Chuanxiong) 川芎 6-9g
hong hua (Flos Carthami Tinctorii) 红花 9-12g
tao ren (Semen Persicae) 桃仁 9-12g
chuan niu xi (Radix Cyathulae Officinalis) 川牛膝 9-15g
zhi ke (Fructus Citri Aurantii) 枳壳 9-12g
jie geng (Radix Platycodi Grandiflori) 桔梗 6-9g
chai hu (Radix Bupleuri) 柴胡 9-12g
gan cao (Radix Glycyrrhizae Uralensis) 甘草 3-6g
gou ji (Rhizoma Cibotii Barometz) 狗脊 12-15g
gu sui bu (Rhizoma Drynariae) 骨碎补 12-18g

Method: Decoction. **Tao ren, hong hua, dan shen, chi shao, chuan xiong, yu jin** and **chuan niu xi** invigorate Blood and eliminate stagnant Blood; **sheng di, dang gui, chi shao** and **chuan xiong** form a modified **SI WU TANG**, the fundamental prescription to nourish and regulate Blood; **chai hu, zhi ke, chi shao** and **gan cao** form a modified **SI NI SAN**, the fundamental prescription to regulate *qi*; **jie geng** and **niu xi** combine rising and descending action to stimulate the flow of *qi* and Blood, and correct the *qi* mechanism; **gou ji** and **gu sui bu** strengthen the Liver, Kidney, teeth and bones. (Source: *Shi Yong Fang Ji Xue*)

Modifications

- With persistent bleeding, add **qian cao gen** (Radix Rubiae Cordifoliae) 茜草根 12-15g.
- To promote healing, add **ru xiang** (Gummi Olibanum) 乳香 6-9g and **mo yao** (Myrrha) 没药 6-9g.
- With pain, add **yan hu suo** (Rhizoma Corydalis Yanhusuo) 延胡索 9-12g, **mo yao** (Myrrha) 没药 6-9g, **ru xiang** (Gummi Olibanum) 乳香 6-9g.
- With Heat in the Liver, add **yu jin** (Tuber Curcumae) 郁金 9-12g.
- With *yang* deficiency or Cold, delete **chai hu** and **jie geng**, and add **zhi fu zi** (Radix Aconiti Carmichaeli Praeparata) 制附子 6-12g (decocted for 30 minutes before the other herbs), **rou gui** (Cortex Cinnamomi Cassiae) 肉桂 3g, **xian ling pi** (Herba Epimedii) 仙灵脾 12-18g and **ba ji tian** (Radix Morindae Officinalis) 巴戟天 9-12g.
- With *yin* deficiency, delete **chai hu, jie geng, chuan xiong** and **zhi ke**, and add **mai dong** (Tuber Ophiopogonis Japonici) 麦冬 9-12g, **yu zhu** (Rhizoma Polygonati Odorati) 玉竹 12-15g, **nu zhen zi** (Fructus Ligustri Lucidi) 女贞子 9-12g and **han lian cao** (Herba Ecliptae Prostratae) 旱连草 9-12g.
- With Blood deficiency, add **shu di** (Radix Rehmanniae Glutinosae Conquitae) 熟地 12-18g, **gou qi zi** (Fructus Lycii) 枸杞子 9-12g and **he shou wu** (Radix Polygoni Multiflori) 何首乌 9-12g.

Patent medicines

Xue Fu Zhu Yu Wan 血府逐瘀丸 (Xue Fu Zhu Yu Wan)
Tong Jing Wan 痛经丸 (Tong Jing Wan)
- the above two formulae can be combined in severe cases

Jian Kang Wan 健康丸 (Sunho Multi Ginseng Tablets)
Sheng Tian Qi Pian 生田七片 (Raw Tian Qi Ginseng Tablets)
Yun Nan Bai Yao 云南白药 (Yunnan Paiyao)
- this famous patent medicine can be used to move Blood and stop bleeding

Topical treatment

ZHI TENG JIU (*Stop Pain Alcohol Extract* 止疼酒).

chuan wu (Radix Aconiti Carmichaeli) 川乌 3g
cao wu (Radix Aconiti Kusnezoffii) 草乌 3g
gao liang jiang (Rhizoma Alpiniae Officinari) 高良姜 3g
xi xin (Herba cum Radice Asari) 细辛 3g
bai zhi (Radix Angelicae Dahuricae) 白芷 3g
neutral spirit (e.g. vodka) 60g

Method: Combine the herbs and warmed alcohol in a container for a few minutes, tip the alcohol off the herbs and use it to rinse the gums and mouth, then spit it out. **Not to be ingested**. Repeat until all the alcohol is used up. Repeat the next day. **Chuan wu** and **cao wu** are excellent for alleviating pain, including neurological pain, however they are very toxic, and may be substituted with **zhi fu zi** (Radix Aconiti Carmichaeli Praeparata) 制附子 6g. (Source: *Zui Xin Fang Ji Shou Ce*)

Acupuncture (select from)

ah shi points .... move *qi* and Blood locally
Bl.17 (*ge shu* -) .... *hui* point for Blood, transforms stagnant Blood
LI.4 (*he gu* -) .... special point for oral diseases
Sp.10 (*xue hai* -) .... regulates and invigorates Blood
Sp.6 (*san yin jiao*) .... strengthens the Spleen, regulates Liver *qi* and invigorates *qi* and Blood
St.36 (*zu san li* -) .... *he* sea point of the Stomach, powerfully invigorates movement of *qi* and Blood and regulates the Stomach
Bl.18 (*gan shu* -) .... *shu* point of the Liver, invigorates Liver *qi* and Blood
Bl.21 (*wei shu* -) .... *shu* point of the Stomach, eliminates stagnant Blood from the Stomach

- with depression, combine LI.4 (*he gu*) and Liv.3 (*tai chong*)
- *Ear points*: liver, mouth, sympathetic, *shen men*, stomach

Clinical notes

- Blood stagnation produces a chronic and difficult condition, where the inflammatory elements and the atrophic aspects are both prominent. Gingivitis or periodontitis of a Blood stagnation type may be diagnosed biomedically as haemochromatosis, Addison's disease, Peutz-Jegher's syndrome, polycythaemia or heavy metal accumulation (bismuth, mercury, lead).
- This pattern takes a long time and persistent treatment to improve, although further deterioration may be prevented. Massaging the gums with an electric toothbrush is useful.
- For dietary recommendations, see p.878, 886.

SUMMARY OF GUIDING FORMULAE FOR GINGIVITIS/ PERIODONTITIS

Stomach Heat/Fire - *Qing Wei Tang* 清胃汤
- with Liver Fire - *Long Dan Xie Gan Tang* 龙胆泻肝汤
- with Toxic Heat - *Huang Lian Jie Du Tang* 黄连解毒汤

Stomach *yin* deficiency with Heat - *Yu Nu Jian* 玉女煎
- with Kidney *yin* deficiency - *Liu Wei Di Huang Wan* 六味地黄丸

Qi and Blood deficiency - *Ba Zhen Tang* 八珍汤
- with Heart and Spleen *qi* deficiency - *Gui Pi Tang* 归脾汤
- with Spleen and Kidney *yang* deficiency - *You Gui Wan* 右归丸 or *Jin Kui Shen Qi Wan* 金匮肾气丸

Blood stagnation - *Xue Fu Zhu Yu Tang* 血府逐瘀汤

11. Haemafecia

Excess patterns

Stomach Heat/Fire

Liver *qi* invading the Stomach, with Heat

Intestinal Wind

Damp Heat in the Large Intestine

Blood stagnation

Deficient patterns

Spleen *qi* deficiency

Spleen and Stomach *yang* deficiency

Stomach *yin* deficiency with Heat

11 HAEMAFECIA

bian xue 便血

Haemafecia (*bian xue*[1]), is a broad term referring to blood, or the digested metabolites of blood, that appears in the stools. The location of the bleeding may be any part of the upper or lower digestive tract. Haemafecia can be subdivided into **melaena** and **haematochezia**. Melaena generally refers to bleeding originating high in the digestive tract, usually from the stomach or duodenum, although the small intestine or ascending colon may be implicated. The stools appear black, tarry and sticky due to the pigments in the digested blood. At least 100-200 millilitres of blood from the upper digestive tract is required before the stools change their appearance.

Haematochezia is the appearance of blood mixed in with, or associated with, the passage of stool. If the source of the bleeding is the distal large intestine or rectum, the blood will usually be fresh red blood. The higher up the digestive tract the source of the bleeding, the darker the blood appears.

Depending on the location of the source of the bleeding, bleeding may or may not be obvious. Blood, or the metabolites of blood digestion, which is not immediately apparent in the stool, may be detected by chemical testing of a stool specimen. This is termed **occult bleeding**. Up to 200ml of blood per day can be lost into the upper gastro-intestinal tract, but may not be visible. When chronic, this occult bleeding can be a cause of severe anaemia and debility.

In the view of Chinese medicine, melaena, haematochezia and chronic occult bleeding are essentially undifferentiated, except in terms of severity and prognosis.

Blood in the stools is an early sign of carcinoma of the colon, and in patients over 40, a high degree of suspicion is warranted. As many as 30% of people with acute gastro-intestinal bleeding are reported to have consumed aspirin or other nonsteroidal anti-inflammatory drugs (NSAIDS), within the previous 24-48 hours.

Significant bleeding from the digestive tract should be considered a medical emergency until proven otherwise, and patients should be assessed by the appropriate medical personnel to exclude conditions not suited to TCM treatment.

AETIOLOGY

External pathogens

The main external pathogens which cause haemafecia are Heat and Cold

[1] Wiseman's 'bloody stool'

that transforms into Heat and Damp Heat. The external Heat lodges in the *yang ming* level (*see* Vol.1), the Stomach and Large Intestine, forcing the reckless movement of Blood, causing it to spill from the vessels.

Damp Heat can be a product of the season, most commonly occurring during hot or humid weather, and more frequent in tropical climates. Damp Heat pathogens can also enter the body with spoiled food.

BOX 11.1 BIOMEDICAL CAUSES OF HAEMAFECIA

Upper gastro-intestinal
- gastric and duodenal ulcers
- gastric and duodenal erosion
- leaking oesophageal varices
- erosive oesophagitis
- vascular malformation
- angioma
- malignancy

Lower gastro-intestinal
- diverticular disease
- ischaemic colitis
- inflammatory bowel disease
  - Crohn's disease
  - ulcerative colitis
- radiation and ischaemic colitis
- angiodysplasia
- colonic carcinoma
- polyps
- haemorrhoids
- anal fissure
- hookworm

Systemic
- leukaemia
- thrombocytopaenia
- polycythaemia
- uraemia
- vasculitis

Medications
- NSAIDs, aspirin
- anticoagulants (warfarin, coumarin)

Caution
- ingested blood from the nose, sinus or oral cavity
- black stools from excess iron ingestion and antacids containing bismuth
- red or dark stools from certain foods, e.g. beetroot and red wine

Diet

Various dietary factors can contribute to haemafecia. Eating spoiled or contaminated food produces acute diarrhoea with bleeding, which in TCM terms may resemble an attack of Damp Heat (*see also* Dysenteric disorder, p.270).

Too much cold natured or raw food weakens Spleen *qi* and *yang*, and disturbs the Spleen's function of holding Blood in the vessels.

Overconsumption in general and excessive consumption of rich, heating or supplementing foods in particular, can lead to the accumulation of food and Damp Heat in the Intestines. Eating large quantities of foods that heat the Stomach and Liver, specifically substances like chilli and spices, alcohol, coffee, chocolate and rich or oily foods, can cause Heat and Damp Heat to accumulate in the Stomach and Intestines.

Eating at odd hours, late at night, while rushing, or in times of stress can disorder the function of the Stomach, contributing to food stagnation (*see*

Table 11.1 *Common haemostatic herbs for gastro-intestinal bleeding*

Bai Ji 白芨 (Rhizoma Bletillae Striatae)	Bai Ji is good for upper gastro-intestinal bleeding and is widely used as a powder for bleeding peptic or duodenal ulcers. It is quite sticky and astringent, and puts a lining over any erosion in the wall of the Stomach and Intestines. Bai Ji is sweet, bitter, astringent and cool, and can be combined with either supplementing or Heat clearing formulae, but is best for chronic patterns. Bai Ji can be used alone for gastric bleeding or gastric ulcers, taken as a powder mixed with a little water or rice porridge. When gastric hyperacidity is a problem, it is combined with cuttlefish bone (Hai Piao Xiao 海螵蛸).
Huai Hua 槐花 (Flos Sophorae Japonicae Immaturus)	Huai Hua is good for Damp Heat patterns of the Large Intestine, especially inflamed and bleeding haemorrhoids and bloody dysenteric disorder. Also used for Liver Heat patterns with red eyes and dizziness.
Di Yu 地榆 (Radix Sanguisorbae Officinalis)	Di Yu is particularly good for Damp Heat patterns causing bleeding from the Large Intestine, including conditions such as Damp Heat diarrhoea with bleeding, bloody dysenteric disorder and bleeding haemorrhoids. Also used for bleeding gastroduodenal ulcers, often with Bai Ji. Di Yu promotes healing of damaged tissues.
Ou Jie 藕节 (Nodus Nelumbinis Nuciferae Rhizomatis)	Ou Jie is a good general astringent herb for bleeding from the Lungs, Stomach and Intestines. Can be used for a variety of patterns depending on the other herbs with which it is combined.
Juan Bai 卷白 (Herba Selaginellae)	Charred Juan Bai is good for rectal bleeding associated with rectal prolapse or haemorrhoids. It is also used for chronic 'Intestinal Wind'. In the raw form it is used to move Blood stasis and treat urinary calculi.
San Qi 三七 (Radix Notoginseng)	An excellent herb for bleeding of all types, but especially good for those associated with Blood stagnation. San Qi has the unique property of being able to stop bleeding without causing Blood stagnation – a common side effect of cold and astringent haemostatic herbs.
Ce Bai Ye 侧柏叶 (Cacumen Biotae Orientalis) Xian He Cao 仙鹤草 (Herba Agrimoniae Pilosae)	Ce Bai Ye and Xian He Cao are all purpose haemostatic herbs, which can be used together or separately for excess, deficient, hot or cold bleeding patterns, depending on the herbs with which they are combined. Used for upper and lower gastro-intestinal haemorrhage. Ce Bai Ye is the cooler of the two, and is preferred in hot patterns.

BOX 11.2 KEY DIAGNOSTIC POINTS

Colour of the blood and location of bleeding

- In general the darker the blood the higher in the gut the source of the bleeding, although be aware that massive bleeding from the upper gastro-intestinal tract that passes rapidly through the gut may appear red.
- bright red blood - anus or rectum
- dark or purplish blood - large and small intestine
- black or tarry blood - stomach or duodenum

Timing and location of the bleeding

- Blood passed before a bowel movement - anus and rectum
- Blood passed after a bowel movement - middle and upper GIT
- Blood on the surface of a formed stool - rectal or anal, haemorrhoids, polyps, fissure

p.3), and the eventual weakening of the Spleen and Stomach.

Emotion

This primarily refers to stress, repressed emotions, in particular frustration, anger and resentment that cause stagnation of Liver *qi*. Even at a mild level, relatively uncomplicated Liver *qi* stagnation can contribute to haemafecia by repeatedly invading the Stomach, disrupting the integrity of the Stomach wall. It is the complications of prolonged *qi* stagnation, however, that more commonly cause bleeding. Repeated invasion by the Liver will damage the Spleen, deplete *qi*, and disrupt the Spleen's ability to hold Blood in the vessels. The weakened Spleen will likely generate Dampness, which may then combine with any Heat in the system, causing Damp Heat.

The prolonged pressure in the system can create Heat, which, depending on duration and the intensity of the aetiological conditions, can develop into stagnant Heat, or the more severe Fire. The Heat can cause Blood to move recklessly, contributing to relatively severe bleeding and/or *yin* damage. Long term *qi* stagnation can also lead to Blood stagnation.

In addition to the emotional factors that upset the Liver, worry, obsessive thinking and prolonged concentration in combination with a sedentary lifestyle and poor diet, will weaken Spleen *qi*, predisposing it to, or inviting, invasion by Liver *qi*, resulting in further damage.

Spleen and Stomach deficiency

The Spleen is responsible for maintaining the integrity of the Blood vessels, that is, Spleen *qi* prevents Blood from leaking out of the vessels. Bleeding of a Spleen *qi* deficiency type tends to be mild, chronic and persistent. *Yang* deficiency haemafecia is usually a chronic condition, although it can be more acute, following gastro-intestinal surgery or sudden excessive ingestion of cold substances and medications.

Overwork, excessive worry or mental activity, irregular dietary habits or prolonged illness progressively weaken Spleen *qi*. The most common causes of Spleen *yang* deficiency are deterioration of Spleen *qi* deficiency, prolonged or excessive consumption of cold raw food and irregular eating habits, or too many cold natured herbs, antibiotics or NSAIDs in the treatment of a febrile disease. Prolonged insult to the Stomach or severely limited food intake, as occurs in famine victims or patients with bulimia and anorexia nervosa, seriously damages the Spleen and Stomach *yang qi*. The damage is aggravated when an irregular diet is combined with sustained mental activity and too much sitting. The Spleen and Stomach can also be weakened following an acute invasion of Cold and/or Dampness. Gastric surgery can also deplete Spleen *yang*, and cause Blood stagnation.

Stomach *yin* deficiency usually follows years of invasion by Liver *qi* or damage from chronic Liver Heat. Stomach *yin* deficiency can also follow an acute febrile disease, such as *yang ming* syndrome. *Yin* damage associated with long term consumption of drugs such as *yang* supplementing substances and amphetamines is becoming more common. Prolonged or excessive vomiting, dehydration, or another chronic Stomach pathology, especially one characterised by Heat, may also be implicated.

Blood stagnation

Blood stagnation is an important cause of haemafecia, especially in older patients. The initial stagnation that eventually gives rise to Blood stagnation may be the result of chronic Liver *qi* stagnation, or chronic food stagnation which, over time, creates Heat and Dampness or Phlegm. By its very nature, *qi* stagnation will ultimately involve Blood stagnation (*qi* leads the Blood). The Heat or Damp Heat produced by chronic food stagnation injures the Intestine by drying and scorching the Intestinal lining and its delicate *luo mai*. Phlegm, being a substantial pathogen and particularly cloying in nature, physically obstructs the circulation of *qi* and Blood at some point. Blood stagnation reflects a physical lesion of the intestine. The common sites of Blood stagnation are the Stomach and distal Large Intestine, however, it can occur anywhere.

Medications

Numerous therapeutic agents, herbal and pharmaceutical, can cause haemafecia. The most common are those that are heating, such as corticosteroids and alcohol, or dispersing, such as nonsteroidal anti-inflammatory drugs (NSAIDS). NSAIDs physically damage the lining of the Stomach. Some *yang* supplementing, or heating herbs, can cause bleeding in sensitive individuals if used inappropriately. Anticoagulants such as coumarin may also be implicated. Medications are so commonly implicated in both acute and chronic bleeding in the digestive tract that a thorough examination of all current and recent medications, supplements and herbs is essential.

Trauma

A trauma to the abdomen and Intestines, either from a previous intestinal illness, surgery, or a penetrating or blunt injury can cause localised Blood stagnation in the form of bruising and bleeding. Once Blood stagnation is present, it will further impede *qi* and Blood circulation, potentially generating the necessary Heat for acute or serious bleeding. Insertion of foreign objects in the rectum may damage the rectal and intestinal mucosa and cause bleeding.

TCM DIFFERENTIAL DIAGNOSIS

- **Dysenteric disorder** (*li ji* 痢疾): a group of patterns characterised by diarrhoea or loose stools with pus and or mucus and/or blood. This type of presentation, while common in true dysentery associated with bacterial or amoebic infection, also occurs in chronic systemic disorders such as ulcerative colitis and Crohn's disease. Haemafecia may occur in the absence of diarrhoea and without mucus or pus in the stools.
- **Haemorrhoids** (*zhi chuang* 痔疮): Haemorrhoids are often associated with bleeding from the rectum. The blood is usually fresh red and in mild cases may be noted on the toilet paper after wiping. There will often be symptoms in the rectal area, such as discomfort or pain, heaviness or protrusion. Haemorrhoids are analysed separately in Chapter 13.

TREATMENT

There are several steps to consider when treating any bleeding disorder. The first step is to stop the bleeding. When the bleeding is severe, the initial focus of treatment is to use first aid or herbs to quickly staunch the bleeding. This can usually be achieved with a styptic formulae (Box 12.2, p.452), or with the use of the patent medicine *Yun Nan Bai Yao* 云南白药 (Yunnan Paiyao).

Once bleeding has ceased, or is under control, the underlying pattern can be dealt with more fully. There are two additional aspects to consider. Any residual Blood outside the vessels is stagnant Blood, which must be removed. Thus, herbs to gently invigorate or regulate Blood are incorporated into the appropriate formula. This is especially important in Heat types of bleeding, as the herbs used to stop bleeding will likely be cold natured and astringent. These herbs congeal Blood. Finally, any *qi* or Blood deficiency that exists as a direct result of Blood loss should be supplemented.

胃中积热

11.1 STOMACH HEAT/FIRE

Pathophysiology

- Stomach Heat can be due to invasion by external pathogens (a kind of *yang ming* syndrome), but more commonly in the case of gastro-intestinal bleeding, the Heat comes from a rich, heating diet, heating medications or drugs. Stagnant Heat from Liver *qi* stagnation may also contribute.
- Once Heat is present in the Stomach and/or Intestines, it can cause bleeding in two ways: First, when Heat is applied to Blood it causes Blood to accelerate and 'move recklessly', and thus spill from the vessels. Second, the Heat can scorch and rupture the delicate *luo mai* of the digestive tract, allowing Blood to escape. The location of the Heat is in the upper gastro-intestinal tract, hence the dark blood or tarry stools.

Clinical features

- dark, purple blood in the stools or tarry, sticky, black stools
- epigastric and abdominal distension, with pain or a burning sensation
- bitter taste in the mouth, acid reflux, heartburn
- dry mouth, thirst with a desire for cold drinks
- halitosis, belching
- tendency to constipation, or dry stools; rarely, diarrhoea
- irritability, restlessness

T red and dry with a thick, dry, yellow coat
P wiry and rapid or slippery and rapid

Treatment principle

Clear Heat and Fire from the Stomach
Cool the Blood and stop bleeding

Prescription

XIE XIN TANG 泻心汤
(*Coptis and Rhubarb Combination*) plus
SHI HUI SAN 十灰散
(*Ten Partially Charred Substance Powder*)

---

da huang (Radix et Rhizoma Rhei) 大黄 6-9g
huang qin (Radix Scutellariae Baicalensis) 黄芩 12-15g
huang lian (Rhizoma Coptidis) 黄连 6-9g
shan zhi zi (Fructus Gardeniae Jasminoidis) 山栀子 9-12g
da ji (Herba seu Radix Cirsii Japonicii) 大蓟 15-30g
xiao ji (Herba Cephalanoplos) 小蓟 15-30g
ce bai ye (Cacumen Biotae Orientalis) 侧柏叶 15-30g
bai ji (Rhizoma Bletillae Striatae) 白芨 15-30g

bai mao gen (Rhizoma Imperatae Cylindricae) 白茅根 15-30g
qian cao gen (Radix Rubiae Cordifoliae) 茜草根 12-15g
mu dan pi (Cortex Moutan Radicis) 牡丹皮 9-12g

Method: Decoction or powder. The styptic ingredients of this formula were traditionally prepared as a powder after being partially burnt, a process thought to improve their haemostatic action. When used in powder form, the powdered herbs should be briefly decocted before ingestion. The uncharred herbs seem to work as well in decoction. **Da Huang**, **huang lian**, **huang qin** and **shan zhi zi** clear Heat and purge Fire; **da ji**, **xiao ji**, **ce bai ye** and **bai mao gen** cool the Blood and stop bleeding; **bai ji** astringes to stop bleeding; **qian cao gen** and **mu dan pi** cool the Blood to stop bleeding, and regulate the Blood to prevent the stagnation that sometimes occurs when using large doses of styptic herbs. (Source: *Zhong Yi Nei Ke Ji Zheng Zheng Zhi*)

Modifications

- When Heat is intense or prolonged, it can 'cook and congeal' Blood, causing Blood stagnation. Blood stagnation is indicated when there are clots of dark blood in the stools, or when abdominal pain is relatively severe. With Blood stagnation, add **san qi fen** (powdered Radix Notoginseng) 三七粉 3-6g to invigorate Blood and stop bleeding.
- With epigastric pain, add **yan hu suo** (Rhizoma Corydalis Yanhusuo) 延胡索 9-12g and **mu xiang** (Radix Aucklandiae Lappae) 木香 9g. With persistent focal gnawing pain and bleeding (suggestive of gastric ulceration), powder equal amounts of **hai piao xiao** (Os Sepiae seu Sepiellae) 海螵蛸, **bai ji** (Rhizoma Bletillae Striatae) 白芨 and **gan cao** (Radix Glycyrrhizae Uralensis) 甘草 and take 3 grams three times daily.
- With nausea, add **zhu ru** (Caulis Bambusae in Taeniis) 竹茹 9-12g, **xuan fu hua** (Flos Inulae) 旋复花 12-15g and **dai zhe shi** (Haematitum) 代赭石 15g.
- With severe thirst, add **shi hu** (Herba Dendrobii) 石斛 12-15g and **tian hua fen** (Radix Trichosanthes Kirilowii) 天花粉 12-15g.
- With constipation or dry stools, add **xuan shen** (Radix Scrophulariae Ningpoensis) 玄参 18-24g, **mai dong** (Tuber Ophiopogonis Japonici) 麦冬 9-12g and **sheng di** (Radix Rehmanniae Glutinosae) 生地 12-18g.

Variations and additional prescriptions

With yin deficiency

- In chronic cases of Stomach Heat, or in the aftermath of a febrile disease, Stomach and Intestinal *yin* and fluids may be damaged. The clinical features are recurrent haemafecia with bright or dark blood, persistent low grade or afternoon fever, irritability, restlessness, dry mouth and throat, ulceration in the mouth, occasional abdominal pain, a thready, rapid pulse and a red, dry tongue with a centrally peeled coat, or no coat. The aim of treatment is to nourish and supplement *yin*, clear

Heat and stop bleeding with **HUANG LIAN E JIAO TANG** (*Coptis and Ass-Hide Gelatin Decoction* 黄连阿胶汤) modified.

huang lian (Rhizoma Coptidis) 黄连 3-6g
huang qin (Radix Scutellariae Baicalensis) 黄芩 9-12g
e jiao (Gelatinum Corii Asini) 阿胶 9-12g
bai shao (Radix Paeoniae Lactiflora) 白芍 12-18g
ji zi huang (egg yolk) 鸡子黄 .... 2 yolks
bai mao gen (Rhizoma Imperatae Cylindricae) 白茅根 15-30g
han lian cao (Herba Ecliptae Prostratae) 旱莲草 12-15g
ou jie (Nodus Nelumbinis Nuciferae Rhizomatis) 藕节 9-12g

Method: Decoction. **E jiao** is melted in the hot strained decoction (*yang hua* 烊化). The egg yolks are stirred into the strained and slightly cooled decoction. **Huang qin** and **huang lian** clear Heat and purge Fire; **bai shao** cools the Liver and astringes *yin*; **e jiao** nourishes Blood and stops bleeding; **ji zi huang** nourishes *yin*; **bai mao gen** and **han lian cao** cool the Blood and stop bleeding; **ou jie** astringes the Intestines and stops bleeding. (Source: *Shi Yong Zhong Yi Nei Ke Xue*)

Severe bleeding precipitating collapse of yang

- If the bleeding is severe, blood loss can lead to sudden collapse of *yang* (a type of *jue zheng* 厥证, Flaccid Collapse Syndrome, hypovolaemic shock). In addition to the appropriate first aid (keeping the patient warm, leg elevation, airway clear etc.), **SHEN FU TANG** (*Ginseng and Prepared Aconite Decoction* 参附汤, p.458) may be administered.

Patent medicines

Huang Lian Jie Du Wan 黄连解毒丸 (Huang Lian Jie Du Wan)
- Damp Heat

Niu Huang Qing Huo Wan 牛黄清火丸 (Niu Huang Qing Huo Wan)
- with constipation

Bei Jing Niu Huang Jie Du Pian 北京牛黄解毒片 (Peking Niu Huang Chieh Tu Pien)
- Damp and Toxic Heat

Sheng Tian Qi Pian 生田七片 (Raw Tian Qi Ginseng Tablets)
- A good general medicine for bleeding. Combine with an appropriate constitutional patent medicine or the primary prescription.

Yun Nan Bai Yao 云南白药 (Yunnan Paiyao)
- The premier medicine for all types of bleeding. Combine with an appropriate constitutional patent medicine or the primary prescription. The red pill that accompanies the powder is only used in severe cases.

Acupuncture (select from)

Ren.12 (*zhong wan* -) .... *mu* point of the Stomach, clears Heat from the Stomach

St.44 (*nei ting* -) .... together these points clear Heat from
LI.4 (*he gu* -) *yang ming*

Sp.10 (*xue hai* -) .... cools the Blood to stop bleeding, and regulates and invigorates Blood
St.37 (*shan ju xu* -) .... lower *he* point of the Large Intestine, clears Heat from the Stomach and Intestines
St.45 (*li dui* ↓) .... clears Heat from the Stomach
LI.11 (*qu chi* -) .... *he* sea point of the Large Intestine, clears Heat and Dampness from *yang ming*
PC.8 (*lao gong* -) .... *rong* spring and Fire point of the Pericardium, clears Heat from the Stomach channel and cools Heart Fire

- with epigastric pain, add the *xi* cleft point St.34 (*liang qiu* -)
- with *yin* deficiency add Bl.21 (*wei shu* +) and Bl.23 (*shen shu* +) to nourish Stomach *yin*
- with vomiting of blood, add the *xi* cleft point PC.4 (*xi men* -)
- With Phlegm Heat, add St.40 (*feng long* -) to transform Phlegm
- For *shao yang* / *yang ming* syndrome, add SJ.5 (*wai guan* -), GB.39 (*xuan zhong* -) and St.25 (*tian shu* -)
- *Ear points*: stomach, duodenum, large intestine, liver, subcortex, *shen men*

Clinical notes

- Stomach Heat type haemafecia may be diagnosed biomedically as bleeding peptic ulcers, dysentery or leaking oesophageal varices.
- This is a relatively common pattern of haemafecia, and in most correctly treated cases the bleeding should stop quickly. The Stomach Heat underlying the bleeding usually responds well to correct treatment. The more prolonged, however, and the greater the degree of *yin* deficiency, the more treatment is required.
- All medications, supplements and herbs should be assessed for their potential in contributing to the haemafecia and removed or reduced if possible.
- For dietary recommendations, see p.882.

肝胃郁热

11.2 LIVER QI INVADING THE STOMACH, WITH STAGNANT HEAT OR FIRE

Pathophysiology

- Liver *qi* invading the Stomach and causing gastro-intestinal bleeding is primarily the result of chronic emotional turmoil and stress. In contrast to the Stomach Heat pattern, which is largely due to an excessively rich or heating diet, this pattern is primarily the result of stress, and consequent disruption to the Liver Stomach axis. There may be dietary complications, but the emotional aspects are the most important. Also described as stagnant Heat in the Liver and Stomach.

Clinical features

- Episodic bleeding of dark, purplish, or occasionally bright red blood from the rectum. The bleeding and pain may be preceded or aggravated by a stressful event or period of emotional turmoil, or may occur premenstrually.
- abdominal, epigastric and hypochondriac distension and/or pain
- bitter taste in the mouth, heartburn, acid reflux
- loss of appetite
- irritability, easy anger
- frontal and temporal headaches
- red, sore eyes
- facial flushing
- dry mouth, thirst
- tendency to constipation, or alternating constipation and diarrhoea

T red, or with red edges or red spots on the edges of the tongue and a thin, yellow coat

P wiry and rapid

Treatment principle

Regulate Liver *qi* and clear Heat from the Liver and Stomach
Cool the Blood and stop bleeding

Prescription

DAN ZHI XIAO YAO SAN 丹栀逍遥散
(*Bupleurum and Paeonia Formula*) modified

chai hu (Radix Bupleuri) 柴胡 9-12g
bai shao (Radix Paeoniae Lactiflora) 白芍 12-18g
dang gui (Radix Angelicae Sinensis) 当归 9-12g
fu ling (Sclerotium Poriae Cocos) 茯苓 12-15g
shan zhi zi (Fructus Gardeniae Jasminoidis) 山栀子 9-12g
mu dan pi (Cortex Moutan Radicis) 牡丹皮 9-12g

gan cao (Radix Glycyrrhizae Uralensis) 甘草 3-6g
sheng di (Radix Rehmanniae Glutinosae) 生地 18-30g
huai hua (Flos Sophora Japonicae Immaturus) 槐花 12-15g
qian cao gen (Radix Rubiae Cordifoliae) 茜草根 12-15g

Method: Decoction. **Chai hu** and **bai shao** soften the Liver and move Liver *qi*; **dang gui** and **bai shao** nourish and regulate Blood; **shan zhi zi** and **mu dan pi** cool the Liver; **mu dan pi** regulates Blood and prevents the cooling styptic herbs from causing Blood stagnation; **mu dan pi**, **sheng di** and **qian cao gen** cool the Blood; **huai hua** clears Heat and stops bleeding; **fu ling** and **gan cao** protect and harmonise the Stomach.

Modifications

- With severe Heat (or Fire) add **long dan cao** (Radix Gentianae Longdancao) 龙胆草 6-9g and **huang qin** (Radix Scutellariae Baicalensis) 黄芩 9-12g.
- With constipation, add **zhi da huang** (processed Radix et Rhizoma Rhei) 制大黄 6-9g.
- With excess gastric acid or heartburn, add **hai piao xiao** (Os Sepiae seu Sepiellae) 海螵蛸 15g and **mu li** (Concha Ostreae) 牡蛎 15-30g, or **huang lian** (Rhizoma Coptidis) 黄连 6g and **wu zhu yu** (Fructus Evodiae Rutaecarpae) 吴茱萸 3g, the latter pair especially when there is nausea or vomiting.
- With damage to *yin* from the stagnant Heat, add **shi hu** (Herba Dendrobii) 石斛 12-15g, **tian hua fen** (Radix Trichosanthes Kirilowii) 天花粉 12-15g and **mai dong** (Tuber Ophiopogonis Japonici) 麦冬 9-12g.
- With severe irritability, manic behaviour or disordered consciousness, add **shui niu jiao** (Cornu Bubali) 水牛角 18-30g and **xuan shen** (Radix Scrophulariae Ningpoensis) 玄参 18-30g.

Variations and additional prescriptions

Qi stagnation with little or no Heat

- Liver *qi* can repeatedly invade the Stomach without generating much Heat. This is a less common cause of haemafecia, as Heat is an important factor in causing reckless movement and consequent spillage of Blood from the vessels. However, the continued insult and damage to the *luo mai* of the Stomach can eventually cause leakage of Blood. The main features are stools that are intermittently tarry and black, epigastric distension and discomfort, acid reflux, heartburn, irritability, hypochondriac ache, general smooth and skeletal muscle tension, dizziness, a wiry pulse and a thin, white tongue coat. The symptoms are worse with stress. The solution is to regulate Liver *qi*, soothe and soften the Liver and stop bleeding with **CHAI HU SHU GAN SAN** (*Bupleurum and Cyperus Formula* 柴胡疏肝散) modified.

  chai hu (Radix Bupleuri) 柴胡 9-12g

bai shao (Radix Paeoniae Lactiflora) 白芍 12-18g
xiang fu (Rhizoma Cyperi Rotundi) 香附 9-12g
zhi ke (Fructus Citri Aurantii) 枳壳 6-9g
chuan xiong (Radix Ligustici Chuanxiong) 川芎 3-6g
gan cao (Radix Glycyrrhizae Uralensis) 甘草 3-6g
bai ji fen (powdered Rhizoma Bletillae Striatae) 白芨粉 12-15g
ce bai ye (Cacumen Biotae Orientalis) 侧柏叶 12-15g

Method: Decoction or as powder. When decocted **bai ji fen** can be taken separately or added to the strained decoction (*chong fu* 冲服). When powdered the dose is 6-9 grams in water before meals. **Chai hu** and **bai shao** soften the Liver and move Liver *qi*; **xiang fu** and **zhi ke** regulate *qi* and alleviate distension; **chuan xiong** regulates *qi* and Blood; **bai ji fen** astringes bleeding; **ce bai ye** cools the Blood and stops bleeding.

Patent medicines

Jia Wei Xiao Yao Wan 加味逍遥丸 (Jia Wei Xiao Yao Wan, Dan Zhi Xiao Yao Wan) - *qi* stagnation with stagnant Heat

Long Dan Xie Gan Wan 龙胆泻肝丸 (Long Dan Xie Gan Wan, Lung Tan Xie Gan Wan) - Liver Fire

Chai Hu Shu Gan Wan 柴胡疏肝丸 (Chai Hu Shu Gan Wan)

Sheng Tian Qi Pian 生田七片 (Raw Tian Qi Ginseng Tablets)
- A good general medicine for bleeding. Combine with an appropriate constitutional patent medicine or the primary prescription.

Yun Nan Bai Yao 云南白药 (Yunnan Paiyao)
- The premier medicine for all types of bleeding. Combine with an appropriate constitutional patent medicine or the primary prescription. The red pill that accompanies the powder is only used in severe cases.

Acupuncture (select from)

Ren.12 (*zhong wan* -) .... *mu* point of the Stomach, clears Heat from the Stomach and regulates the Stomach to stop bleeding

St.25 (*tian shu* -) .... *mu* point of the Large Intestine, regulates Intestinal function

Liv.13 (*zhang men*) .... *mu* point of the Spleen, harmonises the Liver and Spleen and regulates abdominal *qi* flow

ah shi points .... between GB.26 (*dai mai*) and GB.27 (*wu shu*), and St.25 (*tian shu*) and St.30 (*qi chong*)

St.44 (*nei ting* -) .... together these points clear Heat from
LI.4 (*he gu* -) *yang ming*

Liv.2 (*xing jian* -) .... *rong* spring and Fire point of the Liver, cools the Liver and drains Liver Fire

LI.11 (*qu chi* -) .... *he* sea point of the Large Intestine, clears Heat and Dampness from *yang ming*

Sp.10 (*xue hai* -) .... cools the Blood to stop bleeding

- *Ear points*: stomach, liver, large intestine, subcortex, *shen men*

Clinical notes

- Liver *qi* invading the Stomach with stagnant Heat or Fire may be diagnosed biomedically as peptic ulcer disease or leaking oesophageal varices.
- The bleeding will usually respond quite quickly to correct treatment, especially with herbs. The underlying Liver *qi* stagnation responds well to correct treatment, with most patients feeling better quite quickly. For long term results, reduction of stress triggers, stress management and daily exercise are essential to keep the *qi* moving. Acupuncture is of particular benefit for long term results, as over time, it appears to be able to alter and improve the physiological response of the patient to stressors. To achieve this however, at least one and preferably more courses of treatment should be given over some months.
- For dietary recommendations, see p.878, 882.

肠风下血

11.3 INTESTINAL WIND

Pathophysiology

- Intestinal Wind is so called because the bleeding that occurs happens suddenly, and usually without warning. It is associated with lesions in the distal large intestine, rectum or anus, such as vascular malformation, haemorrhoids or polyps. The difference between Intestinal Wind as a cause of haemafecia or associated with haemorrhoids (13.1, p.489) is usually the volume of blood. The larger quantity of blood lost through the rectum, (and thus the definition as haemafecia), is usually associated with a greater degree of heat than is present in the haemorrhoid pattern.

Clinical features

- bleeding of fresh red blood from the bowel, often preceding the bowel motion, but may also follow the passage of stool; the bleeding may be alarmingly copious and sufficient to splash the toilet bowl
- abdominal pain
- burning sensation in the anus and rectum
- dry mouth
- tendency to constipation, dry or difficult stools

T red with a yellow coat

P slippery or thready and rapid

Treatment principle

Clear Heat from the Intestines, cool the Blood to stop bleeding

Prescription

HUAI HUA SAN 槐花散
(*Sophora Japonica Flower Powder*) modified

huai hua (Flos Sophora Japonicae Immaturus) 槐花 9-15g
ce bai ye (Cacumen Biotae Orientalis) 侧柏叶 9-15g
jing jie sui (Herba seu Flos Schizonepetae Tenuifoliae) 荆芥穗 9-12g
zhi ke (Fructus Citri Aurantii) 枳壳 6-9g
di yu (Radix Sanguisorbae Officinalis) 地榆 12-15g
cang zhu (Rhizoma Atractylodis) 苍术 6-9g
dang gui (Radix Angelicae Sinensis) 当归 9-12g
chi xiao dou (Semen Phaseoli Calcarati) 赤小豆 12-15g
san qi fen (powdered Radix Notoginseng) 三七粉 3-6g

Method: Decoction. **Huai hua** and **di yu** cool the Blood and stop bleeding; **ce bai ye** clears Heat and stops bleeding; **jing jie sui** disperses Wind and stops bleeding; **zhi ke** promotes the movement of *qi* and relaxes the Intestines; **dang gui** regulates and nourishes Blood, **san qi fen** regulates Blood and stops bleeding; together the last two herbs help to prevent the cool herbs from causing Blood stagnation; **cang zhu** and **chi xiao dou** strengthen the Spleen, dry Dampness and promote urination. (Source: *Zhong Yi Zhi Liao Yi Nan Za Bing Mi Yao*)

Modifications

- With severe Heat and bleeding, add **huang lian** (Rhizoma Coptidis) 黄连 6-9g and **e jiao** (Gelatinum Corii Asini) 阿胶 9-12g (melted in the hot strained decoction).
- To cool the Blood, add **sheng di** (Radix Rehmanniae Glutinosae) 生地 15-24g and **chi shao** (Radix Paeoniae Rubrae) 赤芍 9-12g.
- With difficult stools or constipation, add **zhi da huang** (processed Radix et Rhizoma Rhei) 制大黄 6-9g and **bai wei** (Radix Cynanchi Baiwei) 白薇 9-12g.
- With *qi* stagnation, abdominal distension or tenesmus, add **mu xiang** (Radix Aucklandiae Lappae) 木香 6-9g.
- With pus mixed in with the blood, add **hong teng** (Caulis Sargentodoxae Cuneatae) 红藤 18-30g and **jin yin hua** (Flos Lonicerae Japonicae) 金银花 18-30g.

Patent medicines

Zhong Guo Zhi Gen Duan 中国痔根断 (Chinese Zhi Gen Duan)
- specific for bleeding from the Intestines from Heat

Huang Lian Jie Du Wan 黄连解毒丸 (Huang Lian Jie Du Wan)
- Damp Heat

Sheng Tian Qi Pian 生田七片 (Raw Tian Qi Ginseng Tablets)
- A good general medicine for bleeding. Combine with an appropriate constitutional patent medicine or the primary prescription.

Yun Nan Bai Yao 云南白药 (Yunnan Paiyao)
- The premier medicine for all types of bleeding. Combine with an appropriate constitutional patent medicine or the primary prescription. The red pill that accompanies the powder is only used in severe cases.

Acupuncture (select from)

Du.1 (*chang jiang* -) .... together these points cool and regulate the
Bl.57 (*cheng shan* -) lower Intestine and rectum, dispel Wind and stop bleeding

Bl.30 (*bai huan shu* -) .... an alternative to Du.1 (*chang jiang*), similar in action although not as strong

St.25 (*tian shu* -) .... *mu* point of the Large Intestine, regulates Intestinal function, clears Heat

ah shi points .... likely to be found between St.25 (*tian shu* -) and St.30 (*qi chong*) on the left, reducing method
Sp.1 (*yin bai* -▲) ....*jing* well point of the Spleen, stops bleeding when treated with rice grain moxa
St.37 (*shang ju xu* -) .... lower *he* point of the Large Intestine, clears Damp Heat and regulates the Intestines
Bl.32 (*ci liao* -) .... clears Damp Heat from the lower *jiao* and the rectal area
er bai (M-UE-29) .... extra point for rectal disease

- with pain in the rectum or lower intestine, add Bl.54 (*zhi bian* -) and Bl.2 (*zan zhu*)
- with severe bleeding, add PC.4 (*xi men* -)
- *Ear points*: large intestine, small intestine, distal segment rectum, subcortex, *shen men*

Clinical notes

- Intestinal Wind type haemafecia may be diagnosed biomedically as intestinal polyps, ulcerative colitis or bleeding haemorrhoids.
- Intestinal Wind usually responds well to correct treatment.

湿热蕴蒸

11.4 DAMP HEAT IN THE LARGE INTESTINE

- with *yin* deficiency

Pathophysiology

- Damp Heat causing haemafecia may be acute or chronic. When acute it is usually due to invasion of an external pathogen. When chronic it is usually due to habitual ingestion of Damp Heat generating substances, such as alcohol and rich or fatty foods. Depending on the location of the Damp Heat, the colour of the blood will vary from dark to plum coloured to fresh red. It can also occur following radiation treatment for tumours of the pelvic basin. *See also* Dysenteric Disorder, p.270 and Haemorrhoids, p.496.
- Damp Heat, due to its sticky lingering nature, has a tendency to become chronic and consume *yin*.

Clinical features

- bleeding of dull, dark, purplish or fresh red blood that may be mixed with the stools or precede or follow a bowel movement
- difficulty passing stools, the patient feels an urge to defecate but only passes a small amount and the bowel movement feels incomplete; the stools may be loose or firm depending on the relative proportions of Dampness and Heat
- tenesmus or a burning sensation in the rectum and anus
- abdominal fullness, distension and/or discomfort
- loss of appetite, dry mouth and throat, sticky sensation in the mouth, bitter taste in the mouth

T greasy, yellow coat

P slippery or soggy and rapid

Treatment principle

Clear Damp Heat from the Intestines
Cool the Blood and stop bleeding

Prescription

DI YU SAN 地榆散
(*Sanguisorba Powder*) modified

di yu (Radix Sanguisorbae Officinalis) 地榆 12-15g
qian cao gen (Radix Rubiae Cordifoliae) 茜草根 12-15g
shan zhi zi (Fructus Gardeniae Jasminoidis) 山栀子 9-12g
huang qin (Radix Scutellariae Baicalensis) 黄芩 9-12g
huang lian (Rhizoma Coptidis) 黄连 6-9g

fu ling (Sclerotium Poria Cocos) 茯苓 12-15g
chi xiao dou (Semen Phaseoli Calcarati) 赤小豆 30g
dang gui (Radix Angelicae Sinensis) 当归 9-12g

Method: Decoction. **Di yu** and **qian cao gen** cool the Blood to stop bleeding; **shan zhi zi**, **huang qin** and **huang lian** clear Damp Heat and eliminate Toxin; **fu ling** and **chi xiao dou** promote urination to drain Dampness; **dang gui** harmonises and nourishes the Blood to prevent Blood stagnation from the cooling herbs. (Source: *Zhong Yi Nei Ke Lin Chuang Shou Ce*)

Modifications

- With copious bleeding, add **huai hua** (Flos Sophora Japonicae Immaturus) 槐花 12-15g and **ce bai ye** (Cacumen Biotae Orientalis) 侧柏叶 12-15g.
- With prominent Dampness (thick tongue coat, fullness in the chest and abdomen, slippery pulse), add **cang zhu** (Rhizoma Atractylodis) 苍术 6-9g.
- With constipation, add **zhi da huang** (processed Radix et Rhizoma Rhei) 制大黄 6-9g.
- With difficult or sluggish stools or tenesmus, add **bing lang** (Semen Arecae Catechu) 槟榔 9-12g and **mu xiang** (Radix Aucklandiae Lappae) 木香 6-9g.
- With abdominal or hypochondriac pain, add **mu xiang** (Radix Aucklandiae Lappae) 木香 6-9g and **yan hu suo** (Rhizoma Corydalis Yanhusuo) 延胡索 9-12g.
- With anal swelling and pain, add one or two of the following herbs: **jin yin hua** (Flos Lonicerae Japonicae) 金银花 18-30g, **lian qiao** (Fructus Forsythia Suspensae) 连翘 9-12g, **ku shen** (Radix Sophorae Flavescentis) 苦参 9-12g, **huang bai** (Cortex Phellodendri) 黄柏 9-12g.

Variations and additional prescriptions

Lingering Damp Heat with mild yin deficiency

- Damp Heat has a tendency to linger and become chronic, especially when promoted by a Damp Hot diet, or if untreated or incorrectly treated. Over time, *yin* and *qi* may be damaged, leading to a mixed pattern of deficiency and excess. Depending on the degree of *yin* deficiency, there are two treatment approaches. The first, outlined here, is suitable for lingering Damp Heat with mild *yin* deficiency. The clinical features are chronic intermittent bleeding or occult blood, a red tongue with a greasy or dry, yellow tongue coat, or little tongue coat, insomnia, nightsweats, fatigue and a thready pulse. The treatment aims to gently clear residual Damp Heat and stop bleeding while supporting *yin* and Blood with **ZHU JU WAN** (*Stop the Chariot Pills* 驻车丸) modified.

    dang gui (Radix Angelicae Sinensis) 当归 9-12g

e jiao (Gelatinum Corii Asini) 阿胶 6-9g
huang lian (Rhizoma Coptidis) 黄连 6-9g
gan jiang (dried Rhizoma Zingiberis Officinalis) 干姜 3g
shi hu (Herba Dendrobii) 石斛 9-12g
bai shao (Radix Paeoniae Lactiflora) 白芍 9-12g
gan cao (Radix Glycyrrhizae Uralensis) 甘草 6-9g
han lian cao (Herba Ecliptae Prostratae) 旱连草 12-15g
di yu (Radix Sanguisorbae Officinalis) 地榆 12-15g

Method: Grind herbs to a fine powder and form into 9-gram pills with water. The dose is one pill 2-3 times daily. May also be decocted with dosages as shown, in which case the **e jiao** is melted before being added to the strained decoction (*yang hua* 烊化). **Dang gui** and **e jiao** nourish yin and Blood; **huang lian** clears Damp Heat; the small quantity of **gan jiang** supports the Spleen and assists elevation of *yang* to balance the bitter cold descent of **huang lian** and thus stimulates the *qi* mechanism and elimination of the residual Damp Heat; **bai shao** and **gan cao** combine sour and sweet to create *yin*, harmonise *ying* and stop pain; **shi hu** nourishes *yin*; **han lian cao** and **di yu** cool the Blood and stop bleeding. (Source: *Zhong Yi Zhi Liao Yi Nan Za Bing Mi Yao*)

Lingering Damp Heat with marked yin deficiency

- The second approach (following on from the previous variation) treats Damp Heat with more severe *yin* damage, which usually follows a severe acute episode that swiftly depletes *yin* and Blood. The treatment focuses on replenishing the *yin* while secondarily clearing residual Damp Heat. The guiding prescription is a mixture of **LIU WEI DI HUANG WAN** (*Rehmannia Six Formula* 六味地黄丸) and **ZHU JU WAN** (*Stop the Chariot Pills* 驻车丸) modified.

shu di (Radix Rehmanniae Glutinosae Conquitae) 熟地 18-24g
shan yao (Radix Dioscoreae Oppositae) 山药 12-15g
shan zhu yu (Fructus Corni Officinalis) 山茱萸 9-12g
fu ling (Sclerotium Poria Cocos) 茯苓 12-15g
ze xie (Rhizoma Alismatis Orientalis) 泽泻 9-12g
mu dan pi (Cortex Moutan Radicis) 牡丹皮 9-12g
dang gui (Radix Angelicae Sinensis) 当归 9-12g
huang lian (Rhizoma Coptidis) 黄连 6-9g
e jiao (Gelatinum Corii Asini) 阿胶 6-9g
gan jiang (dried Rhizoma Zingiberis Officinalis) 干姜 3g
di yu (Radix Sanguisorbae Officinalis) 地榆 9-12g
huai hua (Flos Sophora Japonicae Immaturus) 槐花 9-12g
han lian cao (Herba Ecliptae Prostratae) 旱连草 9-12g

Method: Grind the herbs to powder and form into 9-gram pills with honey. The dose is 2-3 pills daily. May also be decocted with dosage as shown, in which case the **e jiao** is melted before being added to the strained decoction (*yang hua* 烊化). **Shu di** and **shan zhu yu** nourish Liver and Kidney *yin*; **shan yao** strengthens the Spleen and nourishes *yin*, **fu ling**, **ze xie** and **mu dan pi** moderate the cloying tendency of the *yin* supplementing herbs; **dang gui** and **e jiao** nourish yin and Blood; **huang lian** clears Damp Heat; **gan jiang** prevents the bitterness of **huang lian** from damaging *yin* further; **di yu, huai hua** and **han lian cao** cool the Blood and stop bleeding. (Source: *Shi Yong Zhong Yi Nei Ke Xue*)

Patent medicines

Huang Lian Jie Du Wan 黄连解毒丸 (Huang Lian Jie Du Wan)
- Damp Heat

Chuan Xin Lian Kang Yan Pian 穿心莲抗炎片 (Chuan Xin Lian Antiphlogistic Tablets)
- Damp or Toxic Heat

Niu Huang Qing Huo Wan 牛黄清火丸 (Niu Huang Qing Huo Wan)
- Damp Heat with a tendency to constipation or sluggish stools

Zhong Guo Zhi Gen Duan 中国痔根断 (Chinese Zhi Gen Duan)
- specific for bleeding from the Intestines from Heat

Sheng Tian Qi Pian 生田七片 (Raw Tian Qi Ginseng Tablets)
- A good general medicine for bleeding. Combine with an appropriate constitutional patent medicine or the primary prescription.

Yun Nan Bai Yao 云南白药 (Yunnan Paiyao)
- The premier medicine for all types of bleeding. Combine with an appropriate constitutional patent medicine or the primary prescription. The red pill that accompanies the powder is only used in severe cases.

Acupuncture (select from)

St.25 (*tian shu* -) .... together these points regulate Intestinal
Sp.15 (*da heng* -) function and eliminate Dampness and Heat from the Intestines

St.37 (*shang ju xu* -) .... lower *he* point of the Large Intestine, clears Damp Heat and regulates the Intestines

LI.4 (*he gu* -) .... *yuan* point of the Large Intestine, clears Heat from *yang ming* and stops pain

LI.11 (*qu chi* -) .... *he* sea point of the Large Intestine, clears Heat and Dampness from *yang ming*, and regulates *qi* and Blood

ah shi points .... likely to be found between St.25 (*tian shu* -) and St.30 (*qi chong*) on the left, and between St.36 (*zu san li*) and St.39 (*xia ju xu*), reducing method to clear Damp Heat

Bl.57 (*cheng shan* -) .... clears Heat from the lower Intestine and rectum and stops bleeding

Bl.25 (*da chang shu* -) .... *shu* point of Large Intestine, clears Damp Heat

- acupuncture must be given frequently for a good result, 1-2 times daily is appropriate in severe cases.
- with pain in the rectum or lower intestine, add Bl.54 (*zhi bian* -) and Bl.2 (*zan zhu*)
- with high fever add Du.14 (*da zhui* -)
- with nausea add PC.6 (*nei guan*) and Ren.12 (*zhong wan*)
- with tenesmus add Du.1 (*chang qiang* -) and Ren.4 (*guan yuan*)
- with prominent Damp, add Sp.9 (*yin ling quan* -)
- with *yin* deficiency, add Sp.6 (*san yin jiao* +) and Ren.4 (*guan yuan* +)
- *Ear points*: large intestine, small intestine, stomach, kidney, subcortex, *shen men*

Clinical notes

- Damp Heat in the Intestine usually responds quite well to correct treatment, but required persistence of treatment and dietary modification for complete eradication.
- Damp Heat, if incompletely or poorly treated, has a tendency to linger and become recurrent, causing intermittent episodes of bleeding. In between episodes of bleeding in chronic cases, it will often be found that the patient displays elements of *qi* stagnation and/or Spleen deficiency (the primary pathological triad, p.912). A suitable constitutional prescription may be selected on the basis of the patients mix of pathology.
- While Damp Heat remains in the Intestines, the use of astringent herbs and antidiarrhoea agents is contraindicated. Inappropriate use of these substances to stop diarrhoea can lock Damp Heat in. Overenthusiastic or long term use of bitter cold herbs can weaken the Spleen and *yang*, compounding the damage done by the Damp Heat.
- For dietary recommendations, see p.884.

血瘀便血

11.5 BLOOD STAGNATION

Pathophysiology

- Blood stagnation patterns are usually chronic disorders that follow many years of some other pathology, most commonly Liver *qi* stagnation. In the case of bleeding in the bowel, there are several treatment approaches possible depending on where in the bowel the Blood stasis is located; upper, mid or lower digestive tract.
- Bleeding of this type is usually accompanied by pain, and it is the site of the pain that guides the selection of the appropriate prescription. Even if the patient does not experience pain, Blood stagnation type pain will usually be elicited with abdominal palpation.

Clinical features

- bleeding of dark or purple blood from the bowel, or sticky tarry stools, or mixed dark and fresh red blood
- epigastric or abdominal distension and pain; the pain may be intermittent or detected with palpation, but tends to occur or be found in the same place and has a focal, sharp or stabbing quality; pain may be found in the epigastrium, upper abdomen, and left and right lower abdomen
- dark complexion, purplish lips, dark rings around the eyes
- possibly masses beneath the ribs
- purple spider naevi, usually across the cheeks or hypochondriac region; broken vessels on the medial ankle and knee
- possibly haemorrhoids

T purplish or with purple or brown petechial spots with little or no coat; dark and distended sublingual veins

P wiry and thready or choppy

Treatment principle

Invigorate Blood, disperse stagnant Blood
Move *qi* and stop bleeding

Prescription

11.5.1 Stomach and epigastrium Blood stagnation

SHI XIAO SAN 失笑散
(*Break Into a Smile Powder*) plus
DAN SHEN YIN 丹参饮
(*Salvia Decoction*) modified

---

pu huang (Pollen Typhae) 蒲黄 9-12g

chao wu ling zhi (dry fried Excrementum Trogopteri seu Pteromi) 炒五灵脂 9-12g
dan shen (Radix Salviae Miltiorrhizae) 丹参 18-30g
sha ren (Fructus Amomi) 砂仁 6-9g
tan xiang (Lignum Santali Albi) 檀香 6-9g
xiang fu (Rhizoma Cyperi Rotundi) 香附 9-12g
san qi fen (powdered Radix Notoginseng) 三七粉 3-6g

Method: Decoction. **Wu ling zhi** and **pu huang** invigorate Blood and disperse stagnant Blood. An equal mixture of dry fried and unprocessed **pu huang** can be used, as unprocessed **pu huang** can invigorate stagnant Blood, while the dry fried version (**chao pu huang** 炒蒲黄), stops bleeding. **Dan shen** clears Heat, invigorates Blood and breaks up stagnant Blood; **san qi fen** invigorates Blood, disperses stagnant Blood and stops bleeding; **sha ren**, **tan xiang** and **xiang fu** regulate *qi* to assist in moving Blood.

11.5.2 Liver Blood stagnation, with masses

GE XIA ZHU YU TANG 膈下逐瘀汤
(*Drive Out Blood Stasis Below the Diaphragm Decoction*) modified

This prescription is selected when the Liver is involved and there are palpable masses and pain in the upper abdomen.

chao wu ling zhi (dry fried Excrementum Trogopteri seu Pteromi) 炒五灵脂 9-12g
dang gui (Radix Angelicae Sinensis) 当归 9-12g
tao ren (Semen Persicae) 桃仁 9-12g
hong hua (Flos Carthami Tinctorii) 红花 9-12g
chi shao (Radix Paeoniae Rubrae) 赤芍 9-12g
xiang fu (Rhizoma Cyperi Rotundi) 香附 9-12g
wu yao (Radix Linderae Strychnifoliae) 乌药 9-12g
gan cao (Radix Glycyrrhizae Uralensis) 甘草 6-9g
chuan xiong (Radix Ligustici Chuanxiong) 川芎 6-9g
mu dan pi (Cortex Moutan Radicis) 牡丹皮 6-9g
zhi ke (Fructus Citri Aurantii) 枳壳 6-9g
cu yan hu suo (vinegar fried Rhizoma Corydalis Yanhusuo) 醋延胡索 9-12g
san qi fen (powdered Radix Notoginseng) 三七粉 3-6g

Method: Decoction. **San qi fen** is taken separately or added to the strained decoction (*chong fu* 冲服). **Wu ling zhi, dang gui, chuan xiong, chi shao, tao ren** and **hong hua** invigorate Blood and disperse stagnant Blood; **xiang fu, wu yao, zhi ke** and **cu yan hu suo** regulate *qi* and stop pain; **gan cao** protects and harmonises the Stomach; **san qi fen** invigorates Blood, disperses stagnant Blood and stops bleeding. (Source: *Shi Yong Zhong Yi Nei Ke Xue*)

11.5.3 Blood stagnation with Cold, in the lower abdomen

SHAO FU ZHU YU TANG 少腹逐瘀汤
(*Drive Out Blood Stasis in the Lower Abdomen Decoction*) modified

dang gui (Radix Angelicae Sinensis) 当归 9-12g
chi shao (Radix Paeoniae Rubrae) 赤芍 9-12g
pu huang (Pollen Typhae) 蒲黄 9-12g
chao wu ling zhi (dry fried Excrementum Trogopteri seu Pteromi) 炒五灵脂 9-12g
yan hu suo (Rhizoma Corydalis Yanhusuo) 延胡索 9-12g
chuan xiong (Radix Ligustici Chuanxiong) 川芎 6-9g
xiao hui xiang (Fructus Foeniculi Vulgaris) 小茴香 9-12g
mo yao (Myrrha) 没药 6-9g
rou gui (Cortex Cinnamomi Cassiae) 肉桂 3-6g
pao jiang (quick fried Rhizoma Zingiberis Officinalis) 炮姜 3-6g
chao di yu (dry fried Radix Sanguisorbae Officinalis) 炒地榆 12-15g

Method: Decoction. An equal mixture of dry fried and unprocessed **pu huang** can be used, as unprocessed **pu huang** can invigorate stagnant Blood, while the dry fried version (**chao pu huang** 炒蒲黄), stops bleeding. **Dang gui**, **chi shao, wu ling zhi, pu huang, chuan xiong** and **mo yao** invigorate Blood and disperse stagnant Blood; **chuan xiong, xiao hui xiang** and **yan hu suo** regulate *qi* and stop pain; **rou gui** and **pao jiang** warm *yang* and invigorate the circulation of *qi* and Blood; **rou gui** promotes generation of new Blood; **chao di yu** stops bleeding. (Source: *Shi Yong Zhong Yi Nei Ke Xue*)

Modifications (apply to all prescriptions where not already included)

- With severe bleeding add or increase the dose of **san qi** powder to 9g and add **bai ji** (Rhizoma Bletillae Striatae) 白芨 12-15g. Both these herbs can also be taken separately as powder.
- With severe pain add **yan hu suo** (Rhizoma Corydalis Yanhusuo) 延胡索 12-15g, or **ru xiang** (Gummi Olibanum) 乳香 6-9g and **mo yao** (Myrrha) 没药 6-9g.
- With severe *qi* stagnation (distension, belching), add **zhi shi** (Fructus Immaturus Citri Aurantii) 枳实 9-12g and **qing pi** (Pericarpium Citri Reticulatae Viridae) 青皮 9-12g.
- With signs of Heat, add **huang qin** (Radix Scutellariae Baicalensis) 黄芩 9-12g, **huang lian** (Rhizoma Coptidis) 黄连 3-6g and **mu dan pi** (Cortex Moutan Radicis) 牡丹皮 9-12g.
- With Cold, add **gui zhi** (Ramulus Cinnamomi Cassiae) 桂枝 6-9g.
- With *qi* deficiency add **zhi huang qi** (honey fried Radix Astragali Membranacei) 炙黄芪 18-30g, **bai zhu** (Rhizoma Atractylodes Macrocephalae) 白术 12-15g and **huang jing** (Rhizoma Polygonati)

黄精 12-15g.

- With *yin* deficiency, add **sheng di** (Radix Rehmanniae Glutinosae) 生地 12-18g and **sha shen** (Radix Adenophorae seu Glehniae) 沙参 12-15g.
- Most patients with Blood stagnation in the Stomach will have quite impaired digestion, and may have difficulty processing some Blood moving herbs. In most cases it is useful to add some digestion improving herbs, such as **shan zha** (Fructus Crataegi) 山楂 15g and **shen qu** (Massa Fermentata) 神曲 15g.
- When the biomedical diagnosis is cancer, add two or three of the following herbs to enhance the detoxifying, accumulation eliminating action: **bai hua she she cao** (Herba Hedyotidis Diffusae) 白花蛇舌草 30-60g, **ban zhi lian** (Herba Scutellariae Barbatae) 半枝连 15g, **tu fu ling** (Rhizoma Smilacis Glabra) 30g, or **e zhu** (Rhizoma Curcumae Ezhu) 莪术 15g.

Variations and additional prescriptions

Severe Blood stagnation in the Intestines with Heat

- With Blood stagnation in the lower abdomen or left iliac fossa with Heat (severe, fixed lower abdominal pain, dysmenorrhoea, amenorrhoea, fever at night, irritability, restlessness and thirst, urinary difficulty, possible hard to pass tarry stools or constipation and a choppy pulse) the aim of treatment is to drain Heat and break up Blood stasis with **TAO HE CHENG QI TANG** (*Major Rhubarb Combination* 桃核承气汤) modified. This formula can be used for Blood stagnation in the reproductive system or in the Intestine, typically the left lower abdomen or iliac fossa.

  tao ren (Semen Persicae) 桃仁 12-15g
  jiu da huang (wine fried Radix et Rhizoma Rhei)
  酒大黄 9-12g
  gui zhi (Ramulus Cinnamomi Cassiae) 桂枝 6-9g
  mang xiao (Mirabilitum) 芒硝 6-9g
  zhi gan cao (honey fried Radix Glycyrrhizae Uralensis)
  炙甘草 3-6g
  mu dan pi (Cortex Moutan Radicis) 牡丹皮 9-12g
  chi shao (Radix Paeoniae Rubrae) 赤芍 9-12g
  san qi fen (powdered Radix Notoginseng) 三七粉 3-6g

  Method: Decoction. **Mang xiao** is dissolved in the strained decoction (*yang hua* 烊化). **San qi** powder can be taken separately. **Tao ren**, **mu dan pi**, **chi shao** and **jiu da huang** break up stagnant Blood; **jiu da huang** clears Heat and opens the bowels to provide an outlet for the Heat and stagnation; **mang xiao** softens hardness and opens the bowels, **mu dan pi** and **chi shao** cool the Blood; **gui zhi** is warm and dispersing, helping to open the vessels and promote *qi* and Blood circulation; **gan cao** protects and harmonises the Stomach; **san qi fen** invigorates Blood, disperses stagnant Blood and stops bleeding.

  For severe pain, add **sheng pu huang** (Pollen Typhae) 生蒲黄 9-12g and **chao wu ling zhi** (dry fried Excrementum Trogopteri seu Pteromi) 炒五灵脂 9-12g.

Patent medicines

Xue Fu Zhu Yu Wan 血府逐瘀丸 (Xue Fu Zhu Yu Wan)
- *qi* and Blood stagnation

Sheng Tian Qi Pian 生田七片 (Raw Tian Qi Ginseng Tablets)
- A good general medicine for bleeding. Combine with the above constitutional patent medicine or the primary prescription.

Yun Nan Bai Yao 云南白药 (Yunnan Paiyao)
- The premier medicine for all types of bleeding. Combine with the above constitutional patent medicine or the primary prescription. The red pill with the powder is only used in severe cases.

Acupuncture (select from)

St.25 (*tian shu* -) .... *mu* point of the Large Intestine, regulates Intestinal function and invigorates Intestinal *qi* and Blood

Sp.6 (*san yin jiao*) .... invigorates *qi* and Blood, removes obstruction from the *jing luo*

Sp.8 (*di ji* -) .... *xi* cleft point of the Spleen, regulates and invigorates Blood

Sp.10 (*xue hai* -) .... cools the Blood to stop bleeding, regulates and invigorates Blood

Bl.25 (*da chang shu* -) .... *shu* point of Large Intestine, regulates the Intestines and eliminates stagnation

a shi points .... over the site of pain in the abdomen, along the Stomach channel between St.36 (*zu san li*) and St.39 (*xia ju xu*), and along the Urinary Bladder channel between Bl.17 (*ge shu*) and Bl.25 (*da chang shu*)

- congested spider vessels on the legs, especially around the medial knee, ankle and sacral area can be bled with a lancet
- *Ear points*: stomach, duodenum, large intestine, small intestine, liver, adrenal, subcortex, *shen men*

Clinical notes

- Blood stagnation type haemafecia may be diagnosed biomedically as angiodysplasia, leaking oesophageal varices, peptic ulcer disease, diverticulosis, stomach or intestinal cancer or intestinal polyps.
- This pattern can be difficult and may take some months of persistent treatment for a satisfactory result depending on the biomedical diagnosis, although bleeding will often cease within a few weeks. In the case of treatment of cancer TCM offers a useful supportive role.
- For dietary recommendations, see p.886.

脾气不足

11.6 SPLEEN QI DEFICIENCY

Pathophysiology

- *Qi* deficiency type bleeding is always chronic and may be recurrent or intermittent. The blood may be visible or occult.
- The mechanism involves a failure of Spleen *qi* to hold the Blood in the vessels. Blood slowly seeps out into the Intestine mixing with the Intestinal contents. The location of the bleeding is most often relatively high in the digestive tract, hence the dark blood and tarry stools.

Clinical features

- Mild bleeding of dark, purplish blood, or less commonly, red blood preceding or following a bowel movement; or black, tarry, sticky, unformed stools; or occult blood in the stool discovered upon routine testing
- intermittent dull abdominal pain that is alleviated with pressure
- abdominal distension, early satiety, nausea
- loose stools or diarrhoea
- loss of appetite
- waxy pale or sallow complexion
- fatigue, weakness
- shortness of breath with exertion, spontaneous sweating
- dizziness, light headedness
- there may be other signs of bleeding, such as heavy menstrual periods or easy bruising

T pale and swollen, with toothmarks (or pale and thin with significant Blood deficiency)

P thready and weak or moderate

Treatment principle

Strengthen the Spleen, supplement and elevate *qi*
Nourish Blood and stop bleeding

Prescription

11.6.1 With sinking Spleen *qi*

BU ZHONG YI QI TANG 补中益气汤
(*Ginseng and Astragalus Combination*) modified

This prescription is especially good when there is a sensation of heaviness in the anus or prolapse of the rectal mucosa, accompanied by chronic loose stools or diarrhoea.

zhi huang qi (honey fried Radix Astragali Membranacei)
炙黄芪 18-30g

dang shen (Radix Codonopsis Pilosulae) 党参 15-24g
chao bai zhu (dry fried Rhizoma Atractylodes Macrocephalae) 炒白术 12-15g
dang gui (Radix Angelicae Sinensis) 当归 9-12g
chen pi (Pericarpium Citri Reticulatae) 陈皮 6-9g
zhi gan cao (honey fried Radix Glycyrrhizae Uralensis) 炙甘草 6-9g
sheng ma (Rhizoma Cimicifugae) 升麻 3-6g
chai hu (Radix Bupleuri) 柴胡 3-6g
pao jiang (quick fried Rhizoma Zingiberis Officinalis) 炮姜 3-6g
bai ji (Rhizoma Bletillae Striatae) 白芨 12-15g
chao huai hua (dry fried Flos Sophora Japonicae Immaturus) 炒槐花 9-12g
chao di yu (dry fried Radix Sanguisorbae Officinalis) 炒地榆 9-12g

Method: Decoction or powdered and taken in doses of 9-grams as a draft. **Zhi huang qi**, **dang shen** and **chao bai zhu** strengthen the Spleen, supplement *qi* and assist the Spleen in holding Blood in the vessels; **chai hu** and **sheng ma** support the *qi* supplementing herbs in lifting sinking *qi*; **dang gui** supplements Blood; **chen pi** and **gan cao** regulate *qi* and harmonise the middle *jiao*; **pao jiang** warms the Spleen and stops bleeding; **bai ji**, **chao huai hua** and **chao di yu** stop bleeding. (Source: *Shi Yong Zhong Yi Nei Ke Xue*)

11.6.2 With persistent bleeding

GU CHONG TANG 固冲汤
(*Stabilise Gushing Decoction*) modified

This prescription is more astringent than the previous prescription, and is selected when bleeding is persistent or difficult to control. It is used until the bleeding ceases or no more blood can be detected, usually no more than 7-10 days. Once the bleeding has stopped, a less astringent prescription may be selected.

chao bai zhu (dry fried Rhizoma Atractylodes Macrocephalae) 炒白术 18-30g
zhi huang qi (honey fried Radix Astragali Membranacei) 炙黄芪 12-18g
duan long gu (calcined Os Draconis) 煅龙骨 15-24g
duan mu li (calcined Concha Ostraea) 煅牡蛎 15-24g
shan zhu yu (Fructus Corni Officinalis) 山茱萸 18-24g
bai shao (Radix Paeoniae Lactiflora) 白芍 9-12g
hai piao xiao (Os Sepiae seu Sepiellae) 海螵蛸 9-12g
wu bei zi (Galla Rhois Chinensis) 五倍子 1-2g
qian cao gen (Radix Rubiae Cordifoliae) 茜草根 6-9g

e jiao (Gelatinum Corii Asini) 阿胶 6-9g

Method: Decoction. **Long gu** and **mu li** are usually cooked for 30 minutes prior to the other herbs (*xian jian* 先煎). **E jiao** is melted before being added to the strained decoction (*yang hua* 烊化). **Wu bei zi** is powdered and taken with the strained decoction. **Bai zhu** and **huang qi** strengthen the Spleen's function of holding Blood in the vessels and supplement *qi*; **shan zhu yu** and **bai shao** nourish and astringe *yin* and Blood; **e jiao** nourishes *yin* and Blood and stops bleeding; **long gu, mu li, wu bei zi** and **hai piao xiao** powerfully astringe leakage of fluids and stop bleeding; **qian cao gen** invigorates Blood and prevents the astringents from causing Blood stagnation. (Source: *Shi Yong Zhong Yi Nei Ke Xue*)

Modifications

- To increase the styptic action, add **san qi fen** (powdered Radix Notoginseng) 三七粉 3-6g or combine with the patent medicine *Yun Nan Bai Yao* 云南白药 (Yunnan Paiyao).

Variations and additional prescriptions

Heart Blood and Spleen qi deficiency

- If the patient is prone to easy bruising, feels anxious and dizzy, and has trouble sleeping, the formula of choice is **GUI PI TANG** (*Ginseng and Longan Combination* 归脾汤) modified.

zhi huang qi (honey fried Radix Astragali Membranacei) 炙黄芪 18-30g
dang shen (Radix Codonopsis Pilosulae) 党参 15-18g
chao bai zhu (dry fried Rhizoma Atractylodis Macrocephalae) 炒白术 12-15g
fu shen (Sclerotium Poriae Cocos Pararadicis) 茯神 12-15g
dang gui (Radix Angelicae Sinensis) 当归 6-9g
long yan rou (Arillus Euphoriae Longanae) 龙眼肉 9-12g
suan zao ren (Semen Zizyphi Spinosae) 酸枣仁 9-12g
mu xiang (Radix Aucklandiae Lappae) 木香 6-9g
yuan zhi (Radix Polygalae Tenuifoliae) 远志 6-9g
zhi gan cao (honey fried Radix Glycyrrhizae Uralensis) 炙甘草 3-6g
pao jiang (quick fried Rhizoma Zingiberis Officinalis) 炮姜 3-6g
xian he cao (Herba Agrimoniae Pilosae) 仙鹤草 12-15g
san qi fen (powdered Radix Notoginseng) 三七粉 3-6g

Method: Decoction. **Huang qi, dang shen, bai zhu** and **zhi gan cao** strengthen the Spleen, supplement *qi* and assist the Spleen in holding Blood in the vessels; **dang gui, long yan rou** and **huang qi** together supplement Blood; **suan zao ren, long yan rou** and **yuan zhi** nourish the Heart and calm the *shen*; **fu shen** benefits the Spleen and calms the *shen*; **mu xiang** regulates *qi* and aids the Spleen in digesting the Blood supplementing herbs; **pao jiang** warms the Spleen and stops bleeding; **xian he cao** astringes bleeding; **san qi fen** invigorates Blood and stops bleeding.

Patent medicines

Bu Zhong Yi Qi Wan 补中益气丸 (Bu Zhong Yi Qi Wan, Central Qi Pills)

Gui Pi Wan 归脾丸 (Gui Pi Wan, Angelicae Longana Tea, Kwei Be Wan)
- Heart Blood and Spleen *qi* deficiency

Li Zhong Wan 理中丸 (Li Zhong Wan)
- with Cold or Spleen *yang* deficiency

Sheng Tian Qi Pian 生田七片 (Raw Tian Qi Ginseng Tablets)
- A good general medicine for bleeding. Combine with an appropriate constitutional patent medicine or the primary prescription.

Yun Nan Bai Yao 云南白药 (Yunnan Paiyao)
- The premier medicine for all types of bleeding. Combine with an appropriate constitutional patent medicine or the primary prescription. The red pill that accompanies the powder is only used in severe cases.

Acupuncture (select from)

Ren.12 (*zhong wan* +▲) .. *mu* point of the Stomach, warms and strengthens the Spleen and Stomach and supplements *qi*

St.25 (*tian shu* +▲) .... *mu* point of the Large Intestine, regulates Intestinal function

Ren.6 (*qi hai* +▲) .... regulates *qi*, strengthens the Kidneys

St.36 (*zu san li* +▲) .... *he* sea point of the Stomach, powerfully warms and strengthens the Spleen and Stomach, and supplements *qi*

Sp.1 (*yin bai* ▲) ....*jing* well point of the Spleen, a special point for Spleen deficiency bleeding when treated with rice grain moxa

Sp.4 (*gong sun* +) .... *luo* point of the Spleen, master point of *chong mai*, regulates the Spleen and Stomach, stops bleeding; good when there is abdominal pain

Sp.6 (*san yin jiao* +▲) ...... strengthens the Spleen, regulates Liver *qi*, benefits the Kidneys and regulates *qi* and Blood

Bl.20 (*pi shu* +▲) .... *shu* point of the Spleen, warms and strengthens the Spleen and supplements *qi*

Bl.25 (*da chang shu* +▲) .. *shu* point of the Large Intestine, warms and regulates the Intestine

Du.20 (*bai hui* ▲) .... strong moxa to help raise *yang* and astringe the Intestines for difficult to control bleeding

- a moxa box over the abdomen is useful

- with prolapse or a sensation of heaviness in the rectum, add Du.20 (*bai hui* ▲)
- *Ear points*: spleen, stomach, large intestine, small intestine, subcortex, adrenal, *shen men*

Clinical notes

- Spleen *qi* deficiency haemafecia may be diagnosed biomedically as chronic peptic ulcer disease, Crohn's disease, chronic ulcerative colitis, vascular malformation, thrombocytopenia, prolapsing haemorrhoids, intestinal polyps or haemophilia.
- Spleen *qi* deficiency patterns usually respond predictably and fairly quickly to correct treatment. In most cases, the patient should expect to see some improvement within a couple of weeks, then gradual resolution over several months.
- For dietary recommendations, see p.870.

脾胃虛寒

11.7 SPLEEN AND STOMACH YANG DEFICIENCY

Pathophysiology

- Spleen and Stomach *yang* deficiency haemafecia is a chronic pattern, often a deterioration of a chronic Spleen *qi* deficiency pattern. Spleen *yang* deficiency will usually drain Kidney *yang* as the condition progresses.
- The mechanism is associated with the Spleen's failure to keep the Blood inside the vessels. Blood gradually seeps out into the Intestines.

Clinical features

- dark, purplish or pale watery blood preceding, following or mixed with the stool, in which case the stools are unformed, black, tarry or blood streaked; the bleeding may also be occult, detected on routine screening
- persistent, dull abdominal pain that responds favourably to the application of warmth and pressure
- cold intolerance, cold abdomen, cold extremities
- lower abdominal distension
- fatigue, weakness, exhaustion
- waxy, pale or sallow complexion
- loss of appetite, anorexia
- chronic loose stools or diarrhoea; there may be undigested food in the stools; possibly urgent early morning diarrhoea

T pale, wet, and swollen, with toothmarks
P deep, weak and slow

Treatment principle

Warm and supplement Spleen and Stomach *yang*
Nourish the Blood, stop bleeding

Prescription

11.7.1 Relatively severe bleeding

HUANG TU TANG 黄土汤
(*Yellow Earth Decoction*) modified

The focus of this prescription is on stopping the bleeding.

zao xin tu (Terra Flava Usta) 灶心土 30-60g
sheng di (Radix Rehmanniae Glutinosae) 生地 9-15g
chao bai zhu (dry fried Rhizoma Atractylodes Macrocephalae) 炒白术 9-12g
zhi fu zi (Radix Aconiti Carmichaeli Praeparata) 制附子 6-12g
e jiao (Gelatinum Corii Asini) 阿胶 9-12g
chao huang qin (dry fried Radix Scutellariae Baicalensis) 炒黄芩 6-9g

zhi gan cao (honey fried Radix Glycyrrhizae Uralensis)
炙甘草 3-6g
pao jiang (quick fried Rhizoma Zingiberis Officinalis)
炮姜 6-9g
san qi fen (powdered Radix Notoginseng) 三七粉 3-6g

Method: Decoction. **Zao xin tu** is bagged in muslin or cloth and, with **zhi fu zi**, decocted for 30 minutes prior to the other herbs (*xian jian* 先煎). **San qi fen** is taken separately or added to the strained decoction (*chong fu* 冲服), **e jiao** is melted before being added to the strained decoction (*yang hua* 烊化). **Zao xin tu** warms the middle *jiao* and stops bleeding; **zhi fu zi** and **chao bai zhu** warm *yang* and strengthen the Spleen; **sheng di** and **e jiao** nourish *yin*, stop bleeding and prevent the pungent warm herbs from damaging *yin* and Blood; **gan cao** protects the Stomach; **chao huang qin** prevents the pungent warm herbs from generating too much Heat and injuring *yin* and Blood; **pao jiang** warms the middle *jiao* and stops bleeding; **san qi fen** invigorates Blood and stops bleeding. (Source: *Shi Yong Zhong Yi Nei Ke Xue*)

11.7.2 Relatively mild bleeding

FU ZI LI ZHONG WAN 附子理中丸
(*Aconite, Ginseng and Ginger Formula*) modified

This prescription is used when the bleeding is relatively mild or occult. The focus is mainly to warm and strengthen Spleen *yang*. The stools will be loose and intermittently dark or tarry. There may be severe abdominal bloating and loss of appetite.

zhi fu zi (Radix Aconiti Carmichaeli Praeparata) 制附子 9-12g
dang shen (Radix Codonopsis Pilosulae) 党参 15-24g
pao jiang (quick fried Rhizoma Zingiberis Officinalis)
炮姜 6-9g
chao bai zhu (dry fried Rhizoma Atractylodis
Macrocephalae) 炒白术 12-15g
zhi gan cao (honey fried Radix Glycyrrhizae Uralensis)
炙甘草 6-9g
zhi huang qi (honey fried Radix Astragali Membranacei)
炙黄芪 18-30g
dang gui (Radix Angelicae Sinensis) 当归 9-12g
e jiao (Gelatinum Corii Asini) 阿胶 6-9g

Method: Decoction. **Zhi fu zi** is decocted for 30 minutes prior to the other herbs (*xian jian* 先煎); **e jiao** is melted before being added to the strained decoction (*yang hua* 烊化). **Zhi fu zi** warms *yang* and dispels Cold; **dang shen**, **zhi huang qi**, **chao bai zhu** and **zhi gan cao** strengthen the Spleen and supplement *qi*; **pao jiang** warms the middle *jiao* and stops bleeding; **dang gui** and **e jiao** nourish *yin* and Blood; **e jiao** stops bleeding.

Modifications (apply to both prescriptions)

- In most cases, Kidney *yang* will gradually be drained. The features that signal Spleen and Kidney *yang* deficiency include chronic lower back ache, weakness of the legs and knees, urgent diarrhoea first thing in the morning, nocturia and severe cold intolerance. Add **xian ling pi** (Herba Epimedii) 仙灵脾 12-15g, **xian mao** (Rhizoma Curculiginis Orchioidis) 仙茅 9-12g and **bu gu zhi** (Fructus Psoraleae Corylifoliae) 补骨脂 12-15g.

Variations and additional prescriptions

- Once the bleeding has ceased and the *yang* is warmed, care needs to be taken not to injure Blood and *yin* by continuing the primary prescription for too long. A milder Spleen and Stomach *qi* supplementing prescription may be used. Consider **BU ZHONG YI QI TANG** (*Ginseng and Astragalus Combination* 补中益气汤, p.502), or **SI JUN ZI TANG** (*Four Major Herbs Combination* 四君子汤, p.618).

Patent medicines

Fu Zi Li Zhong Wan 附子理中丸 (Fu Tzu Li Chung Wan, Carmichaeli Tea Pills, Li Chung Yuen Medical Pills)
- Spleen *yang* deficiency with severe Cold

Li Zhong Wan 理中丸 (Li Zhong Wan)
- Spleen *yang* deficiency

Sheng Tian Qi Pian 生田七片 (Raw Tian Qi Ginseng Tablets)
- A good general medicine for bleeding. Combine with an appropriate constitutional patent medicine or the primary prescription.

Yun Nan Bai Yao 云南白药 (Yunnan Paiyao)
- The premier medicine for all types of bleeding. Combine with an appropriate constitutional patent medicine or the primary prescription. The red pill that accompanies the powder is only used in severe cases.

Acupuncture (select from)

Ren.12 (*zhong wan* +▲) .. *mu* point of the Stomach, warms and supplements Spleen and Stomach *yang*
St.25 (*tian shu* +▲) .... *mu* point of the Large Intestine, regulates and warms Intestines
Ren.6 (*qi hai* +▲) .... regulates *qi*, strengthens the Kidneys
St.36 (*zu san li* +▲) .... *he* sea point of the Stomach, powerfully warms and strengthens the Spleen and Stomach and supplements *qi*
Sp.1 (*yin bai* ▲) .... *jing* well point of the Spleen, a special point for Spleen deficiency bleeding when treated with rice grain moxa

Sp.4 (*gong sun* +) .... *luo* point of the Spleen, master point of *chong mai*, regulates the Spleen and Stomach, stops bleeding and relieves abdominal pain

Sp.6 (*san yin jiao* +▲) ...... strengthens the Spleen, regulates Liver *qi*, benefits the Kidneys and regulates *qi* and Blood

Bl.20 (*pi shu* +▲) .... *shu* point of the Spleen, warms and supplements Spleen *qi*

Bl.25 (*da chang shu* +▲) .. *shu* point of the Large Intestine, warms and regulates the Intestine

Du.20 (*bai hui* ▲) .... strong moxa to help raise *yang* and astringe the Intestines for difficult to control bleeding or prolapse

- A moxa box over the abdomen is recommended, or strong moxa on Ren.8 (*shen que*), usually on salt. Place a piece of thin cloth over the navel and fill it with salt. Burn large cones of moxa on the salt. The cloth enables quick removal of the salt and prevents burning of the skin.
- with Kidney *yang* deficiency, add Bl.23 (*shen shu* +▲) and Ren.4 (*guan yuan* +▲)
- *Ear points*: spleen, stomach, large intestine, small intestine, adrenal, subcortex, *shen men*

Clinical notes

- Spleen and Stomach *yang* deficiency haemafecia may be diagnosed biomedically as chronic peptic ulcer disease, vascular malformation, Crohn's disease, chronic ulcerative colitis, thrombocytopenia, intestinal polyps, haemorrhoids or haemophilia.
- Spleen *yang* deficiency haemafecia is a chronic condition. The bleeding may clear up relatively quickly, but the *yang* deficiency will usually take a long time (6-12 months) to correct.
- For dietary recommendations, see p.873.

陰虛火旺

11.8 STOMACH YIN DEFICIENCY WITH HEAT

Pathophysiology

- Stomach *yin* deficiency is usually a complication of some other long standing pathology, most commonly Liver *qi* invading the Stomach, or the chronic Heat patterns. It can also be more acute, following damage to Stomach *yin* from a febrile illness, such as *yang ming* syndrome.
- Stomach *yin* is a relatively superficial form of *yin* and in the early stages of depletion may be primarily associated with dryness and fluid damage, rather than the classical deficiency Heat signs and symptoms. In the case of bleeding however, the *yin* depletion is such that significant deficient Heat is usually present.
- The bleeding is the result of the deficient Heat causing Blood to be ejected from the vessels and the thinning and damage of the Stomach lining as the *yin* is depleted.

Clinical features

- black, sticky, tarry or dark dry stools, or tendency to constipation or pellet like stools
- persistent, dull, nagging, epigastric pain
- indeterminate gnawing hunger, heartburn, morning nausea
- general dryness of the skin, mucous membranes and hair, thirst
- facial and malar flushing, nightsweats
- sensation of heat in the palms and soles ('five hearts hot')
- with Kidney *yin* deficiency: dizziness, tinnitus, lower back and knees sore and weak

T slightly red and peeled in the centre, or red and dry with little or no coat; in severe or long standing cases, the tongue may be so denuded of papillae as to resemble a piece of liver (mirror tongue), or have numerous surface cracks or a wide shallow central crack

P thready and rapid

Treatment principle

Nourish *yin* and clear Heat
Cool the Blood and stop bleeding

Prescription

YU NU JIAN 玉女煎
(*Jade Woman Decoction*) modified

shi gao (Gypsum) 石膏 18-30g
sheng di (Radix Rehmanniae Glutinosae) 生地 18-30g
mai dong (Tuber Ophiopogonis Japonici) 麦冬 9-12g

zhi mu (Rhizoma Anemarrhenae Asphodeloides) 知母 9-12g
mu dan pi (Cortex Moutan Radicis) 牡丹皮 9-12g
ce bai ye (Cacumen Biotae Orientalis) 侧柏叶 12-15g
han lian cao (Herba Ecliptae Prostratae) 旱连草 12-15g
qian cao gen (Radix Rubiae Cordifoliae) 茜草根 12-15g

Method: Decoction. **Shi gao** and **zhi mu** clear Heat from the Stomach; **sheng di** cools the Blood and nourishes *yin*; **mai dong** and **han lian cao** clear Heat and nourish *yin*; **mu dan pi** cools the Blood; **ce bai ye** and **qian cao gen** cool the Blood and stop bleeding. (Source: *Xiao Hua Ke Zhuan Bing*)

Modifications

- With severe bleeding, add **bai ji** (Rhizoma Bletillae Striatae) 白芨 12-15g, **zi zhu cao** (Folium Callicarpae) 紫珠草 12-15g, **e jiao** (Gelatinum Corii Asini) 阿胶 9-12g (melted in the hot strained decoction) and **ou jie** (Nodus Nelumbinis Nuciferae Rhizomatis) 藕节12-15g to astringe the Stomach and stop bleeding.
- With *qi* deficiency add **dang shen** (Radix Codonopsis Pilosulae) 党参 15-24g.
- With constipation, add **sheng he shou wu** (unprocessed Radix Polygoni Multiflori) 生何首乌 12-15g and **huo ma ren** (Semen Cannabis Sativae) 火麻仁 9-12g.
- With significant or nagging pain, include herbs that gently move *qi* without damaging *yin*. These include **fo shou** (Fructus Citri Sarcodacylis) 佛手 9-12g, **ba yue zha** (Fructus Akebiae) 八月扎 9-12g, **mei gui hua** (Flos Rosae Rugosae) 玫瑰花 6-9g or **xiang yuan pi** (Pericarpium Citri Medica) 香橼皮 9-12g.
- With acid reflux, heartburn, burning pain and nausea, add **wu zhu yu** (Fructus Evodiae Rutaecarpae) 吴茱萸 1-2g and **huang lian** (Rhizoma Coptidis) 黄连 3-6g, or add **duan wa leng zi** (calcined Concha Arcae) 煅瓦楞子 15g.
- With Kidney *yin* deficiency, combine with the patent medicine *Liu Wei Di Huang Wan* 六味地黄丸 (Liu Wei Di Huang Wan, Six Flavour Tea) or *Zhi Bai Ba Wei Wan* 知柏八味丸 (Zhi Bai Ba Wei Wan, Chih Pai Pa Wei Wan)

Patent medicines

Gu Ben Wan 固本丸 (Gu Ben Wan, Ren Shen Ku Pen Wan)
- Stomach *qi* and *yin* deficiency

Zhi Bai Ba Wei Wan 知柏八味丸 (Zhi Bai Ba Wei Wan, Chih Pai Pa Wei Wan) - with marked deficient Heat symptoms

Sheng Mai San Wan 生脉散丸 (Sheng Mai San Wan)
- Stomach *qi* and *yin* deficiency

Liu Wei Di Huang Wan 六味地黄丸 (Liu Wei Di Huang Wan, Six Flavour Tea) - Kidney *yin* deficiency

Sheng Tian Qi Pian 生田七片 (Raw Tian Qi Ginseng Tablets)
- A good general medicine for bleeding. Combine with an appropriate constitutional patent medicine or the primary prescription.

Yun Nan Bai Yao 云南白药 (Yunnan Paiyao)
- The premier medicine for all types of bleeding. Combine with an appropriate constitutional patent medicine or the primary prescription. The red pill that accompanies the powder is only used in severe cases.

Acupuncture (select from)

Ren.12 (*zhong wan*) .... together these points supplement Stomach *qi* and *yin*
Sp.6 (*san yin jiao* +)
St.36 (*zu san li* +)

St.25 (*tian shu* -) .... *mu* point of the Large Intestine, regulates Intestinal function
Ren.4 (*guan yuan* +) .... meeting point of the *yin* channels, with Sp.6 to supplement the *yin* and *yuan qi* of the body
Bl.25 (*da chang shu* +) ...... *shu* point of the Large Intestine, regulates Intestinal function

Bl.20 (*pi shu* +) .... *shu* points of the Spleen and Stomach respectively, strengthen the Spleen and Stomach and supplement *qi* and *yin*
Bl.21 (*wei shu* +)

Bl.23 (*shen shu* +) .... these points strengthen the source of all inherited *yin*, the Kidney, releasing stored *yin* to support Stomach *yin*
Kid.6 (*zhao hai* +)
Kid.3 (*tai xi* +)

- Patients with *yin* deficiency patterns are often hypersensitive to needles so a gentle approach with few points is recommended to begin with.
- *Ear points*: stomach, kidney, large intestine, distal segment rectum, *shen men*, sympathetic

Clinical notes

- Stomach *yin* deficiency haemafecia may be diagnosed biomedically as bleeding peptic ulcers, atrophic gastritis, chronic colitis, stomach cancer and chronic dysentery.
- This can be a difficult pattern to treat successfully, but may respond reasonably well to prolonged treatment. In long standing cases, 6-12 months of treatment may be necessary for a satisfactory result. More recent cases that follow a febrile illness will usually respond faster.
- For dietary recommendations, see p.876.

SUMMARY OF GUIDING FORMULAE FOR HAEMAFECIA

Excess patterns

Stomach Heat/Fire - *Xie Xin Tang* 泻心汤 plus *Shi Hui San* 十灰散
- with *yin* deficiency - *Huang Lian E Jiao Tang* 黄连阿胶汤

Liver *qi* invading the Stomach with stagnant Heat or Fire - *Dan Zhi Xiao Yao San* 丹栀逍遥散
- with little or no Heat - *Chai Hu Shu Gan San* 柴胡疏肝散

Blood stagnation - *Shi Xiao San* 失笑散 + *Dan Shen Yin* 丹参饮
- with Liver involvement - *Ge Xia Zhu Yu Tang* 膈下逐瘀汤
- in the lower Intestine with Cold - *Shao Fu Zhu Yu Tang* 少腹逐瘀汤
- severe, with Heat - *Tao He Cheng Qi Tang* 桃核承气汤

Intestinal Wind - *Huai Hua San* 槐花散

Damp Heat in the Large Intestine - *Di Yu San* 地榆散
- lingering Damp Heat and mild *yin* deficiency - *Zhu Ju Wan* 驻车丸
- with Liver and Kidney *yin* deficiency - *Liu Wei Di Huang Wan* 六味地黄丸 plus *Zhu Ju Wan* 驻车丸

Deficient patterns

Spleen *qi* deficiency - *Bu Zhong Yi Qi Tang* 补中益气汤
- in persistent cases - *Gu Chong Tang* 固冲汤
- with Heart and Spleen deficiency - *Gui Pi Tang* 归脾汤

Spleen *yang* deficiency - *Huang Tu Tang* 黄土汤
- with severe Spleen *yang* deficiency - *Fu Zi Li Zhong Wan* 附子理中丸

Stomach *yin* deficiency - *Yu Nu Jian* 玉女煎

12. Haematemesis

Excess patterns

Heat in the *ying*/Blood
Stomach Heat/Fire
Damp Heat injuring the Stomach
Liver Fire invading the Stomach
Food stagnation
Blood stagnation

Deficient patterns

Spleen and Stomach *qi* deficiency
Stomach *yin* deficiency with Heat

12 HAEMATEMESIS

tu xue 吐血

Haematemesis is vomiting of blood. The source of the bleeding is usually the upper digestive tract, typically the stomach and oesophagus. The blood may be fresh red, mixed with partially digested food, or dark and lumpy, resembling coffee grounds. Fresh red blood suggests an arterial or variceal source. Dark lumpy blood suggests that the bleeding is sufficiently slow for the blood to linger in the stomach long enough to be digested. Gastric acids convert red haemoglobin to brown haematin.

Bleeding from the gastro-intestinal tract can cause blood to appear in the stools, or to be vomited. In most respects, these disease symptoms (haematemesis and haemafecia) are similar, and indeed there are numerous overlaps. For example, Heat in the Stomach can cause both haematemesis and haemafecia, and usually relates to some pathology of the stomach wall, such as a bleeding gastric or duodenal ulcer.

From a TCM point of view, the difference is one of location and intensity. To force Blood to go up, be ejected through the mouth and appear as haematemesis, a powerful pathogen is required, usually Fire or Toxic Heat. Damp Heat may be sufficiently severe to cause haematemesis, but is more likely to sink into the Large Intestine and cause haemafecia. Similarly, deficiency patterns are more likely to cause haemafecia than haematemesis because the blood tends to seep or leak slowly from the vessels, and without the propelling force of an upward moving pathogen like Heat, descends to appears as haemafecia.

The most common causes of haematemesis are the excess Heat patterns, usually Stomach Heat and/or chronic Liver *qi* stagnation that generates Heat or Fire, or Toxic Heat or Damp Heat.

AETIOLOGY

External pathogens

Invasion of external pathogens directly into the Stomach, or through the surface *tai yang* level into *yang ming*, can cause haematemesis. The most common pathogen is Heat, or Cold that transforms into Heat in the body. Any pathogen can, however, penetrate through the Six Divisions (*liu jing*) or the Four Levels (*wei, qi, ying, xue*) into the Blood (*see* Vol.1). Once the Stomach is heated sufficiently, or Heat has entered the Blood, the Blood is quickened and forced from the vessels.

In addition, in any pattern where violent vomiting is a feature, the wall of the stomach or oesophagus may be breached by the repeated spasm, and blood vessels may burst. This type of haematemesis tends to be a one off event clearly related to another pathology, such as virulent Summerdamp, Summerheat, or Sudden Turmoil Disorder. Eating spoiled or contaminated food can produce severe acute vomiting with bleeding, resembling in TCM terms, an acute invasion of external Damp, Damp Heat or Summerheat.

> **BOX 12.1 SOME BIOMEDICAL CAUSES OF HAEMATEMESIS**
>
> **Stomach**
> - peptic ulcers (most common)
> - vascular lesions
> - gastritis
> - gastric carcinoma
> - hiatus hernia
> - foreign body
> - post operative
> - ingestion of toxins
>
> **Oesophagus**
> - ruptured oesophageal varices
> - reflux oesophagitis
> - Mallory-Weiss tear
> - carcinoma
>
> **Medications**
> - aspirin, NSAID's (common)
> - antiplatelet agents
> - steroids
> - heparin
> - coumarin (warfarin)
>
> **Other**
> - coagulation disorders
>
> **Caution**
> - blood originating from the nasal passage, mouth or pharynx

Diet

A variety of dietary factors can contribute to haematemesis. Over consumption in general, and large quantities of foods that heat the Stomach and Liver, in particular alcohol, chillies and spices, coffee, chocolate and rich, heating or oily foods, can cause Heat and/or Damp Heat or food to accumulate in the Stomach. Haematemesis provoked by alcohol, was noted as far back as 600AD, during the Sui dynasty. Once Heat is resident, Stomach *yin* can easily be damaged.

Overeating repeatedly, or eating large quantities of hard to digest or rich and supplementing foods can cause food stagnation (*see* p.3). Repeated or chronic food stagnation can physically damage the Stomach wall and cause bleeding. In addition, food stagnation frequently leads to the development of Heat or Damp Heat, which can cause the Blood to move recklessly.

In addition to the various dietary factors that can generate too much Heat, habits that damage and deplete Spleen *qi* or *yang* can contribute to haematemesis by disrupting the Spleen's function of holding Blood inside the vessels. Spleen *qi* or *yang* deficiency is uncommon as a primary cause of haematemesis, but will commonly complicate an excess pattern as a secondary effect.

Emotion

Emotional stress is an important contributor to haematemesis. Frustration, anger, bitterness, resentment and repressed emotion can disrupt the distribution of Liver *qi*. As the obstructed *qi* accumulates and the pressure builds, the *qi* seeks an alternative escape route, and will often find it along the controlling cycle, weakening the Spleen and/or Stomach.

Even at a mild level, Liver *qi* stagnation can contribute to bleeding in the gastro-intestinal tract by repeatedly invading the Stomach, and disrupting the integrity of the Stomach wall. However it is the complications of prolonged *qi* stagnation that more commonly contribute to haematemesis. The prolonged pressure created by the stagnation can create Heat which, depending on duration and the intensity of the aetiological conditions, can develop into stagnant Heat or the more severe Fire. Fire rises upwards, can cause Blood to move recklessly, and scorches delicate *luo mai*, thus contributing to relatively severe haematemesis and/or *yin* damage. Liver Fire frequently causes Stomach Fire, as the Fire invades along the controlling cycle.

Long term *qi* stagnation can lead to Blood stagnation.

Other emotions, such as worry, obsessive thinking and prolonged excessive concentration in combination with a sedentary lifestyle and poor diet, can weaken the Spleen, predisposing it to (or inviting) invasion by Liver *qi* resulting in further damage.

Spleen and Stomach deficiency

The Spleen is responsible for maintaining the integrity of the Blood vessels, that is, Spleen *qi* prevents Blood from leaking out of the vessels. Bleeding of a Spleen *qi* deficiency type tends to be mild, chronic and persistent. *Qi* and *yang* deficiency haematemesis is unusual, and generally a chronic condition, although it can follow gastro-intestinal surgery or excessive ingestion of cold substances.

Overwork, excessive worry or mental activity, irregular dietary habits or prolonged illness can weaken Spleen *qi*. The most common causes of Spleen *yang* deficiency are deterioration of Spleen *qi* deficiency, prolonged or excessive consumption of cold, raw food, irregular eating habits, or consumption of too many cold natured herbs or antibiotics in the treatment of a febrile disease. Prolonged insult to the Stomach or severely limited food intake, as occurs in patients with bulimia and anorexia nervosa, seriously damage Spleen and Stomach *yang qi*. The damage is aggravated when an irregular diet is combined with sustained mental activity and too much sitting. The Spleen and Stomach can also be weakened following an acute invasion of Cold and/or Dampness. Gastric surgery can deplete Spleen *yang* and can cause Blood stagnation.

Stomach *yin* deficiency usually follows years of invasion by Liver *qi* or damage from chronic Liver or Stomach Heat. Stomach *yin* deficiency can also follow an acute febrile disease, such as *yang ming* syndrome. Long term consumption of spicy heating foods or drugs, such as *yang* supplementing substances and amphetamines is becoming more common. Prolonged or excessive vomiting, dehydration, or another chronic Stomach pathology, especially one characterised by Heat, may also be implicated.

Blood stagnation

Blood stagnation is an important cause of haematemesis, especially in older patients. Blood stagnation is most commonly the result of chronic Liver *qi* stagnation. It may also be caused by dietary factors that introduce Cold, Heat, Damp Heat and Phlegm, or by trauma. By its very nature, *qi* stagnation will ultimately lead to Blood stagnation as the '*qi* leads the Blood'. Cold retards the circulation if *qi* and Blood. Heat injures the Stomach and Intestine by drying and scorching its delicate *luo mai*. Phlegm and Damp Heat, being substantial pathogens and particularly cloying in nature, physically obstruct the circulation of *qi* and Blood at some point. An acute trauma to the Stomach can also contribute to Blood stagnation and haematemesis. Gastric surgery, a blow to the epigastric region or a penetrating injury from a motor vehicle accident are some examples.

Medications

Numerous therapeutic agents, both herbal or pharmaceutical, can contribute to haematemesis. The most common are nonsteroidal anti-inflammatory drugs (NSAIDs), aspirin, corticosteroids and alcohol. Some *yang* supplementing, or heating herbs, can cause bleeding in sensitive individuals if used inappropriately. Anticoagulants such as coumarin may also be implicated. Medications are so commonly implicated in both acute and chronic bleeding in the digestive tract that a thorough examination of all current and recent medications, supplements and herbs is essential.

TREATMENT

There are several steps to consider when treating any bleeding disorder. The first step is to stop the bleeding. When the bleeding is severe, the initial focus of treatment is to use first aid or herbs to quickly staunch the bleeding. This can usually be achieved with a styptic formulae (Box 12.2, p.452), or with the use of the patent medicine *Yun Nan Bai Yao* 云南白药 (Yunnan Paiyao).

Once bleeding has ceased, or is under control, the underlying pattern can be dealt with more fully. There are two additional aspects to consider. Any residual Blood outside the vessels is stagnant Blood, which must be removed. Thus, herbs to gently invigorate or regulate Blood are incorporated into the appropriate formula. This is especially important in Heat types of bleeding, as the herbs used to stop bleeding will likely be cold natured and astringent. These herbs congeal Blood. Thus the skilful practitioner will need

BOX 12.2 MEASURES TO QUICKLY STOP BLEEDING

Heat types

- Powdered **sheng da huang** 生大黄 (Radix et Rhizoma Rhei) 3g, **bai ji** 白芨 (Rhizoma Bletillae Striatae) 3g and **san qi** 三七 (Radix Notoginseng) 3g can be mixed and taken 3-4 times daily.
- The patent medicine *Yun Nan Bai Yao* 云南白药 (Yunnan Paiyao) taken with a little water.
- Equal quantities of powdered **sheng da huang** 生大黄 (Radix et Rhizoma Rhei) and powdered **hai piao xiao** 海螵蛸 (Os Sepiae seu Sepiellae) can be packed into single or double O gelatin capules and taken 4-6 at a time, 3-4 times daily. Especially good for bleeding with reflux.
- Decoct **sheng di** 生地 (Radix Rehmanniae Glutinosae) 30g in 2 cups of water for 30 minutes then discard the dregs. Add powdered **sheng da huang** 生大黄 (Radix et Rhizoma Rhei) 2g and drink in small doses frequently.
- A decoction of **xian he cao** 仙鹤草 (Herba Agrimoniae Pilosae) 30g, **bai ji** 白芨 (Rhizoma Bletillae Striatae) 30g, **di yu tan** 地榆炭 (charred Radix Sanguisorbae Officinalis) 30g and **huai hua** 槐花 (Flos Sophora Japonicae Immaturus) 15g, sipped frequently until bleeding slows or stops. Then measures may be taken to clear Stomach Heat.

Blood stagnation type

- The patent medicine *Yun Nan Bai Yao* 云南白药 (Yunnan Paiyao) taken with a little water.
- The patent medicine *Sheng Tian Qi Pian* 生田七片 (Raw Tian Qi Ginseng Tablets) taken with a little water.

Deficient types

- The patent medicine *Yun Nan Bai Yao* 云南白药 (Yunnan Paiyao) taken with a little water.
- Powder and mix equal amounts of **bai ji** 白芨 (Rhizoma Bletillae Striatae) and **ce bai ye** 侧柏叶 (Cacumen Biotae Orientalis) and take in doses of 3-6 grams, 3-4 times daily.

to combine treatments from overlapping patterns and be ever mindful of changes in the symptom picture during treatment. Finally, any *qi* or Blood deficiency that exists as a direct result of Blood loss should be supplemented.

Figure 12.1 *Diagnostic strategy for haematemesis*

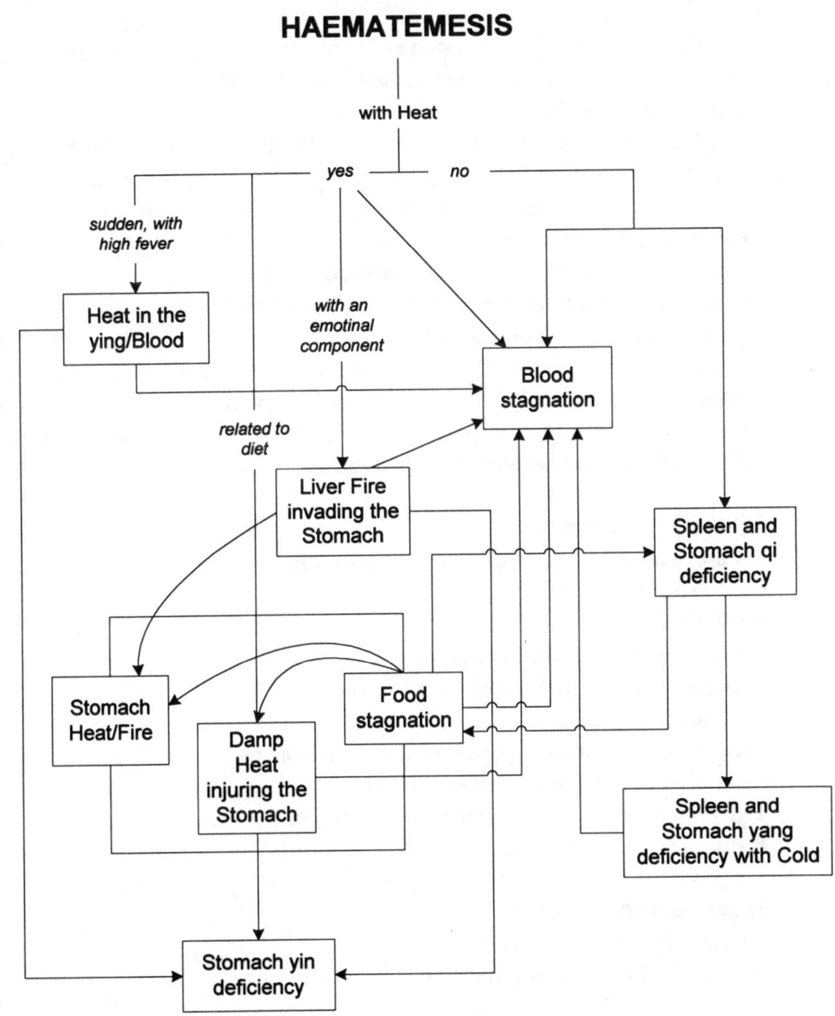

热伤营血

12.1 HEAT IN THE YING/BLOOD

Pathophysiology

- Heat can penetrate to the *ying* and/or Blood level (of the 4 levels, *see* Vol. 1) if *wei qi* is weak or if a pathogen is particularly strong. The pathogen that usually gives rise to haematemesis is Heat, although other pathogens may turn hot once in the body.
- The bleeding occurs because the heated Blood is forcibly ejected from the vessels of the Stomach. The pattern is usually acute, the patient having been relatively well prior to the episode. In cases where there is pre-existing pathology, the patient is likely to have a history of Liver and Stomach Fire, and this pattern represents an acute exacerbation.
- Blood stagnation is a common sequel to this pattern for two reasons. Firstly the severe Heat 'evaporates and congeals' the Blood. Secondly, therapeutic efforts are usually based on swift cessation of the bleeding with large amounts of bitter, cold or astringent substances, which can cool and congeal the Blood. It is common practice to use Blood moving strategies in the aftermath or convalescent stage of febrile illnesses.

Clinical features

- acute, violent vomiting of fresh red blood in a patient with a high fever
- red face, lips and eyes
- dry mouth, thirst
- restlessness, irritability, insomnia
- constipation, or sticky, dark, tarry stools
- concentrated urine
- red or purple subcutaneous bleeding or febrile rashes
- disturbances of consciousness, delirium

T deep red or scarlet, with raised red spots on the edges
P flooding, big and rapid, or thready and rapid

Treatment principle

Clear Heat and Toxic Heat
Cool the Blood to stop bleeding

Prescription

SHUI NIU JIAO DI HUANG TANG 水牛角地黄汤
(*Water Buffalo Horn and Rehmannia Decoction*) modified

shui niu jiao (Cornu Bubali) 水牛角 30g
sheng di (Radix Rehmanniae Glutinosae) 生地 30g
chi shao (Radix Paeoniae Rubrae) 赤芍 12g
mu dan pi (Cortex Moutan Radicis) 牡丹皮 12g

ce bai ye (Cacumen Biotae Orientalis) 侧柏叶 15g
bai mao gen (Rhizoma Imperatae Cylindricae) 白茅根 30g
qian cao gen (Radix Rubiae Cordifoliae) 茜草根 15g

Method: Decoction. **Shui niu jiao** is powdered and decocted for 30 minute before the other herbs are added (*xian jian* 先煎). **Shui niu jiao** clears Fire, cools the Blood and clears Toxic Heat; **sheng di** clears Heat, cools the Blood, stops bleeding and nourishes *yin*; **chi shao** and **mu dan pi** cool the Blood and invigorate the Blood (to assist in preventing Blood stagnation as a result of the Cold substances); **qian cao gen** cools the Blood, stops bleeding and assists in invigorating Blood; **ce bai ye** and **bai mao gen** cool the Blood and stop bleeding. (Source: *Shi Yong Zhong Yi Nei Ke Xue*)

NB. This prescription originally used the horn (**xi jiao** 犀角) of the severely endangered rhinoceros, and was called **Xi Jiao Di Huang Tang**.

Modifications

- With severe bleeding, add **san qi fen** (powdered Radix Notoginseng) 三七粉 6-9g or combine with the patent medicine *Yun Nan Bai Yao* 云南白药 (Yunnan Paiyao).
- With severe fever (and probably in most cases at this stage) herbs such as **da qing ye** (Folium Daqingye) 大青叶 15-24g, **ban lan gen** (Radix Isatidis seu Baphicacanthi) 板蓝根 15-24g and **zi cao** (Radix Lithospermi) 紫草 12-15g are added to enhance the cooling and Toxic Heat clearing effect.
- With Blood stasis (purplish rashes or blood), add **tao ren** (Semen Persicae) 桃仁 6-9g and **dan shen** (Radix Salviae Miltiorrhizae) 丹参 9-12g.

Variations and additional prescriptions

Post acute phase with qi and yin deficiency and Blood stagnation

- During the convalescent phase of this pattern, patients will often suffer the effects of damaged *qi* and *yin*, and stagnant Blood. Suitable prescriptions to clear residual Heat and augment *qi* and *yin* include **ZHU YE SHI GAO TANG** (*Lophatherus and Gypsum Decoction* 竹叶石膏汤, p.835) with the addition of **dan shen** (Radix Salviae Miltiorrhizae) 丹参 12-18g, to invigorate stagnant Blood.

Severe bleeding precipitating collapse of yang

- Severe blood loss can lead to sudden collapse of *yang* (a type of *jue zheng* 厥证). In addition to the appropriate first aid (keeping the patient warm, leg elevation, airway clear etc.), **SHEN FU TANG** (*Ginseng and Prepared Aconite Decoction* 参附汤, p.458) may be administered.

Patent medicines

Niu Huang Qing Huo Wan 牛黄清火丸 (Niu Huang Qing Huo Wan)
Sheng Tian Qi Pian 生田七片 (Raw Tian Qi Ginseng Tablets)
- A good general medicine for bleeding. Combine with an appropriate constitutional patent medicine or the primary prescription.

Yun Nan Bai Yao 云南白药 (Yunnan Paiyao)

- The premier medicine for all types of bleeding. Combine with an appropriate constitutional patent medicine or the primary prescription. The red pill that accompanies the powder is only used in severe cases.

Acupuncture (select from)

PC.3 (*qu ze* ↓) .... *he* sea points of the Pericardium and Urinary
Bl.40 (*wei zhong* ↓) Bladder channel respectively, these points cool the Blood and assist in stopping vomiting when bled

PC.9 (*zhong chong* ↓) .... *jing* well and Wood point of the Pericardium, clears Heat, cools the Blood

LI.11 (*qu chi* -) .... *he* sea point of the Large Intestine, clears Heat and Dampness from *yang ming*, eliminates pathogens

Du.14 (*da zhui* -) .... meeting point of the *yang* channels, excellent for clearing Heat

Du.26 (*ren zhong* -) .... this point is useful in situations of shock due to blood loss

- with unrelenting fever, add *shi xuan* ↓ (M-UE-1)
- with spasms or convulsions, add Du.12 (*shen zhu* -), LI.4 (*he gu* -) and Liv.3 (*tai chong* -)
- with severe nausea, add PC.6 (*nei guan*)
- with severe headache, add *tai yang* ↓ (M-HN-9)
- *Ear points*: stomach, duodenum, *shen men*, lungs, heart, adrenal, subcortex

Clinical notes

- The bleeding in this pattern may be associated with severe infections such as meningococcal meningitis, encephalitis, epidemic haemorrhagic fever and septicaemia, or leukaemic crisis.
- This condition is potentially dangerous and should be managed in hospital.

胃中积热

12.2 STOMACH HEAT/FIRE

Pathophysiology

- Stomach Heat is usually associated with an excessively heating diet, medications or drugs. Stagnant Heat from Liver *qi* stagnation may also contribute.
- The mechanism involves the Blood forcefully ejected from the vessels by the accumulated Heat.

Clinical features

- vomiting, possibly violent, of fresh red or dark purple blood, or blood mixed with undigested food material
- epigastric and abdominal distension and pain or burning sensation
- bitter taste in the mouth, acid reflux, heartburn
- dry mouth, thirst with a desire for cold drinks
- halitosis, belching
- tendency to constipation, or dry stools, or black sticky tarry stools
- irritability, restlessness

T red and dry with a thick, dry, yellow coat
P wiry and rapid or slippery and rapid

Treatment principle

Clear Heat from the Stomach to stop bleeding

Prescription

XIE XIN TANG 泻心汤
(*Coptis and Rhubarb Combination*) plus
SHI HUI SAN 十灰散
(*Ten Partially Charred Substance Powder*) modified

da huang (Radix et Rhizoma Rhei) 大黄 6-9g
huang qin (Radix Scutellariae Baicalensis) 黄芩 12-15g
huang lian (Rhizoma Coptidis) 黄连 6-9g
shan zhi zi (Fructus Gardeniae Jasminoidis) 山栀子 9-12g
da ji (Herba seu Radix Cirsii Japonicii) 大蓟 15-30g
xiao ji (Herba Cephalanoplos) 小蓟 15-30g
ce bai ye (Cacumen Biotae Orientalis) 侧柏叶 15-30g
bai ji (Rhizoma Bletillae Striatae) 白芨 15-30g
bai mao gen (Rhizoma Imperatae Cylindricae) 白茅根 15-30g
qian cao gen (Radix Rubiae Cordifoliae) 茜草根 12-15g
mu dan pi (Cortex Moutan Radicis) 牡丹皮 9-12g

Method: Decoction or powder. The styptic ingredients of this formula were traditionally prepared as a powder after being partially burnt, a process thought to improve their haemostatic action. When powdered, the herbs should be briefly decocted before ingestion. The uncharred herbs seem to work as well in decoction. **Da Huang**, **huang lian**, **huang qin** and **shan zhi zi** clear Heat and purge Fire; **da huang** is an important herb to stop bleeding in the upper body; **da ji**, **xiao ji**, **ce bai ye** and **bai mao gen** cool the Blood and stop bleeding; **bai ji** astringes to stop bleeding; **qian cao gen** and **mu dan pi** cool and regulate the Blood to stop bleeding while preventing Blood stagnation from excessive cooling. (Source: *Zhong Yi Nei Ke Ji Zheng Zheng Zhi*)

Modifications

- When Heat is intense or prolonged, it can 'cook and congeal' Blood, causing Blood stagnation. Blood stagnation is indicated when there are clots of dark blood in the stools or when abdominal pain is relatively severe. With Blood stagnation, add **san qi fen** (powdered Radix Notoginseng) 三七粉 3-6g to invigorate Blood and stop bleeding.
- With Fire, add one or two of the following herbs: **huang qin** (Radix Scutellariae Baicalensis) 黄芩 9-12g, **ban lan gen** (Radix Isatidis seu Baphicacanthi) 板蓝根 12-18g, **zi hua di ding** (Herba cum Radice Violae Yedoensitis) 紫花地丁 9-12g, **pu gong ying** (Herba Taraxaci Mongolici) 蒲公英 15-30g, **lu gen** (Rhizoma Phragmitis Communis) 芦根 24-30g, **si gua luo** (Fasciculus Vascularis Luffae) 丝瓜络 9-12g and **lu dou** (Semen Phaseoli Radiati) 绿豆 9-12g.
- With persistent, focal, gnawing pain and bleeding (suggestive of gastric ulceration), powder equal amounts of **hai piao xiao** (Os Sepiae seu Sepiellae) 海螵蛸, **bai ji** (Rhizoma Bletillae Striatae) 白芨 and **gan cao** (Radix Glycyrrhizae Uralensis) 甘草 and take 3 grams three times daily.
- With excess gastric acid or heartburn, add **hai piao xiao** (Os Sepiae seu Sepiellae) 海螵蛸 15g and **mu li** (Concha Ostreae) 牡蛎 15g.
- With epigastric pain, add **yan hu suo** (Rhizoma Corydalis Yanhusuo) 延胡索 9-12g and **mu xiang** (Radix Aucklandiae Lappae) 木香 6-9g.
- With nausea, add **zhu ru** (Caulis Bambusae in Taeniis) 竹茹 9-12g, **xuan fu hua** (Flos Inulae) 旋复花 12-15g and **dai zhe shi** (Haematitum) 代赭石 15g.
- With severe thirst, add **shi hu** (Herba Dendrobii) 石斛 12-15g and **tian hua fen** (Radix Trichosanthes Kirilowii) 天花粉 12-15g.
- With constipation or dry stools, add **xuan shen** (Radix Scrophulariae Ningpoensis) 玄参 18-24g, **mai dong** (Tuber Ophiopogonis Japonici) 麦冬 9-12g and **sheng di** (Radix Rehmanniae Glutinosae) 生地 12-18g.

Variations and additional prescriptions

Severe bleeding precipitating collapse of yang

- Severe blood loss can lead to sudden collapse of *yang* (a type of *jue zheng* 厥证, Flaccid Collapse Syndrome, hypovolaemic shock). The features are lethargy, confusion, somnolence, copious sweating, cold clammy limbs, pale or ashen complexion, rapid breathing, a weak rapid pulse. The aim of treatment is to rescue and resuscitate *yang*. In addition to the appropriate first aid (keeping the patient warm, leg elevation, airway clear etc.), an injection of **SHEN FU TANG** (*Ginseng and Prepared Aconite Decoction* 参附汤) can be administered if available. Oral administration is avoided to prevent aspiration should vomiting continue.

ren shen (Radix Ginseng) 人参 9-15g
zhi fu zi (Radix Aconiti Carmichaeli Praeparata)
制附子 9-15g

Method: Intramuscular injection or intravenous drip. This prescription is a standard treatment for shock in China. (Source: *Shi Yong Zhong Yi Nei Ke Xue*)

Patent medicines

Huang Lian Jie Du Wan 黄连解毒丸 (Huang Lian Jie Du Wan)
- Stomach Heat, Damp Heat

Niu Huang Qing Huo Wan 牛黄清火丸 (Niu Huang Qing Huo Wan)
- with constipation

Bei Jing Niu Huang Jie Du Pian 北京牛黄解毒片 (Peking Niu Huang Chieh Tu Pien)
- Stomach Heat, Toxic Heat

Sheng Tian Qi Pian 生田七片 (Raw Tian Qi Ginseng Tablets)
- A good general medicine for bleeding. Combine with an appropriate constitutional patent medicine or the primary prescription.

Yun Nan Bai Yao 云南白药 (Yunnan Paiyao)
- The premier medicine for all types of bleeding. Combine with an appropriate constitutional patent medicine or the primary prescription. The red pill that accompanies the powder is only used in severe cases.

Acupuncture (select from)

Ren.12 (*zhong wan* -) .... *mu* point of the Stomach, clears Heat and regulates *qi* and Blood in the Stomach
PC.4 (*xi men* -) .... *xi* point of the Pericardium, for acute bleeding
Sp.4 (*gong sun*) .... *luo* point of the Spleen, master point of *chong mai*, regulates the Spleen and Stomach and stops bleeding

St.44 (*nei ting* -) .... together these points clear Heat from *yang ming*
LI.4 (*he gu* -)

St.45 (*li dui* ↓) .... powerfully clears Heat from the Stomach when bled

PC.8 (*lao gong* -) .... *rong* spring and Fire point of the Pericardium, drains Heat from the Stomach channel and cools Heart Fire

- with epigastric pain, add St.21 (*liang men* -) and the *xi* cleft point St.34 (*liang qiu* -)
- with nausea, add PC.6 (*nei guan* -)
- with constipation, add St.37 (*shang ju xu* -) and St.25 (*tian shu* -)
- with *yin* deficiency add Bl.21 (*wei shu* +) and Bl.23 (*shen shu* +)
- For *shao yang / yang ming* syndrome, add SJ.5 (*wai guan* -), GB.39 (*xuan zhong* -) and St.25 (*tian shu* -)
- *Ear points*: stomach, duodenum, liver, large intestine, adrenal, subcortex, *shen men*

Clinical notes

- Haematemesis associated with Stomach Heat may be diagnosed biomedically as bleeding peptic ulcer, alcoholic liver disease, gastritis, reflux oesophagitis, ruptured oesophageal varices, meningitis or encephalitis.
- Severe haematemesis is a medical emergency and should be managed in hospital. With appropriate dietary and life habit changes, the Stomach Heat that causes the episodic bleeding is relatively easy to clear.
- For dietary recommendations, see p.882.

湿热伤胃

12.3 DAMP HEAT INJURING THE STOMACH

Pathophysiology

- Damp Heat haematemesis is usually associated with chronic ingestion of substances that introduce Damp Heat directly into the body, most commonly alcohol and a diet of rich spicy foods. The bleeding tends to be sporadic, and set against a background of chronic gastro-intestinal complaints of a Damp Heat type.
- There will often be a degree of Liver Blood stagnation associated with this pattern.

Clinical features

- vomiting of copious amounts of fresh red blood, or dark and lumpy coffee ground like material
- epigastric and abdominal fullness, discomfort and pain
- frequent nausea, loss of appetite
- bitter taste in the mouth
- concentrated urine
- tendency to constipation, or sticky, black, tarry stools

T red body with a thick, greasy, yellow coat
P slippery and rapid, or soft and rapid

Treatment principle

Clear Damp Heat from the Stomach
Cool the Blood and stop bleeding

Prescription

ZHI SHI DAO ZHI WAN 枳实导滞丸
(*Immature Bitter Orange Pill to Guide Out Stagnation*) modified

da huang (Radix et Rhizoma Rhei) 大黄 18g
zhi shi (Fructus Immaturus Citri Aurantii) 枳实 9g
shen qu (Massa Fermentata) 神曲 9g
fu ling (Sclerotium Poriae Cocos) 茯苓 6g
huang qin (Radix Scutellariae Baicalensis) 黄芩 6g
huang lian (Rhizoma Coptidis) 黄连 6g
bai zhu (Rhizoma Atractylodes Macrocephalae) 白术 6g
ze xie (Rhizoma Alismatis Orientalis) 泽泻 6g
ce bai ye (Cacumen Biotae Orientalis) 侧柏叶 12g
sheng di (Radix Rehmanniae Glutinosae) 生地 12g

Method: Grind the ingredients into a powder and form into 9 gram pills. The dose is one pill 2-3 times daily. May also be decocted with the quantity of **da huang** reduced by half. **Da huang** clears Heat and alleviates stagnation; **huang qin** and **huang lian** clear Damp Heat; **fu ling** and **ze xie** promote urination and lead Damp Heat out through the Urinary Bladder; **bai zhu** protects the Spleen and dries Dampness; **shen qu** alleviates food stagnation; **ce bai ye** cools the Blood; **sheng di** cools the Blood, nourishes *yin* and assists **ce bai ye** in stopping bleeding. (Source: *Shi Yong Zhong Yi Nei Ke Xue*)

Modifications

- With severe vomiting and bleeding, add **bai mao gen** (Rhizoma Imperatae Cylindricae) 白茅根 30g, **bai ji** (Rhizoma Bletillae Striatae) 白芨 9-15g and **mu dan pi** (Cortex Moutan Radicis) 牡丹皮 9-12g.
- With Blood stagnation, add **pu huang** (Pollen Typhae) 蒲黄 9-12g and **san qi fen** (powdered Radix Notoginseng) 三七粉 3-6g (added to the strained decoction).
- For patients with alcohol problems, add **ge hua** (Flos Puerariae) 葛花 15g.

Patent medicines

Huang Lian Jie Du Wan 黄连解毒丸 (Huang Lian Jie Du Wan)
- Damp Heat, Stomach Heat

Niu Huang Qing Huo Wan 牛黄清火丸 (Niu Huang Qing Huo Wan)
- with constipation

Bei Jing Niu Huang Jie Du Pian 北京牛黄解毒片 (Peking Niu Huang Chieh Tu Pien)
- Stomach Heat, Toxic Heat

Sheng Tian Qi Pian 生田七片 (Raw Tian Qi Ginseng Tablets)
- A good general medicine for bleeding. Combine with an appropriate constitutional patent medicine or the primary prescription.

Yun Nan Bai Yao 云南白药 (Yunnan Paiyao)
- The premier medicine for all types of bleeding. Combine with an appropriate constitutional patent medicine or the primary prescription. The red pill that accompanies the powder is only used in severe cases.

Acupuncture (select from)

Ren.12 (*zhong wan* -) .... *mu* point of the Stomach, clears Damp Heat

LI.11 (*qu chi* -) .... *he* sea point of the Large Intestine, clears Damp Heat from *yang ming* and stops bleeding

LI.4 (*he gu* -) .... together these points clear Heat and Damp
St.44 (*nei ting* -) Heat from *yang ming*

PC.4 (*xi men* -) .... *xi* point of the Pericardium channel, for acute bleeding

St.36 (*zu san li* -) .... *he* sea point of the Stomach, regulates the

Stomach and stops bleeding

St.37 (*shan ju xu* -) .... lower *he* point of the Large Intestine, clears Damp Heat from the Stomach and Intestines

Sp.9 (*yin ling quan* -) .... *he* sea point of the Spleen, promotes urination and drains Damp Heat through the urine

ah shi points .... along the Urinary Bladder channel between Bl.17 (*ge shu*) and Bl.21 (*wei shu*)

- with epigastric pain, add St.21 (*liang men* -) and the *xi* cleft point St.34 (*liang qiu* -)
- with acid reflux or heartburn, palpate the area around LI.10 (*shou san li*) and needle the most tender point
- with *yin* deficiency add Bl.21 (*wei shu* +) and Bl.23 (*shen shu* +)
- For *shao yang* / *yang ming* syndrome, add SJ.5 (*wai guan* -), GB.39 (*xuan zhong* -) and St.25 (*tian shu* -)
- *Ear points*: stomach, duodenum, liver, large intestine, adrenal, subcortex, *shen men*

Clinical notes

- Damp Heat type haematemesis may be diagnosed biomedically as alcoholic liver disease, bleeding oesophageal varices or bleeding peptic ulcers.
- The Damp Heat that gives rise to this type of haematemesis can be difficult to clear, especially if patients persist in unhealthy habits. With appropriate dietary and life habit changes, however, elimination of the Damp Heat and repair to the damaged organ systems may proceed over a period of some months.
- For dietary recommendations, see p.884.

肝火犯胃

12.4 LIVER FIRE INVADING THE STOMACH

Pathophysiology

- When Liver Fire causes haematemesis, the Blood is quickened and forced from the vessels of the Stomach. The key to this pattern is the relationship of the symptoms to emotional stress, and there will often be a history of emotional tension or high stress. In addition, there are frequently elements of Stomach Heat in this pattern, as the development of Liver Fire is aided by overindulgence in heating foods and beverages.

Clinical features

- Vomiting of fresh red or purple blood, or vomitus stained with blood or containing blood clots. Episodes will often be associated with a period of high stress or emotional turmoil.
- hypochondriac distension and pain
- insomnia, restlessness, excessive dreaming
- bitter taste in the mouth
- irritability, easy anger, hot temper
- pounding temporal headaches
- red, sore eyes

T red or with red edges
P wiry and rapid

Treatment principle

Clear Heat from the Liver and Stomach
Cool the Blood and stop bleeding

Prescription

LONG DAN XIE GAN TANG 龙胆泻肝汤
(*Gentiana Combination*) modified

long dan cao (Radix Gentianae Longdancao) 龙胆草 6-9g
huang qin (Radix Scutellariae Baicalensis) 黄芩 9-12g
shan zhi zi (Fructus Gardeniae Jasminoidis) 山栀子 9-12g
sheng di (Radix Rehmanniae Glutinosae) 生地 15-18g
mu dan pi (Cortex Moutan Radicis) 牡丹皮 9-12g
bai mao gen (Rhizoma Imperatae Cylindricae) 白茅根 15-30g
ou jie (Nodus Nelumbinis Nuciferae Rhizomatis) 藕节 15-30g
han lian cao (Herba Ecliptae Prostratae) 旱连草 12-15g
qian cao gen (Radix Rubiae Cordifoliae) 茜草根 12-15g

Method: Decoction. **Long dan cao**, **huang qin** and **shan zhi zi** cool the Liver and purge Fire; **sheng di** and **mu dan pi** cool the Blood; **mu dan pi** prevents the cooling herbs from causing stagnation; **qian cao gen**, **han lian cao** and **bai mao gen** cool the Blood and stop bleeding; **ou jie** astringes to stop bleeding. (Source:

Shi Yong Zhong Yi Nei Ke Xue)

Modifications

- In chronic or recurrent cases there will usually be elements of Blood stagnation; in this case administer **hua rui shi** (Ophicalcitum) 花蕊石 9-12g and **san qi fen** (powdered Radix Notoginseng) 三七粉 3-6g separately as powder.
- With acid reflux or heartburn, add **huang lian** (Rhizoma Coptidis) 黄连 6g and **wu zhu yu** (Fructus Evodiae Rutaecarpae) 吴茱萸 3g.

Patent medicines

Long Dan Xie Gan Wan 龙胆泻肝丸 (Long Dan Xie Gan Wan)

Sheng Tian Qi Pian 生田七片 (Raw Tian Qi Ginseng Tablets)

- A good general medicine for bleeding. Combine with the above constitutional patent medicine or the primary prescription.

Yun Nan Bai Yao 云南白药 (Yunnan Paiyao)

- The premier medicine for all types of bleeding. Combine with the above constitutional patent medicine or the primary prescription. The red pill that accompanies the powder is only used in severe cases.

Acupuncture (select from)

Ren.12 (*zhong wan* -) .... these points used together harmonise the Stomach, stop bleeding and promote the function of the Spleen and Stomach
St.19 (*bu rong* -)
St.21 (*liang men* -)

Liv.13 (*zhang men* -) .... *mu* point of the Spleen and *hui* point of the *zang*, harmonises the Liver and Spleen

PC.8 (*lao gong* -) .... *rong* spring and Fire point of the Pericardium, drains Heat from the Stomach channel and cools Fire

Liv.2 (*xing jian* -) .... *rong* spring and Fire point of the Liver, drains Fire from the Liver and spreads stagnant *qi*

St.44 (*nei ting* -) .... *rong* spring and Water point of the Stomach, clears Heat from *yang ming*, the Stomach and Stomach channel

Sp.4 (*gong sun* -) .... *luo* point of the Spleen, master point of *chong mai*, regulates the Spleen and Stomach, stops bleeding

St.36 (*zu san li* -) .... *he* sea point of the Stomach, regulates the Stomach and stops bleeding

- with severe bleeding, add PC.4 (*xi men* -) or PC.7 (*da ling* -)

- with nausea, add PC.6 (*nei guan* -)
- with epigastric pain, add St.21 (*liang men* -) and the *xi* cleft point St.34 (*liang qiu* -)
- with hypochondriac pain, add GB.34 (*yang ling quan* -) and Liv.14 (*qi men* -)
- *Ear points*: liver, stomach, *shen men*, large intestine, lungs, adrenal, subcortex

Clinical notes

- Liver Fire type haematemesis may be diagnosed biomedically as bleeding oesophageal varices, peptic ulcer disease, acute gastritis, reflux oesophagitis or alcoholic liver disease.
- The bleeding in this pattern will usually respond reasonably quickly to correct treatment, especially with herbs. The underlying Liver *qi* stagnation and Fire can respond well to correct treatment, if modifications are made to diet, lifestyle and attitude. For long term results, reduction of stress triggers, stress management and daily exercise are essential to keep the *qi* moving and prevent development of Heat. Acupuncture is of particular benefit for long term results, as over time, it appears to be able to alter and improve the physiological response of the patient to stressors. To achieve this however, at least one and preferably more courses of treatment should be given over some months.
- For dietary recommendations, see p.878, 882.

积滞伤胃

12.5 FOOD STAGNATION

Pathophysiology

- Food stagnation can contribute to haematemesis by habitually overloading the Stomach, over time weakening the delicate *luo mai* of the Stomach wall. In addition to the physical damage to the Stomach, repeated food stagnation easily causes accumulation of Heat or Damp Heat.
- The key feature of food stagnation patterns is the relationship of the symptoms to the volume of food the patient ingests.
- This is an uncommon form of haematemesis when uncomplicated by Heat.

Clinical features

- Vomiting of fresh red blood or blood streaked undigested food material. The haematemesis may be provoked by a particularly large or indigestible meal.
- abdominal and epigastric pain, fullness and distension, alleviated by belching, vomiting or defecation and worse for pressure and eating
- foul sour belching, flatulence
- loss of appetite, aversion to food
- acid reflux, heartburn
- constipation, sluggish stools or diarrhoea, or black, tarry, sticky stools

T thick, greasy, maybe yellow coat
P slippery, may be rapid

Treatment principle

Alleviate food stagnation
Harmonise the Stomach, stop bleeding
Clear Heat

Prescription

BAO HE WAN 保和丸
(*Citrus and Crategus Formula*) modified

shan zha (Fructus Crataegi) 山楂 18-24g
shen qu (Massa Fermentata) 神曲 12-15g
lai fu zi (Semen Raphani Sativi) 莱服子 9-12g
ban xia (Rhizoma Pinelliae Ternatae) 半夏 9-12g
chen pi (Pericarpium Citri Reticulatae) 陈皮 6-9g
fu ling (Sclerotium Poriae Cocos) 茯苓 12-15g
lian qiao (Fructus Forsythia Suspensae) 连翘 6-9g
qian cao gen (Radix Rubiae Cordifoliae) 茜草根 12-15g
han lian cao (Herba Ecliptae Prostratae) 旱连草 12-15g
mu dan pi (Cortex Moutan Radicis) 牡丹皮 9-12g

chi shao (Radix Paeoniae Rubrae) 赤芍 9-12g
san qi fen (powdered Radix Notoginseng) 三七粉 3-6g

Method: Grind herbs to a powder and form into 9 gram pills with water. The dose is one pill twice daily. May also be decocted with the quantities as shown. **Shan zha** and **shen qu** improve digestion and alleviate food stagnation; **lai fu zi** improves digestion, transforms Phlegm and directs *qi* downwards; **ban xia**, **chen pi** and **fu ling** transform Dampness and harmonise the Stomach; **lian qiao** clears Heat and disperses accumulations; **qian cao gen** and **han lian cao** cool the Blood and stop bleeding; **mu dan pi**, **chi shao** and **san qi** stop bleeding and prevent Blood stagnation. (Source: *Shi Yong Zhong Yi Nei Ke Xue*)

Modifications

- With severe distension or reflux, add **zhi shi** (Fructus Immaturus Citri Aurantii) 枳实 9-12g and **bing lang** (Semen Arecae Catechu) 槟榔 9-12g.
- With constipation, add **zhi da huang** (processed Radix et Rhizoma Rhei) 制大黄 6-9g and **zhi shi** (Fructus Immaturus Citri Aurantii) 枳实 9-12g.

Variations and additional prescriptions

Severe food stagnation and Heat

- In patients with severe stagnation that has generated a degree of Heat, with pain, constipation and a dry, yellow tongue coat, a dose or two of a mild purge, like **TIAO WEI CHENG QI TANG** (*Regulate the Stomach and Order the Qi Decoction* 调胃承气汤) may be useful to quickly clear the Intestines and powerfully direct *qi* and Blood downwards, before proceeding with the main prescription.

sheng da huang (Radix et Rhizoma Rhei) 生大黄 3-9g
mang xiao (Mirabilitum) 芒硝 6-12g
gan cao (Radix Glycyrrhizae Uralensis) 甘草 6g

Method: Decoct the **da huang** and **gan cao**, then dissolve the **mang xiao** into the strained decoction (*hou xia* 后下). The longer the **da huang** is cooked, the less purgative it becomes. **Da huang** and **mang xiao** purge Heat and stagnation; **da huang** can also stop bleeding; **gan cao** protects the Stomach.

Patent medicines

Bao He Wan 保和丸 (Bao He Wan)

Sheng Tian Qi Pian 生田七片 (Raw Tian Qi Ginseng Tablets)

- A good general medicine for bleeding. Combine with the above patent medicine or the primary prescription.

Yun Nan Bai Yao 云南白药 (Yunnan Paiyao)

- The premier medicine for all types of bleeding. Combine with the first patent medicine or the primary prescription. The red pill that accompanies the powder is only used in severe cases.

Acupuncture (select from)

Ren.12 (*zhong wan* -) .... *mu* point of the Stomach, alleviates stagnation and regulates the Stomach

St.36 (*zu san li* -) .... *he* sea point of the Stomach, regulates the Stomach, directs Stomach *qi* downwards and stops bleeding

St.40 (*feng long* -) .... *luo* point of the Stomach, transforms Phlegm and clears stagnant food, Phlegm and Phlegm Heat from the Stomach

LI.10 (*shou san li* -) .... benefits digestion and regulates gastro-intestinal function

PC.6 (*nei guan* -) .... *luo* point of the Pericardium, master point of *yin wei mai*, regulates the middle *jiao*, stops vomiting

Sp.4 (*gong sun* -) .... *luo* point of the Spleen, master point of *chong mai*, stops bleeding

- with Spleen deficiency, add Bl.20 (*pi shu* +)
- with abdominal pain, add Sp.8 (*di ji* -), St.34 (*liang qiu* -) and Sp.4 (*gong sun* -)
- with borborygmus, add Sp.5 (*shang qiu* -)
- with constipation, add St.37 (*shang ju xu* -) and SJ.6 (*zhi gou* -)
- *Ear points*: spleen, stomach, intestines, liver, abdomen

Clinical notes

- Food stagnation, which is a disorder of gluttony and dietary irregularity, is not a common cause of haematemesis. In isolation it needs no treatment other than a sensible approach to diet and eating habits, however if bad habits persist it can become a more entrenched condition requiring treatment.
- The Chinese have long known the benefits of sipping small amounts of certain teas while eating. The action of such teas helps assist digestion, especially of fats, and reduces the risk of food stagnation. European cultures use table wine in much the same way, hence 'a little wine for thy stomach's sake'. Similarly, 'bitters', combinations of bitter herbs and alcohol, are a common accompaniment to food, either as a digestive aid following a meal, or as an aperitive. The bitterness of the herbs assists the descent of Stomach *qi* and dries Damp.

瘀阻胃络

12.6 BLOOD STAGNATION

Pathophysiology

- Blood stagnation haematemesis is a chronic condition, and usually follows another chronic Stomach pathology. The most common precursor is Liver *qi* stagnation repeatedly invading the Stomach and Spleen. Chronic Damp Heat affecting the Liver may also be implicated. Blood stagnation may, however, be more acute, and not necessarily associated with any other pathology, if it follows trauma or gastric surgery. When part of a chronic condition, it almost always appears as a complication of other patterns.
- Blood stagnation patterns manifest a continuum of states, from mild to severe. In mild cases or in the early stages, the movement of Blood is simply sluggish. As the condition deteriorates, Blood comes to a halt at certain points and the classical features appear. Blood stagnation may first manifest when long term gastro-intestinal symptoms such as pain, change from generalised and ill defined to more sharp or localised.

Clinical features

- vomiting of dark or purplish, coffee ground like material
- stools may be black and tarry
- relatively severe, sharp or stabbing epigastric pain, fixed in location and worse with pressure; right sided hypochondriac pain
- dark or purplish spider naevi or broken vessels on the trunk and around the inner ankle and knee
- dark, ashen, sallow or purplish complexion, dark or purplish lips and conjunctiva, dark rings around the eyes
- in women, the menses may be irregular, dark or purple and clotted

T purple or with brown or purple stasis spots, sublingual veins dark and distended

P thready and choppy or wiry

Treatment principle

Invigorate and transform stagnant Blood, stop bleeding
Regulate *qi*, nourish Blood, soften the Liver

Prescription

XUE FU ZHU YU TANG 血府逐瘀汤
(*Achyranthes and Persica Combination*) modified

dang gui (Radix Angelicae Sinensis) 当归 9-12g
sheng di (Radix Rehmanniae Glutinosae) 生地 12-15g
chi shao (Radix Paeoniae Rubrae) 赤芍 9-12g
chuan xiong (Radix Ligustici Chuanxiong) 川芎 6-9g

tao ren (Semen Persicae) 桃仁 9-12g
hong hua (Flos Carthami Tinctorii) 红花 9-12g
chai hu (Radix Bupleuri) 柴胡 6-9g
zhi ke (Fructus Citri Aurantii) 枳壳 9-12g
gan cao (Radix Glycyrrhizae Uralensis) 甘草 3-6g
chuan niu xi (Radix Cyathulae Officinalis) 川牛膝 15-24g
jie geng (Radix Platycodi Grandiflori) 桔梗 3-6g
qian cao gen (Radix Rubiae Cordifoliae) 茜草根 12-15g
san qi fen (powdered Radix Notoginseng) 三七粉 3-6g

Method: Decoction. **Dang gui, sheng di, chuan xiong, chi shao, tao ren** and **hong hua** constitute **TAO HONG SI WU TANG**, the fundamental prescription to nourish, regulate and gently invigorate Blood; **chai hu, zhi ke, gan cao** and **chi shao** constitute **SI NI SAN**, the fundamental prescription to regulate Liver *qi* and move stagnant *qi*; **jie geng** opens up the movement of *qi* through the chest and diaphragm, and can direct *qi* to the upper body; the large dose of **niu xi** leads Blood downwards; together the last two herbs seek to re-establish the correct ascent and descent of *qi* and Blood; **qian cao gen** and **san qi** invigorate Blood and stop bleeding. (Source: *Xiao Hua Ke Zhuan Bing*)

Modifications

- With pain, add either **yan hu suo** (Rhizoma Corydalis Yanhusuo) 延胡索 9-12g, or **ru xiang** (Gummi Olibanum) 乳香 6g and **mo yao** (Myrrha) 没药 6g, or **pu huang** (Pollen Typhae) 蒲黄 9-12g and **chao wu ling zhi** (dry fried Excrementum Trogopteri seu Pteromi) 炒五灵脂 9-12g.
- With persistent, focal, gnawing pain and bleeding, powder equal amounts of **hai piao xiao** (Os Sepiae seu Sepiellae) 海螵蛸 and **sheng da huang** (unprocessed Radix et Rhizoma Rhei) 生大黄 and take 3-6g as powder or in capsules 3-4 times daily.
- With mild signs of Heat, add **mu dan pi** (Cortex Moutan Radicis) 牡丹皮 9-12g and **yu jin** (Tuber Curcumae) 郁金 9-12g.
- With food stagnation, add **shen qu** (Massa Fermentata) 神曲 15g and **shan zha** (Fructus Crataegi) 山楂 15g.
- With *yin* deficiency, delete **chai hu, jie geng, chuan xiong** and **zhi ke**, and add **mai dong** (Tuber Ophiopogonis Japonici) 麦冬 9-12g, **yu zhu** (Rhizoma Polygonati Odorati) 玉竹 12-15g, **nu zhen zi** (Fructus Ligustri Lucidi) 女贞子 9-12g and **han lian cao** (Herba Ecliptae Prostratae) 旱连草 9-12g.
- With *yang* deficiency or Cold, delete **chai hu** and **jie geng**, and add **zhi fu zi** (Radix Aconiti Carmichaeli Praeparata) 制附子 6-12g (decocted for 30 minutes prior to the other herbs), **rou gui** (Cortex Cinnamomi Cassiae) 肉桂 3g, **xian ling pi** (Herba Epimedii) 仙灵脾 12-18g and **ba ji tian** (Radix Morindae Officinalis) 巴戟天 9-12g.
- With Blood deficiency, add **shu di** (Radix Rehmanniae Glutinosae Conquitae) 熟地 12-18g, **gou qi zi** (Fructus Lycii) 枸杞子 9-12g and **he shou wu** (Radix Polygoni Multiflori) 何首乌 9-12g.

Variations and additional prescriptions

With Heat

- Stagnant Blood may be complicated by significant Heat, with sporadic gastro-intestinal bleeding of fresh red blood, a purplish red tongue with a yellow coat and a wiry rapid pulse. The aim of treatment is to clear Heat, cool the Blood and stop bleeding with **DA HUANG HUANG QIN XIE XIN TANG** (*Rhubarb and Scute Decoction to Drain the Epigastrium* 大黄黄芩泻心汤) modified. This formula is used until the bleeding ceases, after which a more general Blood moving formula may be selected.

  da huang (Radix et Rhizoma Rhei) 大黄 6-9g
  huang qin (Radix Scutellariae Baicalensis) 黄芩 9-12g
  huang lian (Rhizoma Coptidis) 黄连 6-9g
  chao pu huang (dry fried Pollen Typhae) 炒蒲黄 9-12g
  e jiao (Gelatinum Corii Asini) 阿胶 6-9g
  di yu tan (charred Radix Sanguisorbae Officinalis)
  地榆炭 12-15g
  bai ji (Rhizoma Bletillae Striatae) 白芨 12-15g
  san qi fen (powdered Radix Notoginseng) 三七粉 3-6g

  Method: Decoction. **San qi** powder is taken separately or added to the strained decoction (*chong fu* 冲服), **e jiao** is melted before being added to the strained decoction (*yang hua* 烊化). **Bai ji** may also be taken as a powder (3g per dose). **Da huang**, **huang qin** and **huang lian** clear Heat; **da huang** stops bleeding; **pu huang** stops bleeding; **di yu** cools the Blood to stop bleeding; **e jiao** nourishes *yin* and Blood and stops bleeding; **bai ji** astringes to stop bleeding; **san qi** invigorates Blood and stops bleeding. (Source: *Shi Yong Zhong Yi Nei Ke Xue*)

With Cold and deficiency

- Blood stagnation may be complicated by deficiency and Cold, in which case the patient presents with vomiting of dark blood, tarry stools, focal stabbing epigastric pain that is worse when pressed, fatigue and weakness, a sallow complexion, cold intolerance, cold extremities and a pale purple tongue. The aim of treatment is to first warm *yang*, strengthen the Spleen and stop bleeding with **HUANG TU TANG** (*Yellow Earth Decoction* 黄土汤, p.438).

Patent medicines

Xue Fu Zhu Yu Wan 血府逐瘀丸 (Xue Fu Zhu Yu Wan)
Tao Hong Si Wu Wan 桃红四物丸 (Tao Hong Si Wu Wan)
- good for mild cases with Blood deficiency

Sheng Tian Qi Pian 生田七片 (Raw Tian Qi Ginseng Tablets)
- A good general medicine for bleeding and Blood stagnation. Combine with an appropriate constitutional patent medicine or the primary prescription.

Yun Nan Bai Yao 云南白药 (Yunnan Paiyao)
- The premier medicine for all types of bleeding. Combine with an appropriate constitutional patent medicine or the primary prescription. The red pill with the powder is used in severe cases.

Acupuncture (select from)

Ren.12 (*zhong wan* -) .... *mu* point of the Stomach, eliminates Blood stagnation and directs Stomach *qi* downwards
St.21 (*liang men* -) .... local point to regulate *qi* and Blood, invigorates stagnant Blood and stops pain
ah shi points .... local points over the epigastrium to invigorate stagnant Blood
PC.6 (*nei guan* -) .... *luo* point of the Pericardium, regulates Liver *qi*, harmonises the middle *jiao* and stops vomiting
PC.4 (*xi men* -) .... *xi* cleft point of the Pericardium, opens the chest, clears Heat and stops bleeding
Sp.10 (*xue hai* -) .... regulates and invigorates Blood, stops bleeding
Sp.4 (*gong sun*) .... *luo* point of the Spleen, master point of *chong mai*, regulates the Spleen and Stomach and stops bleeding
Bl.17 (*ge shu* -).................. *hui* point for Blood, regulates Blood and eliminates stagnant Blood
Bl.21 (*wei shu* -) .... *shu* point for the Stomach, regulates the Stomach and eliminates stagnation from the Stomach

- for severe pain, add LI.4 (*he gu* -) and Liv.5 (*li gou* -)
- with irritability or depression, add Liv.3 (*tai chong*) or Liv.1 (*da dun* ↓) and *yin tang* (M-HN-3)
- *Ear points*: stomach, duodenum, large intestine, small intestine, liver, adrenal, subcortex, *shen men*

Clinical notes

- Blood stagnation type haematemesis may be diagnosed biomedically as stomach cancer, bleeding oesophageal varices, alcoholic liver disease, cirrhosis, perforated peptic ulcer and bleeding peptic ulcer. Endometriosis, in a rare form, can cause cyclical haematemesis.
- Severe bleeding from the digestive tract is a medical emergency and should be treated in hospital.
- This pattern can be difficult and may take some months of persistent treatment for a satisfactory result depending on the biomedical diagnosis, although bleeding will often cease within a few weeks. In the case of treatment of cancer TCM offers a useful supportive role.
- For dietary recommendations, see p.886.

中气虚弱

12.7 SPLEEN AND STOMACH QI DEFICIENCY

- *Yang* deficiency

Pathophysiology

- As a cause of gastro-intestinal bleeding, Spleen and Stomach *qi* deficiency is more likely to give rise to haemafecia than to haematemesis (*see* p.433), as considerable ascending force is required to eject material through the mouth. In *qi* deficiency, the usual bleeding tendency is to slowly leak and sink downwards.
- The mechanism involves a failure of Spleen *qi* to hold the Blood in the vessels. Blood slowly seeps out into the Intestine mixing with the Intestinal contents. The systemic deficiency is usually chronic and the bleeding generally mild and intermittent. The appearance of the blood will vary, depending on how much there is and how long it has remained in the Stomach.
- *Qi* deficiency is usually complicated by varying degrees of Blood deficiency, both from failure of the Spleen to manufacture sufficient Blood and from the chronic Blood loss.

Clinical features

- vomiting of small quantities of pink or blood tinged saliva, pale red or fresh red blood, or purplish or dark clotted blood
- intermittent, dull abdominal pain that is alleviated with pressure and warmth, and worse with cold and when the patient is tired or run down
- tendency to loose stools or diarrhoea or sticky, tarry, black stools; occult haemafecia
- abdominal distension, early satiety, nausea
- loss of appetite
- waxy pale or sallow complexion
- fatigue, weakness, dizziness, light headedness
- shortness of breath with exertion
- spontaneous sweating
- there may be other sites of bleeding, such as heavy menstrual periods and easy bruising

T pale and swollen, with toothmarks (or pale and thin with significant Blood deficiency)

P thready and weak or moderate

Treatment principle

Strengthen the Spleen, supplement *qi* to aid the Spleen's function of holding Blood in the vessels

Nourish Blood and stop bleeding

Prescription

BU ZHONG YI QI TANG 补中益气汤
(*Ginseng and Astragalus Combination*) modified

zhi huang qi (honey fried Radix Astragali Membranacei) 炙黄芪 18-30g
dang shen (Radix Codonopsis Pilosulae) 党参 15-24g
chao bai zhu (dry fried Rhizoma Atractylodes Macrocephalae) 炒白术 12-15g
dang gui (Radix Angelicae Sinensis) 当归 9-12g
chen pi (Pericarpium Citri Reticulatae) 陈皮 6-9g
zhi gan cao (honey fried Radix Glycyrrhizae Uralensis) 炙甘草 6-9g
chai hu (Radix Bupleuri) 柴胡 3-6g
pao jiang (quick fried Rhizoma Zingiberis Officinalis) 炮姜 6-9g
bai ji (Rhizoma Bletillae Striatae) 白芨 12-15g
san qi fen (powdered Radix Notoginseng) 三七粉 3-6g

Method: Decoction or powdered and taken in doses of 9-grams as a draft. **Zhi huang qi**, **dang shen** and **chao bai zhu** strengthen the Spleen, supplement *qi* and assist the Spleen in holding Blood in the vessels; **chai hu** and **sheng ma** support the *qi* supplementing herbs in lifting sinking *qi*; **dang gui** supplements Blood; **chen pi** and **gan cao** regulate *qi* and harmonise the middle *jiao*; **pao jiang** warms the Spleen and stops bleeding; **bai ji** astringes to stop bleeding; **san qi** invigorates Blood and stops bleeding. (Source: *Shi Yong Zhong Yi Nei Ke Xue*)

Modifications

- If the bleeding persists, add other astringent styptic herbs such as **xian he cao** (Herba Agrimoniae Pilosae) 仙鹤草 15-30g, **chao pu huang** (dry fried Pollen Typhae) 炒蒲黄 9-12g and **han lian cao** (Herba Ecliptae Prostratae) 旱连草 9-12g.
- With abdominal pain, add **bai shao** (Radix Paeoniae Lactiflora) 白芍 12-18g.
- With a degree of Kidney *yang* deficiency, add **xian ling pi** (Herba Epimedii) 仙灵脾 15g and **ba ji tian** (Radix Morindae Officinalis) 巴戟天 9-12g and **bu gu zhi** (Fructus Psoraleae Corylifoliae) 补骨脂 9-12g.

Variations and additional prescriptions

Heart Blood and Spleen qi deficiency

- With other sites of bleeding (easy bruising, nosebleeds, bleeding gums, etc.) and signs of Blood deficiency and *shen* disturbance (anxiety, postural dizziness, insomnia), the aim of treatment is to supplement *qi* and Blood, and stop bleeding with **GUI PI TANG** (*Ginseng and Longan Combination* 归脾汤) modified.

zhi huang qi (honey fried Radix Astragali Membranacei) 炙黄芪 18-30g
dang shen (Radix Codonopsis Pilosulae) 党参 15-24g
chao bai zhu (dry fried Rhizoma Atractylodis Macrocephalae) 炒白术 12-15g
fu shen (Sclerotium Poriae Cocos Pararadicis) 茯神 12-15g
dang gui (Radix Angelicae Sinensis) 当归 9-12g
long yan rou (Arillus Euphoriae Longanae) 龙眼肉 9-12g
suan zao ren (Semen Zizyphi Spinosae) 酸枣仁 9-12g
mu xiang (Radix Aucklandiae Lappae) 木香 6-9g
yuan zhi (Radix Polygalae Tenuifoliae) 远志 6-9g
zhi gan cao (honey fried Radix Glycyrrhizae Uralensis) 炙甘草 6-9g
pao jiang (quick fried Rhizoma Zingiberis Officinalis) 炮姜 6-9g
e jiao (Gelatinum Corii Asini) 阿胶 9-12g

Method: Decoction. **E jiao** is melted before being added to the strained decoction (*yang hua* 烊化). **Zhi huang qi**, **dang shen**, **chao bai zhu** and **zhi gan cao** strengthen the Spleen, supplement *qi* and assist the Spleen in holding Blood in the vessels; **dang gui** and **zhi huang qi** powerfully supplement Blood; **suan zao ren**, **long yan rou** and **yuan zhi** nourish the Heart and calm the *shen*; **fu shen** benefits the Spleen and calms the *shen*; **mu xiang** regulates *qi* and aids the Spleen in digesting the Blood supplementing herbs; **pao jiang** warms the Spleen and stops bleeding; **e jiao** nourishes *yin* and Blood and stops bleeding. (Source: *Shi Yong Zhong Yi Nei Ke Xue*)

Spleen yang deficiency

- In elderly, debilitated or susceptible patients, Spleen *yang* may be depleted. Haematemesis of this type is not common, with the blood usually sinking to appear as haemafecia. The mechanism is similar to that of *qi* deficiency, with the addition of cold intolerance. The clinical features are intermittent vomiting of frothy pink tinged saliva, or watery, pale purplish blood. The stools will likely be tarry and black, or loose, sticky and black. Abdominal or epigastric pain is persistent, dull and alleviated by warmth. The patient is pale, thin and has no appetite. The tongue is swollen, pale or bluish and wet. The aim of treatment is to warm Spleen *yang* and stop bleeding with **HUANG TU TANG** (*Yellow Earth Decoction* 黄土汤, p.438).

Patent medicines

Bu Zhong Yi Qi Wan 补中益气丸 (Bu Zhong Yi Qi Wan, Central Qi Pills) - Spleen *qi* deficiency

Gui Pi Wan 归脾丸 (Gui Pi Wan, Angelicae Longana Tea, Kwei Be Wan) - Heart and Spleen *qi* deficiency

Li Zhong Wan 理中丸 (Li Zhong Wan)
- Spleen *yang* deficiency

Fu Zi Li Zhong Wan 附子理中丸 (Carmichaeli Tea Pills, Fu Tzu Li Chung Wan, Li Chung Yuen Medical Pills)
- Spleen *yang* deficiency with severe Cold

Shi Quan Da Bu Wan 十全大补丸 (Shi Quan Da Bu Wan, Ten Flavour Tea) - with Blood deficiency and Cold

Sheng Tian Qi Pian 生田七片 (Raw Tian Qi Ginseng Tablets)
- A good general medicine for bleeding. Combine with an appropriate constitutional patent medicine or the primary prescription.

Yun Nan Bai Yao 云南白药 (Yunnan Paiyao)
- The premier medicine for all types of bleeding. Combine with an appropriate constitutional patent medicine or the primary prescription. The red pill that accompanies the powder is only used in severe cases.

Acupuncture (select from)

Ren.12 (*zhong wan* +▲) .. *mu* point of the Stomach, warms and strengthens the Spleen and Stomach and supplements *qi*

Ren.6 (*qi hai* +▲) .... regulates *qi*, strengthens the Kidneys and supplements *yuan qi*

St.36 (*zu san li* +▲) .... *he* sea point of the Stomach, powerfully warms and strengthens the Spleen and Stomach, supplements *qi* and stops bleeding

Sp.1 (*yin bai* ▲)................*jing* well point of the Spleen, a special point to stop Spleen deficiency bleeding when treated with rice grain moxa

Sp.4 (*gong sun* +) .... *luo* point of the Pericardium, master point of *chong mai*, regulates the Spleen and Stomach, stops bleeding; good when there is abdominal pain

Sp.6 (*san yin jiao* +▲)...... strengthens the Spleen, supplements *qi*, regulates Liver *qi*, benefits the Kidneys and regulates *qi* and Blood

Bl.20 (*pi shu* +▲) .... *shu* point of the Spleen, warms and strengthens the Spleen and supplements *qi*

Bl.21 (*wei shu* + ▲) .... *shu* point of the Stomach, warms and strengthens the Stomach

- A moxa box over the abdomen is useful, and essential for *yang* deficiency. With severe Cold, strong moxa on Ren.8 (*shen que*) over salt, may be applied. Place a piece of thin cloth over the navel and fill

it with salt. Burn large cones of moxa on the salt. The cloth enables quick removal of the salt and prevents burning of the skin.
- with Kidney *yang* deficiency, add Bl.23 (*shen shu* +▲)
- *Ear points*: spleen, stomach, large intestine, small intestine, adrenal, subcortex, *shen men*

Clinical notes

- Spleen *qi/yang* deficiency haematemesis may be diagnosed biomedically as chronic peptic ulcer disease, thrombocytopenia, intestinal polyps or haemophilia.
- The bleeding associated with this pattern will generally cease within a few weeks. The underlying Spleen *qi* and/or *yang* deficiency usually responds reliably and incrementally to correct TCM treatment, but the greater the deficiency, the longer the course or treatment required. Spleen *yang* deficiency may require 6-12 months of treatment.
- For dietary recommendations, see pp.870-873.

陰虛火旺

12.8 STOMACH YIN DEFICIENCY WITH HEAT/FIRE

Pathophysiology

- Stomach *yin* deficiency is usually a complication of some other long standing pathology, most commonly Liver *qi* invading the Stomach, or the chronic Heat patterns. It can also be more acute, following damage to Stomach *yin* from a febrile illness, such as *yang ming* syndrome.
- The vomiting of blood in this pattern is usually the result of several factors. Stomach *yin* deficiency often causes protracted vomiting or dry retching which can rupture Stomach *luo mai*. In chronic *yin* deficiency the Stomach wall is often thinner than normal, making the probability of rupture from repeated vomiting more likely. The deficient Heat compounds the potential for haematemesis by causing Blood to move recklessly and be ejected from the fragile vessels.

Clinical features

- vomiting of fresh red blood that may be copious or scant
- persistent, dull, nagging epigastric pain
- indeterminate gnawing hunger, heartburn, morning nausea
- general dryness of the skin, mucous membranes and hair, thirst
- black, sticky, tarry or dark, dry stools, or tendency to constipation or pellet like stools
- facial and malar flushing
- nightsweats
- sensation of heat in the palms and soles ('five hearts hot')
- with Kidney *yin* deficiency: dizziness, tinnitus, lower back and knees sore and weak

T slightly red and peeled in the centre, or red and dry with little or no coat; in severe or long standing cases, the tongue may be so denuded of papillae as to resemble a piece of liver (mirror tongue) or have numerous surface cracks or a wide shallow central crack

P thready and rapid

Treatment principle

Nourish Stomach *yin*, clear Heat
Cool the Blood, stop bleeding

Prescription

YU NU JIAN 玉女煎
(*Jade Woman Decoction*) modified

shi gao (Gypsum) 石膏 18-30g
sheng di (Radix Rehmanniae Glutinosae) 生地 18-30g

mai dong (Tuber Ophiopogonis Japonici) 麦冬 9-12g
zhi mu (Rhizoma Anemarrhenae Asphodeloides) 知母 9-12g
chuan niu xi (Radix Cyathulae Officinalis) 川牛膝 15-24g
ce bai ye (Cacumen Biotae Orientalis) 侧柏叶 12-15g
bai mao gen (Rhizoma Imperatae Cylindricae) 白茅根 12-18g
han lian cao (Herba Ecliptae Prostratae) 旱连草 12-18g

Method: Decoction. **Shi gao** is decocted for 30 minutes prior to the other herbs (*xian jian* 先煎). **Shi gao** and **zhi mu** clear Heat from the Stomach; **sheng di** cools the Blood and nourishes *yin*; **mai dong** clears Heat and nourishes *yin*; the large quantity of **niu xi** leads the Blood downwards, and prevents the cooling herbs from causing stagnant Blood; **ce bai ye**, **bai mao gen** and **han lian cao** cool the Blood and stop bleeding. (Source: *Shi Yong Zhong Yi Nei Ke Xue*)

Modifications

- With severe bleeding, add **bai ji** (Rhizoma Bletillae Striatae) 白芨 12-15g, **zi zhu cao** (Folium Callicarpae) 紫珠草 12-15g, **e jiao** (Gelatinum Corii Asini) 阿胶 9-12g (melted in the hot strained decoction) and **ou jie** (Nodus Nelumbinis Nuciferae Rhizomatis) 藕节 12-15g to astringe the Stomach and stop bleeding.
- With *qi* deficiency add **dang shen** (Radix Codonopsis Pilosulae) 党参 15-24g.
- With constipation, add **sheng he shou wu** (unprocessed Radix Polygoni Multiflori) 生何首乌 12-15g and **huo ma ren** (Semen Cannabis Sativae) 火麻仁 9-12g.
- With significant or nagging pain, include herbs that gently move *qi* without damaging *yin*. These include **fo shou** (Fructus Citri Sarcodacylis) 佛手 9-12g, **ba yue zha** (Fructus Akebiae) 八月扎 9-12g, **mei gui hua** (Flos Rosae Rugosae) 玫瑰花 6-9g or **xiang yuan pi** (Pericarpium Citri Medica) 香橼皮 9-12g.
- With acid reflux, heartburn, burning pain and nausea, add **wu zhu yu** (Fructus Evodiae Rutaecarpae) 吴茱萸 1-2g and **huang lian** (Rhizoma Coptidis) 黄连 3-6g, or add **duan wa leng zi** (calcined Concha Arcae) 煅瓦楞子 15g.
- With elements of stagnant Blood, add **dan shen** (Radix Salviae Miltiorrhizae) 丹参 9-12g and **san qi fen** (powdered Radix Notoginseng) 三七粉 3-6g.

Patent medicines

Gu Ben Wan 固本丸 (Gu Ben Wan, Ren Shen Ku Pen Wan)
- Spleen and Stomach *yin* and *qi* deficiency

Zhi Bai Ba Wei Wan 知柏八味丸 (Zhi Bai Ba Wei Wan, Chih Pai Pa Wei Wan) - with marked deficient Heat symptoms

Sheng Mai San Wan 生脉散丸 (Sheng Mai San Wan)

- Stomach *qi* and *yin* deficiency

Liu Wei Di Huang Wan 六味地黄丸 (Liu Wei Di Huang Wan, Six Flavour Tea) - Kidney *yin* deficiency

Sheng Tian Qi Pian 生田七片 (Raw Tian Qi Ginseng Tablets)
- A good general medicine for bleeding. Combine with an appropriate constitutional patent medicine or the primary prescription.

Yun Nan Bai Yao 云南白药 (Yunnan Paiyao)
- The premier medicine for all types of bleeding. Combine with an appropriate constitutional patent medicine or the primary prescription. The red pill that accompanies the powder is only used in severe cases.

Acupuncture (select from)

Ren.12 (*zhong wan*) .... together these points nourish Stomach and
Sp.6 (*san yin jiao* +) Kidney *yin*
St.36 (*zu san li* +)

Ren.4 (*guan yuan* +) .... meeting point of the *yin* channels, with Sp.6 to supplement the *yin* and *yuan qi* of the body

Bl.20 (*pi shu* +) .... *shu* points of the Spleen and Stomach
Bl.21 (*wei shu* +) respectively, supplement and replenish Stomach *yin*

Bl.23 (*shen shu* +) .... these points strengthen the source of all
Kid.6 (*zhao hai* +) inherited *yin*, the Kidney, releasing stored *yin* to
Kid.3 (*tai xi* +) support Stomach *yin*

- *Ear points*: stomach, duodenum, oesophagus, adrenal, *shen men*, subcortex

Clinical notes

- Stomach *yin* deficiency haematemesis may be diagnosed biomedically as bleeding peptic ulcers, atrophic gastritis, bleeding oesophageal varices, reflux oeophagitis, stomach cancer.
- This can be a difficult pattern to treat successfully, but may respond reasonably well to prolonged treatment. Although the bleeding may ease relatively quickly, in long standing cases, 6-12 months of treatment may be necessary for a satisfactory constitutional result.
- For dietary recommendations, see p.876.

SUMMARY OF GUIDING FORMULAE FOR HAEMATEMESIS

Excess patterns

Heat in the *ying*/Blood - *Shui Niu Jiao Di Huang Tang* 水牛角地黄汤
- with *qi* and *yin* deficiency during convalescence - *Zhu Ye Shi Gao Tang* 竹叶石膏汤

Stomach Heat/Fire - *Xie Xin Tang* 泻心汤 plus *Shi Hui San* 十灰散
- with severe bleeding and collapsing *yang* - *Shen Fu Tang* 参附汤

Damp Heat injuring the Stomach - *Zhi Shi Dao Zhi Wan* 枳实导滞丸

Liver *qi* invading the Stomach - *Long Dan Xie Gan Tang* 龙胆泻肝汤

Food stagnation - *Bao He Wan* 保和丸
- with severe stagnation and Heat - *Tiao Wei Cheng Qi Tang* 调胃承气汤

Blood stagnation - *Xue Fu Zhu Yu Tang* 血府逐瘀汤
- with Heat - *Da Huang Huang Qin Xie Xin Tang* 大黄黄芩泻心汤
- with Cold and deficiency - *Huang Tu Tang* 黄土汤

Deficient patterns

Spleen and Stomach *qi* deficiency - *Bu Zhong Yi Qi Tang* 补中益气汤
- with Heart Blood and Spleen *qi* deficiency - *Gui Pi Tang* 归脾汤
- with Spleen *yang* deficiency - *Huang Tu Tang* 黄土汤

Stomach *yin* deficiency - *Yu Nu Jian* 玉女煎

13. Haemorrhoids

Excess patterns

Intestinal Wind
Intestinal Dryness
Damp Heat
Blood stagnation

Deficient patterns

Spleen *qi* deficiency
- not holding Blood
- sinking *qi*

Appendix 1 Anal fissure
Appendix 2 Anal abscess
Appendix 3 Anal fistula
Appendix 4 Anal itch

13 HAEMORRHOIDS

zhi chuang 痔疮

Haemorrhoids, colloquially known as piles, are varicosities of the haemorrhoidal veins. They are thought to be due to increased pressure in the venous plexus that drains the rectum and anus, in association with, or independent of, weakness or loss of tone in the venous walls. Haemorrhoids are common, indeed it is estimated that as many as 50% of people will suffer from haemorrhoids by the time they are 50 years old. Haemorrhoids, and the anal disorders that follow, traditionally appear in TCM texts on external medicine or surgery (*wai ke* 外科). Haemorrhoids are, however, commonly seen disorders of the gastro-intestinal tract, and frequently encountered in the TCM clinic, so we include them in this volume.

Haemorrhoids are often asymptomatic, but may cause bleeding or pain, and may protrude. Haemorrhoidal bleeding often follows defecation, and a smear of blood on the toilet paper may be the first sign of their presence. Pain usually occurs only when the haemorrhoids are ulcerated or thrombosed.

There are two broad anatomical categories of haemorrhoids, internal and external. Internal haemorrhoids are located above the dentate line of the anus and are covered by rectal mucosa. External haemorrhoids are located below the dentate line and are covered by squamous epithelium.

Haemorrhoids are classified into three stages, depending on the degree of prolapse and severity. In general, 1st and 2nd degree haemorrhoids are the most amenable to treatment with Chinese medicine.

Figure 13.1 *Classification of haemorrhoids*

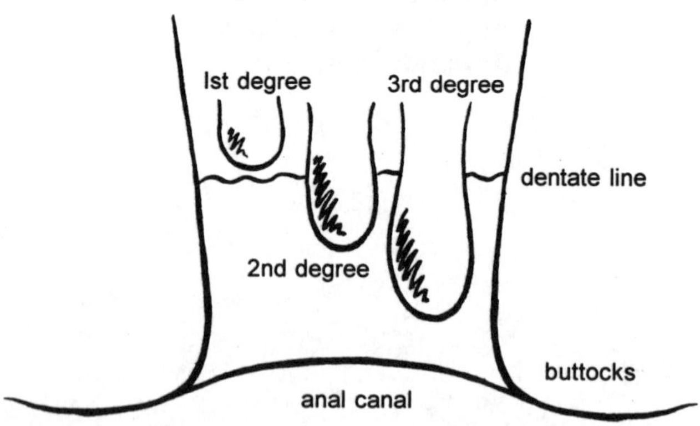

BOX 13.1 SCHEME OF HAEMORRHOID ANALYSIS

The patterns noted here can combine, and various TCM defined haemorrhoid patterns are often seen together. They do not necessarily proceed from early to late stage in a linear fashion.

Stage	TCM description	Characteristics
Early	Intestinal Wind	bleeding of fresh red blood before or after defecation, blood on the toilet paper, generally no pain or prolapse; often no clear systemic pattern
	Dry Intestine	associated with chronic constipation
	Damp Heat	associated with inflammation, pain, swelling and systemic signs of Heat; can be associated with all degrees of haemorrhoids
	Spleen deficiency	loss of muscle tone or failure of the Spleen to hold Blood in the vessels and thus bleeding; 2nd and 3rd degree haemorrhoids that prolapse when standing, walking or with increased intra-abdominal pressure and need manual reduction; with systemic signs of deficiency
Late	Blood stagnation	severe or continuous pain and distension, haemorrhoids may be irreducible or thrombosed; systemic signs of Blood stagnation

Classification of haemorrhoids

Stage I (1st degree): Small, non-protruding haemorrhoids which are characterised mainly by bleeding.

Stage II (2nd degree): Larger haemorrhoids which protrude upon defecation, but are easily reducible or retract spontaneously. Bleeding can also be a feature.

Stage III (3rd degree): Large haemorrhoids which protrude with an increase in abdominal pressure (sneezing, coughing), or with walking, standing and defecation. They may require manual reduction to alleviate discomfort, or be difficult to reduce. Bleeding is a feature.

AETIOLOGY

Bowel habits (constipation, diarrhoea)

Chronic constipation is perhaps the most common cause of haemorrhoids The pressure generated in the rectal veins by an obstructing mass, the stool, weakens the venous walls and increases internal pressure within the haemorrhoidal plexus, causing a ballooning of the veins. Lack of dietary fibre and a sedentary life are the common predisposing factors in the Western world, however, there are many causes of constipation (*see* Constipation, p.164).

Chronic diarrhoea, especially when frequent, may contribute to haemorrhoids by directly weakening the anal and rectal area through the repeated downward pressure of the diarrhoea. In addition, chronic diarrhoea, by definition involves weakness of the Spleen and thus implies already weakened muscle tone. The ongoing diarrhoea compounds the existing weakness.

Diet

Diet can contribute to haemorrhoids in several ways:

- by engendering Damp Heat that lodges in the Intestines (and Liver system)
- by weakening the Spleen, and thus the Spleen's ability to hold the Blood in the vessels and maintain muscle tone, or by causing diarrhoea
- by causing constipation.

Overeating, eating irregularly or at odd hours, especially late at night, weakens Spleen and Stomach *qi* and leads to food stagnation. Too much cold natured or raw food weakens Spleen *qi* and *yang*. Overconsumption in general and excessive consumption of rich and hot natured foods and alcohol in particular, can lead to the accumulation and stagnation of food (*see* p.3) and Damp Heat in the Intestines.

Biomechanics

A sedentary occupation or lifestyle restricts the free circulation of *qi* and Blood through the seat and hence the anal area. Prolonged standing, jarring exercise, such as long distance running, or exertion while carrying hefty loads, may exhaust *qi* and weaken the Spleen, leading to loss of muscle tone and prolapse of the haemorrhoidal veins. Any activity that causes a significant or prolonged increase in abdominal pressure, for example chronic cough or lifting heavy weights, may contribute to the generation of haemorrhoids.

Haemorrhoids frequently occur during pregnancy due to the pressure of the growing foetus on the pelvic circulation, as well as the tremendous pressure on the anus and rectum that occur during labour.

Emotion

Emotions contribute to the formation of haemorrhoids mostly through the effects of prolonged Liver *qi* stagnation, as follows:

- repeated invasion by stagnant Liver *qi* weakens the Spleen, damages *qi* and leads to build-up of Dampness
- long term pressure from stagnation may generate stagnant Heat, which may then contribute to forming Damp Heat in those with pre-existing Damp
- stagnant *qi* retards the movement of Blood
- stagnation of *qi* or Damp Heat in the Liver can contribute to back pressure in the portal system and increased venous pressure in the rectal veins and haemorrhoidal plexus.

In addition, excessive worry, mental strain or prolonged concentration may deplete Spleen *qi*. The damage is aggravated when an irregular diet is combined with sustained mental activity and too much sitting.

Failure of Lung *qi* to descend properly as a result of severe grief, sadness or loss can also contribute to haemorrhoids by hindering the descent of Large Intestine *qi* and thereby contributing to constipation.

TREATMENT

Treatment of simple haemorrhoids is often successful with Chinese herbal medicine, acupuncture and dietary modification. The key feature of long term success with haemorrhoids is to combine constitutional treatment with local treatment.

Constipation should be addressed with a change of diet or with the addition of a stool bulking agent, such as psyllium husks. If constipation persists, appropriate treatments as detailed in Chapter 5 should be added. Medications should not be taken within an hour of the patient ingesting psyllium.

The surgical option, including ligation, cryotherapy, injection and sphincterotomy, should be considered when conservative treatment fails. This is especially the case for haemorrhoids that are severe, persistently painful, or irreducible. While the surgical option is excellent for producing quick relief in such cases, TCM treatment is still strongly indicated to address the constitutional components of the pattern, and thus prevent a recurrence, or a shifting of the manifestation of the pattern to another site.

BOX 13.2 GENERAL GUIDELINES FOR PREVENTION AND TREATMENT OF ANORECTAL DISORDERS

Squatting during defecation

- In some patients the pressure applied to the buttocks by the rim of the toilet seat is sufficient to occlude the anus and increase the force required to defecate completely. This can be avoided by adopting the squatting position during defecation. The squatting position opens the anal sphincter, gently increases intra-abdominal downwards pressure, and facilitates easy evacuation. There are readily available commercial platform devices that fit around the average western toilet to aid squatting. The position can take a little getting used to, but the effort is definitely worth it for those with persistent anorectal disorders or constipation.

Anal exercises

- This is a type of modified *qi gong* exercise, and works to tone the anal sphincter and rectal tissues, improve local blood circulation and aid evacuation. The exercise simply involves clenching and drawing upwards of the anus at regular intervals for several minutes at a time. The clenching may be co-ordinated with the breathing. While inhaling deeply using the abdominal muscles, relax the anus. On the outbreath the abdomen and the anus are contracted. This is repeated as often as possible. These exercises can be performed at any time and in any position, seated, standing or prone.

Exercise

- Regular exercise is especially important for those in sedentary or immobile occupations. Prolonged sitting impedes the local circulation of *qi* and Blood. Standing still for long periods weakens the Spleen and Kidneys. Gentle exercises are best for those with prolapsing haemorrhoids as the relentless pounding of running, or the increase in abdominal pressure that can occur with weight training, may aggravate an existing disorder.

Diet

- A diet that promotes a healthy bowel habit is essential. Avoidance of aggravating and constipating foods is recommended. Drinking plenty of water and ensuring adequate intake of dietary fibre in the form of vegetables and fruits (cooked for those with Spleen deficiency) is important.

Sexual activity

- Sexual activity should be limited for the duration of treatment as it may increase local pressure and aggravate the existing condition.

Constipation and diarrhoea

- Prompt treatment of constipation and diarrhoea is essential. This may require ensuring the patient has a supply of some mild laxative on hand when travelling or in a situation where constipation is more likely.

Anal hygiene

- Washing the anal area with warm water after bowel movement is recommended, especially for anal fissures and fistulae. This cleans the area thoroughly and promotes circulation. Use of toilet paper is not only relatively unhygienic, but may abrade the delicate mucosa, aggravate inflammation and inhibit healing.

肠风下血

13.1 INTESTINAL WIND

Pathophysiology

- Intestinal Wind is a term that describes mild haemorrhoids which are not accompanied by constitutional signs and symptoms. In situations where there are constitutional signs and symptoms, they tend to be of a Heat type, and as such tend to cause significant bleeding, and thus are classified as haemafecia (p.420).

Clinical features

- bleeding of fresh blood prior to, or following defecation, or with blood on the stool or on the toilet paper
- absence of pain, itch, distension or swelling

T unremarkable
P unremarkable

Treatment principle

Dispel Wind from the Intestines
Cool the Blood and stop bleeding

Prescription

HUAI JIAO WAN 槐角丸
(*Sophora Japonica Fruit Pill*)

huai jiao (Fructus Sophorae Japonicae) 槐角 120g
di yu (Radix Sanguisorbae Officinalis) 地榆 60g
fang feng (Radix Ledebouriellae Divaricatae) 防风 60g
dang gui (Radix Angelicae Sinensis) 当归 60g
zhi ke (Fructus Citri Aurantii) 枳壳 60g
huang qin (Radix Scutellariae Baicalensis) 黄芩 60g

Method: Grind the herbs to a fine powder and form into 9 gram pills with water. The dose is one pill twice daily. May also be decocted with an 80-90% reduction in quantities. **Huai jiao** and **di yu** cool the Blood and stop bleeding; **fang feng** dispels Wind and relaxes the Intestines; **dang gui** nourishes and regulates Blood; **zhi ke** regulates *qi* and, with the **dang gui**, prevents the cooling herbs from causing Blood stagnation; **huang qin** clears Heat and stops bleeding. (Source: *Shi Yong Fang Ji Xue*)

Modifications

- With copious bleeding, add **hai piao xiao** (Os Sepiae seu Sepiellae) 海螵蛸 15g and **san qi fen** (powdered Radix Notoginseng) 三七粉 3-6g.

Topical treatment

- In persistent cases, an astringent ointment can be directly applied to tone the rectal tissue and stop bleeding. Most suitable for cases that do not respond, or that respond slowly. Dissolve **ming fan** (Alumen) 明矾 3g in a little water and mix with 30g of a suitable carrier such as sorbolene or vaseline. The resulting ointment can be placed on sterile gauze and inserted in the anal canal, covering the haemorrhoid.

Patent medicines

Yi Zi Tang 乙字汤 (Cimicifuga Combination)
Zhong Guo Zhi Gen Duan 中国痔根断 (Chinese Zhi Gen Duan)
- this medicine is specific for bleeding haemorrhoids

Yun Nan Bai Yao 云南白药 (Yunnan Paiyao)
- the premier medicine for all types of bleeding. It is used in addition to the main formula. The red pill that accompanies the powder is only used in severe cases.

Acupuncture (select from)

Du.1 (*chang qiang* -) .... *luo* point of the *du* channel, an important point for haemorrhoids
Bl.30 (*bai huan shu* -) .... an alternative to Du.1 (*chang qiang*), similar in action although not as strong
er bai (M-UE-29) .... extra point for bleeding haemorrhoids
Bl.57 (*cheng shan* -) .... special point for haemorrhoids (especially with Du.1), regulates the lower Intestine and rectum, dispels Wind and stops bleeding
Sp.1 (*yin bai* -▲) .... *jing* well point, stops bleeding
St.37 (*shang ju xu* -) .... lower *he* point of the Large Intestine, clears Damp Heat and regulates the Intestines
Bl.32 (*ci liao* -) .... clears Heat from the lower *jiao* and the rectal area

- with severe bleeding, add PC.4 (*xi men* -) and Sp.10 (*xue hai* -)
- magnets can be applied to Du.2 (*yao shu*)
- *Ear points*: haemorrhoids, large intestine, distal segment rectum, *shen men*

Blood letting

This method is suitable for the excess haemorrhoid patterns. Search the lumbosacral area for small red or purple spots that blanch with pressure. Select 3-5 spots per treatment, sterilise them and bleed with a lancet or three edged needle. Apply cups over the puncture sites and draw a few millilitres of blood. This can be repeated once or twice a week for a few weeks.

Clinical notes

- Intestinal Wind is a common form of early stage haemorrhoids and responds rapidly to correct TCM treatment.

肠燥痔疮

13.2 INTESTINAL DRYNESS

Pathophysiology

- Haemorrhoids associated with Intestinal dryness are usually the result of chronic constipation and repeated straining, which puts pressure on the rectal circulation. The main focus of treatment is to treat the constipation by keeping the stools soft, relieving pressure on the anorectal area, and allowing the haemorrhoids to resolve.
- The dryness may be constitutional and is common in patients with a *yang* excess or hot constitution. It may also be acquired, following a febrile disease or chronic dryness of the Lungs, from smoking or respiratory disease.
- This pattern may be considered to be a type of 'Intestinal Wind'.

Clinical features

- Haemorrhoids with bleeding of fresh red blood that may precede or follow defecation. If the bleeding precedes defecation, it may be copious and forcefully ejected from the anus. The haemorrhoids may protrude (2nd degree), but are usually easily reduced. There may be pain, fullness or distension associated with defecation.
- chronic tendency to constipation, dry stools, straining or sluggish incomplete bowel movements
- thirst, dry skin

T unremarkable, or dry or with a dry, yellow coat over the root of the tongue
P possible thready or rapid

Treatment principle

Moisten the Intestines, soften the stools

Prescription

QIN JIAO BAI ZHU WAN 秦艽白术丸
(*Gentiana Macrophylla and Atractylodes Macrocephala Pill*)

qin jiao (Radix Gentianae Qinjiao) 秦艽 30g
dang gui wei (tail of Radix Angelicae Sinensis) 当归尾 30g
tao ren (Semen Persicae) 桃仁 30g
zao jiao zi (charred Fructus Gleditsiae Sinensis) 皂荚子 30g
di yu (Radix Sanguisorbae Officinalis) 地榆 30g
bai zhu (Rhizoma Atractylodes Macrocephalae) 白术 15g
chao zhi shi (dry fried Fructus Immaturus Citri Aurantii)
炒枳实 15g
ze xie (Rhizoma Alismatis Orientalis) 泽泻 15g

Method: Grind the herbs to powder and form into 6-gram pills with water or honey. The dose is one pill three times daily on an empty stomach. May also be decocted with a 50% reduction in quantities. **Qin jiao** clears Damp Heat while lubricating the bowel; **dang gui wei** and **tao ren** regulate the Blood and moisten the Intestine; **zao jiao zi** is acrid, warm and dispersing, lubricates the bowel and reinforces the laxative action of the **qin jiao**; **di yu** cools the Blood and stops bleeding; **bai zhu** strengthens the Spleen and dries Dampness; **zhi shi** directs *qi* downward and breaks up *qi* and food accumulation; **ze xie** promotes urination and provides an outlet for the Heat. (Source: *Shi Yong Fang Ji Xue*)

Variations and additional prescriptions

Chronic constipation

- Not uncommonly, patients will have chronic or recurrent haemorrhoids with few, if any, constitutional symptoms other than a chronic tendency to constipation or straining at stool. Additional prescriptions to consider to soften and facilitate the passage of stools are **MA ZI REN WAN** (*Apricot Seed and Linum Formula* 麻子仁丸, p.174), **RUN CHANG WAN** (*Moisten the Intestines Pill* 润肠丸 p.192), **ZENG YE TANG** (*Increase the Fluids Decoction* 增液汤, p.200) or **ZENG YE CHENG QI TANG** (*Increase the Fluids and Order the Qi Decoction* 增液承气汤, p.512), or **LIU MO TANG** (*Six Milled Herb Decoction* 六磨汤, p.19). Herbs to stop bleeding may be added, specifically **huai hua** (Flos Sophora Japonicae Immaturus) 槐花 and **di yu** (Radix Sanguisorbae Officinalis) 地榆, or in severe cases, combine with **HUAI HUA SAN** (*Sophora Japonica Flower Powder* 槐花散, p.496).

Haemorrhoids in robust, yang excess patients

- For robust patients with a *yang* excess constitution and significant Heat and dryness contributing to the constipation, copious bleeding and anal irritation, the emphasis shifts to clearing Heat from the Intestines, cooling the Blood and moistening *yin* with **LIANG XUE DI HUANG TANG** (*Rehmannia Decoction to Cool the Blood* 凉血地黄汤).

  sheng di (Radix Rehmanniae Glutinosae) 生地 18-24g
  dang gui (Radix Angelicae Sinensis) 当归 9-12g
  huang qin (Radix Scutellariae Baicalensis) 黄芩 9-12g
  tian hua fen (Radix Trichosanthes Kirilowii) 天花粉 9-12g
  di yu (Radix Sanguisorbae Officinalis) 地榆 12-15g
  huai hua (Flos Sophora Japonicae Immaturus) 槐花 12-15g
  chi shao (Radix Paeoniae Rubrae) 赤芍 9-12g
  zhi ke (Fructus Citri Aurantii) 枳壳 9-12g
  huang lian (Rhizoma Coptidis) 黄连 3-6g
  gan cao (Radix Glycyrrhizae Uralensis) 甘草 3-6g
  jing jie (Herba seu Flos Schizonepetae Tenuifoliae) 荆芥 ... 6-9g
  sheng ma (Rhizoma Cimicifugae) 升麻 3-6g

  Method: Decoction. **Sheng di** and **chi shao** cool the Blood; **tian hua fen** and **sheng di** clear Heat and generate fluids; **huang qin** and **huang lian** clear Damp

Heat; **di yu** and **huai hua** cool the Blood and stop bleeding; **zhi ke** regulates *qi* and prevents the cooling herbs from causing stagnation; **jing jie** dispels Wind and stops bleeding; **sheng ma** elevates *qi*.

Liver Fire

- For patients with constipation and haemorrhoids associated with Liver Heat or Fire (irritable, easily angered, red face and eyes, dizziness, concentrated urine, hypochondriac pain, a wiry, rapid pulse, and red edged tongue with a thick, dry coat) consider **DANG GUI LONG HUI WAN** (*Tangkuei, Gentiana Longdancao, and Aloe Pill* 当归龙荟丸, p.175).

Topical treatment

Jin Wan Hong 京万红 (Ching Wan Hung) - ointment
See p.490.

Patent medicines

Run Chang Wan 润肠丸 (Run Chang Wan, Fructus Persica Compound Pills, Smooth Tea Pills)
- a useful laxative formula for Heat type constipation

Chen Xiang Hua Qi Wan 沉香化气丸 (Chen Xiang Hua Qi Wan)
- constipation with *qi* stagnation

Gu Ben Wan 固本丸 (Gu Ben Wan, Ren Shen Ku Pen Wan)
- to nourish *yin* and moisten dryness

Jing Wan Hong 京万红 (Ching Wan Hung)
- topical ointment

Acupuncture (select from)

SJ.6 (*zhi gou* -) .... *jing* river and Fire point of the *san jiao*, spreads *qi* and disperses accumulation in the Intestines

St.25 (*tian shu* -) .... together these points regulate Intestinal
Sp.15 (*da heng* -) function and eliminate Dampness and Heat

Bl.57 (*cheng shan* -) .... special point for haemorrhoids, regulates the lower Intestine and rectum, dispels Wind and stops bleeding

St.37 (*shang ju xu* -) .... lower *he* point of the Large Intestine, clears Heat and regulates the Intestines

Bl.25 (*da chang shu* -) .... *shu* point of Large Intestine, clears Damp Heat

Kid.6 (*zhao hai* +) .... nourishes and moistens dryness and *yin*

- with Heat add LI.11 (*qu chi*) and LI.4 (*he gu* -)
- with Heat in the Liver, add Liv.2 (*xing jian* -)

- with severe bleeding, add *er bai* (M-UE-29) and PC.4 (*xi men* -)
- with severe pain, add Du.1 (*chang qiang*) and SI.5 (*yang gu* -)
- magnets can be applied to Du.2 (*yao shu*)
- *Ear points*: constipation area, haemorrhoids, large intestine, distal segment rectum, *shen men*, *san jiao*

Blood letting

See p.490.

Clinical notes

- The main feature of treatment is control of the constipation. Once the bowels move freely, the haemorrhoids will often spontaneously resolve. In long term cases there may be complications, such as Blood stagnation.
- For dietary recommendations, see pp.874, 876, 887.

湿热内蕴

13.3 DAMP HEAT

Pathophysiology

- The Damp Heat pattern generally corresponds to inflamed internal haemorrhoids. The Damp Heat from the diet, or Damp Heat created by Liver and Spleen dysfunction, sinks to the lower *jiao*, irritating the tissues of the rectum and anus, contributing to swelling, redness and pain.
- Another presentation of 'Intestinal Wind'.

Clinical features

- Haemorrhoids with bleeding of fresh red or plum coloured blood which may precede or follow defecation, or may coat the stool; the bleeding is often copious. The haemorrhoids may be swollen and painful and may protrude following defecation (2nd or 3rd degree) but will reduce spontaneously or will be able to be manually reduced.
- itch, discomfort, distension, burning, irritation and/or pain in the anus
- tenesmus
- abdominal distension
- thirst
- concentrated urine
- tendency to constipation or sluggish loose stools

T red body or red edges, with a greasy, yellow coat, especially over the root
P wiry and rapid, or slippery and rapid

Treatment principle

Clear Damp Heat from the Intestines
Cool the Blood and stop bleeding

Prescription

HUAI HUA SAN 槐花散
(*Sophora Japonica Flower Powder*) modified

huai hua (Flos Sophora Japonicae Immaturus) 槐花 12-15g
ce bai ye (Cacumen Biotae Orientalis) 侧柏叶 9-12g
jing jie sui (Herba seu Flos Schizonepetae Tenuifoliae) 荆芥穗 9-12g
zhi ke (Fructus Citri Aurantii) 枳壳 9-12g
huang bai (Cortex Phellodendri) 黄柏 9-12g
huang qin (Radix Scutellariae Baicalensis) 黄芩 9-12g
huang lian (Rhizoma Coptidis) 黄连 6-9g

Method: Decoction or powdered and taken in doses of 9-grams as a draft. **Huai hua** clears Damp Heat from the Intestines, cools the Blood and stops bleeding; **ce bai ye** cools the Blood, stops bleeding and reinforces the effect of the **huai hua**; **jing jie sui** dispels Wind and stops bleeding; **zhi ke** regulates *qi* and prevents the cooling herbs from causing Blood stagnation; **huang bai** clears Damp Heat from the lower *jiao*. (Source: *Zhong Yi Zhi Liao Yi Nan Za Bing Mi Yao*)

Modifications

- With copious bleeding, add **di yu** (Radix Sanguisorbae Officinalis) 地榆 12-15g and **hai piao xiao** (Os Sepiae seu Sepiellae) 海螵蛸 15g.
- With Heat in the Liver (red, sore eyes, irritability, red edges on the tongue), add **long dan cao** (Radix Gentianae Longdancao) 龙胆草 6g, **shan zhi zi** (Fructus Gardeniae Jasminoidis) 山栀子 9-12g and **qing dai** (Pulverata Indigo) 青黛 1-3g.
- With severe pain, add **yan hu suo** (Rhizoma Corydalis Yanhusuo) 延胡索 9-12g.
- With tenesmus, add **mu xiang** (Radix Aucklandiae Lappae) 木香 6-9g.

Topical treatment

Jin Wan Hong 京万红 (Ching Wan Hung) - ointment

A wash may also be used when itching, burning and local irritation are present. Boil 30 grams each of **ku shen** (Radix Sophorae Flavescentis) 苦参, **she chuang zi** (Fructus Cnidii Monnieri) 蛇床子, **huang bai** (Cortex Phellodendri) 黄柏 and **da huang** (Radix et Rhizoma Rhei) 大黄 in 2-3 litres of water for 30 minutes. Discard the herb residue and use the remaining water to soak the affected area once or twice daily, in a sitzbath or suitable bowl.

Patent medicines

Zhong Guo Zhi Gen Duan 中国痔根断 (Chinese Zhi Gen Duan)
- Damp Heat with bleeding

Yi Zi Tang 乙字汤 (Cimicifuga Combination)
- with constipation

Huang Lian Jie Du Wan 黄连解毒丸 (Huang Lian Jie Du Wan)
- Damp Heat

Chuan Xin Lian Kang Yan Pian 穿心莲抗炎片 (Chuan Xin Lian Antiphlogistic Tablets)
- combine with one of the above patent medicines for severe Heat

Jing Wan Hong 京万红 (Ching Wan Hung)
- topical ointment

Acupuncture (select from)

Du.1 (*chang qiang* -) .... best local point for haemorrhoids, but can be quite uncomfortable when there is significant inflammation

Bl.30 (*bai huan shu* -) .... an alternative to Du.1 (*chang qiang*), similar in action although not as strong

Bl.57 (*cheng shan* -) .... special point for haemorrhoids, regulates the lower Intestine and rectum, dispels Wind and stops bleeding

St.37 (*shang ju xu* -) .... lower *he* point of the Large Intestine, clears Damp Heat and regulates the Intestines

er bai (M-UE-29) .... extra point for bleeding haemorrhoids

Bl.32 (*ci liao* -) .... clears Damp Heat from the lower *jiao* and the rectal area

LI.11 (*qu chi* -) .... *he* sea point of the Large Intestine, clears Damp Heat from the Intestines

- with swelling and pain add Bl.58 (*fei yang* -), Bl.30 (*bai huan shu* -) and Bl.54 (*zhi bian* -)
- with severe Heat, add St.44 (*nei ting* -) and LI.4 (*he gu* -)
- with Heat in the Liver, add Liv.2 (*xing jian* -)
- magnets can be applied to Du.2 (*yao shu*)
- *Ear points*: haemorrhoids, large intestine, distal segment rectum, *shen men*

Blood letting

See p.490.

Clinical notes

- This is a common presentation of haemorrhoids, when they become inflamed and painful.
- While acupuncture is successful in reducing the swelling and pain of the haemorrhoids, the resolution of the systemic Damp Heat is best addressed with herbs and diet.
- Change of diet is imperative for any long term resolution of the haemorrhoids. For dietary recommendations, see p.884.

气不摄血

13.4 SPLEEN QI DEFICIENCY NOT HOLDING BLOOD

Pathophysiology

- Spleen *qi* deficiency not holding the Blood in the vessels is associated with persistent bleeding, rather than painful or prolapsing haemorrhoids. In contrast to the Intestinal Wind pattern, there are clear signs of constitutional deficiency.

Clinical features

- Haemorrhoids with bleeding of pale or fresh red blood; the volume of blood is usually relatively scant, but may on occasion be copious. There may be little protrusion of haemorrhoids, and little distension or discomfort.
- pale, lustreless or sallow complexion
- fatigue and lethargy
- poor appetite, abdominal distension, early satiety
- loose stools
- postural dizziness, light-headedness, blurred vision
- forgetfulness, poor memory, poor concentration
- insomnia, palpitations, with or without anxiety
- anxiety, phobias, panic attacks
- there may be other sites of bleeding, such as heavy menstrual periods or easy bruising

T pale and swollen, with toothmarks (or pale and thin with significant Blood deficiency)

P thready and weak or hollow

Treatment principle

Strengthen the Spleen's function of holding Blood in the vessels
Stop bleeding

Prescription

GUI PI TANG 归脾汤
(*Ginseng and Longan Combination*) modified

zhi huang qi (honey fried Radix Astragali Membranacei) 炙黄芪 18-30g
dang shen (Radix Codonopsis Pilosulae) 党参 15-24g
chao bai zhu (dry fried Rhizoma Atractylodes Macrocephalae) 炒白术 12-15g
fu ling (Sclerotium Poria Cocos) 茯苓 12-15g
dang gui (Radix Angelicae Sinensis) 当归 9-12g
mu xiang (Radix Aucklandiae Lappae) 木香 6-9g

chen pi (Pericarpium Citri Reticulatae) 陈皮 6-9g
xian he cao (Herba Agrimoniae Pilosae) 仙鹤草 15-30g
zhi huang jing (processed Rhizoma Polygonati) 制黄精 18-30g

Method: Decoction. **Dang shen, zhi huang qi, bai zhu** and **fu ling** strengthen the Spleen to control bleeding and supplement *qi*; **dang gui** nourishes Liver and Heart Blood; **mu xiang** and **chen pi** regulate *qi* and harmonise the Stomach; **xian he cao** astringes to stop bleeding; **huang jing** supplements *qi* and benefits the lower *yin*. (Source: *Zhong Yi Zhi Liao Yi Nan Za Bing Mi Yao*)

Variations and additional prescriptions

Yin and Blood deficiency

- Patients with chronic bleeding may eventually suffer *yin* and Blood deficiency. In addition to the bleeding and possibly painful haemorrhoids and signs and symptoms of Blood deficiency, patients experience signs of deficient Heat (flushing, nightsweats, thirst and dryness and a red, dry or pink tongue). The aim of treatment is to nourish *yin* and Blood, regulate Blood, ease bowel movements and stop pain with **ZHI LOU WAN** (*Fistula Pill* 痔漏丸).

shu di (Radix Rehmanniae Glutinosae Conquitae) 熟地 24g
shan zhu yu (Fructus Corni Officinalis) 山茱萸 15g
shan yao (Radix Dioscoreae Oppositae) 山药 15g
fu ling (Sclerotium Poria Cocos) 茯苓 12g
mu dan pi (Cortex Moutan Radicis) 牡丹皮 9g
bai shao (Radix Paeoniae Lactiflora) 白芍 9g
rou cong rong (Herba Cistanches Deserticolae) 肉苁蓉 12g
he shou wu (Radix Polygoni Multiflori) 何首乌 12g
chun gen pi (Cortex Ailanthi Altissimae) 椿根皮 9g

Method: Grind all the herbs to a fine powder and form into 9-gram pills with honey. The dose is one pill 2-3 times daily. May also be decocted with quantities as shown. **Shu di** supplements Kidney *yin* and nourishes Blood, **shan zhu yu** nourishes Liver *yin* and astringes; **shan yao** strengthens the Spleen and supplements *qi*; **fu ling** strengthens the Spleen and calms the *shen*; **mu dan pi** regulates the Blood and clears deficient Heat–these five herbs make up the bulk of **LIU WEI DI HUANG WAN** (*Rehmannia Six Formula* 六味地黄丸), the base prescription for all Liver and Kidney *yin* deficiency patterns; **bai shao** softens the Liver, nourishes Blood and astringes *yin*; **rou cong rong** warms *yang*, moistens the Intestines and gently promotes bowel movement; **he shou wu** nourishes *yin* and Blood; **chun gen pi** astringes the Intestines and stops bleeding. (Source: *Zui Xin Fang Ji Shou Ce*)

Topical treatment

See p.490.

Patent medicines

Gui Pi Wan 归脾丸 (Gui Pi Wan, Angelicae Longana Tea, Kwei Be Wan)
- Heart and Spleen deficiency

Shi Quan Da Bu Wan 十全大补丸 (Shi Quan Da Bu Wan, Ten Flavour Tea) - *qi* and Blood deficiency with Cold

Cong Rong Bu Shen Wan 苁蓉补肾丸 (Cong Rong Bu Shen Wan) - with a tendency to constipation

Acupuncture (select from)

Ren.12 (*zhong wan* +▲) .. *mu* point of the Stomach, warms and strengthens the Spleen and Stomach and supplements *qi*

St.25 (*tian shu* +▲) .... *mu* point of the Large Intestine, regulates Intestinal function

St.36 (*zu san li* +▲) .... *he* sea point of the Stomach, powerfully warms and strengthens the Spleen and Stomach and supplements *qi*

Sp.1 (*yin bai* ▲) .... *jing* well point of the Spleen, a special point for Spleen deficiency bleeding when treated with rice grain moxa

Sp.3 (*tai bai* +) .... *yuan* and *shu* stream point of the Spleen, strengthens and regulates the Spleen and Stomach, eliminates Damp; especially good for deficiency type haemorrhoids when combined with Sp.1 (*yin bai*)

Sp.6 (*san yin jiao* +▲) ...... strengthens the Spleen, regulates Liver *qi*, benefits the Kidneys, regulates *qi* and Blood

Bl.20 (*pi shu* +▲) .... *shu* point of the Spleen, warms and strengthens the Spleen and supplements *qi*

Bl.25 (*da chang shu* -) .... *shu* point of Large Intestine, regulates Intestinal function

- a moxa box over the abdomen is useful
- with prolapse or a sensation of heaviness in the rectum, add Du.20 (*bai hui* ▲)
- with anxiety or insomnia, add Ht.7 (*shen men*) and PC.6 (*nei guan*)
- *Ear points*: spleen, stomach, haemorrhoids, large intestine, distal segment rectum, *shen men*

Clinical notes

- Spleen *qi* deficiency type haemorrhoids are always chronic and will usually take 3-9 months of treatment to fully resolve and rebuild *qi* and Blood, although the bleeding should stop within a few weeks.
- For dietary recommendations, see p.870, 874.

气虚下陷

13.5 SPLEEN QI DEFICIENCY, SINKING QI

Pathophysiology

- This pattern corresponds with a reducible protrusion of second or third degree haemorrhoids, most commonly in older patients with poor muscle tone, or patients (often children) with chronic diarrhoea. The main feature is the prolapsing nature of the haemorrhoids.

Clinical features

- Haemorrhoids that easily protrude with defecation, coughing, sneezing, prolonged standing or walking. The haemorrhoids can be manually reduced, and may only spontaneously reduce when the patient is lying down. There may be bleeding of variable quantities of pale or fresh red blood, and discomfort, distension or fullness in the anal region. There may be a history of chronic diarrhoea.
- intermittent, dull, abdominal pain that is alleviated with warmth and pressure
- abdominal distension, early satiety
- tendency to loose stools or diarrhoea; occasionally sluggish bowels
- loss of appetite
- waxy, pale or sallow complexion
- fatigue, weakness
- shortness of breath with exertion
- spontaneous sweating

T pale and swollen, with toothmarks (or thin with Blood deficiency)
P thready and weak or moderate

Treatment principle

Strengthen the Spleen and Lungs, supplement *qi*
Promote the elevation of *yang qi*
Stop bleeding

Prescription

BU ZHONG YI QI TANG 补中益气汤
(*Ginseng and Astragalus Combination*)

zhi huang qi (honey fried Radix Astragali Membranacei) 炙黄芪 18-30g
dang shen (Radix Codonopsis Pilosulae) 党参 15-24g
chao bai zhu (dry fried Rhizoma Atractylodes Macrocephalae) 炒白术 12-15g
sheng ma (Rhizoma Cimicifugae) 升麻 9-12g
chai hu (Radix Bupleuri) 柴胡 9-12g
dang gui (Radix Angelicae Sinensis) 当归 6-9g

chen pi (Pericarpium Citri Reticulatae) 陈皮 6-9g
zhi gan cao (honey fried Radix Glycyrrhizae Uralensis)
炙甘草 6-9g

Method: Decoction or powdered and taken in doses of 9-grams as a draft. **Huang qi**, **dang shen** and **bai zhu** strengthen the Spleen, supplement *qi* and assist the Spleen in holding Blood in the vessels; **chai hu** and **sheng ma** support the *qi* supplementing herbs in lifting sinking *qi*; **dang gui** supplements Blood; **chen pi** and **gan cao** regulate *qi* and harmonise the middle *jiao*. (Source: *Shi Yong Zhong Yi Nei Ke Xue*)

Modifications

- With bleeding, add one or two of the following herbs: **pao jiang** (quick fried Rhizoma Zingiberis Officinalis) 炮姜 3-6g, **bai ji** (Rhizoma Bletillae Striatae) 白芨 12-15g, **chao huai hua** (dry fried Flos Sophora Japonicae Immaturus) 炒槐花 9-12g, **chao di yu** (dry fried Radix Sanguisorbae Officinalis) 炒地榆 9-12g.
- With anal distension and pain, add **zhi ke** (Fructus Citri Aurantii) 枳壳 9-12g and **mu xiang** (Radix Aucklandiae Lappae) 木香 6-9g.
- With Cold or elements of *yang* deficiency, add **zhi fu zi** (Radix Aconiti Carmichaeli Praeparata) 制附子 6-9g (decocted for 30 minutes prior to the other herbs).
- With diarrhoea, add **chao yi ren** (dry fried Semen Coicis Lachryma-jobi) 炒苡仁 15g, **chao bian dou** (dry fried Semen Dolichos Lablab) 炒扁豆 12-15g and **chao shan yao** (dry fried Radix Dioscoreae Oppositae) 炒山药 15-18g.
- With sluggish stools, add **huo ma ren** (Semen Cannabis Sativae) 火麻仁 9-12g, **hu tao ren** (Semen Juglandis Regiae) 胡桃仁 12-15g and **rou cong rong** (Herba Cistanches Deserticolae) 肉苁蓉 18-24g.

Variations and additional prescriptions

Spleen yang deficiency

- Patients with prolapsing haemorrhoids and relatively severe Spleen *yang* deficiency, will benefit from a few weeks treatment with a powerful and focused *yang* warming prescription. The aim of treatment is to warm *yang*, strengthen the Spleen and elevate Spleen *yang qi* with **FU ZI LI ZHONG WAN** (*Aconite, Ginseng and Ginger Formula* 附子理中丸) modified.

zhi fu zi (Radix Aconiti Carmichaeli Praeparata) 制附子 9-15g
gan jiang (Rhizoma Zingiberis Officinalis) 干姜 9-12g
dang shen (Radix Codonopsis Pilosulae) 党参 15-24g
chao bai zhu (dry fried Rhizoma Atractylodis
Macrocephalae) 炒白术 12-15g
zhi gan cao (honey fried Radix Glycyrrhizae Uralensis)
炙甘草 6-9g

zhi huang qi (honey fried Radix Astragali Membranacei) 炙黄芪 18-30g
zhi ke (Fructus Citri Aurantii) 枳壳 9-12g

Method: Grind herbs into powder and form into 3-gram pills with honey. The dose is one pill 2-3 times daily on an empty stomach. May also be prepared as a decoction, in which case **zhi fu zi** is cooked for 30 minutes prior to the other herbs (*xian jian* 先煎). **Zhi fu zi** and **gan jiang** warm Spleen *yang* and disperse Cold; **dang shen**, **chao bai zhu**, **zhi gan cao** and **huang qi** strengthen the Spleen and supplement *qi*; **huang qi** and **zhi ke** elevate *yang qi*.

Persistent diarrhoea with bleeding and prolapsing haemorrhoids

- In patients with persistent chronic diarrhoea and bleeding haemorrhoids associated with Spleen *yang* deficiency, the aim of treatment is to warm and supplement Spleen and Stomach *yang*, nourish the Blood and stop bleeding with **HUANG TU TANG** (*Yellow Earth Decoction* 黄土汤, p.438).

Topical treatment

See p.490.

Patent medicines

Bu Zhong Yi Qi Wan 补中益气丸 (Bu Zhong Yi Qi Wan, Central Qi Pills)

Fu Zi Li Zhong Wan 附子理中丸 (Fu Tzu Li Chung Wan, Carmichaeli Tea Pills, Li Chung Yuen Medical Pills)
- *yang* deficiency; may be combined with the above patent medicine

Cong Rong Bu Shen Wan 苁蓉补肾丸 (Cong Rong Bu Shen Wan)
- with a tendency to sluggish bowels

Acupuncture (select from)

Du.1 (*chang qiang* -) .... *luo* point of the *du* channel, an important point for toning the local tissues

Bl.30 (*bai huan shu* -) .... an alternative to Du.1 (*chang qiang*), similar in action although not as strong

Du.20 (*bai hui* ▲) .... raises *yang qi* when strongly moxaed

Ren.6 (*qi hai*) .... needle obliquely downwards with a 3-inch needle from Ren.6 (*qi hai*) towards Ren.3 (*zhong ji*). The needle is twirled to anchor it, then raised towards the sternum creating a lifting sensation in the lower abdomen. It can be taped (in its lifted position) in place for the duration of the treatment.

Ren.12 (*zhong wan* +▲) .. *mu* point of the Stomach, warms and strengthens the Spleen and Stomach and supplements *qi*

St.25 (*tian shu* +▲) .... *mu* point of the Large Intestine, regulates Intestinal function

St.36 (*zu san li* +▲) .... *he* sea point of the Stomach, powerfully warms and strengthens the Spleen and Stomach and supplements *qi*

Sp.6 (*san yin jiao* +▲)...... strengthens the Spleen, regulates Liver *qi*, benefits the Kidneys and regulates *qi* and Blood

Bl.20 (*pi shu* +▲) .... *shu* point of the Spleen, warms and strengthens the Spleen and supplements *qi*

Bl.25 (*da chang shu* +) ...... *shu* point of Large Intestine, regulates Intestinal function

- a moxa box over the lower abdomen is useful
- with bleeding, add Sp.1 (*yin bai* ▲) and Sp.3 (*tai bai* +)
- *Ear points*: spleen, prolapse, haemorrhoids, large intestine, distal segment rectum, *shen men*

Clinical notes

- Spleen *qi* or *yang* deficiency type haemorrhoids are always chronic and will usually take 3-9 months of treatment to fully resolve, although the sensation of prolapse should resolve quite quickly, usually within a few weeks.
- For dietary recommendations, see p.870-873.

血瘀痔疮

13.6 BLOOD STAGNATION

Pathophysiology

- Blood stagnation haemorrhoids are chronic, and are characterised by continuous or severe pain. They may develop from one of the previously described pathologies, or they may be associated with chronic Liver *qi* stagnation. As the movements of *qi* and Blood are intimately linked, *qi* stagnation retards Blood circulation, in this case, Blood circulation in the portal system. The resulting stagnation in the haemorrhoidal and rectal veins causes thrombosed haemorrhoids.

Clinical features

- Haemorrhoids with relatively severe or continuous anal pain, protrusion, distension and swelling, aggravated during defecation; the haemorrhoids appear dark or purple and may be quite large. Bleeding may be fresh red or plum coloured.
- dark or purplish spider naevi or broken vessels around the inner ankle and knee
- pain in the iliac fossae with palpation, especially left around St.27
- hypochondriac pain, tension or discomfort under the ribs
- dry mouth and throat with no desire to drink
- dry, scaly skin
- dull, sallow or darkish complexion, dark rings around the eyes
- dark or purplish lips and conjunctiva

T purplish or with purple or brown petechial spots with little or no coat; sublingual vessels are distended and dark

P thready and choppy

Treatment principle

Invigorate Blood, disperse and eliminate stagnant Blood

Regulate *qi*, stop bleeding and pain

Prescription

HUO XUE SAN YU TANG 活血散瘀汤

(*Decoction to Regulate Blood and Disperse Stagnant Blood*)

dang gui wei (tail of Radix Angelicae Sinensis) 当归尾 12-15g
mu dan pi (Cortex Moutan Radicis) 牡丹皮 9-12g
jiu da huang (wine fried Radix et Rhizoma Rhei)
酒大黄 6-9g
chi shao (Radix Paeoniae Rubrae) 赤芍 9-12g
tao ren (Semen Persicae) 桃仁 9-12g
hong hua (Flos Carthami Tinctorii) 红花 9-12g

su mu (Lignum Sappan) 苏木 9-12g
zhi ke (Fructus Citri Aurantii) 枳壳 9-12g
gua luo ren (Semen Trichosanthis) 瓜蒌仁 12-15g
bing lang (Semen Arecae Catechu) 槟榔 9-12g

Method: Decoction. **Dang gui wei**, **tao ren** and **hong hua** regulate Blood and eliminate stagnant Blood; **mu dan pi** and **chi shao** cool and invigorate the Blood and eliminate stagnant Blood; **jiu da huang** breaks up stagnant Blood and opens the bowels; **su mu** invigorates Blood; **zhi ke** regulates *qi*; **gua lou ren** moistens the Intestines; **bing lang** regulates *qi*, directs *qi* downwards and eases defecation. (Source: *Shi Yong Zhong Yi Wai Ke Xue*)

Variations and additional prescriptions

Severe Blood stagnation with constipation and pain

- With relatively severe constipation and pain, the aim of treatment is to open the bowels, soften hardness and break up Blood stagnation with **TAO HE CHENG QI TANG** (*Major Rhubarb Combination* 桃核承气汤) modified.

tao ren (Semen Persicae) 桃仁 12-15g
jiu da huang (wine fried Radix et Rhizoma Rhei) 酒大黄 .. 9-12g
mang xiao (Mirabilitum) 芒硝 6-9g
gui zhi (Ramulus Cinnamomi Cassiae) 桂枝 6-9g
zhi gan cao (honey fried Radix Glycyrrhizae Uralensis) 炙甘草 3-6g
chi shao (Radix Paeoniae Rubrae) 赤芍 9-12g
sheng pu huang (Pollen Typhae) 生蒲黄 9-12g
chao wu ling zhi (dry fried Excrementum Trogopteri seu Pteromi) 炒五灵脂 9-12g
san qi fen (powdered Radix Notoginseng) 三七粉 3-6g

Method: Decoction. **Mang xiao** is dissolved in the strained decoction (*yang hua* 烊化). **San qi** powder can be taken separately. **Tao ren** and **chi shao** invigorate Blood and eliminate stagnant Blood; **jiu da huang** breaks up stagnant Blood and opens the bowels; **gui zhi** opens and unblocks the channels to clear a path for eliminating the stagnant Blood; the saltiness of **mang xiao** softens hardness and disperses accumulated stools and stagnant Blood; **sheng pu huang** and **chao wu ling zhi** eliminate stagnant Blood and stop pain; **san qi** invigorates Blood and stops bleeding; **zhi gan cao** protects the Stomach and moderates the harsh nature of the other herbs.

Qi and Blood stagnation

- Blood stagnation frequently follows years of Liver *qi* stagnation. Patients so afflicted may initially suffer chronic intermittent haemorrhoids that gradually get worse, with generalised signs of Blood stagnation and *qi* stagnation. The haemorrhoids are swollen and painful, worse for stress, and may be irreducible. The aim of treatment is to move *qi* and Blood with **XUE FU ZHU YU TANG** (*Achyranthes and*

Persica Combination 血府逐瘀汤) modified.

dang gui (Radix Angelicae Sinensis) 当归 9-12g
sheng di (Radix Rehmanniae Glutinosae) 生地 12-15g
chi shao (Radix Paeoniae Rubrae) 赤芍 9-12g
chuan xiong (Radix Ligustici Chuanxiong) 川芎 6-9g
tao ren (Semen Persicae) 桃仁 9-12g
hong hua (Flos Carthami Tinctorii) 红花 9-12g
chai hu (Radix Bupleuri) 柴胡 6-9g
gan cao (Radix Glycyrrhizae Uralensis) 甘草 3-6g
chuan niu xi (Radix Cyathulae Officinalis) 川牛膝 12-15g
zhi ke (Fructus Citri Aurantii) 枳壳 9-12g
jie geng (Radix Platycodi Grandiflori) 桔梗 3-6g
di yu (Radix Sanguisorbae Officinalis) 地榆 9-15g
huai hua (Flos Sophora Japonicae Immaturus) 槐花 9-15g

Method: Decoction. **Dang gui**, **sheng di**, **chuan xiong**, **chi shao**, **tao ren** and **hong hua** constitute a variation of **TAO HONG SI WU TANG**, the fundamental prescription to nourish, regulate and invigorate Blood; **chai hu**, **zhi ke**, **gan cao** and **chi shao** constitute a variation of **SI NI SAN**, the fundamental prescription to regulate Liver *qi* and move stagnant *qi*; **jie geng** opens up the movement of *qi* through the chest and diaphragm, and can direct *qi* to the upper body; **niu xi** invigorates Blood and leads Blood downwards. Together these last two herbs seek to re-establish the correct ascent and descent of *qi* and Blood; **di yu** and **huai hua** cool the Blood and stop bleeding.

Following haemorrhoidectomy

- If the patient does require surgery, constitutional treatment to move the Blood stagnation is still strongly indicated. An appropriate prescription, based on the degree of Blood stagnation and the nature of the patient, may be selected. Consider **XUE FU ZHU YU TANG** (*Achyranthes and Persica Combination* 血府逐瘀汤, above), **GUI ZHI FU LING WAN** (*Cinnamon and Hoelen Formula* 桂枝茯苓丸, p.909) or **TAO HONG SI WU TANG** (*Dang Gui Four Combination with Persica and Carthamus* 桃红四物汤, p.910).

Topical treatment

Jin Wan Hong 京万红 (Ching Wan Hung)
See also p.490.

Patent medicines

Tong Jing Wan 痛经丸 (Tong Jing Wan)
- relatively severe Blood stagnation, with pain

Xue Fu Zhu Yu Wan 血府逐瘀丸 (Xue Fu Zhu Yu Wan)
- *qi* and Blood stagnation

Sheng Tian Qi Pian 生田七片 (Raw Tian Qi Ginseng Tablets)

- a good medicine for bleeding with Blood stagnation, combine with the above patent medicines

Jing Wan Hong 京万红 (Ching Wan Hung)
- topical application

Acupuncture (select from)

Du.1 (*chang qiang* -) .... *luo* point of the *du* channel, opens up the flow of *qi* and Blood through the *ren* and *du* channels, the main point for stagnant Blood haemorrhoids

Bl.57 (*cheng shan* -) .... special point for haemorrhoids, regulates the lower Intestine and rectum, stops bleeding and pain

Bl.30 (*bai huan shu* -) .... special point for rectal diseases, an alternative to Du.1 for sensitive patients

Bl.25 (*da chang shu* -) .... *shu* point of the Large Intestine, eliminates stagnation and regulates the Intestine

Bl.32 (*ci liao* -) .... clears Blood stagnation from the lower *jiao* and the rectal area

St.37 (*shang ju xu* -) .... lower *he* point of the Large Intestine, regulates the Intestines

er bai (M-UE-29) .... extra point for bleeding haemorrhoids

Sp.8 (*di ji* -) .... *xi* cleft point of the Spleen, regulates and invigorates Blood

Sp.10 (*xue hai* -) .... regulates and invigorates Blood, stops bleeding

LI.4 (*he gu* -) ....*yuan* point, stops pain, invigorates *qi* and Blood

- *Ear points*: haemorrhoids, large intestine, distal segment rectum, *shen men*

Blood letting

This technique (*see* p.490) is especially good when there is Blood stagnation. Ideally several millilitres of dark blood should be drawn. As the condition improves, the drawn blood should become fresh red.

Clinical notes

- Blood stagnation type haemorrhoids can be difficult to treat successfully with TCM alone and usually require a combined WM and TCM approach. Surgery is often the best solution, however the patient will definitely do better if the constitutional aspects of the pattern are dealt with at the same time.
- For dietary recommendations, see p.886.

SUMMARY OF GUIDING FORMULAE FOR HAEMORRHOIDS

Intestinal Wind - *Huai Jiao Wan* 槐角丸

Intestinal dryness - *Qin Jiao Bai Zhu Wan* 秦艽白术丸
- with chronic constipation - *Ma Zi Ren Wan* 麻子仁丸, *Run Chang Wan* 润肠丸, *Zeng Ye Tang* 增液汤, *Zeng Ye Cheng Qi Tang* 增液承气汤 or *Liu Mo Tang* 六磨汤
- in robust, *yang* excess patients - *Liang Xue Di Huang Tang* 凉血地黄汤
- with Liver Fire - *Dang Gui Long Hui Wan* 当归龙荟丸

Damp Heat - *Huai Hua San* 槐花散

Spleen *qi* deficiency not holding Blood - *Gui Pi Tang* 归脾汤
- with *yin* and Blood deficiency - *Zhi Lou Wan* 痔漏丸

Spleen *qi* deficiency with sinking *qi* - *Bu Zhong Yi Qi Tang* 补中益气汤
- with *yang* deficiency - *Fu Zi Li Zhong Wan* 附子理中丸

Blood stagnation - *Huo Xue San Yu Tang* 活血散瘀汤
- severe, with constipation and pain - *Tao He Cheng Qi Tang* 桃核承气汤
- with *qi* stagnation - *Xue Fu Zhu Yu Tang* 血府逐瘀汤

A13.1 Appendix: Anal Fissure

gang lie 肛裂

An anal fissure is a longitudinal tear or ulceration in the stratified squamous epithelium of the anal canal, below the dentate line (Fig. 13.2.1, p.520). Fissures usually occur in patients with a history of constipation and repeated straining at stool.

Anal fissures may seem a minor lesion, but they can cause bleeding, excruciating pain, and contribute to significant misery, as the patient dreads the moment of evacuation.

AETIOLOGY

Any condition that causes dry stools, and the straining that accompanies chronic constipation, can lead to an anal fissure. In addition, local trauma from insertion of a foreign object, or anal intercourse, can damage the anal epithelium.

TREATMENT

Treatment is based upon maintaining a soft stool so as to avoid repeatedly opening the fissure and keeping the area scrupulously clean. This means washing the anus with soap and water after defecation and avoiding the use of toilet paper as much as possible.

BOX A13.1 GENERAL MANAGEMENT RULES

1. Washing the anal area with warm water after bowel movement is recommended. This cleans the area thoroughly and promotes circulation. Use of toilet paper is not only relatively unhygienic, but may abrade the delicate mucosa, aggravate inflammation and inhibit healing. After washing, dry thoroughly with a soft towel or hair dryer–do not rub.
2. Keep bowel movements soft and regular. A diet with plenty of fibre, bulking material and lots of water helps to keep the stool soft.
3. Scratching the area should be avoided as much as possible, if necessary wearing soft cotton gloves to bed.
4. When bathing, very hot water, excessive showering and scrubbing should be avoided.
5. Use a bland cleansing cream rather than soap; avoid perfumed agents and talcum powder.
6. Loose clothing, boxer shorts or no underwear allows air to circulate to keep the area dry.
7. In obese patients, the buttocks can be strapped apart with adhesive tape to allow air flow over the anal area.

From a TCM perspective there are a few approaches. The rational treatment strategy is based on keeping the stools moist and soft, firstly by manipulating the diet, and secondly by adding appropriate gentle laxatives, with a tertiary strategy of clearing Heat or Damp Heat, and/or nourishing *yin* and Blood. The various patterns that cause constipation with dry stools are the most likely to contribute to anal fissures.

It is reasonable to persist with treatment for 4-6 weeks. If there has been no appreciable result after that time then the surgical option should be considered.

A13.1.1 HEAT/FIRE

Pathophysiology

- Heat dries the stools and makes them hard and difficult to pass. The hard stool can abrade or stretch the anal canal causing a tear in the mucosa.

Clinical features

- focal anal pain, aggravated during defecation
- dry hard stools or constipation, the stools may be streaked with fresh red blood
- thirst, dry mouth

T red or red edges and a dry, yellow coat, especially on the root
P wiry and rapid

Treatment principle

Clear Heat and Fire from the Intestine
Soften the stool and stop pain

Prescription

ZENG YE CHENG QI TANG 增液承气汤
(*Increase the Fluids and Order the Qi Decoction*) modified

da huang (Radix et Rhizoma Rhei) 大黄 6-9g
mang xiao (Mirabilitum) 芒硝 6-9g
sheng di (Radix Rehmanniae Glutinosae) 生地 15-18g
xuan shen (Radix Scrophulariae) 玄参 15-18g
mai dong (Tuber Ophiopogonis Japonici) 麦冬 12-15g
di yu (Radix Sanguisorbae Officinalis) 地榆 12-15g
huai hua (Flos Sophora Japonicae Immaturus) 槐花 12-15g

Method: Decoction. **Da huang** and **mang xiao** purge the Intestines and clear Heat; **xuan shen**, **sheng di** and **mai dong** nourish *yin* and moisten dryness; the saltiness of **xuan shen** and **mang xiao** also softens a hard stool; **di yu** and **huai hua** clear Heat, cool the Blood and stop bleeding. (Source: *Zhong Yi Zhi Liao Yi Nan Za Bing Mi Yao*)

Topical therapies

Applied after washing and drying the anus

- *Jing Wan Hong* 京万红 (Ching Wan Hung) - topical ointment
- *Gang Lie Gao* 肛裂膏 (Fissure Ointment), made from grinding equal quantities of **hu zhang** (Radix et Rhizoma Polygoni Cuspidati) 虎杖, **long gu** (Os Draconis) 龙骨 and **bai ji** (Rhizoma Bletillae Striatae) 白芨 into a fine powder and mixing the powder with vaseline.

Wash, sitzbath

The anal area can be bathed in a lukewarm decoction of **mang xiao** (Mirabilitum) 芒硝 30g and **huai jiao** (Fructus Sophorae Japonicae) 槐角 15g, boiled in 2 litres of water until reduced by 25%. 10 days for a course.

Patent medicines

Qing Fei Yi Huo Pian 清肺抑火片 (Ching Fei Yi Huo Pien)
Niu Huang Qing Huo Wan 牛黄清火丸 (Niu Huang Qing Huo Wan)
Run Chang Wan 润肠丸 (Run Chang Wan, Fructus Persica Compound Pills, Smooth Tea Pills)
Jing Wan Hong 京万红 (Ching Wan Hung) - topical ointment

Acupuncture (select from)

SJ.6 (*zhi gou* -) .... *jing* river and Fire point of the *san jiao*, spreads *qi* and disperses accumulation in the Intestines

St.25 (*tian shu* -) .... together these points regulate Intestinal
Sp.15 (*da heng* -) function and eliminate Heat

Du.1 (*chang qiang* -) .... best local point for anal disease
Bl.30 (*bai huan shu* -) .... special point for rectal and anal diseases, alternative to Du.1
Bl.57 (*cheng shan* -) .... special point for anal diseases, regulates the lower Intestine and rectum, dispels Wind and stops bleeding
St.37 (*shang ju xu* -) .... lower *he* point of the Large Intestine, clears Heat and regulates the Intestines
Bl.25 (*da chang shu* -) .... *shu* point of Large Intestine, clears Heat
Kid.6 (*zhao hai* +) .... nourishes and moistens dryness and *yin*

- with systemic Heat add LI.11 (*qu chi*) and LI.4 (*he gu* -)
- with Heat in the Liver, add Liv.2 (*xing jian* -)
- with severe bleeding, add *er bai* (M-UE-29) and PC.4 (*xi men* -)

- with severe pain, add Du.1 (*chang qiang*) and SI.5 (*yang gu* -)
- magnets can be applied to Du.2 (*yao shu*)
- *Ear points*: anus, haemorrhoids, constipation area, large intestine, distal segment rectum, *shen men*

Clinical notes

- In many cases, simply by softening the stools and reducing the mechanical pressure on the lesion, the fissure will resolve.
- Diet is an essential feature of treatment. See p.882 for recommendations. Make sure water consumption is adequate.

A13.1.2 DAMP HEAT

Pathophysiology

- When Damp Heat complicates an anal fissure, it usually relates to an aggravation or infection of an existing lesion.

Clinical features

- Focal anal pain, aggravated during defecation; accompanied by itch, discomfort, distension, burning, tenesmus and irritation; the stools may be blood streaked. There may be pus as well, or evidence of a discharge in between bowel movements.
- the stools may be dry and hard, or soft, sluggish, difficult to expel and foul smelling
- abdominal distension
- thirst
- concentrated urine
- tendency to constipation or sluggish, or loose stools

T red body or red edges, with a greasy, yellow coat, especially over the root
P wiry and rapid, or slippery and rapid

Treatment principle

Clear Damp Heat from the Intestine
Ease and promote bowel movements

Prescription

ZENG YE CHENG QI TANG 增液承气汤
(*Increase the Fluids and Order the Qi Decoction*) modified

da huang (Radix et Rhizoma Rhei) 大黄 6-9g
mang xiao (Mirabilitum) 芒硝 6-9g
sheng di (Radix Rehmanniae Glutinosae) 生地 15-18g
xuan shen (Radix Scrophulariae) 玄参 15-18g

mai dong (Tuber Ophiopogonis Japonici) 麦冬 12-15g
di yu (Radix Sanguisorbae Officinalis) 地榆 12-15g
huai hua (Flos Sophora Japonicae Immaturus) 槐花 12-15g
jin yin hua (Flos Lonicerae Japonicae) 金银花 12-15g
lian qiao (Fructus Forsythia Suspensae) 连翘 9-12g
ku shen (Radix Sophorae Flavescentis) 苦参 9-12g
di fu zi (Fructus Kochiae Scopariae) 地肤子 9-12g
sheng yi ren (Semen Coicis Lachryma-jobi) 生苡仁 15-24g
huang bai (Cortex Phellodendri) 黄柏 9-12g
cang zhu (Rhizoma Atractylodis) 苍术 9-12g

Method: Decoction. **Da huang** and **mang xiao** purge the Intestines and clear Heat; **xuan shen**, **sheng di** and **mai dong** nourish *yin* and moisten dryness; the saltiness of **xuan shen** and **mang xiao** also softens a hard stool; **di yu** and **huai hua** clear Heat, cool the Blood and stop bleeding; **jin yin hua** and **lian qiao** clear Toxic Heat; **ku shen** and **di fu zi** clear Damp Heat and stop itching; **sheng yi ren** clears Damp Heat; **huang bai** and **cang zhu** constitute **ER MIAO SAN**, and are particularly indicated for Damp Heat in the lower *jiao*. (Source: *Zhong Yi Zhi Liao Yi Nan Za Bing Mi Yao*)

Topical therapies

Applied after washing and drying the anus:

- *Jing Wan Hong* 京万红 (Ching Wan Hung) - topical ointment
- *Gang Lie Gao* 肛裂膏 (Fissure Ointment), made from grinding equal quantities of **hu zhang** (Radix et Rhizoma Polygoni Cuspidati) 虎杖, **long gu** (Os Draconis) 龙骨 and **bai ji** (Rhizoma Bletillae Striatae) 白芨 into a fine powder and mixing the powder with vaseline.
- A wash can be used when itching, burning and local irritation are present. Boil 30 grams each of **ku shen** (Radix Sophorae Flavescentis) 苦参, **she chuang zi** (Fructus Cnidii Monnieri) 蛇床子, **huang bai** (Cortex Phellodendri) 黄柏 and **da huang** (Radix et Rhizoma Rhei) 大黄 in 2-3 litres of water for 30 minutes. Discard the herb residue and use the remaining water to soak the affected area once or twice daily, in a sitzbath or suitable bowl.

Patent medicines

Long Dan Xie Gan Wan 龙胆泻肝丸 (Long Dan Xie Gan Wan, Lung Tan Xie Gan Wan) - Damp Heat in the Liver

Bei Xie Sheng Shi Wan 萆解胜湿丸 (Bi Xie Sheng Shi Wan)
- Damp Heat, with Damp greater than Heat

Huang Lian Jie Du Wan 黄连解毒丸 (Huang Lian Jie Du Wan)
- Heat greater than Damp

Niu Huang Qing Huo Wan 牛黄清火丸 (Niu Huang Qing Huo Wan)
- with constipation

Jing Wan Hong 京万红 (Ching Wan Hung)
- topical ointment

Acupuncture (select from)

St.25 (*tian shu* -) .... together these points regulate Intestinal
Sp.15 (*da heng* -) function and eliminate Damp Heat

Du.1 (*chang qiang* -) .... best local point for anal disease, but can be quite uncomfortable, especially when there is significant inflammation
Bl.30 (*bai huan shu* -) .... special point for rectal and anal diseases, alternative to Du.1
Bl.57 (*cheng shan* -) .... special point for anal diseases, regulates the lower Intestine and rectum, dispels Wind and stops bleeding
St.37 (*shang ju xu* -) .... lower *he* point of the Large Intestine, clears Damp Heat and regulates the Intestines
Bl.31-34 (*ba liao* -) .... clears Damp Heat from the lower *jiao* and the rectal area, select the most tender
LI.11 (*qu chi* -) .... *he* sea point of the Large Intestine, clears Damp Heat from the Intestines

- with redness, swelling and pain add Bl.58 (*fei yang* -) and Bl.54 (*zhi bian* -)
- with perineal itch, add Sp.10 (*xue hai* -)
- with Damp Heat in the Liver, add Liv.2 (*xing jian* -)
- magnets can be applied to Du.2 (*yao shu*)
- *Ear points*: constipation area, anus, haemorrhoids, large intestine, distal segment rectum, *shen men*

Clinical notes

- For dietary recommendations see p.884.

A13.1.3 BLOOD AND YIN DEFICIENCY

Pathophysiology

- Blood and *yin* deficiency can give rise to chronic constipation due to lack of nutrition and moisture in the Large Intestine. Repeated straining or abrasion of the anal canal during defecation can tear the mucosa causing fissures. Fissures can be compounded by the thinness of rectal tissues as a result of the depleted *yin* and Blood.

Clinical features

- focal anal pain, aggravated during defecation

- chronic constipation with dry stools that may be pellet or button like
- generalised dryness–skin, hair, eyes, mouth and throat
- generalised signs of Blood and *yin* deficiency: insomnia, postural dizziness, blurring vision, palpitations, fatigue

T pale or pink with a thin or absent coat
P thready and weak

Treatment principle

Nourish the Blood and *yin*
Moisten the Intestines and open the bowels

Prescription

RUN CHANG BU XUE WAN 润肠补血丸
(*Moisten the Intestines and Supplement Blood Pill*)

you dang gui (oily Radix Angelicae Sinensis) 油当归 15g
cu bai shao (vinegar fried Radix Paeoniae Lactiflorae) 醋白芍 30g
shu di (Radix Rehmanniae Glutinosae Conquitae) 熟地 30g
yu li ren (Semen Pruni) 郁李仁 12g
huo ma ren (Semen Cannabis Sativae) 火麻仁 12g

Method: Grind herbs to a powder and form into 9-gram pills with honey. The dose is one pill 2-3 times daily. May also be decocted with a slight reduction in quantities. **You dang gui** effectively lubricates the bowel while nourishing Blood; **cu bao shao** nourishes Blood and softens the Liver; **shu di** supplements *yin* and Blood; **yu li ren** and **huo ma ren** moisten and lubricate the bowel. **Huo ma ren** may be unavailable in some countries. An alternative herb is **hu ma ren** (Semen Lini) 胡麻仁.

Patent medicines

Run Chang Wan 润肠丸 (Run Chang Wan, Fructus Persica Compound Pills) plus one of the following if necessary:

Gui Pi Wan 归脾丸 (Gui Pi Wan, Angelicae Longana Tea, Kwei Be Wan)
- especially good when there are *shen* disturbances

Ba Zhen Wan 八珍丸 (Ba Zhen Wan, Women's Precious Pills)
- *qi* and Blood deficiency

Dang Gui Ji Jing 当归鸡精 (Tang Kuei Essence of Chicken)
- especially good postpartum with quite severe (and acute) Blood deficiency

Acupuncture (select from)

Du.1 (*chang qiang* -) .... best local point for invigorating local circulation of *qi* and Blood
Bl.30 (*bai huan shu* -) .... special point for rectal and anal diseases,

alternative to Du.1

St.25 (*tian shu*) .... *mu* point of the Large Intestine, regulates Intestinal function

Ren.4 (*guan yuan* +) .... meeting point of the *yin* channels on the abdomen, nourishes *yin* systemically especially when combined with Sp.6

Sp.6 (*san yin jiao* +▲)...... strengthens the Spleen, supplements *yin* and Blood, benefits the Kidneys and invigorates *qi* and Blood

St.36 (*zu san li* +▲) .... *he* sea point of the Stomach, powerfully warms and strengthens the Spleen and Stomach and supplements *qi* to create *yin* and Blood

Sp.10 (*xue hai* +) .... regulates and invigorates Blood

Bl.20 (*pi shu* +▲) .... *shu* point for the Spleen and Kidney
Bl.23 (*shen shu* +▲) respectively, warm and supplement to promote the creation of *yin* and Blood

Bl.25 (*da chang shu*) .... *shu* point of Large Intestine, regulates the Intestines

- with Kidney *yin* deficiency, add Kid.6 (*zhao hai* +)
- magnets can be applied to Du.2 (*yao shu*)
- *Ear points*: constipation area, anus, haemorrhoids, large intestine, distal segment rectum, *shen men*

Clinical notes

- In most cases, simply by softening the stools and reducing the mechanical pressure on the lesion, the fissure will resolve.
- Even though the fissure may resolve after 4-6 weeks, the chronic constipation that causes the fissure can take a long time to cure, especially if the patient has been taking bitter stimulant laxatives, such as senna and cascara. In recent cases, caused by haemorrhage or childbirth, some weeks to a couple of months is usually long enough for satisfactory results; in elderly patients and those with chronic problems, one to two years may be required to restore health and enable an easy bowel movement without a laxative formula.
- Increasing the consumption of *yin* and Blood moistening foods may be helpful. These include black sesame seeds, walnuts, pine nuts, honey, apricots and bananas. The Chinese like to mix a variety of these foods together in cakes and biscuits for prolonged use. These foods are suitable for all chronic dry types of constipation.
- For dietary recommendations see pp.874-876.

A13.2 Appendix: Anorectal Abscess

gang men yong 肛门痈

An anorectal abscess[1] is a collection of pus in the tissues around the anus and rectum. In TCM terms, an anorectal abscess is attributed to a localised collection of Toxic Heat, usually associated with an intense concentration of Damp Heat that has sunk into the lower *jiao*.

In TCM terms there are two types, acute and chronic. Acute abscesses often resolve spontaneously, usually within 7-10 days, but may recur. Depending on the severity of the initial condition and the general constitution of the patient, an acute abscess may go on to become chronic or to form a fistula. Chronic abscesses linger for more than two or three weeks. They may be encapsulated, or periodically open to the exterior through a thin drainage channel. They will sometimes exude a watery discharge.

TCM treatment is certainly worthwhile, and is effective in many acute and chronic cases. Resistant and unresponsive cases will require surgical drainage.

AETIOLOGY

Damp and Toxic Heat

Acute abscesses are associated with an intense accumulation of Damp Heat, or by definition, Toxic Heat. The line between Damp Heat and Toxic Heat is one of locality and degree. Toxic Heat is a focal aggregation of Damp Heat that breaks down the local tissue to form pus. Toxic Heat can also cause specific systemic symptoms, such as fever and chills or rigors, malaise, anorexia and nausea as the *zheng qi* does battle with the pathogenic Heat.

Accumulation of Damp Heat and predisposition to abscess formation occurs in patients with diets rich in Damp Heat inducing foods and liquids, in particular greasy and spicy foods, meats and alcohol. It can also be associated with chronic retention of Damp Heat in the Large Intestine as a result of organ system dysfunction, specifically Spleen weakness. This creates Dampness that sinks downwards and stagnates, over time generating Heat. The Spleen weakness may have its roots in Liver *qi* invasion, irregular dietary habits or Spleen damaging foods and substances. Once focal Damp Heat is present, it obstructs the circulation of *qi* and Blood, causing pain. Local trauma to the anus and rectum may also cause localised blockage to *qi* and Blood, allowing Damp Heat to collect. Abscess formation is also noted to occur in sedentary men with hairy buttocks, as ingrown hairs form a convenient focus to attract pre-existing Damp Heat.

In immunocompromised patients, those with pre-existing weakness of

---

[1] Wiseman's 'Anal welling-abscess'

Figure 13.2.1. *Anorectal abscess, fissure and fistula*

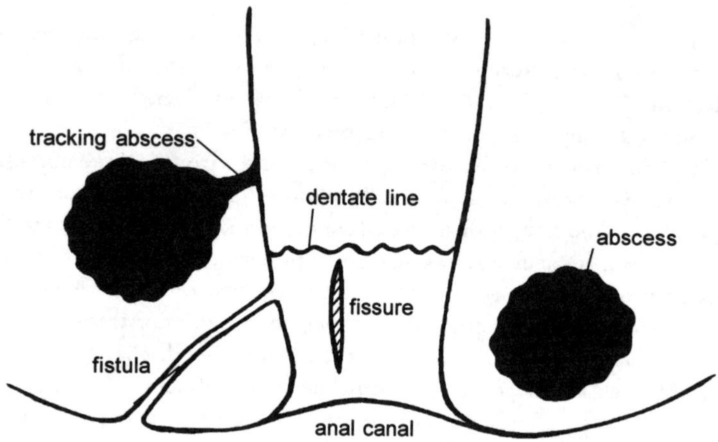

the Lungs, Spleen and Kidney, the elderly or frail, the *zheng qi* may be insufficient to expel the pathogen and repair the damaged area, so that an acute abscess may become chronic.

DIFFERENTIAL DIAGNOSIS

Thrombosed haemorrhoid: can be acutely painful and feel swollen, but usually lacks any systemic signs and symptoms of Toxic Heat (fever, chills etc.). Thrombosed haemorrhoids usually bleed.

TREATMENT

In acute cases 10-20 days of treatment is usually quite sufficient. Aggressive treatment is warranted because of the tendency of abscesses to form fistulae which can be difficult to treat. Treatment should continue for a period of time (1-3 weeks) following resolution of the abscess, to clear away any residual Damp or Toxic Heat, so as to prevent a recurrence. In chronic cases treatment needs to be prolonged, first to clear the lingering pathogen, and second to strengthen the patient's *zheng qi* to overcome the pathogen, prevent recurrence and repair the damaged area. Depending on the degree of deficiency, satisfactory treatment may take several months and should continue well after the abscess has resolved, to rebuild the patients *qi* and *yin*.

A13.2.1 ACUTE ABSCESS (TOXIC HEAT)

Pathophysiology

- Toxic Heat represents the acute phase of abscess formation. There are two stages in the life of an abscess: the developing focus of infection and suppuration, and healing following rupture. Normally once an abscess has ruptured, healing proceeds. However in weak or deficient patients this process may be disrupted. If this occurs the healing may be slow, or a chronic abscess or a fistula may form.

Clinical features

- Acute anorectal abscess; the features vary slightly depending on the depth of the abscess. Shallow abscesses can be painful, with progressive localised throbbing pain around the anus, and swelling, redness and tenderness. Deep abscesses may be less painful but tend to have more systemic manifestations of Toxic Heat.
- malaise, loss of appetite, nausea, fever and chills or rigors, lower abdominal pain (deeper abscess)
- constipation, concentrated urine

T yellow, greasy coat on the root; with systemic Heat, red body
P slippery, flooding and rapid

Treatment principle

Clear Toxic Heat
Reduce swelling and stop pain

Prescription

WAI BA FANG 外八方
(*External Formula for All Points of the Compass*)

This prescription is good for deep abscesses with less localised pain and more of the systemic signs of Toxic Heat.

zi hua di ding (Herba cum Radice Violae Yedoensitis) 紫花地丁 15-30g
pu gong ying (Herba Taraxaci Mongolici cum Radice) 蒲公英 15-30g
jin yin hua (Flos Lonicerae Japonicae) 金银花 15-30g
chi shao (Radix Paeoniae Rubrae) 赤芍 12-15g
ban zhi lian (Herba Scutellariae Barbatae) 半枝连 12-15g
huang qin (Radix Scutellariae Baicalensis) 黄芩 9-12g
ye ju hua (Flos Chrysanthemi Indici) 野菊花 9-12g

Method: Decoction. **Zi hua di ding, pu gong ying, jin yin hua, ban zhi lian** and **ye ju hua** clear Toxic Heat, **chi shao** cools the Blood and eliminates Blood stagnation; **huang qin** clears Damp Heat. (Source: *Zhong Yi Zhi Liao Yi Nan Za Bing Mi Yao*)

XIAN FANG HUO MING YIN 仙方活命饮 (*Sublime Formula for Sustaining Life*) modified

This prescription can be used interchangeably with the above prescription, although it is directed more towards shallow abscesses. The main difference is that this prescription has herbs to aid in the discharge of pus and invigorate Blood. It is effective once pus has formed and there is significant pain.

jin yin hua (Flos Lonicerae Japonicae) 金银花 15-30g
tian hua fen (Radix Trichosanthis Kirilowii) 天花粉 12-15g
dang gui (Radix Angelicae Sinensis) 当归 9-12g
chi shao (Radix Paeoniae Rubrae) 赤芍 9-12g
zhe bei mu (Bulbus Fritillariae Thunbergii) 浙贝母 9-12g
bai zhi (Radix Angelicae Dahuricae) 白芷 9-12g
chao zao jiao ci (dry fried Spina Gleditsiae Sinensis) 炒皂角刺 9-12g
ru xiang (Gummi Olibanum) 乳香 6-9g
mo yao (Myrrha) 没药 6-9g
fang feng (Radix Ledebouriellae Divaricatae) 防风 6-9g
chen pi (Pericarpium Citri Reticulatae) 陈皮 6-9g
gan cao (Radix Glycyrrhizae Uralensis) 甘草 3-6g
chuan niu xi (Radix Cyathulae Officinalis) 川牛膝 12-15g
wang bu liu xing (Semen Vaccariae Segetalis) 王不留行 ... 9-12g

Method: Decoction. **Jin yin hua** clears Toxic Heat; **tian hua fen** and **zhe bei mu** clear Heat, transform Phlegm and reduce swelling; **dang gui**, **chi shao**, **ru xiang** and **mo yao** regulate and invigorate Blood and eliminate Blood stagnation; **ru xiang** and **mo yao** are especially good for pain; **bai zhi** and **fang feng** dispel Wind and Damp, and reduce superficial swelling; **zao jiao ci** and **bai zhi** open up areas of accumulation and aid in the discharge of pus; **chen pi** regulates *qi*; **gan cao** clears Toxins and protects the Stomach; **chuan niu xi** invigorates Blood and directs the action of the prescription to the lower body; **wang bu liu xing** invigorates Blood and unblocks the channels.

NB: **Wang bu liu xing** is substituted for **chuan shan jia** (Squama Manitis) 穿山甲, the scales of the endangered pangolin that appeared in the original prescription.

Modifications

- With constipation, add **zhi da huang** (processed Radix et Rhizoma Rhei) 制大黄 6-9g and **mang xiao** (Mirabilitum) 芒硝 6-9g.
- With Heat in the Blood, add **mu dan pi** (Cortex Moutan Radicis) 牡丹皮 9-12g and **sheng di** (Radix Rehmanniae Glutinosae) 生地 15-18g.

- In cases with severe focal anal pain and swelling and significant systemic Toxic Heat signs and symptoms, combine both prescriptions.

Variations and additional prescriptions

With recurrent abscesses

- Patients with recurrent abscesses may benefit from a low dose of a Damp Heat or Toxic Heat clearing prescription for 6-8 weeks in between episodes, to clear any residual Damp or Toxic Heat from the Large Intestine. Patent medicines such as *Huang Lian Jie Du Wan* 黄连解毒丸 (Huang Lian Jie Du Wan), *Wu Wei Xiao Du Wan* 五味消毒丸 (Wu Wei Xiao Du Wan), *Chuan Xin Lian Kang Yan Pian* 穿心莲抗炎片 (Chuan Xin Lian Antiphlogistic Tablets) or *Huang Lian Su Pian* 黄连素片 (Tabellae Berberini) are suitable, administered at ¼ - ½ of the standard dose.

Patent medicines

Niu Huang Qing Huo Wan 牛黄清火丸 (Niu Huang Qing Huo Wan)
- with constipation

Huang Lian Jie Du Wan 黄连解毒丸 (Huang Lian Jie Du Wan)
- Damp and Toxic Heat

Wu Wei Xiao Du Wan 五味消毒丸 (Wu Wei Xiao Du Wan)
- Toxic Heat

Huang Lian Su Pian 黄连素片 (Tabellae Berberini)
- Damp Heat

Chuan Xin Lian Kang Yan Pian 穿心莲抗炎片 (Chuan Xin Lian Antiphlogistic Tablets)
- Toxic Heat, this medicine is often combined with one of the above patent medicines to enhance the Toxic Heat clearing action

Acupuncture (select from)

Bl.30 (*bai huan shu* -) .... local point for anal disorders

Bl.57 (*cheng shan* -) .... special point for rectal disorders, regulates the lower Intestine and rectum, dispels Wind and stop bleeding

Bl.40 (*wei zhong* ↓) .... clears Heat and cools the Blood

Du.12 (*shen zhu* -) .... special points for superficial abscesses and
Du.10 (*ling tai* -) sores

St.37 (*shang ju xu* -) .... lower *he* point of the Large Intestine, clears Damp Heat and regulates the Intestines

LI.4 (*he gu* -) .... *yuan* point of the Large Intestine, clears Heat from *yang ming*, stops pain and invigorates *qi* and Blood

LI.11 (*qu chi* -) .... *he* sea point of the Large Intestine, clears Damp Heat from the Intestines

- *Ear points*: anus, large intestine, distal segment rectum, *shen men*

Clinical notes

- Herbs are the treatment of choice for abscesses. In general, TCM treatment is effective for acute abscesses. Severe or unresponsive abscesses may need to be surgically lanced and drained.
- For dietary recommendations, see p.882.

A13.2.2 CHRONIC ABSCESS

A13.2.2.1 Yin Deficiency with lingering Damp or Toxic Heat

Pathophysiology

- Chronic abscesses may develop in patients with a pre-existing *yin* deficiency, or following an illness characterised by severe Heat that scorches *yin*. The *zheng qi* is unable to completely expel the remaining pathogen and an equilibrium is reached. These abscesses can persist for lengthy periods.
- In China, *yin* deficiency chronic abscess is often associated with tuberculosis.

Clinical features

- Chronic anorectal abscess with a mild degree of local swelling, heat and pain; the skin over the lesion is relatively normal in colour, or slightly darker than the surrounding tissue; on palpation the lesion feels soft and spongy.
- there may be sporadic watery or purulent discharge from the lesion
- nightsweats, afternoon fever, recurrent low grade fever, lingering fever
- insomnia, restlessness at night, flushing
- dry mouth, lips and throat
- tendency to constipation

T red with a thin, greasy coat
P thready and rapid

Treatment principle

Nourish *yin* and clear residual Damp/Toxic Heat
Aid in discharge of pus

Prescription

ZHU YE HUANG QI TANG 竹叶黄芪汤
(*Lophatherus and Astragalus Decoction*)

This prescription is used for a chronic abscess with residual *yin* deficiency and Damp Heat following a high fever. This pattern occurs in the few weeks following the acute phase of the abscess.

sheng di (Radix Rehmanniae Glutinosae) 生地 15-24g
mai dong (Tuber Ophiopogonis Japonici) 麦冬 9-12g
shi hu (Herba Dendrobii) 石斛 9-12g
huang qi (Radix Astragali Membranacei) 黄芪 12-18g
dang gui (Radix Angelicae Sinensis) 当归 9-12g
dan zhu ye (Herba Lophatheri Gracilis) 淡竹叶 6-9g
shi gao (Gypsum) 石膏 15-30g

huang lian (Rhizoma Coptidis) 黄连 3-6g
zi hua di ding (Herba cum Radice Violae Yedoensitis) 紫花地丁 15-24g
jin yin hua (Flos Lonicerae Japonicae) 金银花 15-24g
zao jiao ci (Spina Gleditsiae Sinensis) 皂角刺 9-12g
gan cao (Radix Glycyrrhizae Uralensis) 甘草 6-9g

Method: Decoction. **Sheng di, mai dong** and **shi hu** nourish *yin* and generate fluids; **huang qi** supplements *qi* to aid in discharge of pathogens; **shi gao** and **dan zhu** ye clear Heat from the *qi* level and *yang ming*; **huang lian, jin yin hua** and **zi hua di ding** clear residual Toxic Heat; **zao jiao ci** assists **huang qi** in discharging pus and opening the abscess; **gan cao** clears Toxins and protects the Stomach. (Source: *Zhong Yi Zhi Liao Yi Nan Za Bing Mi Yao*)

YANG YIN QING RE TANG 养阴清热汤
(*Decoction to Nourish Yin and Clear Heat*)

This prescription is used for a chronic abscess associated with a severe *yin* deficiency.

dang gui (Radix Angelicae Sinensis) 当归 9-12g
bai shao (Radix Paeoniae Lactiflorae) 白芍 12-15g
shu di (prepared Radix Rehmanniae Glutinosae) 熟地 12-18g
huang bai (Cortex Phellodendri) 黄柏 9-12g
ze xie (Rhizoma Alismatis Orientalis) 泽泻 9-12g
di gu pi (Cortex Lycii Chinensis) 地骨皮 9-12g
qing hao (Herba Artemesiae Annuae) 青蒿 15-24g
lu xian cao (Herba Pyrola Rotundifolia) 鹿衔草 15-30g
sha shen (Radix Adenophorae seu Glehniae) 沙参 12-15g
tian dong (Tuber Asparagi Cochinchinensis) 天冬 12-15g

Method: Decoction. **Dang gui, bai shao** and **shu di** nourish *yin* and supplement the Blood; **sha shen** and **tian dong** nourish *yin* and generate fluids; **lu xian cao, huang bai** and **ze xie** clear Heat, Toxin and Dampness; **di gu pi** and **qing hao** reach deep into the *yin* to clear Heat. (Source: *Zhong Yi Zhi Liao Yi Nan Za Bing Mi Yao*)

Topical ointment

CHONG HE GAO (*Flush and Harmonise Ointment* 冲和膏)

chao zi jing pi (dry fried Cortex Cercis Chinensis) 炒紫荆皮 150g
du huo (Radix Angelicae Pubescentis) 独活 90g
chi shao (Radix Paeoniae Rubrae) 赤芍 60g
shi chang pu (Rhizoma Acori Graminei) 石菖蒲 45g
bai zhi (Radix Angelicae Dahuricae) 白芷 30g

Method: Grind the herbs to a fine powder and mix into a paste with shallot (scallion) juice or yellow wine. Apply to the abscess as often as practical. (Source: *Shi Yong Zhong Yi Wai Ke Xue*)

Patent medicines

Zhi Bai Ba Wei Wan 知柏八味丸 (Zhi Bai Ba Wei Wan, Chih Pai Pa Wei Wan) plus *Chuan Xin Lian Kang Yan Pian* 穿心蓮抗炎片 (Chuan Xin Lian Antiphlogistic Tablets)

Acupuncture (select from)

Bl.30 (*bai huan shu* -) .... local point for anal and rectal disorders
Bl.57 (*cheng shan* -) .... special point for rectal disorders, regulates the lower Intestine and rectum, dispels Wind and stops bleeding
Bl.40 (*wei zhong* ↓) .... clears Heat and cools the Blood

Ren.4 (*guan yuan* +) .... meeting point of the *yin* channels, with Sp.6 to
Sp.6 (*san yin jiao* +) benefit the *yin* and *yuan qi* of the body

Bl.20 (*pi shu* +) .... *shu* points of the Spleen and Stomach
Bl.21 (*wei shu* +) respectively to bolster *yin*

St.36 (*zu san li* +) .... *he* sea point of the Stomach, strengthens the Spleen and Stomach and supplements *qi* and *yin*
Kid.3 (*tai xi* +) .... *yuan* and *shu* stream point of the Kidney, nourishes *yin*
Kid.6 (*zhao hai* +) .... master point of *yin qiao mai*, supplements *yin*

- *Ear points*: anus, haemorrhoids, large intestine, distal segment rectum, *shen men*

A13.2.2.2 Qi and Blood Deficiency with residual pathogen

Pathophysiology

- Chronic abscess of a *qi* and Blood deficient type develops in patients with *qi* and Blood deficiency patterns, often the debilitated or elderly. Following the acute phase, the *zheng qi* is simply insufficient to completely expel the pathogen and, instead of being eliminated, it reaches an equilibrium state with the *zheng qi*. This containment process, however, is energetically demanding, and the patient tends to weaken further over time, enabling the pathogen to periodically re-exert itself.

Clinical features

- Chronic anorectal abscess without a head; often little or no pain or awareness of swelling; the skin over the lesion may be indurated and is relatively normal in colour, or may be slightly darker than the surrounding tissue; on palpation the lesion feels flaccid and empty.

- may be occasional thin watery discharge
- pale or lustreless complexion
- fatigue, weakness
- loss of appetite
- spontaneous sweating
- loose stools

T pale with toothmarks, and a thick, white or yellow coat over the root
P weak, thready, soft

Treatment principle

Supplement *qi* and Blood
Aid discharge of pus

Prescription

TUO LI TOU NONG SAN 托里透脓散
(*Powder to Support the Interior While Discharging Pus*)

huang qi (Radix Astragali Membranacei) 生黄芪 18-30g
dang shen (Radix Codonopsis Pilosulae) 党参 15-24g
chao bai zhu (dry fried Rhizoma Atractylodes Macrocephalae) 炒白术 12-15g
dang gui (Radix Angelicae Sinensis) 当归 9-12g
zao jiao ci (Spina Gleditsiae Sinensis) 皂角刺 6-9g
bai zhi (Radix Angelicae Dahuricae) 白芷 6-9g
sheng ma (Rhizoma Cimicifugae) 升麻 3-6g
qing pi (Pericarpium Citri Reticulatae Viridae) 青皮 3-6g
gan cao (Radix Glycyrrhizae Uralensis) 甘草 3-6g

Method: Decoction. **Huang qi**, **dang shen**, **chao bai zhu** and **gan cao** strengthen the Spleen and supplement *qi*; **huang qi** powerfully augments *wei qi* and, in association with **zao jiao ci**, opens up and promotes movement of *qi* through areas of obstruction; **dang gui** nourishes and regulates Blood; **bai zhi** aids in the discharge of pus; **sheng ma** assists in elevating and invigorating Spleen *qi*; **qing pi** regulates and breaks up stagnant *qi*. (Source: *Shi Yong Fang Ji Xue*)

Modifications

- With residual Toxic Heat, add **lian qiao** (Fructus Forsythia Suspensae) 连翘 12g and **jin yin hua** (Flos Lonicerae Japonicae) 金银花 15g.
- If the abscess ruptures and continues to discharge a thin or watery exudate, delete **bai zhi** and add **rou gui** (Cortex Cinnamomi Cassiae) 肉桂 3g and **lu jiao jiao** (Cornu Cervi Gelatinum) 鹿角胶 12g.

Topical ointment

See p.526.

Patent medicines

Shi Quan Da Bu Wan 十全大补丸 (Shi Quan Da Bu Wan, Ten Flavour Tea)
Ba Zhen Wan 八珍丸 (Ba Zhen Wan, Women's Precious Pills)
Chuan Xin Lian Kang Yan Pian 穿心莲抗炎片 (Chuan Xin Lian Antiphlogistic Tablets)
- add to one of the above patent medicines to assist in clearing Toxic Heat

Acupuncture (select from)

Bl.30 (*bai huan shu* -) .... local point for anal and rectal disorders
Bl.57 (*cheng shan* -) .... special point for rectal disorders, regulates the lower Intestine and rectum and stops bleeding
Bl.25 (*da chang shu* ▲)..... *shu* point of the Large Intestine
Ren.4 (*guan yuan* +▲)..... meeting point of the *yin* channels, with Sp.6 to supplement the *yuan qi* of the body
Sp.6 (*san yin jiao*) .... strengthens the Spleen, regulates Liver *qi*, supplements *qi* and drains Dampness
Ren.12 (*zhong wan* +▲) .. *mu* point of the Stomach, warms and strengthens the Spleen and Stomach
St.36 (*zu san li* +▲) .... *he* sea point of the Stomach, powerfully warms and strengthens the Spleen and Stomach and supplements *qi*
Bl.20 (*pi shu* +▲) .... *shu* point of the Spleen, warms and strengthens the Spleen and supplements *qi*

- *Ear points*: anus, large intestine, distal segment rectum, *shen men*

Clinical notes

- Chronic abscesses can be difficult, and if not treated consistently, may form a fistula which can be resistant to treatment. *Qi* and Blood deficiency type chronic abscesses tend to respond somewhat better to treatment than *yin* deficiency chronic abscesses, but both types usually need reasonably lengthy treatment to resolve completely.

A13.3 Appendix: Anorectal Fistula

gang lou 肛瘘

An anorectal fistula is a tube like tract that forms a continuous opening between the anal canal and the perianal skin on the buttock. Some fistulae have multiple openings. Most commonly they are the sequelae of an incompletely resolved anorectal abscess and, as such, are the end phase of an abscess. Fistulas are difficult to treat satisfactorily with TCM alone due to their anatomy and location. Because they open into the anal canal they are subject to repeated contamination with faecal matter and subsequent reinfection. Small openings or a tortuous path can inhibit adequate drainage.

Fistulae are characterised by their chronicity and by discharge of thick or thin material, pain and itching. There are three main patterns, Damp Heat, *qi* and Blood deficiency and *yin* deficiency.

AETIOLOGY

Accumulation of an intense focus of Damp and Toxic Heat in the tissues around the anus, as for anorectal abscess. As the Toxic Heat damages more tissue and the abscess expands, it begins to track towards an external surface,

Figure A13.3.1 *Fistula formation*

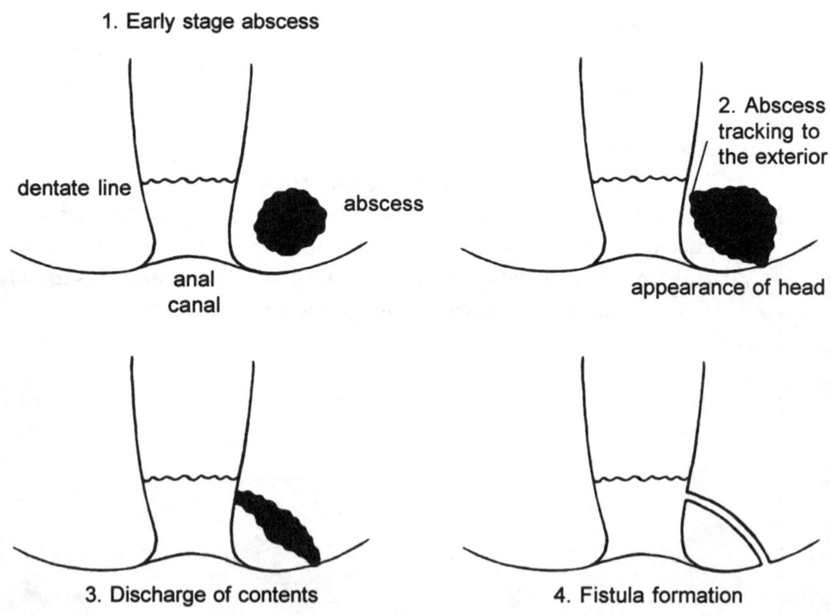

where the contents of the abscess are discharged. If the patient's *zheng qi* is compromised, or if the location of the fistula opening is such that reinfection occurs, the lesion will fail to heal and become chronic. Severe Damp Heat, which is complicated by *qi* and Blood stagnation, can also cause fistulae formation, sometimes without forming an abscess first. This is sometimes seen in patients with chronic diarrhoea, abdominal pain or dysenteric disorder.

TREATMENT

Treatment of fistulae with TCM are often unsatisfactory, but worth trying. TCM treatment is useful however, in assisting in recovery and healing after surgery, in preparing a patient for surgery, and for correcting any predisposing imbalances that may have contributed to fistula formation.

湿热肛瘘

A13.3.1 DAMP HEAT

Pathophysiology

- Damp Heat type fistulae are usually associated with the post acute phase of an acute anorectal abscess, where the pathogen is still evident and there are clear features of excess. The residual Damp (Toxic) Heat continues to smoulder, causing on-going suppuration and discharge.

Clinical features

- Anorectal fistula with discharge of thick yellow, malodorous material. There may be relatively severe pain and itching around the anus.
- feverishness, afternoon fever
- bitter taste in the mouth
- thirst or dry mouth with little desire to drink
- heaviness in the body, lethargy
- loss of appetite
- concentrated urine
- constipation or sluggish stools

T greasy, yellow coat
P wiry or slippery

Treatment principle

Clear Damp Heat, promote urination to clear Heat

Prescription

BEI XIE SHEN SHI TANG 萆解渗湿汤
(*Dioscorea Hypoglauca Decoction to Leach Out Dampness*)

bei xie (Rhizoma Dioscoreae Hypoglaucae) 萆解 9-12g
huang bai (Cortex Phellodendri) 黄柏 9-12g
chi fu ling (Sclerotium Poria Cocos Rubrae) 赤茯苓 12-15g
ze xie (Rhizoma Alismatis Orientalis) 泽泻 9-12g
yi ren (Semen Coicis Lachryma-jobi) 苡仁 18-30g
mu dan pi (Cortex Moutan Radicis) 牡丹皮 9-12g
chi shao (Radix Paeoniae Rubrae) 赤芍 9-12g
che qian cao (Herba Plantaginis) 车前草 15-30g

Method: Decoction. **Bei xie** and **huang bai** clear Damp Heat from the lower *jiao*; **chi fu ling**, **ze xie**, **yi ren** and **che qian cao** promote urination and clear Heat; **chi shao** and **mu dan pi** invigorate Blood and cool the Blood. (Source: *Zhong Yi Zhi Liao Yi Nan Za Bing Mi Yao*)

Modifications

- With severe residual Toxic Heat, add **huang qin** (Radix Scutellariae Baicalensis) 黄芩 9-12g, **huang lian** (Rhizoma Coptidis) 黄连 3-6g, **jin**

yin hua (Flos Lonicerae Japonicae) 金银花 18-30g and **pu gong ying** (Herba Taraxaci Mongolici cum Radice) 蒲公英 18-30g.

- With itching, add **di fu zi** (Fructus Kochiae Scopariae) 地肤子 9-12g and **bai xian pi** (Cortex Dictamni Dasycarpi Radicis) 白藓皮 9-12g.
- With constipation, add **da huang** (Radix et Rhizoma Rhei) 大黄 6-9g and **mang xiao** (Mirabilitum) 芒硝 6-9g.
- With discomfort in the rectal area, or tenesmus, add **mu xiang** (Radix Aucklandiae Lappae) 木香 6-9g and **bing lang** (Semen Arecae Catechu) 槟榔 9-12g.

Patent medicines

Bi Xie Sheng Shi Wan 萆解胜湿丸 (Bi Xie Sheng Shi Wan)
Long Dan Xie Gan Wan 龙胆泻肝丸 (Long Dan Xie Gan Wan, Lung Tan Xie Gan Wan)
- Damp Heat affecting the Liver

Huang Lian Jie Du Wan 黄连解毒丸 (Huang Lian Jie Du Wan)
- Damp Heat

Chuan Xin Lian Kang Yan Pian 穿心莲抗炎片 (Chuan Xin Lian Antiphlogistic Tablets)
- can be added to any other patent medicine to augment the Toxic Heat clearing action

Acupuncture (select from)

Du.1 (*chang qiang*) .... local points for anorectal disorders, invigorate
Ren.1 (*hui yin*) the circulation of *qi* and Blood locally

Bl.30 (*bai huan shu* -) .... local point for anal and rectal disorders, alternative to Du.1 for sensitive patients
Bl.25 (*da chang shu* -) .... *shu* point of the Large Intestine
Bl.57 (*cheng shan* -) .... special point for anorectal disorders, regulates the lower Intestine and rectum, dispels Wind and stops bleeding
Bl.40 (*wei zhong* ↓) .... clears Heat and cools the Blood
LI.4 (*he gu* -) .... *yuan* point of the Large Intestine, clears Heat from *yang ming*, stops pain, activates the dispersing function of the Lungs and invigorates *qi* and Blood
LI.11 (*qu chi* -) .... *he* sea point of the Large Intestine, clears Damp Heat from the Intestines

Ear points: anus, large intestine, distal segment rectum, *shen men*

气血两虚

A13.3.2 QI AND BLOOD DEFICIENCY

Pathophysiology

- *Qi* and Blood deficiency fistulae mostly occur in debilitated or elderly patients with insufficient *zheng qi* to expel the pathogen.

Clinical features

- Anorectal fistula with discharge of small amounts of thin, grey or watery material that is not particularly malodorous; the surrounding skin is dark or purplish. There is usually no obvious swelling and little or no pain, but there may be itching.
- pale or lustreless complexion
- fatigue, weakness
- loss of appetite
- spontaneous sweating
- loose stools

T pale with toothmarks, (or thin with significant Blood deficiency), with little or no coat or a thickish, white or yellow coat over the root

P deep, thready, weak, deficient

Treatment principle

Supplement *qi* and Blood
Clear residual Damp Heat

Prescription

BA ZHEN TANG 八珍汤
(*Ginseng and Dang Gui Eight Combination*) modified

dang shen (Radix Codonopsis Pilosulae) 党参 15-24g
chao bai zhu (dry fried Rhizoma Atractylodes Macrocephalae) 炒白术 12-15g
fu ling (Sclerotium Poriae Cocos) 茯苓 12-15g
zhi gan cao (honey fried Radix Glycyrrhizae Uralensis) 炙甘草 6-9g
shu di (Radix Rehmanniae Glutinosae Conquitae) 熟地 12-15g
dang gui (Radix Angelicae Sinensis) 当归 9-12g
chi shao (Radix Paeoniae Rubrae) 赤芍 9-12g
chuan xiong (Radix Ligustici Chuanxiong) 川芎 9-12g
huang bai (Cortex Phellodendri) 黄柏 9-12g
hu zhang (Radix et Rhizoma Polygoni Cuspidati) 虎杖 15-30g

Method: Decoction. **BA ZHEN TANG** supplements and regulates *qi* and Blood to augment *zheng qi*, and aids in expulsion of any residual pathogen; **chi shao** is substituted for the usual **bai shao** to invigorate Blood; **huang bai** and **hu zhang** clear Damp Heat. (Source: *Zhong Yi Zhi Liao Yi Nan Za Bing Mi Yao*)

Modifications

- With severe *qi* deficiency, add **huang qi** (Radix Astragali Membranacei) 黄芪 18-30g.
- With Damp (copious white or grey discharge), add **cang zhu** (Rhizoma Atractylodis) 苍术 12-15g and **bei xie** (Rhizoma Dioscoreae Hypoglaucae) 萆解 9-12g.
- With persistent discharge of a thin or watery exudate, add **rou gui** (Cortex Cinnamomi Cassiae) 肉桂 3g and **lu jiao jiao** (Cornu Cervi Gelatinum) 鹿角胶 12g (melted in the hot strained decoction).

Patent medicines

Shi Quan Da Bu Wan 十全大补丸 (Shi Quan Da Bu Wan, Ten Flavour Tea)
Ba Zhen Wan 八珍丸 (Ba Zhen Wan, Women's Precious Pills)
Wu Ji Bai Feng Wan 乌鸡白凤丸 (Wu Chi Pai Feng Wan)
Chuan Xin Lian Kang Yan Pian 穿心莲抗炎片 (Chuan Xin Lian Antiphlogistic Tablets) - a small dose can be added to any other patent medicine if there is significant residual pathogen

Acupuncture (select from)

Du.1 (*chang qiang*) .... local points for anorectal disorders, invigorate
Ren.1 (*hui yin*) the circulation of *qi* and Blood locally

Bl.30 (*bai huan shu* -) .... local point for anal and rectal disorders, alternative to Du.1 for sensitive patients
Bl.57 (*cheng shan* -) .... special point for rectal disorders, regulates the lower Intestine and rectum, dispels Wind and stops bleeding
Bl.25 (*da chang shu* ▲) ..... *shu* point of the Large Intestine

Ren.4 (*guan yuan* +▲) ..... meeting point of the *yin* channels, with Sp.6 to
Sp.6 (*san yin jiao* +) supplement the *yuan qi* of the body

Ren.12 (*zhong wan* +▲) .. *mu* point of the Stomach, warms and strengthens the Spleen and Stomach and supplements *qi*
St.36 (*zu san li* +▲) .... *he* sea point of the Stomach, powerfully warms and strengthens the Spleen and Stomach and supplements *qi*
Bl.20 (*pi shu* +▲) .... *shu* point of the Spleen, warms and strengthens the Spleen and supplements *qi*

Ear points: anus, large intestine, distal segment rectum, *shen men*

肝肾阴虚

A13.3.3 LIVER AND KIDNEY YIN DEFICIENCY

Pathophysiology

- Chronic Liver and Kidney *yin* deficiency type fistulae may develop in patients with a pre-existing *yin* deficiency, or following an illness characterised by severe or protracted Damp or Toxic Heat that burns up the *yin*. The *zheng qi* is unable to completely expel the remaining pathogen and an equilibrium is reached. These lesions can persist for lengthy periods.
- In China, *yin* deficiency chronic fistulae are often associated with tuberculosis.

Clinical features

- Anorectal fistula with discharge of small amounts of thin or thick material that may or may not be offensive. The anal area may be irritated and itch.
- nightsweats, afternoon fever, recurrent low grade fever, lingering fever
- insomnia, restlessness at night, flushing
- dry mouth, lips and throat
- tendency to constipation

T red with a thin greasy coat

P thready and rapid

Treatment principle

Nourish and supplement Liver and Kidney *yin*
Clear residual Damp/Toxic Heat
Aid in discharge of pus

Prescription

LIU WEI DI HUANG WAN 六味地黄丸
(*Rehmannia Six Formula*) modified

shu di (Radix Rehmanniae Glutinosae Conquitae) 熟地 15-24g
shan yao (Radix Dioscoreae Oppositae) 山药 15-18g
shan zhu yu (Fructus Corni Officinalis) 山茱萸 15-18g
mu dan pi (Cortex Moutan Radicis) 牡丹皮 9-12g
mai dong (Tuber Ophiopogonis Japonici) 麦冬 12-15g
yu zhu (Rhizoma Polygonati Odorati) 玉竹 9-15g
huang qi (Radix Astragali Membranacei) 黄芪 18-30g
zhi mu (Rhizoma Anemarrhenae Asphodeloidis) 知母 9-12g

Method: Decoction. **Shu di, shan yao** and **shan zhu yu** nourish Liver and Kidney *yin*; **mu dan pi** and **zhi mu** nourish *yin* and cool the Blood; **huang qi, yu zhu** and **mai dong** supplement *qi* and *yin*. (Source: *Zhong Yi Zhi Liao Yi Nan Za Bing Mi Yao*)

Modifications

- With residual Toxic Heat, add **lian qiao** (Fructus Forsythia Suspensae) 连翘 12g and **jin yin hua** (Flos Lonicerae Japonicae) 金银花 15g.
- With residual Damp Heat, add **bei xie** (Rhizoma Dioscoreae Hypoglaucae) 萆解 9-12g and **yi ren** (Semen Coicis Lachryma-jobi) 苡仁 18-30g.
- With itching, add **di fu zi** (Fructus Kochiae Scopariae) 地肤子 9-12g and **bai xian pi** (Cortex Dictamni Dasycarpi Radicis) 白藓皮 9-12g.

Patent medicines

Zhi Bai Ba Wei Wan 知柏八味丸 (Zhi Bai Ba Wei Wan, Chih Pai Pa Wei Wan)

Chuan Xin Lian Kang Yan Pian 穿心莲抗炎片 (Chuan Xin Lian Antiphlogistic Tablets) - a small dose can be added to any other patent medicine if there is significant residual pathogen

Acupuncture (select from)

Du.1 (*chang qiang*) .... local points for anorectal disorders, invigorate
Ren.1 (*hui yin*) the circulation of *qi* and Blood locally
Bl.30 (*bai huan shu* -) .... local point for anal and rectal disorders, alternative to Du.1 for sensitive patients
Ren.4 (*guan yuan* +) .... meeting point of the *yin* channels, with Sp.6 to
Sp.6 (*san yin jiao* +) supplement the *yin* and *yuan qi* of the body
Bl.30 (*bai huan shu* -) .... local point for anal disorders
Bl.57 (*cheng shan* -) .... special point for rectal disorders, regulates the lower Intestine and rectum, dispels Wind and stops bleeding
Bl.40 (*wei zhong* ↓) .... clears Heat and cools the Blood
St.36 (*zu san li* +) .... strengthens the Spleen and supplements *qi* and *yin*
Bl.20 (*pi shu* +) .... *shu* points of the Spleen and Stomach
Bl.21 (*wei shu* +) respectively to supplement *yin*
Kid.3 (*tai xi* +) .... *yuan* and *shu* stream point of the Kidney, supplements *yin*
Kid.6 (*zhao hai* +) .... supplements *yin*

Ear points: anus, large intestine, distal segment rectum, kidney, *shen men*

Clinical notes (all patterns)

- Difficult to treat satisfactorily. If there is no appreciable result after a few weeks of treatment, it is unlikely that TCM treatment will be effective. Surgical referral is recommended, but TCM treatment to promote healing and build *qi*, Blood and *yin* is useful.

A13.4 Appendix: Anal Itch

gang men sao yang 肛门瘙痒

Anal itching (or pruritus ani) refers to anal itching in the absence of any demonstrable anal pathology such as fistulae, ulcerated haemorrhoids or fissures. For itching associated with one of these pathologies, see the relevant section of the text.

From a biomedical point of view, the common causes of anal itching are noted in Box A13.4. Anal itching is however, frequently idiopathic.

AETIOLOGY

In all types of itching, it is usually Wind and, to a lesser extent, Dampness, that is the major causative factor. Itching is one of the cardinal symptoms of Wind. Wind is able to gain access to the superficial tissues through direct invasion, or can be created by a local or systemic deficiency.

Wind Heat

Wind Heat is associated with a direct invasion of Wind and Heat into the superficial layers of the body and Lungs. The Large Intestine and anus may be affected due to their close relationship, being a *yin yang zang fu* pair. Due to the dynamics of Wind Heat, (light, airy, rising and expansive), it usually affects the upper body. Anal itching is a relatively uncommon manifestation, but can occur as a result of the general dryness of skin and mucous membranes engendered by Heat affecting the Lungs.

Damp Heat

Damp Heat is a common cause of anal itching, because Damp Heat has a tendency to sink downwards and settle at the lowest point of the lower *jiao*. It causes itching by clogging and heating the local tissues. The local circulation of *qi* and Blood is impeded, and a type of localised Wind is engendered. Damp Heat is usually fed by consumption of Damp or Heating foods, such as greasy, rich or spicy foods and alcohol. It can also be created internally by organ system dysfunction, such as a disruption to the relationship between the Liver and Spleen. Liver *qi* stagnation can overcontrol the Spleen, which is weakened, and in turn creates Dampness. The Damp can then be acted upon by the Heat or Fire that is so often the by-product of chronic *qi* stagnation.

In addition, a Damp Heat Intestinal environment provides an ideal nursery for the incubation and growth of parasites of various kinds, including worms yeasts and fungi.

Blood deficiency

Blood deficiency is a common cause of chronic itching, and is characterised by dryness of the skin and itching that is aggravated by overexertion or bleeding, and by cold or dry weather.

Blood deficiency patterns are common in women with heavy menstrual periods and following gestation, childbirth and breastfeeding. Blood deficiency also occurs in patients with inadequate protein intake or Spleen deficiency, and in those who suffer excessive Blood loss through haemorrhage.

BOX A13.4 SOME CAUSES OF ANAL ITCHING

- atopic dermatitis and eczema, or psoriasis
- contact dermatitis, from chemicals, soaps, cleaning agents, perfumed toilet paper and topical anaesthetics
- allergy (citrus, Vitamin C, beer, coffee, chillies, cola drinks)
- parasites (pinworms, candida, scabies, nits)
- following oral antibiotics
- chronic diarrhoea with excoriation
- poor or obsessive personal hygiene
- excessively warm or tight clothing
- obesity
- climate
- fissure, fistula, haemorrhoids (see relevant section)

Systemic

- diabetes mellitus
- liver disease
- Crohn's disease

Parasites

Parasites, in particular pinworms, are a common cause of anal itch. They tend to occur in families in contact with animals, in those who travel to humid climates or in those who are exposed to less than sanitary conditions. They may, however, appear in patients with no identifiable transmission source. Yeast and fungal infections can also cause anal itching. Parasites tend to thrive in a Damp or Damp Heat internal environments.

TREATMENT

Local causes, such as fissure, fistula and haemorrhoids must be excluded or treated appropriately. All the obvious measures, such as identification of contact irritants, allergen and hygiene issues should be considered. Potentially irritant foods should be eliminated. See Box A13.1, p.511, for more management guidelines.

风热肛门瘙痒

13.4.1 WIND HEAT

Pathophysiology

- The mechanism of Wind Heat type anal itching is explained by the relationship between the Lungs and the Large Intestine. Wind Heat easily invades the Lungs causing dryness. The Heat and dryness may then be transmitted to the Large Intestine as the *yang* partner of the Lungs, and thus the anus.

Clinical features

- Intermittent, sporadic or acute anal itching; the local tissues tend to be dry, and may appear normal or slightly red; the itch may be aggravated or initiated during periods of dry or windy weather.
- In some cases, the episodes of itching may be accompanied by dryness of the mouth and nasal mucous membranes, cough, frontal headaches or dry, scratchy throat, but in others there may be no clear pattern.

T possibly red tipped, thin, white or yellowish coat
P possibly floating and/or slightly rapid

Treatment principle

Clear Wind Heat, supplement the Blood, stop itch

Prescription

XIAO FENG ZHI YANG TANG 消风止痒汤
(*Decoction to Eliminate Wind and Stop Itching*)

fang feng (Radix Ledebouriellae Divaricatae) 防风 9-12g
jing jie (Herba seu Flos Schizonepetae Tenuifolia) 荆芥 9-12g
niu bang zi (Fructus Arctii Lappae) 牛蒡子 9-12g
chan tui (Periostracum Cicadae) 蝉蜕 9-12g
ku shen (Radix Sophorae Flavescentis) 苦参 9-12g
bai xian pi (Cortex Dictamni Dasycarpi Radicis) 白藓皮 ... 9-12g
chi fu ling (Sclerotium Poriae Cocos Rubrae) 赤茯苓 12-15g
dang gui (Radix Angelicae Sinensis) 当归 9-12g
sheng di (Radix Rehmanniae Glutinosae) 生地 12-18g
zhi mu (Rhizoma Anemarrhenae Asphodeloides) 知母 9-12g
chuan xiong (Radix Ligustici Chuanxiong) 川芎 6-9g
gan cao (Radix Glycyrrhizae Uralensis) 甘草 3-6g

Method: Decoction. **Fang feng, jing jie, niu bang zi** and **chan tui** dispel Wind Heat and clear the exterior; **chan tui, ku shen** and **bai xian pi** stop itch; **chi fu ling** promotes urination to clear any lurking Damp Heat; **dang gui, sheng di** and **chuan xiong** nourish and regulate Blood, and are used on the basis of the principle that 'where the Blood flows, Wind cannot tarry'; **zhi mu** clears Heat from the *qi* level, nourishes *yin* and moistens dryness; **gan cao** clears Heat and harmonises the actions of the other herbs.

Modifications

- With severe itch, add **di fu zi** (Fructus Kochiae Scopariae) 地肤子 9-12g.
- With sluggish or dry stools, increase the dose of **niu bang zi** to 15g.

Patent medicines

Lian Qiao Bai Du Pian 连翘败毒片 (Lien Chiao Pai Tu Pien)
Yin Qiao Jie Du Pian 银翘解毒片 (Yin Chiao Chieh Tu Pien, Yin Chiao Plus)

Topical therapies

Wash the anal area in a decoction of **pu gong ying** (Herba Taraxaci Mongolici cum Radice) 蒲公英 30g, **ye ju hua** (Flos Chrysanthemi Indici) 野菊花 20g, **ai ye** (Folium Artemesiae Argyi) 艾叶 15g, **ming fan** (Alumen) 明矾 10g and **chuan jiao** (Pericarpium Zanthoxyli Bungeani) 川椒 10g.

Acupuncture (select from)

LI.11 (*qu chi* -) .... *he* sea point of the Large Intestine, clears Wind Heat and Damp Heat from the Lungs and Intestines
SI.3 (*hou xi* -) .... *shu* stream point of the Small Intestine, master point of the *du mai*, dispels Wind
Bl.30 (*bai huan shu* -) .... local point for anal diseases
Bl.57 (*cheng shan* -) .... special point for anal diseases, regulates the lower Intestine, rectum and anus, and dispels Wind
Sp.10 (*xue hai* -) .... regulates and invigorates Blood, dispels Wind
GB.31 (*feng shi* -) .... dispels Wind, stops itch

- with redness, swelling and pain add Bl.58 (*fei yang* -) and Bl.54 (*zhi bian* -); in severe cases add Du.1 (*chang qiang* -)
- with cough or sore throat, add LI.4 (*he gu* -) and Du.14 (*da zhui* -Ω)
- *Ear points*: large intestine, lower portion of rectum, *shen men*, adrenal

Clinical notes

- Anal itching of this type is often considered idiopathic, as no specific biomedical cause can be discovered. It generally responds well to TCM treatment.
- For dietary recommendations, see p.882.

湿热肛门瘙痒

13.4.2 DAMP HEAT

Pathophysiology

- Damp Heat type anal itch is usually associated with Damp Heat that originates from the diet, or disharmony between the Liver and Spleen. The Damp Heat sinks downwards into the Large Intestine. There will often be yeast overgrowth or parasites associated with this pattern.

Clinical features

- Acute, or more usually chronic, anal itching with relatively severe itching and irritation that tends to be worse at night and when stressed, and may be at times unbearable. The buttocks and anal area tend to be sweaty or moist, and the anus and surrounding tissues may appear red and swollen. The area of itching may involve other structures in the area, buttocks, scrotum, perineum or vulva. There may be a serous exudate.
- restless sleep or sleep often broken by itching
- irritability, short temper
- temporal headaches, stress headaches
- bitter taste in the mouth
- red complexion and eyes
- tendency to sluggish stools
- concentrated urine
- may be overweight, with a strong body odour and a glistening sheen to the skin

T thick, greasy, yellow coat on the root, may be red body or with red edges
P slippery and rapid

Treatment principle

Clear Damp Heat from the Liver system
Stop itch

Prescription

LONG DAN XIE GAN TANG 龙胆泻肝汤
(*Gentiana Combination*) modified

long dan cao (Radix Gentianae Longdancao) 龙胆草 6-9g
shan zhi zi (Fructus Gardeniae Jasminoides) 山栀子 9-12g
ze xie (Rhizoma Alismatis Orientalis) 泽泻 9-12g
che qian zi (Semen Plantaginis) 车前子 12-15g
huang bai (Cortex Phellodendri) 黄柏 9-12g
cang zhu (Rhizoma Atractylodis) 苍术 9-12g
di fu zi (Fructus Kochiae Scopariae) 地肤子 9-12g
ku shen (Radix Sophorae Flavescentis) 苦参 9-12g

bai xian pi (Cortex Dictamni Dasycarpi Radicis) 白藓皮 ... 9-12g
yi ren (Semen Coicis Lachryma-jobi) 苡仁 15-30g

Method: Decoction. **Long dan cao** clears and drains Heat and Damp Heat from the Liver; **shan zhi zi** and **huang bai** assist **long dan cao** in clearing Damp Heat from the lower *jiao*; **cang zhu** and **huang bai** make up **Er Miao San**, a standard combination for clearing Damp Heat from the lower body; **di fu zi**, **ku shen** and **bai xian pi** clear Damp Heat from the skin and stop itch; **ze xie**, **che qian zi** and **yi ren** promote urination to provide an outlet for the Damp Heat; **yi ren** protects the Stomach from the bitter cold herbs.

Modifications

- With severe itch and Dampness, add **xu chang qing** (Herba cum Radice Cynanchum Paniculatum) 徐长卿 12-15g and **tu fu ling** (Rhizoma Smilacis Glabrae) 土茯苓 18-30g.
- With sleep disturbance, add **ye jiao teng** (Caulis Polygoni Multiflori) 夜交藤 12-18g, **zhen zhu mu** (Concha Margaritaferae) 珍珠母 15-30g and **mu li** (Concha Ostreae) 牡蛎 15-30g, the latter two cooked for 30 minutes before the other herbs.
- With Spleen deficiency, add **fu ling** (Sclerotium Poriae Cocos) 茯苓 12-15g and substitute **bai zhu** (Rhizoma Atractylodes Macrocephalae) 白术 9-12g for **cang zhu**.
- With constipation, add **da huang** (Radix et Rhizoma Rhei) 大黄 6-9g.
- With Heat in the Blood, add **chi shao** (Radix Paeoniae Rubrae) 赤芍 9-12g.
- With damage to *yin*, add **sheng di** (Radix Rehmanniae Glutinosae) 生地 15-18g.
- With suspected parasites, add **bai bu** (Radix Stemonae) 百部 12-15g, **bing lang** (Semen Arecae Catechu) 槟榔 9-12g and **da huang** (Radix et Rhizoma Rhei) 大黄 3-6g.

Patent medicines

Long Dan Xie Gan Wan 龙胆泻肝丸 (Long Dan Xie Gan Wan, Lung Tan Xie Gan Wan)
- Damp Heat in the Liver

Ming Mu Shang Qing Pian 明目上清片 (Ming Mu Shang Ching Pien)
- with severe itch

Bei Xie Sheng Shi Wan 萆解胜湿丸 (Bi Xie Sheng Shi Wan)
- Damp Heat, with Damp greater than Heat

Jing Wan Hong 京万红 (Ching Wan Hung)
- soothing topical ointment

Topical therapies

The anal area can be bathed in a decoction of **huang bai** (Cortex Phellodendri) 黄柏 15g, **wu bei zi** (Galla Rhois Chinensis) 五倍子 15g,

ma chi xian (Herba Portulacae Oleraceae) 马齿苋 30g, **cang zhu** (Rhizoma Atractylodis) 苍术 15g and **tu fu ling** (Rhizoma Smilacis Glabrae) 土茯苓 15g.

Acupuncture (select from)

St.25 (*tian shu* -) .... *mu* point of the Large Intestine, regulates Intestinal function and clears Damp Heat
St.37 (*shang ju xu* -) .... lower *he* point of the Large Intestine, clears Damp Heat and regulates the Intestines
Bl.57 (*cheng shan* -) .... special point for anal diseases, regulates the lower Intestine and rectum, dispels Wind
GB.31 (*feng shi* -) .... dispels Wind, stops itch
Sp.10 (*xue hai* -) .... cools the Blood, dispels Wind and stops itch
Liv.5 (*li gou* -) .... *luo* point of the Liver, clears Damp Heat from the Liver and lower *jiao*
Liv.2 (*xing jian* -) .... *rong* spring and Fire point of the Liver, cools the Liver and drains Liver Fire
Bl.31-34 (*ba liao* -) .... clears Damp Heat from the lower *jiao* and the rectal area, select the most tender
LI.11 (*qu chi* -) .... *he* sea point of the Large Intestine, clears Damp Heat from the Intestines

- with severe redness and swelling, add Bl.58 (*fei yang* -) and Bl.30 (*bai huan shu* -)
- with severe itch, add Du.1 (*chang qiang* -) and Liv.8 (*qu quan* -)
- with temporal headaches, add GB.34 (*yang ling quan* -)
- magnets can be applied to Du.2 (*yao shu*)
- *Ear points*: large intestine, lower portion of rectum, Liver, *shen men*, adrenal

Clinical notes

- Damp Heat type anal itching may be diagnosed biomedically as fungal or candida infection of the anal area, or eczema, psoriasis or dermatitis.
- When *Candida albicans* is the pathogen, topical treatment with an antifungal cream may be necessary, in addition to the systemic treatment, as it can be persistent.
- For dietary recommendations, see p.884.

血虚生风

13.4.3 BLOOD DEFICIENCY (GENERATING WIND)

Pathophysiology

- Blood deficiency causes itching by not filling the vessels and tissues of the anus, creating a local vacuum and thus engendering the local movement of Wind.

Clinical features

- Chronic anal itching that is mild during the day, but worse at night, when fatigued, during cold dry weather or following a menstrual period. The local tissues tend to be quite dry and may appear scaly or thickened. The itching may interrupt sleep and make the patient anxious about going to bed. The lack of sleep aggravates the deficiency, creating a vicious cycle. The area of itching may involve other structures in the area, buttocks, scrotum, perineum or vulva.
- postural dizziness
- insomnia, anxiety, palpitations
- fatigue, weakness
- pale complexion, conjunctivae, lips, nails

T pale, or with pale edges and little or no coat
P thready

Treatment principle

Nourish and supplement Blood, dispel Wind, stop itch

Prescription

SI WU XIAO FENG SAN 四物消风散
(*Eliminate Wind Powder with the Four Substances*)

sheng di (Radix Rehmanniae Glutinosae) 生地 12-18g
dang gui (Radix Angelicae Sinensis) 当归 9-12g
chuan xiong (Radix Ligustici Chuanxiong) 川芎 6-9g
bai shao (Radix Paeoniae Lactiflorae) 白芍 12-18g
chi shao (Radix Paeoniae Rubrae) 赤芍 9-12g
fang feng (Radix Ledebouriellae Divaricatae) 防风 9-12g
jing jie (Herba seu Flos Schizonepetae Tenuifolia) 荆芥 9-12g
bai ji li (Fructus Tribuli Terrestris) 白蒺藜 12-15g
he shou wu (Radix Polygoni Multiflori) 何首乌 12-15g
ji xue teng (Radix et Caulis Jixueteng) 鸡血藤 18-30g

Method: Decoction. **Sheng di, dang gui, chuan xiong, bai shao** and **he shou wu** nourish Blood and *yin*, and moisten dryness, eliminating the basis of the internal Wind; **fang feng** and **jing jie** dispel Wind; **bai ji li** calms the Liver, dispels Wind and stops itch; **ji xue teng** supplements Blood and promotes movement of Blood dispeling Wind.

Modifications

- With severe itch, add **xu chang qing** (Herba cum Radice Cynanchum Paniculatum) 徐长卿 12-15g and **bai xian pi** (Cortex Dictamni Dasycarpi Radicis) 白藓皮 9-12g.
- With insomnia or anxiety, add **bai zi ren** (Semen Biotae Orientalis) 柏子仁 9-12g, **ye jiao teng** (Caulis Polygoni Multiflori) 夜交藤 18-30g and **he huan pi** (Cortex Albizziae Julibrissin) 合欢皮 12-15g.

Variations and additional prescriptions

- With *yin* and Blood deficiency, and a degree of *yang* deficiency (fairly common in menopausal women), anal itching may be accompanied by vulval itching and clear signs of *shen* and sleep disturbance. Anxiety becomes a major feature, as the patient frets about the aggravation of the itch at night and its effect on sleep. The aim of treatment is to nourish Blood and *yin*, support *yang* and calm the *shen* with **GUI PI TANG** (*Ginseng and Longan Combination* 归脾汤) modified.

  zhi huang qi (honey fried Radix Astragali Membranacei) 黄芪 15-18g
  dang shen (Radix Codonopsis Pilosulae) 党参 12-15g
  dang gui (Radix Angelicae Sinensis) 当归 12-15g
  bai shao (Radix Paeoniae Lactiflorae) 白芍 12-18g
  fu shen (Sclerotium Poria Cocos Pararadicis) 茯神 12-15g
  yuan zhi (Radix Polygalae Tenuifoliae) 远志 6-9g
  chao suan zao ren (dry fried Semen Zizyphi Spinosae) 酸枣仁 12-18g
  zhi gan cao (honey fried Radix Glycyrrhizae Uralensis) 炙甘草 3-6g
  zhi mu (Rhizoma Anemarrhenae Asphodeloides) 知母 9-12g
  ze xie (Rhizoma Alismatis Orientalis) 泽泻 9-12g
  xian mao (Rhizoma Curculiginis Orchioidis) 仙茅 9-12g
  xian ling pi (Herba Epimedii) 仙灵脾 12-15g
  huang bai (Cortex Phellodendri) 黄柏 9-12g

  Method: Decoction. **Zhi huang qi, dang shen** and **zhi gan cao** strengthen the Spleen and supplement *qi* to generate Blood; **dang gui** and **bai shao** nourish Blood and soften the Liver to eliminate internal Wind; **fu shen, yuan zhi** and **chao suan zao ren** nourish the Heart and calm the *shen*; **xian mao** and **xian ling pi** supplement and warm Kidney *yang*; **zhi mu, huang bai** and **ze xie** nourish Kidney *yin* and cool the Liver; **zhi gan cao** harmonises the middle *jiao*.

Patent medicines

Gui Pi Wan 归脾丸 (Gui Pi Wan, Angelicae Longana Tea, Kwei Be Wan)
Shi Quan Da Bu Wan 十全大补丸 (Shi Quan Da Bu Wan, Ten Flavour Tea)

Ba Zhen Wan 八珍丸 (Ba Zhen Wan, Women's Precious Pills)
Wu Ji Bai Feng Wan 乌鸡白凤丸 (Wu Chi Pai Feng Wan)
Dang Gui Ji Jing 当归鸡精 (Tangkwei Essence of Chicken)

Topical therapies

The anal area can be bathed in a decoction of **dang gui** (Radix Angelicae Sinensis) 当归 15g, **she chuang zi** (Fructus Cnidii Monnieri) 蛇床子 15g, **ku shen** (Radix Sophorae Flavescentis) 苦参 30g, **di fu zi** (Fructus Kochiae Scopariae) 地肤子 15g and **bai xian pi** (Cortex Dictamni Dasycarpi Radicis) 白藓皮 15g.

Acupuncture (select from)

Bl.30 (*bai huan shu*) .... local point for anal disorders
Bl.57 (*cheng shan*) .... special point for rectal disorders, regulates the lower Intestine and rectum and dispels Wind
Ren.4 (*guan yuan* +▲) ..... meeting point of the *yin* channels, with Sp.6 to benefit *yuan qi* and Blood
Ren.12 (*zhong wan* +▲) .. *mu* point of the Stomach, warms and strengthens the Spleen and Stomach to supplement and generate Blood
St.36 (*zu san li* +▲) .... *he* sea point of the Stomach, powerfully warms and strengthens the Spleen and Stomach and supplements *qi*
Sp.10 (*xue hai*) .... regulates and invigorates Blood, dispels Wind and stops itch
GB.31 (*feng shi* -) .... dispels Wind and stops itch
Sp.6 (*san yin jiao* +) .... strengthens the Spleen to nourish Blood, regulates Liver *qi*, benefits the Kidneys and invigorates *qi* and Blood
Bl.20 (*pi shu* +▲) .... *shu* point of the Spleen, warms and strengthens the Spleen and supplements *qi* and Blood

- *Ear points*: large intestine, lower portion of rectum, *shen men*, adrenal

Clinical notes

- Blood deficiency anal itch is a chronic pattern that primarily affects women over 40, and will most likely be diagnosed biomedically as idiopathic pruritus or pruritus associated with menopause.
- Blood deficiency anal itching respond satisfactorily to prolonged treatment, with herbs and diet as the main therapies.
- For dietary recommendations, see p.874.

虫积肛门瘙痒

13.4.4 PARASITES

Pathophysiology

- Intestinal parasites are a quite common cause of anal itching, especially in children and in warmer climates.
- The term 'worm' (*chong* 虫) has several connotations in TCM. It can refer to the visible variety of worm, such as the pin or thread worms that most commonly cause itching, the larger inhabitant of the intestines such as tape and round worms, and to blood parasites like schistosomes. *Chong* can also refer to the 'invisible' variety of parasite, manifesting in conditions which we may describe as 'candidiasis', *gu* syndrome, or any of a number of patterns due to the lingering persistence of some obstinate pathogenic influence (*fu xie* 伏邪). These may be chronic viral, bacterial or fungal infections.
- Depending on the type of 'worm' infestation, the approach will be different. For the large and visible variety, vermicidal drugs can be used for a relatively short period of time to kill the worms, perhaps then followed by a Spleen supplementing prescription to restore the digestion. For the invisible variety, treatment needs to be prolonged and flexible, slowly altering the internal environment to make it hostile to the invader, while gently strengthening *zheng qi*. This can be a complex business, as too much supplementation can strengthen the pathogen, and too much pathogen clearing can damage *zheng qi*.

Clinical features

- Anal itching, most commonly in children, but may occur in adults. This is often the only symptom, but in some cases may be accompanied by one or more of the following–
- intermittent abdominal pain of variable intensity, usually around the umbilicus
- persistent abdominal distension, flatulence
- ravenous hunger or loss of appetite, craving for odd foods, multiple food sensitivities
- tooth grinding at night, itching of the nose
- dark rings under the eyes, blue or purple spots or lines in the sclera
- scaly white spots on the face and neck (*chong ban* 虫斑), small red papules on the inside of the lips and upper surface of the tongue
- there will often be some objective evidence such as worms (or worm parts or eggs) in the stools
- in chronic cases there may be signs of *qi* and Blood deficiency such as emaciation, sallow complexion, fatigue, lethargy, dizziness, insomnia, pale tongue and weak pulse

Treatment principle

Kill worms

Prescription

ZHUI CHONG WAN 追虫丸
(*Pursue Parasites Pill*)

This prescription is a broad spectrum vermicide. It should not be used for more than a week or two, and then always followed by an appropriate Spleen supplementing prescription, or *qi* and Blood supplementing prescription.

bing lang (Semen Arecae Catechu) 槟榔 9-12g
lei wan (Sclerotium Omphaliae Lapidescens) 雷丸 6-9g
shi jun zi (Fructus Quisqualis Indicae) 使君子 9-12g
ku lian gen pi (Cortex Meliae Radicis) 苦楝根皮 9-12g
mu xiang (Radix Aucklandiae Lappae) 木香 6-9g
qian niu zi (Semen Pharbitidis) 牵牛子 6-9g
zhi ke (Fructus Citri Aurantii) 枳壳 9-12g
hou po (Cortex Magnoliae Officinalis) 厚朴 9-12g

Method: Decoction. **Bing lang, lei wan, shi jun zi, ku lian gen pi** and **qian niu zi** kill worms; **mu xiang** regulates middle *jiao qi*; **qian niu zi** unblocks the bowels to assist in the expulsion of the dead worms; **zhi ke** and **hou po** regulate *qi* and direct *qi* downwards.

Enema

An enema prepared from 5-6 good sized garlic cloves boiled in 200ml of water for a few minutes is useful in resistant or recurrent cases. Cool the liquid to body temperature and retain for 15-30 minutes.

Topical therapies

See p.543.

Patent medicines

Fei Zi San 肥仔散 (Baby Fat Powder)

- This is a effective treatment for intestinal parasites, but it needs to be continued for a least 2 weeks to be effective in the long term. The adult dose is four vials daily.

Acupuncture

The strategy with acupuncture in parasite infestations is to strengthen and regulate the digestive system and *zheng qi* so as to make the environment as inhospitable as possible to the parasite. However, the direct application of vermicidal herbs is necessary in most cases. A general Spleen and Stomach strengthening strategy, such as that outlined below, may be adopted.

Ren.12 (*zhong wan* +▲) .. *mu* point of the Stomach, strengthens the Spleen and Stomach, harmonises the Stomach

Liv.13 (*zhang men* -) .... *mu* point of the Spleen and *hui* point of the *zang*, strengthens the Spleen, improves digestion and promotes Liver function

St.25 (*tian shu*) .... *mu* point of the Large Intestine, regulates Intestinal function

St.36 (*zu san li* +▲) .... *he* sea point of the Stomach, powerfully strengthens the Spleen and Stomach, supplements *qi* and corrects the *qi* mechanism

Sp.3 (*tai bai*) ....*yuan*, *shu* stream and Earth point of the Spleen, strengthens the Spleen, supplements *qi* and transforms Dampness

Sp.6 (*san yin jiao*) .... strengthens the Spleen, supplements *qi*, regulates Liver *qi* and benefits the Kidneys

Bl.20 (*pi shu* +) .... *shu* point of the Spleen, strengthens the Spleen and supplements *qi*

Bl.21 (*wei shu* +) .... *shu* point of the Stomach, benefits the Stomach and regulates the *qi* mechanism

- *Ear points*: spleen, stomach, intestines, abdomen

Clinical notes

- The most likely culprits are pinworms or candidiasis. Worms in general are a relatively common clinical presentation in the West, and respond well to appropriate treatment. Estimates of chronic infestation run as high as 10% of the population and may well be even higher in some rural or pet loving populations. Parasites are worth considering in otherwise baffling cases where there is no direct evidence of parasites, but standard therapies based on sound diagnoses have failed. TCM treatment is also excellent for strengthening the system to prevent reinfection. In the case of worms, the whole family, including animals, should be treated to avoid re-transmission.
- When *Candida albicans* is the pathogen, topical treatment with an antifungal cream may be necessary, in addition to the systemic treatment, as candida can be persistent. Dietary modification is usually essential as well, and treatment may be lengthy. *See also* p.95.

14. Halitosis

Stomach Heat
Lung Heat
Food stagnation

14 HALITOSIS

kou chou 口臭

Halitosis is bad breath. The most common and important cause of halitosis is poor oral hygiene. Dental and oral causes should be eliminated before commencing TCM treatment. However, it should be noted that it is usually underlying Stomach pathology, that contributes to oral disease and halitosis.

It is important to ensure the patient does in fact have halitosis, as noted by a loved one or friend. Cases of psychogenic halitosis are not uncommon, and are often associated with anxiety states and disturbances of the *shen*.

Halitosis caused by pathology of the Stomach and/or Lung is the bad breath analysed in this chapter, and should be distinguished from odours related to certain metabolic disorders. These include diabetes (acetone), hepatic failure (foetid) and renal failure (uriniferous). Patients with halitosis as a feature of these systemic disorders will most likely present with one or more of the major symptoms of that condition, and will be analysed from the appropriate TCM disease-symptom.

AETIOLOGY

Poor oral hygiene

The most common cause of halitosis is poor oral hygiene, and before any treatment is instituted, steps must be taken to identify and correct this. Disorders of the mouth and gums are often associated with TCM defined pathologies, in particular Stomach Heat, and can be analysed and treated according to the patterns described in this chapter. *See also* Chapter 10. Gingivitis and Periodontitis and Chapter 25. Tooth abscess.

Diet

The most important aspects of the diet that contribute to pathological halitosis are those that heat the Stomach or cause food stagnation. The actual mechanism of the halitosis may be related to the rising of 'fermented' Stomach *qi* to the mouth, or the inflammatory influence of the Heat on the structures of the oral cavity.

A diet rich in spicy, hot or oily foods, coffee and alcohol, heats the Stomach. Similarly, an excess of supplementing herbs, in particular those that warm *yang*, may also cause build-up of Heat in the Stomach.

Eating more food than the Spleen and Stomach can cope with, either because of simple overeating or because the Spleen is already weak, can lead to accumulation of undigested or partly digested materials in the Stomach.

Overeating, eating irregularly or at odd hours, especially late at night, weakens Spleen and Stomach *qi* and leads to food stagnation (*see also* p.3).

Too much cold natured or raw food weakens Spleen *qi* and *yang* and dampens down digestive Fire, setting the scene for further stagnation and accumulation. Overconsumption in general, and excessive consumption of rich heating foods in particular, can lead to the accumulation of Damp Heat in the Intestines.

Halitosis (at least to some olfactory senses) can also be caused directly by certain foods, the classic culprits being members of the onion family. Garlic is the most frequently cited offender. This is non-pathological halitosis.

BOX14.1 SOME BIOMEDICAL CAUSES OF HALITOSIS (# indicates common)

Gastro-intestinal
- poor oral hygiene#
- gingivitis#
- dental disease/infection#
- dietary habits#
- smoking/alcohol#
- chronic mouth breathing (from allergy, nasal blockage, etc.)
- xerostomia
- severe constipation or faecal impaction
- poor gastric motility

Respiratory
- lung abscess
- bronchiectasis
- nasal and sinus infection
- tuberculosis
- tonsillar abscess

Metabolic
- diabetes (acetone, sweet)
- hepatic failure
- uraemia (foetid/ammoniac)

Other
- dehydration
- Sjogren's syndrome
- drugs (especially those that decrease saliva or upset the gut)
- pharyngeal pouch
- malignancy of the lung, nose, stomach or oropharynx
- systemic infection

Emotion

Emotions which cause Liver *qi* stagnation, and consequent invasion of the Stomach, can contribute to halitosis. Liver *qi* stagnation is caused by repressed emotion, frustration, anger and resentment. These emotions, especially when chronically unexpressed, can gradually lead to the development of stagnant Heat which may affect the Stomach.

Liver *qi* stagnation can also disrupt Spleen function and digestive efficiency. Spleen weakness and inefficient digestion will contribute to the pathological residue, Dampness, which in turn may obstruct *qi* circulation and generate Heat. Spleen weakness may predispose a patient to food stagnation.

Lung Heat

Any process that generates Heat in the Lungs can contribute to halitosis, the most common being smoking. External pathogens, typically Wind Cold or Wind Heat can invade the Lungs and Lung system and lodge there, cooking and congealing fluids into Phlegm. Accumulation of Phlegm and Phlegm Heat in the sinuses and nasopharynx can cause halitosis.

DIAGNOSIS

Local, dietary and psychogenic causes should be excluded before TCM analysis of halitosis. Eliminate dental disease or lack of oral hygiene as possible causes. If the source of the halitosis originates from the Lung system (including the sinuses and throat), or is associated with disturbances of the *shen*, the condition may be better analysed in other sections of the text (*see* Sinusitis, Lung Abscess and Sore throat or Anxiety, all in Volume 1).

胃热口臭

14.1 STOMACH HEAT

Pathophysiology

- Stomach Heat is the most common cause of halitosis, and the most common cause of the Stomach Heat is diet, in particular, a diet rich in heating, spicy or oily foods and alcohol.
- The clinical picture can vary quite a lot depending on the intensity of the Heat. In mild cases, the Heat may be focused in the Stomach, with few systemic signs of Heat; in severe cases there will be clear manifestations of systemic Heat, in addition to the specific Stomach Heat signs and symptoms. Although the basic pathology is the same or similar, the different presentations require different treatment strategies. There are several commonly used prescriptions.

Clinical features

- halitosis
- thirst, with a desire for cold fluids
- dry mouth and lips
- bleeding gums
- frequent hunger or voracious appetite
- ulcerations of the mouth, redness and swelling of the gums
- possible fever, or afternoon fever
- frontal headaches
- red complexion and lips
- tendency to constipation, hard dry stools; rarely, diarrhoea
- concentrated urine

T red, with a dry or greasy yellow coat
P rapid, possibly slippery, wiry or thready

Treatment principle

Clear Heat, Fire or Damp Heat from the Stomach and Spleen

Prescription

14.1.1 With severe and systemic Heat

XIE XIN TANG 泻心汤
(*Coptis and Rhubarb Combination*)

This prescription is used for relatively severe cases with systemic manifestations of Heat (fever, constipation, concentrated urine, flushed complexion), in addition to those specific to Stomach Heat.

da huang (Radix et Rhizoma Rhei) 大黄 6-9g
huang lian (Rhizoma Coptidis) 黄连 3-9g

huang qin (Radix Scutellariae Baicalensis) 黄芩 6-12g

Method: Decoction. The main herb, **da huang**, clears Heat and drains Fire by purging; **huang lian** and **huang qin** clear Damp Heat and drain Fire. (Source: *Shi Yong Zhong Yi Nei Ke Xue*)

14.1.2 With mild systemic Heat

QING WEI SAN 清胃散
(*Clear the Stomach Powder*)

This prescription is indicated for accumulated Heat in the Stomach and Stomach channel, with mild systemic Heat (facial flushing, feverishness). In addition to the halitosis there may be toothache, swelling of the cheeks and headaches.

huang lian (Rhizoma Coptidis) 黄连 3-6g
sheng di (Radix Rehmanniae Glutinosae) 生地 12-18g
mu dan pi (Cortex Moutan Radicis) 牡丹皮 9-12g
dang gui (Radix Angelicae Sinensis) 当归 9-12g
sheng ma (Rhizoma Cimicifugae) 升麻 3-6g

Method: Decoction. The main herb, bitter and cold **huang lian** clears Heat from the Stomach and directs Stomach *qi* and turbid *qi* downward; pungent, sweet, cool and elevating **sheng ma** encourages the ascent of clear *qi*, clears Toxic Heat from the Stomach and balances the descending nature of **huang lian**; together this pair, one ascending, one descending, clear Heat without drying, and correct the *qi* mechanism; **mu dan pi** cools the Blood and disperses stagnant Blood; **sheng di** cools the Blood and nourishes *yin*; **dang gui** nourishes and regulates Blood and protects it against the drying effects of the Heat. (Source: *Shi Yong Zhong Yi Nei Ke Xue*)

14.1.3 Heat focused in the Stomach

XIE HUANG SAN 泻黄散
(*Drain the Yellow Powder*)

This elegant prescription uses both cooling and dispersing herbs to reveal, and then clear, the hidden Heat that afflicts the Stomach and Spleen. Systemic manifestations of Heat are reduced or absent. There may be mouth ulcers.

shi gao (Gypsum) 石膏 15-30g
shan zhi zi (Fructus Gardeniae Jasminoidis) 山栀子 9-12g
fang feng (Radix Ledebouriellae Divaricatae) 防风 9-12g
huo xiang (Herba Agastaches seu Pogostemi) 藿香 9-15g
gan cao (Radix Glycyrrhizae Uralensis) 甘草 3-6g

Method: Decoction. **Shi gao** is decocted for 30 minutes prior to the other herbs (*xian jian* 先煎). **Shi gao** clears Heat from the Spleen and Stomach; **shan zhi zi** clears Heat from all three *jiao* through the urine and enters the Heart to relieve irritability; **fang feng**, being pungent, warm and light in nature, aids in dispersal of smouldering Stomach Heat by chasing it up and out, enabling the cooling herbs to clear and drain it; **huo xiang's** fragrant nature revives the Spleen and invigorates the *qi* mechanism, it also assists **fang feng** in uncovering the smouldering Heat so it can be cleared; **gan cao** harmonises and protects the Stomach. (Source: *Zui Xin Fang Ji Shou Ce*)

14.1.4 Damp Heat and *yin* deficiency

GAN LU YIN 甘露饮
(*Sweet Dew Decoction*)

This prescription clears Damp Heat and nourishes Stomach *yin*, and is indicated in chronic patterns of Damp Heat in the Stomach with a degree of damage to Stomach *yin*. The features are halitosis, throat pain, oral ulceration and gum swelling, a red tongue with a patchy, greasy tongue coat, perhaps peeled in the centre, and a slippery or thready and rapid pulse.

sheng di (Radix Rehmanniae Glutinosae) 生地 9-15g
shu di (Radix Rehmanniae Glutinosae Conquitae) 熟地 9-15g
mai dong (Tuber Ophiopogonis Japonici) 麦冬 9-12g
tian dong (Tuber Asparagi Cochinchinensis) 天冬 9-12g
shi hu (Herba Dendrobii) 石斛 6-9g
zhi ke (Fructus Citri Aurantii) 枳壳 6-9g
pi pa ye (Folium Eriobotryae) 枇杷叶 6-12g
yin chen (Herba Artemisiae Yinchenhao) 茵陈 9-12g
huang qin (Radix Scutellariae Baicalensis) 黄芩 9-12g
gan cao (Radix Glycyrrhizae Uralensis) 甘草 3-6g

Method: Decoction. **Sheng di, shu di, mai dong, tian dong** and **shi hu** nourish *yin* and generate fluids to restrain and cool Heat; **huang qin** and **yin chen** clear Damp Heat; **pi pa ye** and **zhi ke** harmonise the Stomach and direct *qi* downwards; **gan cao** benefits the throat and protects the Stomach. (Source: *Shi Yong Zhong Yi Nei Ke Xue*)

Modifications (suitable to all prescriptions)

- If excessive consumption of alcohol is responsible for generating the Heat, the addition of **ge hua** (Flos Puerariae) 葛花 12g may be useful. This can also be taken separately as a tea.

Patent medicines

Huang Lian Jie Du Wan 黄连解毒丸 (Huang Lian Jie Du Wan)
- Damp Heat

Niu Huang Qing Huo Wan 牛黄清火丸 (Niu Huang Qing Huo Wan)
- with constipation

Bei Jing Niu Huang Jie Du Pian 北京牛黄解毒片 (Peking Niu Huang Chieh Tu Pien)
- Damp and Toxic Heat

Qing Fei Yi Huo Pian 清肺抑火片 (Ching Fei Yi Huo Pien)
- Lung and Stomach Heat

Acupuncture (select from)

Ren.12 (*zhong wan* -) .... *mu* point of the Stomach, reducing method clears Heat from the Stomach

St.44 (*nei ting* -) .... together these points clear Heat from *yang*
LI.4 (*he gu* -) *ming* when reduced; they also have a special effect on oral diseases

PC.8 (*lao gong* -) .... *rong* spring and Fire point of the Pericardium, drains Heat from the Stomach channel and cools Heart Fire
LI.11 (*qu chi* -) .... *he* sea point of the Large Intestine, clears Heat and Dampness from *yang ming*
St.45 (*li dui* ↓) .... powerfully clears Heat from the Stomach
- *Ear points*: stomach, duodenum, abdomen, *shen men*, sympathetic

Clinical notes

- This pattern usually responds well to correct treatment in association with appropriate dietary modifications.
- For dietary recommendations, see p.882-885.

肺热口臭

14.2 LUNG HEAT

Pathophysiology

• Lung Heat can give rise to halitosis in several ways. The Heat can affect different parts of the Lung system, the Lungs themselves (as in bronchitis, abscess or bronchiectasis), the sinuses or the throat. See the relevant section in Volume 1 of this series for more detail.

Clinical features

• halitosis accompanied by one or more of the following–
  • dry, hacking cough with scanty, hard to expectorate sputum, or with sticky, yellow or green sputum
  • sore throat that appears swollen and red, perhaps with a white or yellow exudate
  • sticky, yellow or green purulent and malodorous mucus discharge from the nose, or nasal congestion

In addition there may be
• high, low or afternoon fever with or without sweating
• chest tightness and pain, sensation of heat in the chest
• red complexion and nose
• dry mouth and thirst, hoarse voice
• reduction or loss of sense of smell, nasal voice
• shortness of breath, laboured breathing or wheezing
• constipation
T red or with a red tip, dry or greasy, yellow coat
P rapid, and large in the distal position, possibly slippery or thready

Treatment principle

Clear Heat from the Lungs (throat, sinuses)

Prescription

14.2.1 Heat in the Lungs

XIE BAI SAN 泻白散
(*Clear the White Powder*)

This prescription is selected when there is Heat in the Lungs causing dry cough. The cough and fever tend to be worse in the afternoon as Lung *yin* is frequently injured by the Heat.

sang bai pi (Cortex Mori Albae Radicis) 桑白皮 12-15g
di gu pi (Cortex Lycii Chinensis) 地骨皮 12-15g
zhi gan cao (honey fried Radix Glycyrrhizae Uralensis)
炙甘草 3-6g

jing mi (Semen Oryzae) 粳米 15g

Method: Decoction. **Sang bai pi** clears Heat from the Lungs, directs Lung *qi* downwards and stops cough and wheezing; **di gu pi** clears both excess and deficient Heat from the Lungs; **zhi gan cao** and **jing mi** harmonise the other herbs and protect the Stomach. (Source: *Shi Yong Zhong Yi Nei Ke Xue*)

14.2.2 Severe Heat/Phlegm Heat in the Lungs

WEI JING TANG 苇茎汤
(*Reed Decoction*)

This is the representative prescription for Lung abscess, characterised by cough with copious foul smelling, yellow-green, purulent sputum.

lu gen (Rhizoma Phragmitis Communis) 芦根 30-60g
dong gua ren (Semen Benincasae Hispidae) 冬瓜仁 15-30g
yi ren (Semen Coicis Lachryma-jobi) 苡仁 15-30g
tao ren (Semen Persicae) 桃仁 9-12g

Method: Decoction. **Lu gen** (also known as **wei jing**) clears Heat from the Lungs, promotes discharge of pus and resolves Lung abscess; **dong gua ren** clears Heat, transforms Phlegm Heat, promotes discharge of pus and the clearance of pathogens through the bowel; **yi ren** promotes discharge of pus and clears Damp Heat; **tao ren** regulates Blood, eliminates stagnant Blood and lubricates the Intestines, and with **dong gua ren**, promotes discharge of pathogens through the bowel. (Source: *Shi Yong Zhong Yi Nei Ke Xue*)

14.2.3 Toxic Heat in the throat

PU JI XIAO DU YIN 普济消毒饮
(*Universal Benefit Decoction to Eliminate Toxin*)

This prescription is selected for Lung Heat or Toxic Heat affecting the throat.

huang qin (Radix Scutellariae Baicalensis) 黄芩 6-12g
huang lian (Rhizoma Coptidis) 黄连 3-9g
ban lan gen (Radix Isatidis seu Baphicacanthi) 板蓝根 9-15g
lian qiao (Fructus Forsythia Suspensae) 连翘 9-12g
xuan shen (Radix Scrophulariae Ningpoensis) 玄参 12-18g
jiang can (Bombyx Batryticatus) 僵蚕 3-9g
ma bo (Fructificatio Lasiosphaerae seu Calvatiae) 马勃 2-3g
niu bang zi (Fructus Arctii Lappae) 牛蒡子 9-15g
chen pi (Pericarpium Citri Reticulatae) 陈皮 3-6g
jie geng (Radix Platycodi Grandiflori) 桔梗 3-6g
sheng ma (Rhizoma Cimicifugae) 升麻 3-6g
chai hu (Radix Bupleuri) 柴胡 3-9g
bo he (Herba Mentha Haplocalycis) 薄荷 3-6g
gan cao (Radix Glycyrrhizae Uralensis) 甘草 3-6g

Method: Decoction. **Bo he** is added just before the end of cooking (*hou xia*

后下), **ma bo** is usually cooked in a muslin bag (*bao jian* 包煎). **Huang lian** and **huang qin** clear Heat from the upper body; **ban lan gen, lian qiao** and **ma bo** clear Toxic Heat; **jiang can, niu bang zi, sheng ma, bo he** and **chai hu** clear Wind Heat; **sheng ma** and **chai hu** also conduct the action of the other herbs to the head; **xuan shen** cools the Blood; **xuan shen, gan cao, jie geng, niu bang zi** and **ma bo** collectively have a powerful effect on clearing Heat from the throat and stopping pain; **chen pi** regulates *qi*. (Source: *Shi Yong Zhong Yi Nei Ke Xue*)

14.2.4 Heat in the sinuses

CANG ER ZI SAN 苍耳子散
(*Xanthium Formula*)

This prescription is selected for Heat accumulating in the sinuses and nasal cavity, with yellow-green nasal discharge and frontal headache.

cang er zi (Fructus Xanthii Sibirici) 苍耳子 9g
xin yi hua (Flos Magnoliae) 辛夷花 9g
bai zhi (Radix Angelicae Dahuricae) 白芷 30g
bo he (Herba Mentha Haplocalycis) 薄荷 15g

Method: Grind the herbs to a fine powder and take in 6-gram doses after eating, traditionally taken with shallot (cong bai) soup. **Cang er zi** and **xin yi hua** are the main herbs to dispel Wind from the nose and unblock the nasal passages; **bai zhi** clears the exterior, opens the orifices and stops pain; **bo he** dispels Wind Heat. (Source: *Shi Yong Zhong Yi Nei Ke Xue*)

14.2.5 Chronic Phlegm Heat in the Lung system

QING QI HUA TAN WAN 清气化痰丸
(*Clear the Qi and Transform Phlegm Pill*)

This prescription is appropriate for more chronic disorders of the Lung system, with Phlegm Heat. The Phlegm may or may not be visible or able to be expelled, depending on its viscosity and location (for example, Phlegm Heat in the sinuses doesn't always produce obvious congestion). In addition to the halitosis, there may be nausea, insomnia, palpitations and anxiety. The tongue coat is greasy and yellow.

gua lou (Fructus Trichosanthis) 瓜楼 30g
huang qin (Radix Scutellariae Baicalensis) 黄芩 30g
chen pi (Pericarpium Citri Reticulatae) 陈皮 30g
chao zhi shi (dry fried Fructus Immaturus Citri Aurantii)
炒枳实 30g
xing ren (Semen Pruni Armeniacae) 杏仁 30g
fu ling (Sclerotium Poriae Cocos) 茯苓 30g
jiang ban xia (ginger fried Rhizoma Pinelliae Ternatae)
姜半夏 45g
dan nan xing (Pulvis Arisaemae cum Felle Bovis)
胆南星 45g

Method: Grind the herbs to a fine powder and form into 9-gram pills with water or ginger juice. The dose is one pill twice 2-3 times daily. May also be decocted with an 70%-80% reduction in quantities. **Gua lou** clears and transforms Phlegm Heat; **huang qin** clears Heat from the Lung system; **chen pi** and **zhi shi** regulate *qi* and transform Phlegm; **fu ling** strengthens the Spleen and leaches out Damp; **xing ren** assists the descent of Lung *qi*; **ban xia** and **dan nan xing** transform Phlegm. (Source: *Shi Yong Fang Ji Xue*)

Patent medicines

Qing Fei Yi Huo Pian 清肺抑火片 (Ching Fei Yi Huo Pien) - Lung and Stomach Heat

Qing Qi Hua Tan Wan 清气化痰丸 (Qing Qi Hua Tan Wan, Clean Air Tea, Pinellia Expectorant Pills) - chronic Phlegm Heat

Bei Jing Niu Huang Jie Du Pian 北京牛黄解毒片 (Peking Niu Huang Chieh Tu Pien) - commonly used for early stage febrile disorder with sore throat, mouth ulcers, conjunctivitis, otitis and suppurative skin infections

Chuan Xin Lian Kang Yan Pian 穿心莲抗炎片 (Chuan Xin Lian Antiphlogistic Tablets) - all Toxic Heat patterns

Niu Huang Qing Huo Wan 牛黄清火丸 (Niu Huang Qing Huo Wan) - severe cases

Shuang Liao Hou Feng San 双料喉风散 (Superior Sore Throat Powder) - for topical use in the throat and sinuses

Acupuncture (select from)

Lungs

Lu.5 (*chi ze* -) .... *he* sea and Water point of the Lungs, clears Lung Heat, directs Lung *qi* downwards and stops cough

Lu.6 (*kong zui* -) .... *xi* cleft point of the Lungs, clears Lung Heat, directs Lung *qi* downwards and stops bleeding and pain

LI.11 (*qu chi* -) .... *he* sea point of the Large Intestine, clears Heat and Dampness from *yang ming* and systemically, dispels Wind and regulates *qi* and Blood

Bl.13 (*fei shu* -) .... *shu* point of the Lungs, clears Heat

Du.14 (*da zhui* -) .... meeting point of the *yang* channels, clears Heat

Lu.1 (*zhong fu*) .... *mu* point of the Lungs, clears Heat from the Lungs

- in severe cases, add Du.12 (*shen zhu* -) and Du.10 (*ling tai* -)
- with Phlegm Heat, add St.40 (*feng long* -)
- with constipation, add SJ.6 (*zhi gou* -) and St.25 (*tian shu* -)
- with severe Heat, bleed Lu.11 (*shao shang* ↓) and LI.1 (*shang yang* ↓)
- *Ear points*: lungs, throat, trachea

Throat

LI.4 (*he gu* -) .... *yuan* point of the Large Intestine, dispels Wind Heat, clears Heat from the Lungs and throat, stops pain and activates the dispersing function of the Lungs

Lu.10 (*yu ji*) .... *rong* spring and Fire point of the Lungs, clears Heat from the Lungs and benefits the throat

LI.11 (*qu chi* -) .... *he* sea point of the Large Intestine, clears Heat and Dampness from *yang ming* and systemically, dispels Wind and regulates *qi* and Blood

Lu.11 (*shao shang* ↓) .... *jing* well and Wood point of the Lungs, clears Heat from the Lungs, dispels Wind Heat and benefits the throat

Du.14 (*da zhui* -) .... meeting point of the *yang* channels, clears Heat

Ren.22 (*tian tu*) .... clears Heat from the throat and directs Lung *qi* downwards

- *Ear points*: lungs, throat, tonsils ↓

Sinuses

yin tang (M-HN-3) .... local points to open the nose
GB.14 (*yang bai* -)
LI.20 (*ying xiang* -)

Du.23 (*shang xing*) .... special point for opening the nose

GB.20 (*feng chi* -) .... disperses Wind and Heat, opens the nose

LI.4 (*he gu* -) .... *yuan* point of the Large Intestine, dispels Wind Heat, clears Heat from the Lungs, opens the nose and activates the dispersing function of the Lungs

LI.11 (*qu chi* -) .... *he* sea point of the Large Intestine, clears Heat and Dampness from *yang ming*, dispels Wind

Ear points: lungs, nose

Clinical notes

- The various manifestations of the Lung Heat pattern generally respond reasonably well to correct treatment, plus avoidance of heating foods and tobacco. In severe cases, and in the elderly, frail or debilitated, concurrent use of antibiotics may be necessary to quickly cool the Heat. Herbs and acupuncture support the swift action of the antibiotics, and finish the job by expelling the pathogen, clearing residual Phlegm, strengthening resistance and nourishing damaged *yin*.
- For dietary recommendations, see p.882-885.

食滞口臭

14.3 FOOD STAGNATION

Pathophysiology

- Food stagnation is a common cause of halitosis, as many people in the western world (and increasingly in Asia) consume more food than their digestive systems can process.

Clinical features

- halitosis
- sour, foul belching
- acid reflux, heartburn
- flatulence, indigestion
- epigastric distension, fullness, discomfort and pain which is relieved by vomiting and belching, and worse for pressure and eating
- no appetite
- nausea and vomiting with undigested food
- constipation, sluggish, foul stools or diarrhoea that relieves the pain

T thick, greasy, white or yellow coat
P slippery and full

Treatment principle

Soothe the Liver, clear heat
Harmonise the Stomach

Prescription

BAO HE WAN 保和丸
(*Citrus and Crategus Formula*)

chao shan zha (dry fried Fructus Crataegi) 炒山楂 18-24g
chao shen qu (dry fried Massa Fermentata) 炒神曲 12-15g
chao lai fu zi (dry fried Semen Raphani Sativi)
炒莱服子 9-12g
ban xia (Rhizoma Pinelliae Ternatae) 半夏 9-12g
fu ling (Sclerotium Poriae Cocos) 茯苓 12-15g
chen pi (Pericarpium Citri Reticulatae) 陈皮 6-9g
lian qiao (Fructus Forsythia Suspensae) 连翘 6-9g

Method: Grind herbs to a powder and form into 9-gram pills with water. The dose is one pill 2-3 times daily. May also be decocted with the quantities as shown. **Shan zha, shen qu** and **lai fu zi** improve digestion and alleviate food stagnation; **ban xia** and **chen pi** eliminate Phlegm; **lian qiao** disperses accumulations and clears Heat; **fu ling** strengthens the Spleen. (Source: *Shi Yong Zhong Yi Nei Ke Xue*)

Modifications

- With severe distension, add **zhi shi** (Fructus Immaturus Citri Aurantii)

枳实 9-12g and **hou po** (Cortex Magnoliae Officinalis) 厚朴 9-12g.

- If the stagnation is associated with excessive meat consumption, double the dose of **shan zha**.
- If starchy carbohydrate rich foods, such as noodles and grains, are the cause of the stagnation, increase the dose of **lai fu zi**.
- With severe nausea or vomiting, add **sheng jiang** (Rhizoma Zingiberis Officinalis) 生姜 9-12g.
- With Heat in the Stomach, add **lu gen** (Rhizoma Phragmitis Communis) 芦根 15-30g and **huang lian** (Rhizoma Coptidis) 黄连 3-6g.
- With Cold in the Stomach, delete **lian qiao**, and add **gan jiang** (Rhizoma Zingiberis Officinalis) 干姜 6-9g and **sha ren** (Fructus Amomi) 砂仁 6-9g.
- With Liver *qi* stagnation, add **fo shou** (Fructus Citri Sarcodactylis) 佛手 9-12g, and **mei gui hua** (Flos Rosae Rugosae) 玫瑰花 6-9g.
- With Spleen deficiency, add **chao bai zhu** (dry fried Rhizoma Atractylodes Macrocephalae) 炒白术 12-15g.
- With constipation, add **da huang** (Radix et Rhizoma Rhei) 大黄 6-9g and **bing lang** (Semen Arecae Catechu) 槟榔 9-12g.

Variations and additional prescriptions

With Damp Heat

- For more chronic cases, with significant digestive disruption and the generation of Damp Heat or Phlegm Heat, the correct treatment is to guide stagnation downward, clear Heat and dispel Dampness with **ZHI SHI DAO ZHI WAN** (*Immature Bitter Orange Pill to Guide out Stagnation* 枳实导滞丸, p.181).

With parasites

- Foul breath in children may be associated with accumulated food and parasites. Uncommon in the developed word, this pattern is a form of childhood nutritional impairment (*gan ji* 疳积), usually associated with poverty, malnutrition and poor sanitation. The features are halitosis with intermittent abdominal pain, tooth grinding, restlessness at night, anal itch, abdominal bloating, indigestion, loss of appetite or desire for unusual or uncharacteristic foods, emaciation and a sallow complexion. The treatment aims to kill the parasites, reduce accumulation, strengthen the Spleen and clear Heat with **FEI ER WAN** (*Fat Baby Pill* 肥儿丸).

chao shen qu (dry fried Massa Fermentata) 炒神曲 30g
bing lang (Semen Arecae Catechu) 槟榔 12g
huang lian (Rhizoma Coptidis) 黄连 30g
shi jun zi (Fructus Quisqualis Indicae) 使君子 15g

rou dou kou (Semen Myristicae Fragrantis) 肉豆蔻 15g
chao mai ya (dry fried Fructus Hordei Vulgaris Germinantus) 炒麦芽 15g
mu xiang (Radix Aucklandiae Lappae) 木香 6g

Method: Grind all the herbs to a fine powder. The dose is 3 grams, once or twice daily for children, half dose for infants, on an empty stomach. Although traditionally formed into pills with pig bile, the powdered form is easier to administer to children, disguised in apple sauce or some other sweet medium. The main to herbs to reduce accumulation and kill parasites are **shen qu** and **bing lang**; **chao mai ya** and **shi jun zi** strengthen the Spleen, harmonise the middle *jiao* and assist the main herbs in expelling parasites; **huang lian** clears Heat from the Stomach and drains downwards; **rou dou kou** strengthens the Spleen and eliminates Dampness; **mu xiang** regulates digestive *qi*. (Source: *Zui Xin Fang Ji Shou Ce*)

Patent medicines

Bao He Wan 保和丸 (Bao He Wan)
Chen Xiang Hua Qi Wan 沉香化气丸 (Chen Xiang Hua Qi Wan)
- with constipation

Jian Pi Wan 健脾丸 (Jian Pi Wan)
- with Spleen deficiency

Xiang Lian Wan 香连丸 (Xiang Lian Wan)
Zi Sheng Wan 资生丸 (Zi Sheng Wan, Zi Sheng Stomachic Pills)
Mu Xiang Shun Qi Wan 木香顺气丸 (Mu Xiang Shun Qi Wan)
- with *qi* stagnation

Fei Zi San 肥仔散 (Baby Fat Powder)
- for parasites

Acupuncture (select from)

Ren.12 (*zhong wan* -) .... *mu* point of the Stomach, reducing method clears Heat and alleviates stagnation
St.36 (*zu san li* -) .... *he* sea point of the Stomach, regulates and strengthens the Stomach and stops vomiting
St.44 (*nei ting* -) .... *rong* spring and Water point of the Stomach, clears Heat from the Stomach and alleviates food stagnation
St.40 (*feng long* -) .... *luo* point of the Stomach, transforms Phlegm and clears Heat and Phlegm from the Stomach
LI.10 (*shou san li* -) .... benefits digestion and regulates gastro-intestinal function
PC.8 (*lao gong* -) .... *rong* spring and Fire point of the Pericardium, drains Heat from the Stomach channel and cools Heart Fire

- with nausea, add PC.6 (*nei guan* -)
- with epigastric or abdominal pain, add Sp.4 (*gong sun* -)

- with constipation, add SJ.6 (*zhi gou* -) and St.25 (*tian shu* -)
- with diarrhoea, add St.37 (*shan ju xu*)
- *Ear points*: spleen, stomach, intestines, liver, abdomen

Clinical notes

- This is mostly a disorder of gluttony and dietary irregularity, although parasites may be implicated in some cases. In isolation it generally needs no treatment other than a sensible approach to diet and eating habits. However if bad habits persist it can become a more serious problem.
- The Chinese have long known the benefits of sipping small amounts of certain teas while eating. The action of such teas helps assist digestion, especially of fats, and reduces the risk of food stagnation. European cultures use table wine in much the same way, hence 'a little wine for thy stomach's sake'. Similarly, 'bitters', combinations of bitter herbs and alcohol, are a common accompaniment to food, either as a digestive aid following a meal, or as an aperitive. The bitterness of the herbs assists the descent of Stomach *qi* and dries Damp.

SUMMARY OF GUIDING FORMULAE FOR HALITOSIS

Stomach Heat - *Xie Xin Tang* 泻心汤
- with mild systemic Heat - *Qing Wei San* 清胃散
- with mouth ulcers - *Xie Huang San* 泻黄散
- with Damp Heat - *Gan Lu Yin* 甘露饮

Lung Heat - *Xie Bai San* 泻白散
- with acute Phlegm Heat in the Lungs - *Wei Jing Tang* 苇茎汤
- with Toxic Heat in the throat - *Pu Ji Xiao Du Yin* 普济消毒饮
- in the sinuses - *Cang Er Zi San* 苍耳子散
- with chronic Phlegm Heat - *Qing Qi Hua Tan Wan* 清气化痰丸

Food stagnation - *Bao He Wan* 保和丸
- with Damp Heat - *Zhi Shi Dao Zhi Wan* 枳实导滞丸
- with parasites in children - *Fei Er Wan* 肥儿丸

15. Hiccough

Excess patterns

Cold in the Stomach
Stomach Heat/Fire
Food stagnation
Liver *qi* invading the Stomach
Phlegm Damp
Blood stagnation

Deficient patterns

Spleen and Kidney *yang* deficiency
Stomach *yin* deficiency

15 HICCOUGH

e ni 呃逆

Hiccoughs are repeated, involuntary, spasmodic contractions of the diaphragm, followed by a sudden closure of the glottis which produces the characteristic sound. Hiccoughs can occur alone or as part of some other condition.

Most cases of hiccough are rarely more than an annoyance. They tend to be self limiting and require no treatment other than the simple measures outlined in Box 15.2, p.572. Treatment is required when hiccoughs go on too long without respite, are recurrent, or endanger the patient in some way, usually by physical exhaustion. This can occur in elderly patients or in those who are already debilitated in some way. Persistent hiccoughs sometimes occur in the end stage of a chronic or serious illness, as Stomach *qi* begins to decline precipitously and becomes too feeble to descend. This is considered to be a poor prognostic sign.

Chinese medicine views hiccoughs simply as rebellious Stomach *qi*. Numerous factors can contribute to this rebellion, and these can be broadly classed into two groups–excess and deficiency. Excess patterns are due to external or internal pathogens which accumulate at the level of the Stomach, and obstruct the descent of Stomach *qi*. The deficient patterns are due to the fact that Stomach *yang qi* or *yin* is too weak to descend on its own–*qi* begins to accumulate in the Stomach and at some point rebels upwards as hiccoughs.

AETIOLOGY

Diet

Consumption of cold natured foods and fluids, or an excess of cooling herbs or medications used to treat a hot disease, can cause contraction of the Stomach and subsequent obstruction and rebellion of Stomach *qi*. Too much cold natured or raw food weakens Spleen *qi* and *yang*.

Eating irregularly or at odd hours, especially late at night, weakens Spleen and Stomach *qi* and leads to food stagnation (*see also* p.3). Eating more food than the Spleen and Stomach can cope with, either because of simple overeating or because the Spleen is already weak, will obstruct the *qi* mechanism and the descent of middle *jiao qi*.

Phlegm Damp is generated by overindulgence in Phlegm or Damp producing foods and eating habits that weaken Spleen *qi*. Repeated courses of antibiotics can also damage Spleen *qi*, allowing the generation and accumulation of Dampness. Foods that can weaken the Spleen if consumed in excess include dairy products, fatty, sweet or raw foods, and alcohol. Once the

Spleen is weak, inefficient digestion allows accumulation of Dampness, which over time congeals into Phlegm. In the presence of Heat, Damp may be condensed to form Phlegm in a shorter time.

BOX 15.1 SOME BIOMEDICAL CAUSES OF HICCOUGH

Neurological
- medullary tumours
- alcoholism
- postoperative
- phrenic nerve irritation

Gastro-intestinal
- oesophagitis
- peptic ulcer
- hiatus hernia
- cholecystitis
- hepatomegaly

Respiratory
- diaphragmatic pleurisy
- pneumonia

Other
- subphrenic abscess
- pregnancy
- uraemia
- neurosis
- diaphragmatic irritation
- overconsumption of alcohol and food

Emotion

Frustration, anger, resentment, prolonged emotional turmoil, repressed emotions and stress disrupt the circulation of Liver *qi*. These emotions, or repressed emotions, can cause spasms and tension in the smooth muscle of the gastro-intestinal tract and diaphragm. Patients with chronic *qi* stagnation type digestive problems will often note that stress and tension affects the digestive system, causing a knot in the stomach, hiccoughs, loss of appetite, etc. Hiccoughs associated with Liver *qi* stagnation tend to be paroxysmal, and are usually related to the patient's emotional state.

When the smooth movement of Liver *qi* is impeded, it finds alternative pathways. In the case of hiccoughs, stagnant *qi* is discharged horizontally via the controlling (*ke* 克) cycle, disrupting the descent of Stomach *qi*.

There are several consequences of Liver *qi* invading the Stomach. When *qi* stagnates for any length of time, the resulting pressure can generate Heat. Chronic Heat in the Stomach will eventually consume Stomach *yin*. Stagnant *qi* can disrupt the Spleen, weakening it, and contributing to the development of Phlegm Damp.

Spleen and Stomach deficiency

Spleen and Stomach *qi*, *yang* or *yin* deficiency can give rise to hiccoughs if the *qi* mechanism fails. Prolonged or excessive consumption of cold raw food and irregular eating habits, too many cold natured herbs or antibiotics in the treatment of a febrile disease or general anaesthetic and upper abdominal surgery can damage *yang*. The Spleen and Stomach can also be weakened following a direct invasion of external Cold and/or Dampness. Prolonged insult to the Stomach or severely limited food intake, as occurs in patients

BOX 15.2 SIMPLE METHODS TO STOP ACUTE HICCOUGHS (in descending order of usefulness)

- strong finger nail pressure on LI.1 *shang yang*
- nipping the skin over the shoulder (C3, 4 innervation)
- strong pressure over the sternoclavicular junction (above the phrenic nerve)
- deep breath holding, or rebreathing deeply into a paper bag
- sneezing
- pressure on the eyeballs
- carotid sinus massage
- drinking a glass of water quickly
- ice in the mouth
- sipping rice vinegar
- clove cigarettes

with bulimia and anorexia nervosa, can seriously damage Spleen and Stomach *yang* and *qi*. Excessive mental strain or prolonged concentration may deplete Spleen *qi*. The damage is aggravated when an irregular diet is combined with sustained mental activity and too much sitting.

Stomach *yin* deficiency may follow a febrile disease or long term consumption of spicy heating foods or drugs, such as steroids, amphetamines and *yang* supplementing substances. Stomach *yin* can be damaged following prolonged or excessive vomiting, or another chronic Stomach pathology, especially one characterised by Heat or *qi* stagnation.

Spleen and Stomach deficiency may also be constitutional. In patients with a component of inherited weakness, there will often be a history of recurrent gastro-intestinal disturbances since childhood.

Blood stagnation

Hiccoughs caused by Blood stagnation are relatively uncommon, although they may occur in older patients as a result of trauma, gastric surgery or following overenthusiastic use of styptic herbs to quell bleeding from the gastro-intestinal system. Blood stagnation may also follow other long term pathology, in particular, chronic *qi* stagnation.

胃中寒冷

15.1 COLD IN THE STOMACH

Pathophysiology

- Hiccoughs due to Cold in the Stomach are usually due to ingestion of an excess of cold natured substances, typically cold drinks. Hiccoughs of this type may also occur post-operatively, as abdominal surgery, general anaesthetics and the opening of the abdominal wall in a cold surgical theatre can introduce Cold directly to the organs and structures of the abdominal cavity. The Cold constricts the Stomach and diaphragm and disrupts the *qi* mechanism, preventing the descent of Stomach *qi*, which then rises rebelliously as a hiccough.

Clinical features

- loud, resonant, sometimes violent hiccough that is aggravated by cold and ameliorated by heat
- discomfort in epigastrium
- reduced appetite, no thirst, or desire for warming drinks

T white coat
P moderate

Treatment principle

Warm the middle *jiao* and dispel Cold
Redirect Stomach *qi* downwards, stop hiccoughs

Prescription

DING XIANG SAN 丁香散
(*Clove Powder*) modified

ding xiang (Flos Caryophylli) 丁香 3-6g
shi di (Calyx Diospyros Kaki) 柿蒂 9-12g
gao liang jiang (Rhizoma Alpiniae Officinari) 高良姜 6-9g
zhi gan cao (honey fried Radix Glycyrrhizae Uralensis) 炙甘草 3-6g
xiang fu (Rhizoma Cyperi Rotundi) 香附 9-12g
chen pi (Pericarpium Citri Reticulatae) 陈皮 9-12g

Method: Decoction. **Ding xiang** and **gao liang jiang** warm the Stomach, dispel Cold and redirect Stomach *qi* downwards; **shi di** stops hiccoughs; **zhi gan cao** harmonises the Stomach and supplements *qi*; **xiang fu** regulates *qi*; **chen pi** dries and transforms Phlegm Damp and regulates *qi*; the last two herbs are included to regulate and correct the *qi* mechanism. (Source: *Zhong Yi Nei Ke Shou Ce*)

Modifications

- With severe Cold, add **wu zhu yu** (Fructus Evodiae Rutaecarpae) 吴茱萸 3-6g and **rou gui** (Cortex Cinnamomi Cassiae) 肉桂 3g.

- With *qi* and Phlegm stagnation (epigastric and abdominal distension and fullness, foul belching and a thick, greasy tongue coat) add **ban xia** (Rhizoma Pinelliae Ternatae) 半夏 9-12g, **hou po** (Cortex Magnoliae Officinalis) 厚朴 9-12g and **zhi shi** (Fructus Immaturus Citri Aurantii) 枳实 9-12g.
- With Wind Cold exterior symptoms (muscle aches, chilliness, floating pulse), add **huo xiang** (Herba Agastaches seu Pogostemi) 藿香 12-15g, **zi su ye** (Folium Perillae Frutescentis) 紫苏叶 9-12g and **jing jie** (Herba seu Flos Schizonepetae Tenuifolia) 荆芥 9-12g.

Patent medicines

Fu Zi Li Zhong Wan 附子理中丸 (Fu Tzu Li Chung Wan, Carmichaeli Tea Pills, Li Chung Yuen Medical Pills)
Li Zhong Wan 理中丸 (Li Zhong Wan)

Acupuncture (select from)

Ren.12 (*zhong wan* -▲) .... *mu* point of the Stomach, warms and regulates the Stomach, disperses Cold and directs Stomach *qi* downwards
PC.6 (*nei guan*) .... *luo* point of the Pericardium, master point of *yin wei mai*, regulates the middle *jiao* and stops hiccough
St.36 (*zu san li* +▲) .... *he* sea point of the Stomach, powerfully warms and regulates the Spleen and Stomach and corrects the *qi* mechanism
Ren.17 (*shan zhong* ▲) .... *hui* point for *qi*, directs rebellious *qi* downward and benefits the diaphragm
Ren.22 (*tian tu*) .... directs Lung *qi* downwards, thus aiding descent of Stomach *qi*
Bl.17 (*ge shu* -▲) .... *shu* point for the diaphragm, regulates diaphragm function

- A moxa box or strong moxa stick over the Stomach is useful. Cupping over the upper *shu* points and *ah shi* points in the mid thoracic area may also be useful.
- *Ear points*: diaphragm, sympathetic, stomach, liver, spleen (embedding needles may be used in stubborn cases)

Clinical notes

- When acute, Stomach Cold type hiccoughs may be rapidly corrected with herbs, acupuncture and moxa. Acupuncture can be given once or twice daily. When they have persisted for some time, it can take some days of treatment to resolve the hiccoughs.
- For dietary recommendations, see p.873.

胃火上逆

15.2 STOMACH HEAT/FIRE

Pathophysiology

- Stomach Heat type hiccoughs can be the result of an external invasion of Heat, or Cold that transforms into Heat, lodging in the Stomach (i.e. the *yang ming* level), or the result of an overly heating diet.
- When associated with an external invasion, the hiccoughs are acute and usually accompanied by other signs of an acute pathogenic invasion. The hiccoughs may persist for some time as a result of complications of the external Heat attack.
- When associated with a heating diet, alcohol or too many warm supplementing herbs or drinks, the hiccoughs tend to be somewhat more chronic or recurrent, and are obviously related to diet.

Clinical features

- loud, strong, continuous hiccoughs
- halitosis
- thirst, dry lips and mouth
- irritability, restlessness
- tendency to constipation; rarely, diarrhoea
- concentrated urine

T dry, yellow or yellowy brown tongue coat
P rapid or slippery and rapid

Treatment principle

Clear Heat and Fire from the Stomach, stop hiccoughs

Prescription

ZHU YE SHI GAO TANG 竹叶石膏汤
(*Lophatherus and Gypsum Decoction*) modified

This formula is used when an external pathogen has lodged in the Stomach, or the patient is left with lingering Heat and hiccoughs in the aftermath of a febrile illness. There is no constipation and no abdominal pain with palpation.

dan zhu ye (Herba Lophatheri Gracilis) 淡竹叶 12-15g
shi gao (Gypsum) 石膏 15-30g
mai dong (Tuber Ophiopogonis Japonici) 麦冬 6-15g
ban xia (Rhizoma Pinelliae Ternatae) 半夏 6-9g
dang shen (Radix Codonopsis Pilosulae) 党参 12-15g
jing mi (Semen Oryzae) 粳米 9-15g
gan cao (Radix Glycyrrhizae Uralensis) 甘草 3-6g
shi di (Calyx Diospyros Kaki) 柿蒂 9-12g

zhu ru (Caulis Bambusae in Taeniis) 竹茹 9-12g

Method: Decoction. **Shi gao** is decocted for 30 minute prior to the other herbs (*xian jian* 先煎). **Dan zhu ye** and **shi gao** clear Heat from the Stomach and alleviate irritability; **mai dong** nourishes Stomach *yin* and clears Heat; **ban xia** directs Stomach *qi* downwards; **dang shen** supplements *qi*, generates fluids and with **gan cao** and **jing mi**, prevents the cold herbs from damaging the Spleen and Stomach; **shi di** stops hiccoughs; **zhu ru** clears Heat and directs Stomach *qi* downwards. (Source: *Shi Yong Zhong Yi Nei Ke Xue*)

Modifications

- With damage to Stomach *yin*, delete **zhu ru** and add **sha shen** (Radix Adenophorae seu Glehniae) 沙参 12-15g, **tian hua fen** (Radix Trichosanthis Kirilowii) 天花粉 12-15g and **shi hu** (Herba Dendrobii) 石斛 12-15g.

Variations and additional prescriptions

With constipation

- When there is constipation (*yang ming fu* syndrome), **XIAO CHENG QI TANG** (*Minor Rhubarb Combination* 小承气汤) modified, may be used to rapidly clear Heat and stools through *yang ming* and redirect Stomach *qi* downwards.

da huang (Radix et Rhizoma Rhei) 大黄 6-9g
zhi shi (Fructus Immaturus Citri Aurantii) 枳实 12-15g
hou po (Cortex Magnoliae Officinalis) 厚朴 12-15g
shi di (Calyx Diospyros Kaki) 柿蒂 9-12g
zhu ru (Caulis Bambusae in Taeniis) 竹茹 9-12g

Method: Decoction. **Da huang** clears and purges Heat through the bowels; **zhi shi** and **hou po** regulate *qi* and alleviate accumulated Heat; **shi di** stops hiccoughs; **zhu ru** clears Heat and directs Stomach *qi* downwards. (Source: *Zhong Yi Nei Ke Shou Ce*)

Heat and Cold mixtures

- When Stomach Heat has transformed from a pre-existing Cold pathogen, there will often be mixtures of Hot and Cold symptoms, such as loud hiccoughs with waterbrash, irritating thirst, epigastric fullness and distension, a watery splash with epigastric palpation and loud borborygmus. Consider **SHENG JIANG XIE XIN TANG** (*Fresh Ginger Decoction to Drain the Epigastrium* 生姜泻心汤) modified.

sheng jiang (Rhizoma Zingiberis Officinalis Recens)
生姜 12-15g
ban xia (Rhizoma Pinelliae Ternatae) 半夏 9-12g
huang qin (Radix Scutellariae Baicalensis) 黄芩 9-12g
huang lian (Rhizoma Coptidis) 黄连 3-6g
dang shen (Radix Codonopsis Pilosulae) 党参 12-18g

zhi gan cao (honey fried Radix Glycyrrhizae Uralensis) 炙甘草 6-9g
gan jiang (dried Rhizoma Zingiberis Officinalis) 干姜 3-6g
da zao (Fructus Zizyphi Jujubae) 大枣 4pce
shi di (Calyx Diospyros Kaki) 柿蒂 9-12g

Method: Decoction. **Sheng jiang** as the main herb, warms and harmonises the Stomach, and with **ban xia** directs rising Stomach *qi* downwards; **huang qin** and **huang lian**, bitter and cold, clear Heat; **gan jiang**, pungent, hot and dispersing, warms Spleen and Stomach *yang*, dispels Cold and balances the bitter coldness of the previous two herbs–bitter and descending combined with pungent and opening neatly clears hidden Heat and corrects the *qi* mechanism; **dang shen**, **zhi gan cao** and **da zao** strengthen the Spleen, supplement *qi* and prevent the dispersing action of the principal herbs from injuring the Spleen and Stomach *qi* and *yin*; **shi di** stops hiccoughs. (Source: *Zhong Yi Nei Ke Shou Ce*)

Persistent hiccoughs from Phlegm Heat

- Following an external invasion of Heat, or Cold that transforms into Heat, into *yang ming* (Stomach and Intestines), fluids and *yin* are often dried and damaged (by the Heat itself or by vomiting), or congealed into Phlegm Heat which blocks the *qi* mechanism. The resulting persistent hiccoughs can be loud and paroxysmal or weak and intermittent, depending on the degree of accompanying deficiency. They may be accompanied by nausea or dry retching, restlessness, insomnia, palpitations and loss of appetite. The tongue is red and tender with a greasy, yellow coat, possibly somewhat thinner in the middle. The pulse may be rapid and slippery, soft, soggy or thready. The treatment aims to clear and transform Phlegm Heat, direct Stomach *qi* downwards and stop hiccoughs with **JU PI ZHU RU TANG** (*Tangerine Peel and Bamboo Shavings Decoction* 橘皮竹茹汤) modified.

chen pi (Pericarpium Citri Reticulatae) 陈皮 9-12g
zhu ru (Caulis Bambusae in Taeniis) 竹茹 9-12g
sheng jiang (Rhizoma Zingiberis Officinalis Recens) 生姜 6-9g
dang shen (Radix Codonopsis Pilosulae) 党参 12-18g
gan cao (Radix Glycyrrhizae Uralensis) 甘草 6-9g
da zao (Fructus Zizyphi Jujubae) 大枣 4pce
gua luo ren (Semen Trichosanthis) 瓜蒌仁 12-18g
shi di (Calyx Diospyros Kaki) 柿蒂 9-12g
ban xia (Rhizoma Pinelliae Ternatae) 半夏 9-12g
fu ling (Sclerotium Poria Cocos) 茯苓 12-15g

Method: Decoction. **Chen pi** transforms Phlegm, harmonises the Stomach, regulates middle *jiao qi* and corrects the *qi* mechanism; **zhu ru** clears Phlegm Heat from the Stomach, directs Stomach *qi* downwards and stops hiccough; **sheng jiang** warms and harmonises the Stomach and prevents damage to the Spleen by the cooling herbs; **dang shen**, **gan cao**, **fu ling** and **da zao**, strengthen the Spleen and supplement *qi*, as well as preventing the regulating herbs from damaging *qi*; **gua lou ren** clears and transforms Phlegm Heat; **shi di** stops hiccough; **ban xia** transforms Phlegm and directs rising Stomach *qi* downwards.

Patent medicines

Huang Lian Jie Du Wan 黄连解毒丸 (Huang Lian Jie Du Wan)
- Damp Heat

Ming Mu Shang Qing Pian 明目上清片 (Ming Mu Shang Ching Pien)
Wen Dan Wan 温胆丸 (Wen Dan Wan)
- Phlegm Heat

Niu Huang Qing Huo Wan 牛黄清火丸 (Niu Huang Qing Huo Wan)
- with constipation

Acupuncture (select from)

Ren.12 (*zhong wan* -) .... *mu* point of the Stomach, clears Heat from the Stomach and directs Stomach *qi* downwards
PC.6 (*nei guan* -) .... *luo* point of the Pericardium, master point of *yin wei mai*, regulates the middle *jiao* and stops hiccough
St.36 (*zu san li* -) .... *he* sea point of the Stomach, regulates the Spleen and Stomach and corrects the *qi* mechanism
St.44 (*nei ting* -) .... *rong* spring and Water point of the Stomach, clears Heat from *yang ming*, the Stomach and Stomach channel
Bl.17 (*ge shu* -) .... *shu* point for the diaphragm, regulates diaphragm function
Ren.17 (*shan zhong*) .... *hui* point for *qi*, directs rebellious *qi* downward and benefits the diaphragm

- with severe Heat, add LI.4 (*he gu* -) and LI.11 (*qu chi* -)
- with constipation, add SJ.6 (*zhi gou* -) and St.25 (*tian shu* -)
- with Phlegm Heat, add St.40 (*feng long* -) and PC.5 (*jian shi*)
- *Ear points*: diaphragm, sympathetic, stomach, liver, spleen, *shen men*

Clinical notes

- Stomach Heat type hiccoughs may occur following an acute infection, surgery, or may be associated with conditions such as acute or chronic gastritis.
- Acute episodes usually respond well to frequent acupuncture (1-2 times daily), but chronic conditions may require long term herb therapy, in addition to dietary changes.
- For dietary recommendations, see p.882-885.

饮食停滞

15.3 FOOD STAGNATION

Pathophysiology

- Food stagnation type hiccoughs are related to overeating or drinking. In the West, a tendency to food stagnation is often combined with weakness of Spleen and Stomach *qi*, so the onset may be gradual, rather than manifest as an acute event. As the pattern progresses, the deficiency will become more and more prominent.
- The mechanism is simple obstruction to the natural descent of Stomach *qi* by food so that Stomach *qi* ascends spasmodically. The Heat or Damp Heat produced by chronic food stagnation or overconsumption injures the Stomach and diaphragm by drying, scorching and contracting the delicate *luo mai*.

Clinical features

- Loud acute hiccoughs which may be associated with acid reflux, heartburn or waterbrash. The hiccoughs may be initiated or aggravated by eating or drinking and ameliorated by vomiting.
- sour belching, flatulence
- epigastric and abdominal fullness and distension
- nausea and vomiting

T thick greasy coat
P slippery

Treatment principle

Relieve food stagnation and harmonise the Stomach
Redirect Stomach *qi* downward

Prescription

BAO HE WAN 保和丸
(*Citrus and Crategus Formula*) modified

chao shan zha (dry fried Fructus Crataegi) 炒山楂 18-24g
chao shen qu (dry fried Massa Fermentata) 炒神曲 12-15g
chao lai fu zi (dry fried Semen Raphani Sativi)
炒莱服子 9-12g
ban xia (Rhizoma Pinelliae Ternatae) 半夏 9-12g
fu ling (Sclerotium Poriae Cocos) 茯苓 12-15g
chen pi (Pericarpium Citri Reticulatae) 陈皮 6-9g
lian qiao (Fructus Forsythia Suspensae) 连翘 6-9g
zhu ru (Caulis Bambusae in Taeniis) 竹茹 9-12g
zhi shi (Fructus Immaturus Citri Aurantii) 枳实 9-12g

Method: Grind herbs to a powder and form into 9-gram pills with water. The dose is one pill 2-3 times daily. May also be decocted with quantities as shown. **Shan zha**, **shen qu**, **chao lai fu zi** and **chao mai ya** improve digestion and alleviate food stagnation; **chao lai fu zi** also directs *qi* downwards; **ban xia** and **chen pi** harmonise the Stomach, resolve Phlegm and promote the movement of *qi*; **fu ling** strengthens the Spleen and leaches out Damp; **zhu ru** clears Heat and directs Stomach *qi* downwards; **zhi shi** regulates *qi* and promotes descent of Stomach *qi*. (Source: *Zhong Yi Nei Shou Ce*)

Modifications

- With constipation, add **bing lang** (Semen Arecae Catechu) 槟榔 9-12g and **da huang** (Radix et Rhizoma Rhei) 大黄 3-6g.
- With a degree of Heat (greasy, yellow tongue coat), add **huang lian** (Rhizoma Coptidis) 黄连 3-6g.
- With Cold in the Stomach, add **gan jiang** (Rhizoma Zingiberis Officinalis) 干姜 6-9g and **sha ren** (Fructus Amomi) 砂仁 6-9g.
- With Spleen deficiency, add **chao bai zhu** (dry fried Rhizoma Atractylodes Macrocephalae) 炒白术 12-15g.

Variations and additional prescriptions

Resistant cases

- In resistant cases with persistent hiccoughs, a few doses of a mild purge, such as **TIAO WEI CHENG QI TANG** (*Regulate the Stomach and Order the Qi Decoction* 调胃承气汤, p.468) may be useful to powerfully redirect *qi* downwards and clear the stagnation through the bowel.

Patent medicines

Bao He Wan 保和丸 (Bao He Wan)
Liu He Bao He Wan 六合保和丸 (Bo Wo Yuen Medical Pills)
Jian Pi Wan 建脾丸 (Jian Pi Wan)
- with Spleen deficiency
Chen Xiang Hua Qi Wan 沉香化气丸 (Chen Xiang Hua Qi Wan)
- with constipation
Mu Xiang Shun Qi Wan 木香顺气丸 (Mu Xiang Shun Qi Wan)
- with *qi* stagnation

Acupuncture (select from)

Ren.12 (*zhong wan* -) .... *mu* point of the Stomach, clears and alleviates food stagnation in the Stomach
Ren.14 (*ju que* -) .... pacifies the Stomach and benefits the diaphragm
Ren.17 (*shan zhong*) .... *hui* point for *qi*, directs rebellious *qi* downward and benefits the diaphragm
PC.6 (*nei guan* -) .... *luo* point of the Pericardium, regulates the middle *jiao* and stops hiccough

St.36 (*zu san li* -) .... *he* sea point of the Stomach, regulates the Spleen and Stomach and corrects the *qi* mechanism

St.44 (*nei ting* -) .... *rong* spring and Water point of the Stomach, clears Heat from the Stomach and alleviates food stagnation

St.40 (*feng long* -) .... *luo* point of the Stomach, transforms Phlegm and clears Heat and food stagnation from the Stomach

LI.10 (*shou san li* -) .... benefits digestion and regulates gastro-intestinal function

- with constipation, add SJ.6 (*zhi gou* -), Sp.14 (*fu jie* -) and St.25 (*tian shu* -)
- with Spleen deficiency, add Sp.4 (*gong sun*) and Bl.20 (*pi shu* +)
- with severe abdominal bloating add St.25 (*tian shu* -) and Ren.6 (*qi hai*)
- *Ear points*: diaphragm, sympathetic, stomach, liver, spleen

Clinical notes

- Because this is largely an event associated with overindulgence and irregular dietary habits, a change in the patient's eating habits should be enough to cure the problem and prevent recurrence. Herbs and acupuncture can stop acute episodes and speed up removal of food stagnation.
- The Chinese have long known the benefits of sipping small amounts of certain teas while eating. The action of such teas helps assist digestion, especially of fats, and reduces the risk of food stagnation. European cultures use table wine in much the same way, hence 'a little wine for thy stomach's sake'. Similarly, 'bitters', combinations of bitter herbs and alcohol, are a common accompaniment to food, either as a digestive aid following a meal, or as an aperitive. The bitterness of the herbs assists the descent of Stomach *qi* and dries Damp.

肝气犯胃

15.4 LIVER QI INVADING THE STOMACH

Pathophysiology

- Liver *qi* invading the Stomach disrupts the functional integrity of the Stomach and interrupts the natural descent of Stomach *qi*, which then ascends as hiccoughs. The hiccoughs will be triggered or aggravated by an emotional upset or sudden stressful situation.
- Liver *qi* stagnation type hiccoughs are frequently complicated by stagnant Heat and/or Phlegm accumulation.

Clinical features

- Paroxysmal or continuous hiccoughs that have a clear emotional component; they may be triggered or aggravated when the patient is under emotional stress, and relieved when the patient is relaxed and calm.
- epigastric, abdominal and/or hypochondriac fullness, distension or discomfort
- loss of appetite, mild nausea
- belching, borborygmus, flatulence
- irritability

T unremarkable, or with a greasy coat and red edges
P wiry or slippery, and/or rapid

Treatment principle

Direct Stomach *qi* downwards to stop hiccoughs
Harmonise the Stomach and Liver, regulate Liver *qi*

Prescription

XUAN FU DAI ZHE TANG 旋复代赭汤
(*Inula and Haematite Decoction*) modified

dai zhe shi (Haematitum) 代赭石 15-30g
xuan fu hua (Flos Inulae) 旋复花 12-15g
sheng jiang (Rhizoma Zingiberis Officinalis Recens) 生姜 12-15g
ban xia (Rhizoma Pinelliae Ternatae) 半夏 9-12g
chuan lian zi (Fructus Meliae Toosendan) 川楝子 9-12g
yu jin (Tuber Curcumae) 郁金 9-12g
dao dou zi (Semen Canavalia gladiata) 刀豆子 30g

Method: Decoction. **Xuan fu hua** is decocted in a cloth bag (*bao jian* 包煎). **Xuan fu hua** and **dai zhe shi** are the main herbs and together forcefully drive down rising Stomach *qi*; **xuan fu hua** transforms Phlegm, **dai zhe shi** weighs down rising Stomach *qi*; **ban xia** and **sheng jiang** harmonise the Stomach and transform Phlegm; **chuan lian zi** regulates Liver *qi* and stops pain; **yu jin** regulates Liver *qi* and Blood and stops pain; **dao dou zi** directs Stomach *qi* downwards and stops hiccough. (Source: *Zhong Yi Nei Ke Shou Ce*)

Modifications

- With Phlegm accumulation (greasy tongue coat, epigastric fullness, nausea) add **chen pi** (Pericarpium Citri Reticulatae) 陈皮 6-9g and **fu ling** (Sclerotium Poria Cocos) 茯苓 12-15g.
- With stagnant Heat (bitter taste in the mouth, red edges on the tongue, restlessness and irritability) add **huang lian** (Rhizoma Coptidis) 黄连 3-6g and **zhu ru** (Caulis Bambusae in Taeniis) 竹茹 9-12g.
- With a degree of Spleen deficiency (loss of appetite and loose stools), add **dang shen** (Radix Codonopsis Pilosulae) 党参 15-24g, **da zao** (Fructus Zizyphi Jujubae) 大枣 4pce and **gan cao** (Radix Glycyrrhizae Uralensis) 甘草 6-9g.

Patent medicines

Mu Xiang Shun Qi Wan 木香顺气丸 (Mu Xiang Shun Qi Wan)
- with food stagnation

Chai Hu Shu Gan Wan 柴胡疏肝丸 (Chai Hu Shu Gan Wan)
- Liver invading the Spleen and Stomach

Chen Xiang Hua Qi Wan 沉香化气丸 (Chen Xiang Hua Qi Wan)
- with constipation

Shu Gan Wan 舒肝丸 (Shu Gan Wan, Shu Kan Wan)
- with pain

Jia Wei Xiao Yao Wan 加味逍遥丸 (Jia Wei Xiao Yao Wan, Dan Zhi Xiao Yao Wan) - with stagnant Heat

Acupuncture (select from)

PC.6 (*nei guan* -) .... *luo* point of the Pericardium, master point of *yin wei mai*, regulates the middle *jiao* and stops hiccough

Liv.3 (*tai chong* -) .... *yuan*, *shu* and Earth point of the Liver, regulates Liver *qi*, pacifies the Liver and stops spasms

Ren.12 (*zhong wan* -) .... *mu* point of the Stomach, clears Heat from the Stomach and directs Stomach *qi* downwards

Liv.14 (*qi men* -) .... *mu* point of the Liver, harmonises the Liver and Spleen

St.36 (*zu san li*) .... *he* sea point of the Stomach, regulates the Spleen and Stomach and corrects the *qi* mechanism

Bl.17 (*ge shu* -) .... *shu* point for the diaphragm, regulates diaphragm function

Ren.17 (*shan zhong*) .... *hui* point for *qi*, directs rebellious *qi* downward and benefits the diaphragm

- with Heat, add Liv.2 (*xing jian* -)
- with hypochondriac distension or pain, add GB.34 (*yang ling quan* -) and SJ.6 (*zhi gou* -)
- with Phlegm, add St.40 (*feng long* -) and Sp.3 (*tai bai*)
- with plum stone throat, add PC.5 (*jian shi* -) and St.40 (*feng long* -)
- with abdominal distension, add St.25 (*tian shu* -) and Ren.6 (*qi hai* -)
- *Ear points*: diaphragm, liver, sympathetic, stomach, spleen

Clinical notes

- Acupuncture is helpful in relieving this type of hiccough. Treatment should be frequent, once or twice daily.
- For dietary recommendations, see p.878.

痰湿内阻

15.5 PHLEGM DAMP

Pathophysiology

- Phlegm Damp and Liver *qi* stagnation frequently coexist, and can in some patients be difficult to distinguish. The presence of Phlegm in the Stomach disrupts the *qi* mechanism; Liver *qi* stagnation can retard the movement of fluids which can congeal into Phlegm. The difference is often one of degree, and one or other pathology will tend to be dominant. In both cases, the patient is usually relatively robust, or at least, not exhausted by the hiccoughing.

Clinical features

- continuous hiccoughs, possibly initiated or aggravated by eating certain foods, such as cold or raw substances, dairy products or sugar
- epigastric and abdominal fullness, distension and stuffiness
- rattling sputum in the chest or sinuses
- loss of appetite
- borborygmus
- sticky sensation in the mouth, or dry mouth with no desire to drink
- nausea and/or vomiting
- dizziness or vertigo, foggy-headedness
- greasy skin, musty body odour
- tendency to obesity, pear shape
- palpitations

T thick, greasy, white coat; the tongue body may be flabby and pale
P slippery, wiry, moderate

Treatment principle

Harmonise the Stomach and stop hiccoughs
Transform Phlegm and redirect *qi* downwards

Prescription

ER CHEN TANG 二陈汤
(*Citrus and Pinellia Combination*) modified

ban xia (Rhizoma Pinelliae Ternatae) 半夏 9-12g
chen pi (Pericarpium Citri Reticulatae) 陈皮 9-12g
fu ling (Sclerotium Poria Cocos) 茯苓 12-15g
gan cao (Radix Glycyrrhizae Uralensis) 甘草 6-9g
sheng jiang (Rhizoma Zingiberis Officinalis Recens) 生姜 9-12g
wu yao (Radix Linderae Strychnifoliae) 乌药 9-12g
mu xiang (Radix Aucklandiae Lappae) 木香 9-12g

ding xiang (Flos Caryophylli) 丁香 3-6g
shi di (Calyx Diospyros Kaki) 柿蒂 9-12g

Method: Decoction. **Ban xia** transforms Phlegm, dries Damp, directs rising Stomach *qi* downwards and stops nausea and vomiting; **chen pi** transforms Phlegm and dries Damp, regulates middle *jiao qi* and corrects the *qi* mechanism; **fu ling** strengthens the Spleen and leaches out Damp; **zhi gan cao** strengthens the Spleen and harmonises the Stomach; **wu yao** and **mu xiang** regulate *qi*; **ding xiang** warms the Stomach, dispels Cold and redirects Stomach *qi* downwards; **shi di** stops hiccoughs. (Source: *Zhong Yi Nei Ke Shou Ce*)

Modifications

- With severe epigastric bloating and fullness, add **hou po** (Cortex Magnoliae Officinalis) 厚朴 9-12g and **zhi ke** (Fructus Citri Aurantii) 枳壳 9-12g.
- With signs of Heat (bitter taste in the mouth, indeterminate gnawing hunger), add **huang lian** (Rhizoma Coptidis) 黄连 3-6g and **zhu ru** (Caulis Bambusae in Taeniis) 竹茹 9-12g.

Patent medicines

Er Chen Wan 二陈丸 (Er Chen Wan, Pinellia-Pachyma Compound Pills)
Xiang Sha Liu Jun Zi Wan 香砂六君子丸 (Xiang Sha Liu Jun Wan, Aplotaxis-Ammomum Pills, Six Gentlemen Tea Pills)
- with Spleen *qi* deficiency
Wen Dan Wan 温胆丸 (Wen Dan Wan)
- Phlegm Heat
Fu Zi Li Zhong Wan 附子理中丸 (Fu Tzu Li Chung Wan, Carmichaeli Tea Pills, Li Chung Yuen Medical Pills)
- Spleen *yang* deficiency with thin Phlegm
Xiang Sha Yang Wei Wan 香砂养胃丸 (Xiang Sha Yang Wei Wan, Hsiang Sha Yang Wei Wan) - with *qi* stagnation

Acupuncture (select from)

PC.6 (*nei guan* -) .... *luo* point of the Pericardium, master point of *yin wei mai*, regulates the middle *jiao* and the *qi* mechanism
PC.5 (*jian shi* -) .... *jing* river point of the Pericardium, transforms Phlegm and harmonises the Stomach
Ren.12 (*zhong wan* -) .... *mu* point of the Stomach, clears pathogens, directs Stomach *qi* downwards and harmonises the Stomach
Bl.17 (*ge shu*) .... *shu* point for the diaphragm, regulates diaphragm function
St.40 (*feng long* -) .... *luo* point of the Stomach, transforms Phlegm and clears Heat and Phlegm from the Stomach

Sp.3 (*tai bai*) .... *yuan*, *shu* stream and Earth point of the Spleen, strengthens the Spleen and supplements *qi* to transforms Dampness

- with Spleen deficiency, add St.36 (*zu san li* +) and Liv.13 (*zhang men* +)
- with Liver *qi* stagnation, add Liv.3 (*tai chong*)
- with foggy-headedness, add GB.20 (*feng chi*) and Bl.62 (*shen mai*)
- with Cold Phlegm, apply moxa cones to Bl.20 (*pi shu* ▲) and Bl.21 (*wei shu* ▲)
- with muscle aches and heaviness, add Sp.21 (*da bao*)
- with fluid retention and oedema, add Sp.9 (*yin ling quan* -) and Sp.6 (*san yin jiao*)
- with somnolence, add Kid.6 (*zhao hai*) and Bl.62 (*shen mai*)
- with abdominal distension, add St.25 (*tian shu*) and Sp.15 (*da heng*)
- *Ear points*: diaphragm, stomach, spleen, liver, sympathetic

Clinical notes

- Acupuncture will usually quickly improve Phlegm Damp hiccoughs, but dietary changes and herbs will help reduce Phlegm.
- For dietary recommendations, see p.880.

瘀血阻滞

15.6 BLOOD STAGNATION

Pathophysiology

- Blood stagnation type hiccoughs can be acute or chronic. When acute they may follow trauma. The traumatic incident may be physical, such as abdominal surgery or a motor vehicle accident, or emotional. Acute Blood stagnation may also follow overenthusiastic use of styptic herbs to quell bleeding from the gastro-intestinal system. In acute cases, there may be few of the classical systemic signs and symptoms.
- When chronic, there will usually be a long history of digestive problems, typically Liver *qi* stagnation or accumulation of pathogens that over time, block the movement of Blood. Blood stagnation frequently coexists with other patterns and pathogens, such as Liver *qi* stagnation, various deficiencies, Phlegm, Heat and Cold.
- Stagnant Blood causes hiccoughs by physically obstructing the descent of Stomach *qi* and disrupting the function of the diaphragm.

Clinical features

- chronic, persistent, intractable hiccoughs that may cause focal stabbing pain in the epigastrium; pain is worse with pressure
- the epigastrium is firm and resists palpation; a mass may be palpable
- irritability, short temper, depression, mood swings
- low grade fever at night
- fixed, sharp pains, particularly in the head and upper body
- dry, scaly skin
- insomnia, restlessness at night, feverishness at night
- broken vessels or spider naevi on the face, trunk, inner knee and ankle
- purplish lips, sclera, conjunctivae and nail beds, dark rings under the eyes

T in acute cases, the tongue body may be unremarkable; in chronic cases it may be dark or purple with brown or purple stasis spots (perhaps in the centre) and a thin, white coat; the sublingual veins are distended and dark

P choppy, wiry or intermittent

Treatment principle

Invigorate Blood circulation and eliminate stagnant Blood
Harmonise the Stomach and stop hiccoughs

Prescription

XUE FU ZHU YU TANG 血府逐瘀汤
(*Achyranthes and Persica Combination*) modified

sheng di (Radix Rehmanniae Glutinosae) 生地 15-18g
dang gui (Radix Angelicae Sinensis) 当归 9-12g

tao ren (Semen Persicae) 桃仁 9-12g
hong hua (Flos Carthami Tinctorii) 红花 9-12g
chi shao (Radix Paeoniae Rubrae) 赤芍 9-12g
zhi ke (Fructus Citri Aurantii) 枳壳 9-12g
chai hu (Radix Bupleuri) 柴胡 6-9g
chuan niu xi (Radix Cyathulae Officinalis) 川牛膝 12-18g
xuan fu hua (Flos Inulae) 12-15g

Method: Decoction. **Xuan fu hua** may be decocted in a cloth bag (*bao jian* 包煎). **Sheng di** cools the Blood and nourishes *yin*; **dang gui** regulates and nourishes Blood; **tao ren**, **hong hua** and **chi shao** invigorate Blood and eliminate stagnant Blood; **zhi ke** and **chai hu** regulate *qi*; **chuan niu xi** invigorates Blood and directs *qi* and Blood downwards; **xuan fu hua** directs *qi* downward. (Source: *Zhong Yi Nei Ke Shou Ce*)

Modifications

- With a tendency to Heat, add **mu dan pi** (Cortex Moutan Radicis) 牡丹皮 9-12g and **zhu ru** (Caulis Bambusae in Taeniis) 竹茹 9-12g.
- With a tendency to Cold, add **bai dou kou** (Fructus Amomi Kravanh) 白豆蔻 6-9g, **ding xiang** (Flos Caryophylli) 丁香 3-6g and **ban xia** (Rhizoma Pinelliae Ternatae) 半夏 9-12g.
- With *qi* deficiency add **huang qi** (Radix Astragali Membranacei) 黄芪 18-30g, **chao bai zhu** (dry fried Rhizoma Atractylodes Macrocephalae) 炒白术 12-15g and **huang jing** (Rhizoma Polygonati) 黄精 15-18g.
- With *yin* deficiency, add **sha shen** (Radix Adenophorae seu Glehniae) 沙参 9-12g.
- With pain, add **yan hu suo** (Rhizoma Corydalis Yanhusuo) 延胡索 9-12g, or **ru xiang** (Gummi Olibanum) 乳香 6-9g and **mo yao** (Myrrha) 没药 6-9g.
- With *qi* stagnation (distension, belching), substitute **zhi shi** (Fructus Immaturus Citri Aurantii) 枳实 9-12g for **zhi ke**, and add **qing pi** (Pericarpium Citri Reticulatae Viridae) 青皮 9-12g.
- If the hiccoughs follow a traumatic injury add **san qi fen** (powdered Radix Notoginseng) 三七粉 3-6g and **wang bu liu xing** (Semen Vaccariae Segetalis) 王不留行 6-9g. Where there is extensive bruising, add **zhi da huang** (processed Radix et Rhizoma Rhei) 制大黄 6-9g and **gui zhi** (Ramulus Cinnamomi Cassiae) 桂枝 9g.

Patent medicines

Xue Fu Zhu Yu Wan 血府逐瘀丸 (Xue Fu Zhu Yu Wan)

Acupuncture (select from)

Ren.12 (*zhong wan* -) .... *mu* point of the Stomach, clears stagnant Blood, directs Stomach *qi* downwards and harmonises the Stomach

St.21 (*liang men* -) .... local point to promotes function of the Spleen and Stomach and alleviates distension
Liv.13 (*zhang men* -) .... *mu* point of the Spleen, *hui* point for the *zang*, relieves stagnation and assists the *qi* mechanism
Bl.17 (*ge shu* -) .... *shu* point for the diaphragm, *hui* point for Blood, transforms stagnant Blood and regulates diaphragm function
Bl.18 (*gan shu* -) .... *shu* point of the Liver, invigorates Liver *qi* and Blood
Bl.21 (*wei shu* -) .... *shu* point of the Stomach, eliminates Stagnant Blood from the Stomach
Du.8 (*jin suo* -) .... special point for spasms
St.34 (*liang qiu* -) .... *xi* cleft point of the Stomach, stops pain
Sp.10 (*xue hai* -) .... regulates and invigorates Blood
Sp.6 (*san yin jiao*) .... strengthens the Spleen, regulates Liver *qi*, benefits the Kidneys, invigorates *qi* and Blood and removes obstruction from the *jing luo*
Sp.4 (*gong sun*) .... *luo* point of the Spleen, master point of *chong mai*, regulates the Spleen and Stomach and stops pain
LI.10 (*shou san li*) .... benefits digestion and regulates gastro-intestinal function
ah shi points .... over focal pain

- with nausea and vomiting, add PC.6 (*nei guan*)
- with irritability or depression, add Liv.3 (*tai chong*) or Liv.1 (*da dun* ▲)
- for severe pain, add LI.4 (*he gu* -) and Liv.5 (*li gou* -)
- *Ear points*: diaphragm, liver, sympathetic, stomach, *shen men*

Clinical notes

- Hiccoughs associated with Blood stagnation are often difficult to resolve, and may require persistent treatment for a satisfactory result.
- For dietary recommendations, see p.886.

脾肾阳虚

15.7 SPLEEN AND KIDNEY YANG DEFICIENCY

Pathophysiology

- *Yang* deficiency hiccoughs are due to serious functional weakness of the Spleen, and its partner organ, the Stomach. The *qi* mechanism fails, subverting the natural descent of Stomach *qi* and ascent of Spleen *qi*. The accumulated *qi* ascends pathologically as weak and persistent hiccoughs. In addition to the accumulation of *qi*, the deficient *yang* contributes to build up of pathological Cold, which compounds the lack of correct *qi* movement and aggravates the tendency of the diaphragm to contract and spasm.
- Hiccoughs associated with Spleen and Kidney *yang* deficiency are most common in the elderly, the seriously debilitated, or following a general anaesthetic. Patients with this type of hiccough can deteriorate quickly as their remaining *yang qi* is consumed by the persistent diaphragm muscle spasm.

Clinical features

- prolonged, continuous weak hiccoughs with a low sound; the patient is exhausted by the hiccoughs, gradually growing weaker and weaker; the patient may have trouble catching breath between hiccoughs
- hypersalivation or vomiting of thin watery fluids
- epigastric and abdominal discomfort or pain that is eased with warmth and pressure
- mental and physical exhaustion, depression
- soft voice, reluctance to speak
- pale, sallow complexion
- loss of appetite
- chronic loose stools or watery diarrhoea with undigested food
- cold intolerance and extremities
- weak, aching lower back and legs
- frequent urination or nocturia

T pale or bluish and swollen with toothmarks and a thin, white coat
P deep, thready and weak

Treatment principle

Warm and supplement Spleen and Kidney *yang*
Harmonise the Stomach, redirect Stomach *qi* downwards and stop hiccoughs

Prescription

FU ZI LI ZHONG WAN 附子理中丸
(*Aconite, Ginseng and Ginger Formula*) modified

zhi fu zi (Radix Aconiti Carmichaeli Praeparata) 制附子 9-15g
gan jiang (Rhizoma Zingiberis Officinalis) 干姜 9-12g
dang shen (Radix Codonopsis Pilosulae) 党参 15-24g
chao bai zhu (dry fried Rhizoma Atractylodis Macrocephalae) 炒白术 12-15g
zhi gan cao (honey fried Radix Glycyrrhizae Uralensis) 炙甘草 6-9g
ding xiang (Flos Caryophylli) 丁香 3-6g
bai dou kou (Fructus Amomi Kravanh) 白豆蔻 6-9g

Method: Decoction. **Zhi fu zi** is cooked for 30 minutes prior to the other herbs (*xian jian* 先煎), **bai dou kou** is added a few minutes before the end of cooking (*hou xia* 后下). **Zhi fu zi** and **gan jiang** powerfully warm the Spleen and Stomach, invigorate function of the *qi* mechanism and dispel Cold; **gan jiang** resolves thin congested fluids; **dang shen** supplements *qi* and strengthens the Spleen; **chao bai zhu** strengthens the Spleen and dries Dampness; **zhi gan cao** supplements *qi* and harmonises the Stomach; **ding xiang** and **bai dou kou** warm the Stomach, promote the movement of *qi*, ease the diaphragm and stop hiccoughs and vomiting. (*Shi Yong Zhong Yi Nei Ke Xue*)

Modifications

- With nausea, reflux or heartburn, add **wu zhu yu** (Fructus Evodiae Rutaecarpae) 吴茱萸 3-6g and **gui zhi** (Ramulus Cinnamomi Cassiae) 桂枝 6-9g.
- Too many bitter herbs are avoided as they may aggravate *yang qi* dispersal. However, if the above prescription is slow to have effect or does not appear to be working, add **shi di** (Calyx Diospyros Kaki) 柿蒂 9-12g.

Variations and additional prescriptions

To restore Spleen and Kidney yang

- Once the hiccoughs have subsided, the focus of treatment may shift to strengthening both Spleen and Kidney *yang* by combining the above prescription with **JIN KUI SHEN QI WAN** (*Rehmannia Eight Formula* 金匮肾气丸, p.724).

Patent medicines

Fu Zi Li Zhong Wan 附子理中丸 (Fu Tzu Li Chung Wan, Carmichaeli Tea Pills, Li Chung Yuen Medical Pills)
- Spleen *yang* deficiency with Cold

Li Zhong Wan 理中丸 (Li Zhong Wan)
- Spleen *yang* deficiency

Jin Kui Shen Qi Wan 金匮肾气丸 (Fu Gui Ba Wei Wan, Sexoton Pills, Golden Book Tea) - Kidney *yang* deficiency

Acupuncture (select from)

Ren.12 (*zhong wan* +▲) .. *mu* point of the Stomach, warms and regulates the Stomach and Spleen and directs Stomach *qi* downwards

Ren.4 (*guan yuan* ▲) .... these points warm Kidney *yang* and *yuan*
Ren.6 (*qi hai* ▲) *qi* and aid the Kidneys in anchoring the dissipating *yang*

PC.6 (*nei guan*) .... *luo* point of the Pericardium, master point of *yin wei mai*, regulates the middle *jiao*

St.36 (*zu san li* +▲) .... *he* sea point of the Stomach, powerfully warms and strengthens the Spleen and Stomach and supplements *qi*

Bl.17 (*ge shu* ▲) .... *shu* point of the diaphragm, regulates diaphragm function

Bl.20 (*pi shu* +▲) .... *shu* point of the Spleen, warms and supplements Spleen *qi* and *yang*

- a moxa box over the abdomen is useful
- with severe Kidney *yang* deficiency, add Bl.23 (*shen shu* +▲) and Du.4 (*ming men* +▲)
- *Ear points*: diaphragm, stomach, spleen, sympathetic, adrenal

Clinical notes

- Hiccoughs associated with *yang* deficiency are often intractable, and may occur following upper abdominal surgery or trauma in weak or debilitated patients. Frequent treatment may be necessary to alleviate the hiccoughs, and some months of constitutional treatment necessary to rebuild Spleen and Kidney *yang*.
- For dietary recommendations, see p.873.

胃阴不足

15.8 STOMACH YIN DEFICIENCY

Pathophysiology

- Stomach *yin* deficiency hiccoughs may be acute or chronic. When acute, the hiccoughs often follow a severe febrile illness, such as *yang ming* syndrome, that has damaged Stomach *yin*. When chronic there will generally be a long history of digestive problems. Chronic Liver *qi* invasion of the Stomach, chronic Stomach Heat, an excessively hot or spicy diet, or a familial tendency to digestive weakness, are frequently found.

Clinical features

- short, rapid hiccoughs which come in paroxysms or clusters
- vague, dull or burning epigastric discomfort which is worse when the stomach is empty, and may improve with pressure.
- dry mouth, lips and throat
- thirst with desire for cool drinks
- mild nausea, and in severe cases dry retching
- poor appetite, or indeterminate gnawing hunger with no real desire to eat
- constipation or dry stools

T slightly red and peeled in the centre, or red and dry with little or no coat; in severe or long standing cases, the tongue may be so denuded of papillae as to resemble a piece of liver (mirror tongue), or have numerous surface cracks or a wide shallow central crack.

P thready and rapid

Treatment principle

Nourish and supplement Stomach *yin*, and clear Heat
Harmonise the Stomach, redirect Stomach *qi* downwards and stop hiccoughs

Prescription

YI WEI TANG 益胃汤
(*Benefit the Stomach Decoction*) modified

sha shen (Radix Adenophorae seu Glehniae) 沙参 12-15g
sheng di (Radix Rehmanniae Glutinosae) 生地 15-18g
mai dong (Tuber Ophiopogonis Japonici) 麦冬 9-12g
yu zhu (Rhizoma Polygonati Odorati) 玉竹 9-12g
shi hu (Herba Dendrobi) 石斛 9-12g
pi pa ye (Folium Eriobotryae Japonicae) 枇杷叶 9-12g
shi di (Calyx Diospyros Kaki) 柿蒂 9-12g
zhu ru (Caulis Bambusae in Taeniis) 竹茹 9-12g
dao dou zi (Semen Canavalia gladiata) 刀豆子 30g

Method: Decoction. **Sha shen, sheng di, mai dong, yu zhu** and **shi hu** nourish Stomach *yin*; **pi pa ye** and **zhu ru** clear Heat and direct Stomach *qi* downwards; **shi di** and **dao dou zi** stop hiccoughs. (Source: *Zhong Yi Nei Ke Shou Ce*)

Modifications

- With *qi* deficiency (swollen, slightly reddish tongue with multiple surface cracks, loss of appetite), add **shan yao** (Radix Dioscoreae Oppositae) 山药 15-18g and **dang shen** (Radix Codonopsis Pilosulae) 党参 15-24g.
- With acid reflux or heartburn, add **hai piao xiao** (Os Sepiae seu Sepiellae) 海螵蛸 15g, or **wu zhu yu** (Fructus Evodiae Rutaecarpae) 吴茱萸 1-3g and **huang lian** (Rhizoma Coptidis) 黄连 3-6g if there is significant Heat.
- With food stagnation, add **mai ya** (Fructus Hordei Vulgaris Germinantus) 麦芽 15-30g and **ji nei jin** (Endothelium Corneum Gigeriae Galli) 鸡内金 12g.
- With significant deficiency Heat, add **zhi mu** (Rhizoma Anemarrhenae Asphodeloides) 知母 9-12g and **xuan shen** (Radix Scrophulariae) 玄参 18-24g.
- With hypo-acidity, add **wu mei** (Fructus Pruni Mume) 乌梅 9-12g, **shi hu** (Herba Dendrobi) 石斛 9-12g and **shan zha** (Fructus Crataegi) 山楂 15g.
- With stagnant *qi*, add **mei gui hua** (Flos Rosae Rugosae) 玫瑰花 6-9g and **fo shou** (Fructus Citri Sarcodacylis) 佛手 9-12g, or consider **YI GUAN JIAN** (*Linking Decoction* 一贯煎, p.78).
- With stagnant Blood (intermittent stabbing pain, or a focal area that is painful with pressure), add **dan shen** (Radix Salviae Miltiorrhizae) 丹参 12-18g and **tao ren** (Semen Persicae) 桃仁 9-12g.
- With constipation, add **sheng he shou wu** (unprocessed Radix Polygoni Multiflori) 生何首乌 12-15g and **huo ma ren** (Semen Cannabis Sativae) 火麻仁 9-12g.

Patent medicines

Gu Ben Wan 固本丸 (Gu Ben Wan, Ren Shen Ku Pen Wan)
- Stomach and Spleen *yin* and *qi* deficiency

Sheng Mai San Wan 生脉散丸 (Sheng Mai San Wan)
- *qi* and *yin* deficiency

Shen Ling Bai Zhu Wan 参苓白术丸 (Shen Ling Bai Zhu Wan)
- good for mild *yin* and *qi* deficiency

Liu Wei Di Huang Wan 六味地黄丸 (Liu Wei Di Huang Wan, Six Flavour Tea)

Mai Wei Di Huang Wan 麦味地黄丸 (Mai Wei Di Huang Wan, Ba Xian Chang Shou Wan)
- A small dose of one of the last two patent formulae may be

combined with the principle formula when there is Kidney *yin* deficiency.

Acupuncture (select from)

Ren.12 (*zhong wan* +) .... *mu* point of the Stomach, nourishes Stomach *yin*, regulates the Stomach and directs Stomach *qi* downwards
PC.6 (*nei guan*) .... *luo* point of the Pericardium, master point of *yin wei mai*, regulates the middle *jiao*
St.36 (*zu san li* +) .... *he* sea point of the Stomach, powerfully strengthens the Spleen and Stomach and supplements *qi* and *yin*
Bl.17 (*ge shu* -) .... *shu* point for the diaphragm, regulates diaphragm function
Bl.20 (*pi shu* +) .... *shu* point of the Spleen, supplements Spleen *qi* and *yin*
Bl.21 (*wei shu* +) .... *shu* point of the Stomach, supplements Stomach *qi* and *yin*
Kid.3 (*tai xi* +) .... *yuan* point of the Kidney, nourishes *yin*
Kid.9 (*zhu bin* +) .... *xi* point of *yin wei mai*, with PC.6 (*nei guan*) can direct weak Stomach *qi* downwards

- with deficient Heat, add St.43 (*xian gu* -) and Kid.2 (*ran gu*)
- *Ear points*: diaphragm, stomach, spleen, sympathetic, liver

Clinical notes

- When chronic, this can be a difficult problem to resolve fully, and will require persistent treatment for success. The hiccoughs may be controlled in the short term, however, the underlying Stomach *yin* deficiency will generally need some months of treatment, particularly herbal medicine.
- For dietary recommendations, see p.876.

SUMMARY OF GUIDING FORMULAE FOR HICCOUGH

Excess patterns

Cold in the Stomach - *Ding Xiang San* 丁香散

Stomach Heat/Fire - *Zhu Ye Shi Gao Tang* 竹叶石膏汤
- with constipation - *Xiao Cheng Qi Tang* 小承气汤
- mixed Heat and Cold - *Sheng Jiang Xie Xin Tang* 生姜泻心汤
- Phlegm Heat - *Ju Pi Zhu Ru Tang* 橘皮竹茹汤

Food stagnation - *Bao He Wan* 保和丸

Liver *qi* invading the Stomach - *Xuan Fu Dai Zhe Tang* 旋复代赭汤

Phlegm Damp - *Er Chen Tang* 二陈汤

Blood stagnation - *Xue Fu Zhu Yu Tang* 血府逐瘀汤

Deficient patterns

Spleen and Kidney *yang* deficiency - *Fu Zi Li Zhong Wan* 附子理中丸

Stomach *yin* deficiency - *Yi Wei Tang* 益胃汤

16. Indeterminate Gnawing Hunger

Stomach Heat
Liver *qi* invading the Stomach
Stomach (and Liver) *yin* deficiency
Stomach *qi* deficiency
Blood stagnation
Food stagnation

16 INDETERMINATE GNAWING HUNGER

cao za 嘈杂

Indeterminate gnawing hunger[1] is a sensation of nagging discomfort in the pit of the stomach that simulates hunger and pain, without clearly being either. The stomach feels empty and uncomfortable and the patient feels the need to eat as if eating would give relief, but when offered food does not want to ingest it.

Indeterminate gnawing hunger can be somewhat vague and difficult to describe. There is no suitable word or phrase in common English. Some western patients explain: 'I can't describe it but my stomach just doesn't feel right'. Any such vague epigastric malaise should prompt consideration of indeterminate gnawing hunger. One reasonably consistent feature to be noted is the tendency of patients to wake in the middle of the night with nagging epigastric discomfort, drink a little milk or eat some bland food and gain temporary relief.

Indeterminate gnawing hunger is almost always chronic. Heat, the most common cause of indeterminate gnawing hunger, may be excess, deficient or mixed. The most common patterns are Stomach Heat and/or Stomach *yin* deficiency, perhaps with the complication of Phlegm. The dynamic relationship between the various patterns is often seen as a progression of pathology. It may proceed from chronic *qi* stagnation that invades the Stomach, to the generation of stagnant Heat that damages Stomach *yin*.

Some patients will have been diagnosed with 'indigestion' or 'dyspepsia', and in fact there are many aetiological and therapeutic similarities. Indigestion and dyspepsia are umbrella terms for a set of upper abdominal symptoms, one of which may be indeterminate gnawing hunger. Indeterminate gnawing hunger may, however, occur in isolation.

AETIOLOGY

External pathogens

External pathogens, either Heat or Cold transforming into Heat may invade the Stomach and Intestines, drying the Stomach and damaging *yin*. This type of indeterminate gnawing hunger is not uncommon, and may be observed following a severe febrile illness, such as *yang ming* syndrome, or Heat in the Blood.

---

[1]Wiseman's 'Clamouring Stomach'

Diet

A diet rich in Heat producing foods directly introduces Heat into the Stomach and may lead to indeterminate gnawing hunger. In addition, there are certain groups of food that are especially aggravating to people prone to indeterminate gnawing hunger and heartburn. These include acid foods like the citrus family, tomatoes, uncooked peppers and capsicums, radishes, onions and garlic. Excessive consumption of Damp generating, sweet or cold, raw foods can clog the digestion and generate food stagnation that may generate Heat. Eating more food than the Spleen and Stomach can cope with, either because of simple overeating or because the Spleen is already weak, will obstruct *qi* mechanism. The resulting increase in pressure from the accumulated *qi* can generate Heat.

BOX 16.1 SOME BIOMEDICAL CAUSES OF INDETERMINATE GNAWING HUNGER

- peptic ulcer disease
- chronic gastritis
- chronic atrophic gastritis
- gastro-oesophageal reflux
- motility disorder
- alcohol abuse
- gall bladder disease
- Zollinger-Ellison syndrome
- neoplasm of the stomach
- NSAIDs, aspirin

Skipping meals, eating at odd hours, eating too late at night, or while under stress can disorder the function of the Stomach, contributing to *qi* stagnation, food stagnation and Heat generation (*see* p.3), and the eventual weakening of the Spleen and Stomach. Once the *qi* mechanism is obstructed by unprocessed food, various complications can arise to further disrupt the Stomach, most typically the generation of Dampness, Phlegm and Heat.

Some pharmaceutical drugs are notorious for causing indeterminate gnawing hunger, in particular aspirin and nonsteroidal anti-inflammatory drugs (NSAIDs). Other drugs that have a Heating nature as defined in TCM, such as steroids, *yang* supplementing substances and amphetamines, may also be problematic.

Emotion

Liver *qi* stagnation, which invades the Stomach and generates stagnant Heat, is a common component of indeterminate gnawing hunger.

Liver *qi* stagnation is usually the result of repression of emotion, typically frustration, resentment and anger. These emotions, expressed or unexpressed, can cause spasm and tension in the smooth muscle of the Stomach. Aggravation or initiation of the epigastric discomfort is clearly related to the patient's emotional state and stress levels.

In addition to the emotional factors that upset the Liver, worry, obsessive thinking and prolonged concentration in combination with a sedentary or studious lifestyle and poor diet, will weaken middle *jiao qi*, predisposing it to (or inviting) invasion by Liver *qi* resulting in further damage. The weakened

Spleen produces Dampness that can then be congealed into Phlegm and Phlegm Heat.

TREATMENT

Treatment usually needs to be quite lengthy for good results as the problem is usually quite chronic and gastric lining may be damaged. This can be rebuilt, but it takes time. The time required to alleviate the main complaint will vary from patient to patient, but in long standing cases, it can take weeks to months before symptomatic relief is achieved, so diligence and encouragement are essential. The exception is the pattern that follows a febrile illness, which usually resolve quite quickly.

胃热嘈杂

16.1 STOMACH HEAT

Heat is the most common cause of indeterminate gnawing hunger. The Heat may be the result of several distinct or mixed processes, such as consumption of Heating foods and drinks, the constraining effect of an overbearing Liver, Heat created by stagnation of Dampness or Phlegm or an invasion of the Stomach by external pathogenic Heat.

In practice, excess Heat patterns are frequently complicated by deficiency of *yin* and/or fluids, especially when chronic . Even though the patient may at first appear quite robust, some level of Stomach deficiency will often be revealed as treatment progresses.

胃肝郁热

16.1.1 Stagnant Heat in the Stomach and Liver

Pathophysiology

- This type of Heat is caused by constraint of Liver *qi* and invasion of the Stomach by Liver *qi*. A heating diet and overeating contribute to the pattern, which is frequently complicated by *yin* deficiency and food stagnation. When prolonged, Blood stagnation may intervene.
- This is a common pattern of indeterminate gnawing hunger, and usually corresponds to a relatively early stage in the evolution of the disorder. As the Heat clears, the underlying Liver *qi* stagnation will come to the fore, and the focus of treatment will need to shift. *See* 16.2, p.609.

Clinical features

- frequent indeterminate gnawing hunger, aggravated or initiated by heating foods and/or increase in stress levels
- may be vague epigastric discomfort or burning, acid reflux and heartburn, sour belching
- may be vomiting of sour fluids first thing in the morning
- bitter taste in the mouth
- thirst with desire for cold fluids, dry mouth
- irritability, easy anger, hot temper
- tendency to constipation; rarely, diarrhoea

T red or with red edges and a dry or yellow coat

P wiry and/or slippery, possibly rapid

Treatment principle

Clear stagnant Heat from the Stomach and Liver

Harmonise the Liver and Stomach

Regulate *qi*, nourish and protect *yin*

Prescription

DAN ZHI XIAO YAO SAN 丹栀逍遥散
(*Bupleurum and Paeonia Formula*) modified

chai hu (Radix Bupleuri) 柴胡 9-12g
bai shao (Radix Paeoniae Lactiflora) 白芍 12-24g
dang gui (Radix Angelicae Sinensis) 当归 9-12g
fu ling (Sclerotium Poriae Cocos) 茯苓 12-15g
bai zhu (Rhizoma Atractylodes Macrocephalae) 白术 9-12g
mu dan pi (Cortex Moutan Radicis) 牡丹皮 9-12g
shan zhi zi (Fructus Gardeniae Jasminoidis) 山栀子 9-12g
zhi gan cao (honey fried Radix Glycyrrhizae Uralensis) 炙甘草 6-9g
bo he (Herba Mentha Haplocalycis) 薄荷 6-9g
huang lian (Rhizoma Coptidis) 黄连 3-6g
wu zhu yu (Fructus Evodiae Rutaecarpae) 吴茱萸 1-2g

Method: Decoction. **Bo he** is added towards the end of cooking (*hou xia* 后下). **Chai hu** and **bai shao** regulate and move Liver *qi*; **fu ling**, **bai zhu** and **zhi gan cao** strengthen the Spleen; **fu ling** leaches out Damp and promotes urination; **bai zhu** dries Damp; **dang gui** and **bai shao** nourish Blood and soften the Liver; **bai shao** and **zhi gan cao** alleviate spasms and stop pain; **shan zhi zi** and **mu dan pi** cool the Liver and clear stagnant Heat; **bo he** clears Heat and alleviates Liver *qi* constraint; **huang lian** and **wu zhu yu** clear Heat from the Liver and Stomach and alleviate gnawing hunger.

Modifications

- With severe Heat, add **lian qiao** (Fructus Forsythia Suspensae) 连翘 9-12g and **pu gong ying** (Herba Taraxaci Mongolici) 蒲公英 15-30g.
- With food stagnation, add **shan zha** (Fructus Crataegi) 山楂 15g and **shen qu** (Massa Fermentata) 神曲 15g.
- With constipation, add **da huang** (Radix et Rhizoma Rhei) 大黄 6-9g and **zhi shi** (Fructus Immaturus Citri Aurantii) 枳实 9-12g.
- To assist in regulating *qi* without damaging *qi* and *yin*, mild *qi* regulating herbs such as **fo shou** (Fructus Citri Sarcodacylis) 佛手 9-12g, **ba yue zha** (Fructus Akebiae) 八月扎 9-12g and **xiang yuan pi** (Pericarpium Citri Medica) 香橼皮 9-12g may be added.

Patent medicines

Jia Wei Xiao Yao Wan 加味逍遥丸 (Jia Wei Xiao Yao Wan, Dan Zhi Xiao Yao Wan)
- Liver *qi* stagnation with stagnant Heat

Wei Te Ling 胃特灵 (Wei Te Ling Stomach Sedative)
- an antacid formula that can be combined with the appropriate constitutional formula for symptomatic relief of reflux

Xiang Lian Wan 香莲丸 (Xiang Lian Wan)
- this patent can be combined with the appropriate constitutional formula for symptomatic relief of reflux

Bao He Wan 保和丸 (Bao He Wan)
- add a small dose with food stagnation

Acupuncture (select from)

Ren.12 (*zhong wan* -) .... *mu* point of the Stomach, clears Heat from the Stomach, regulates Stomach *qi* and harmonises the Stomach
Ren.10 (*xia wan* -) .... local point for Stomach disorders
PC.8 (*lao gong* -) .... *rong* spring and Fire point of the Pericardium, drains Heat from the Stomach channel and cools the Blood

St.44 (*nei ting* -) .... together these points clear Heat from
LI.4 (*he gu* -) the Stomach

Liv.2 (*xing jian* -) .... *rong* spring and Fire point of the Liver, cools the Liver and regulates *qi*
LI.11 (*qu chi* -) .... *he* sea point of the Large Intestine, clears Heat and Dampness from *yang ming*
LI.10 (*shou san li*) .... benefits digestion and regulates gastro-intestinal function

- with severe Heat, add St.45 (*li dui* ↓)
- with constipation, add SJ.6 (*zhi gou* -) and St.25 (*tian shu* -)
- with nausea, add PC.6 (*nei guan*)
- *Ear points:* liver, stomach, spleen, *shen men*, subcortex, sympathetic

痰热嘈杂

16.1.2 Phlegm Heat, following febrile illness

Pathophysiology

- Phlegm Heat in the Stomach can be associated with the remnants of a febrile illness that has damaged the Stomach and congealed *yin* fluids into Phlegm. It may also be due to chronic overeating and consequent food stagnation which creates Phlegm Heat. As in the previous pattern, a diet rich in greasy, fatty, sweet and/or heating foods and alcohol is a potent contributor. The main difference between this pattern and the previous pattern is the relationship of symptoms to the emotional state and stress levels of the patient; here the patient may be anxious, but unlike the previous pattern, increasing stress is of negligible influence on the development or aggravation of the symptoms.

Clinical features

- indeterminate gnawing hunger
- nausea, vomiting of sour fluids, worse in the morning
- bitter taste in the mouth
- mild thirst
- anxiety, nervousness, timidity
- palpitations, tachycardia
- insomnia, sleeplessness, restlessness
- dizziness or vertigo
- fullness in the chest with copious sputum

T thick, greasy, yellow coat
P wiry and/or slippery, possibly rapid

Treatment principle

Clear Heat and transform Phlegm
Cool the Stomach and Gallbladder, regulate *qi*

Prescription

WEN DAN TANG 温胆汤
(*Bamboo and Hoelen Combination*)

zhu ru (Caulis Bambusae in Taeniis) 竹茹 12-15g
zhi shi (Fructus Immaturus Citri Aurantii) 枳实 9-12g
ban xia (Rhizoma Pinelliae Ternatae) 半夏 9-12g
chen pi (Pericarpium Citri Reticulatae) 陈皮 6-9g
fu ling (Sclerotium Poria Cocos) 茯苓 12-15g
sheng jiang (Rhizoma Zingiberis Officinalis Recens)
生姜 6-9g
gan cao (Radix Glycyrrhizae Uralensis) 甘草 3-6g

Method: Decoction. **Zhu ru** clears Phlegm Heat from the Stomach and Gallbladder; **zhi shi** breaks up stagnant *qi*, directs *qi* downwards and alleviates distension; **ban xia** transforms Phlegm, dries Damp and directs rising Stomach *qi* downwards; **chen pi** transforms Phlegm and dries Damp, regulates middle *jiao qi* and corrects the *qi* mechanism; **fu ling** strengthens the Spleen and leaches out Damp; **gan cao** strengthens the Spleen and harmonises the Stomach; **sheng jiang** assists the other herbs in stopping nausea and vomiting. (Source: *Shi Yong Zhong Yi Nei Ke Xue*)

Modifications

- With severe Heat, add **huang lian** (Rhizoma Coptidis) 黄连 3-6g and **shan zhi zi** (Fructus Gardeniae Jasminoides) 山栀子 9-12g.
- With severe Phlegm Heat (thick, yellow, greasy coat, fuzzy-headedness, dizziness), add **tian zhu huang** (Concretio Silicea Bambusae Textillis) 天竺黄 9-12g, **zhu li** (Succus Bambusae) 竹沥 9-12g and **dan nan xing**

(Pulvis Arisaemae cum Felle Bovis) 胆南星 3-6g.

- With food stagnation, add **shen qu** (Massa Fermentata) 神曲 15g, **shan zha** (Fructus Crataegi) 山楂 15g, **mai ya** (Fructus Hordei Vulgaris Germinantus) 麦芽 15-30g and **chao lai fu zi** (dry fried Semen Raphani Sativi) 炒莱服子 9-12g.
- With palpitations, panic attacks or severe anxiety, add **zhen zhu mu** (Concha Margaritaferae) 珍珠母 15-30g, **duan long gu** (calcined Os Draconis) 煅龙骨 15-30g or **duan mu li** (calcined Concha Ostreae) 煅牡蛎 15-30g.
- With constipation, add **da huang** (Radix et Rhizoma Rhei) 大黄 6-9g and **gua lou ren** (Semen Trichosanthis) 栝楼仁 12-15g.
- With discomfort, fullness or a sense of tightness in the chest, add **gua lou** (Fructus Trichosanthis) 瓜蒌 15-24g.

Patent medicines

Wen Dan Wan 温胆丸 (Wen Dan Wan)
- Phlegm Heat

Bao He Wan 保和丸 (Bao He Wan)
- add a small dose with food stagnation

Acupuncture (select from)

Ren.12 (*zhong wan* -) .... *mu* point of the Stomach, clears Phlegm Heat and harmonises the Stomach

St.40 (*feng long* -) .... *luo* point of the Stomach, transforms Phlegm and clears Heat, stagnant foodand Phlegm from the Stomach

GB.40 (*qiu xu* -) ....*yuan* point of the Gallbladder, benefits the Gallbladder and regulates Liver *qi*

Sp.3 (*tai bai*) ....*yuan*, *shu* stream and Earth point of the Spleen, strengthens the Spleen and transforms Dampness

St.44 (*nei ting* -) .... *rong* spring and Water point of the Stomach, clears Heat from *yang ming*, the Stomach and Stomach channel

PC.8 (*lao gong* -) .... *rong* spring and Fire point of the Pericardium, drains Heat from the Stomach channel, cools the Blood and clears Heart Fire

St.36 (*zu san li* -) .... *he* sea point of the Stomach, powerfully regulates and supplements *qi* and corrects the *qi* mechanism

LI.11 (*qu chi* -) .... *he* sea point of the Large Intestine, clears Heat and Dampness from *yang ming*

- with severe Heat, add St.45 (*li dui* ↓) and SJ.2 (*ye men* -)
- with anxiety, add Ht.7 (*shen men*) and Kid.4 (*da zhong*)
- with constipation, add SJ.6 (*zhi gou* -) and St.25 (*tian shu* -)
- with nausea, add PC.6 (*nei guan*)
- with food stagnation, add St.25 (*tian shu* -)
- *Ear points:* liver, stomach, subcortex, sympathetic, *shen men*

Clinical Notes

- Liver and Stomach stagnant Heat is a common pattern in stressed individuals who tend to eat on the run, miss meals and eat poorly. It may be diagnosed as gastritis or peptic ulcer disease. The Phlegm Heat pattern may be associated with disorders such as chronic gastritis, peptic ulcer disease, post febrile disease or neurosis.
- Both types of indeterminate gnawing hunger respond well to treatment. In the latter pattern treatment needs to continue until all signs of Phlegm are cleared, in particular, until the tongue coat becomes normal. The Liver *qi* stagnation that gives rise to stagnant Heat often has an good prognosis, particularly if the source of external stress can be resolved. Acupuncture and herbs are certainly among the best and most reliable treatments. Treatment to regulate *qi* usually needs to be prolonged (3 months+) and must be combined with appropriate relaxation and stress management techniques, or other forms of *qi* mobilising activity. Particularly useful is walking, swimming, yoga or *tai ji chuan*, although all exercise is beneficial.
- The use of slippery elm powder, before meals or bed, can be of assistance in lining the Stomach and easing discomfort. Mint tea is good for gently cooling Heat.
- For dietary recommendations, see p.882-885.

肝气犯胃

16.2 LIVER QI INVADING THE STOMACH

Pathophysiology

- Indeterminate gnawing hunger caused by Liver *qi* invading the Spleen is a common precursor to the more chronic and common Heat patterns, stagnant Heat in the Liver and Stomach and *yin* deficiency. The history will often elicit a prolonged tendency towards tension, pain or knots in the Stomach, or other stress induced upper digestive tract upsets. This pattern is also described as Liver and Stomach disharmony.
- The repeated invasion by stagnant *qi* causes spasm and functional disorder in the Stomach. When the Stomach is in a tense state, vague epigastric discomfort occurs, which may be temporarily relieved by eating, and thus bringing *qi* into the Stomach. The background tension remains however, and as digestion finishes and middle *jiao qi* moves on the sensation returns.
- Chronic Liver *qi* invading the Spleen will often be complicated by another pathology. In addition to the Heat patterns noted above, *qi* stagnation can give rise to Blood stagnation, Damp or Phlegm Damp accumulation, *qi* deficiency and food stagnation.

Clinical features

- Indeterminate gnawing hunger that has a clear relationship to the emotional state of the patient, and is aggravated or initiated by stress. The indeterminate gnawing hunger may be slightly relieved by eating a little, but tends to recur quickly.
- hypochondriac and epigastric tenderness, ache, pain, fullness or discomfort
- epigastric and abdominal bloating
- alternating constipation and loose stools
- loss of appetite, frequent sighing and belching, morning nausea
- fullness or tightness in the chest
- irritability, moodiness, depression, anxiety, 'a worrier'
- dizziness, tension headaches
- irregular menstruation, premenstrual breast tenderness
- shoulder and neck tension
- cold fingers and toes

T unremarkable or darkish, with a thin white or yellow coat
P wiry, maybe thready

Treatment principle

Harmonise the Liver and Stomach
Regulate and invigorate Liver *qi*, ease the Stomach

Prescription

CHAI HU SHU GAN SAN 柴胡疏肝散
(*Bupleurum and Cyperus Formula*) modified

chai hu (Radix Bupleuri) 柴胡 9-12g
bai shao (Radix Paeoniae Lactiflorae) 白芍 12-24g
zhi ke (Fructus Citri Aurantii) 枳壳 9-12g
chuan xiong (Radix Ligustici Chuanxiong) 川芎 6-9g
chen pi (Pericarpium Citri Reticulatae) 陈皮 9-12g
xiang fu (Rhizoma Cyperi Rotundi) 香附 9-12g
zhi gan cao (honey fried Radix Glycyrrhizae Uralensis)
炙甘草 3-6g
huang lian (Rhizoma Coptidis) 黄连 3-6g
wu zhu yu (Fructus Evodiae Rutaecarpae) 吴茱萸 1-3g

Method: Decoction. **Chai hu** regulates and invigorates Liver *qi* and relieves *qi* constraint; **bai shao** softens the Liver and nourishes *yin* and Blood thus preventing excessive dispersal of, and damage to, *qi* and Liver *yin* by **chai hu**, and with **gan cao**, eases spasms and tension in the Stomach; **zhi shi** breaks up stagnant *qi*, directs *qi* downwards, it's descending action neatly balancing the ascending nature of **chai hu** thus facilitating the correct functioning of the *qi* mechanism; **gan cao** harmonises the Stomach and strengthens the Spleen; **chuan xiong** and **xiang fu** regulate *qi* and Blood; **chen pi** regulates *qi* and corrects the *qi* mechanism; **huang lian** clears Heat from the Liver and Stomach; **wu zhu yu** is pungent and warm and promotes movement of *qi*; together these last two herbs clear stagnant Heat, alleviate heartburn and ease the sensation of gnawing hunger.

Modifications

- With severe heartburn and hyperacidity, add **hai piao xiao** (Os Sepiae seu Sepiellae) 海螵蛸 15g and **duan wa leng zi** (calcined Concha Arcae) 煅瓦楞子 15g.
- With bloating and distension, add **zhi shi** (Fructus Immaturus Citri Aurantii) 枳实 9-12g and **jie geng** (Radix Platycodi Grandiflori) 桔梗 6-9g.
- With nausea, add **ban xia** (Rhizoma Pinelliae Ternatae) 半夏 9-12g and **sheng jiang** (Rhizoma Zingiberis Officinalis Recens) 生姜 6-9g.
- With Phlegm Damp (thick tongue coat, heaviness, bloating, foggy headedness) add **cang zhu** (Rhizoma Atractylodis) 苍术 12-15g and **hou po** (Cortex Magnoliae Officinalis) 厚朴 9-12g.
- With Blood deficiency, add one or two of the following herbs: **dang gui** (Radix Angelicae Sinensis) 当归 9-12g, **ji xue teng** (Radix et Caulis Jixueteng) 鸡血藤 15-18g, **gou qi zi** (Fructus Lycii) 枸杞子 9-12g or **e jiao** (Gelatinum Corii Asini) 阿胶 6-9g.
- With *qi* deficiency, add **dang shen** (Radix Codonopsis Pilosulae) 党参 15-24g and **chao bai zhu** (dry fried Rhizoma Atractylodes Macrocephalae) 炒白术 12-15g.

- With mild signs of *yin* deficiency, add **sheng di** (Radix Rehmanniae Glutinosae) 生地 12-15g, **mai dong** (Tuber Ophiopogonis Japonici) 麦冬 9-12g and **shan yao** (Radix Dioscoreae Oppositae) 山药 15-18g.
- With mild signs of Blood stagnation (occasional stabbing pain), add **dan shen** (Radix Salviae Miltiorrhizae) 丹参 12-18g.
- With epigastric pain, add **yu jin** (Tuber Curcumae) 郁金 9-12g, **yan hu suo** (Rhizoma Corydalis Yanhusuo) 延胡索 9-12g or **fo shou** (Fructus Citri Sarcodactylis) 佛手 9-12g.
- Prolonged or severe *qi* stagnation will often generate Heat, especially when the diet tends to be heating. With a degree of stagnant Heat, add **shan zhi zi** (Fructus Gardeniae Jasminoidis) 山栀子 9-12g and **mu dan pi** (Cortex Moutan Radicis) 牡丹皮 9-12g. *See also* **DAN ZHI XIAO YAO SAN** (*Bupleurum and Paeonia Formula* 丹栀逍遥散, p.604).
- With excessive belching or sighing, add two or three of the following herbs: **bai dou kou** (Fructus Amomi Kravanh) 白豆蔻 6-9g, **mei gui hua** (Flos Rosae Rugosae) 玫瑰花 6-9g, **chen xiang** (Lignum Aquilariae) 沉香 3-6g and **xuan fu hua** (Flos Inulae) 旋复花 12-15g.
- If the patient is tense and uptight, add **he huan pi** (Cortex Albizziae Julibrissin) 合欢皮 15g, **suan zao ren** (Semen Zizyphi Spinosae) 酸枣仁 15g and **mu li** (Concha Ostreae) 牡蛎 15-30g. In most cases it is valuable to add some *shen* calming herbs.
- With food stagnation and a tendency to constipation, add **hou po** (Cortex Magnoliae Officinalis) 厚朴 12-15g, **bing lang** (Semen Arecae Catechu) 槟榔 9-12g and **shan zha** (Fructus Crataegi) 山楂 15g.

Variations and additional prescriptions

Complex or confusing patterns with multiple pathology

- In patients with chronic or complicated patterns, it can be difficult to determine the main pathology as there will often be elements of several, such as *qi* and food stagnation, Dampness, Heat and stagnant Blood. The approach in these cases is to initially use a mild, yet broad spectrum, prescription to clear the picture. The treatment aims to clear all potential stagnations and harmonise the Stomach with a combination of **YUE JU WAN** (*Escape Restraint Pill* 越鞠丸, p.17) and **ZUO JIN WAN** (*Left Metal Pill* 左金丸, p.117).

For women

- Liver *qi* stagnation is frequently complicated by Blood deficiency, especially in women. In addition to the primary complaint, there may be menstrual disorders, and increase of symptoms before menstruation, sleep disturbance and anxiety states. The aim of treatment is to soothe the Liver, harmonise the Stomach, nourish Blood and strengthen the

Spleen and Stomach with **XIAO YAO SAN** (*Bupleurum and Dang Gui Formula* 逍遥散, p.159) plus **ZUO JIN WAN** (*Left Metal Pill* 左金丸, p.117).

Patent medicines

Chai Hu Shu Gan Wan 柴胡疏肝丸 (Chai Hu Shu Gan Wan)
Shu Gan Wan 舒肝丸 (Shu Gan Wan, Shu Kan Wan)
- with epigastric pain

Xiao Yao Wan 逍遥丸 (Xiao Yao Wan, Hsiao Yao Wan, Bupleurum Sedative Pills)
Jia Wei Xiao Yao Wan 加味逍遥丸 (Jia Wei Xiao Yao Wan, Dan Zhi Xiao Yao Wan)
- with stagnant Heat

Wei Te Ling 胃特灵 (Wei Te Ling Stomach Sedative)
- combine with the appropriate constitutional formula for symptomatic relief of heartburn

Acupuncture (select from)

Ren.12 (*zhong wan*) .... *mu* point of the Stomach, alleviates stagnation, strengthens and regulates the Stomach
Liv.13 (*zhang men* -) .... *mu* point of the Spleen and *hui* point of the *zang*, harmonises the Liver, Spleen and Stomach
PC.6 (*nei guan*) .... *luo* point of the Pericardium, master point of *yin wei mai*, spreads Liver *qi*, regulates and harmonises the middle *jiao* and stimulates the *qi* mechanism
Liv.3 (*tai chong* -) ....*yuan*, *shu* and Earth point of the Liver, regulates and spreads Liver *qi* and Blood and pacifies rising *yang*
GB.34 (*yang ling quan* -) ... *he* sea point of the Gallbladder, regulates Liver *qi* and harmonises the Liver and Stomach
St.36 (*zu san li*) .... *he* sea point of the Stomach, powerfully regulates and supplements *qi* and harmonises the Stomach
LI.10 (*shou san li* -) .... good for regulating *qi* in the epigastrium, often tender in Stomach disorders

Bl.18 (*gan shu*) .... *shu* points of the Liver, Gallbladder and
Bl.19 (*dan shu*) Stomach respectively, move Liver *qi* and
Bl.21 (*wei shu*) harmonise the Stomach

- with lateral headaches and neck tension, add GB.34 (*yang ling quan*)

and GB.21 (*jian jing* -)
- with hypochondriac pain, add Liv.14 (*qi men* -)
- with Gallbladder involvement or morning vomiting of sour fluids, add GB.24 (*ri yue*), GB.40 (*qiu xu* -), and *dan nang xue* (M-LE-23)
- with Heat in the Liver, add Liv.2 (*xing jian* -)
- with Spleen deficiency, add Bl.20 (*pi shu* +)
- with Phlegm or plum stone throat, add PC.5 (*jian shi* -), St.40 (*feng long* -) and Sp.3 (*tai bai*)
- with dizziness, add GB.20 (*feng chi* -)
- In most cases, points to calm the *shen* should be added: select one or two points from Ht.7 (*shen men*), *yin tang* (M-HN-3), Du.19 (*hou ding*), Du. 24 (*shen ting*)
- *Ear points*: liver, stomach, subcortex, sympathetic, *shen men*

Clinical Notes

- Liver *qi* invading the Stomach type indeterminate gnawing hunger may be diagnosed biomedically as nervous stomach, chronic gastritis, hiatus hernia or peptic ulcer disease.
- Liver *qi* stagnation patterns generally have a good prognosis, particularly if the source of external stress can be resolved. Acupuncture and herbs are certainly among the best and most reliable treatments. Treatment to regulate *qi* usually needs to be prolonged (3 months+) and must be combined with appropriate relaxation and stress management techniques, or other forms of *qi* mobilising activity. Particularly useful is walking, swimming, yoga or *tai ji chuan*, although all exercise is beneficial.
- The use of slippery elm powder, before meals or bed, can be of assistance in lining the Stomach and easing discomfort.
- For dietary recommendations, see p.878.

胃肝阴虚

16.3 STOMACH (LIVER) YIN DEFICIENCY

Pathophysiology

- Stomach *yin* (± Liver *yin*) deficiency is an important and common pattern of indeterminate gnawing hunger. It is usually the result of chronic stagnant Liver and/or Stomach Heat, or prolonged Liver invasion of the Stomach. The emphasis of the pattern will vary somewhat depending on the aetiology. When diet is the main aetiology, Stomach Heat is likely to be primary. When there is an emotional component to the problem, Liver pathology may be the main feature.
- Stomach *yin* deficiency often represents a physical deterioration of the stomach lining itself, and thus treatment usually needs to be quite prolonged for satisfactory results.

Clinical features

- Intermittent episodes of mild but persistent indeterminate gnawing hunger which tend to be worse towards the end of the day or during the evening. The patient may wake during the night (often around 1-4am) with epigastric discomfort which may be relieved by eating.
- mild, dull epigastric burning sensation or pain
- acid reflux, heartburn, vague nausea
- general dryness of mucous membranes and skin, thirst, dry mouth, lips and throat
- tendency to dry stools or constipation

T red and dry with little or no coat, or red and peeled or cracked in the centre; in some cases the only tongue sign is a peeled centre

P thready and wiry, possibly rapid

Treatment principle

Nourish and supplement Stomach (and Liver) *yin*

Regulate *qi* and harmonise the Stomach

Prescription

16.3.1 Stomach *yin* deficiency

YI WEI TANG 益胃汤

(*Benefit the Stomach Decoction*) modified

This prescription is selected when the Stomach *yin* deficiency is largely uncomplicated.

sha shen (Radix Adenophorae seu Glehniae) 沙参 12-15g
mai dong (Tuber Ophiopogonis Japonici) 麦冬 12-15g
sheng di (Radix Rehmanniae Glutinosae) 生地 15-18g

shi hu (Herba Dendrobii) 石斛 12-15g
bai shao (Radix Paeoniae Lactiflora) 白芍 12-24g
gan cao (Radix Glycyrrhizae Uralensis) 甘草 3-6g

Method: Decoction. **Sha shen, mai dong, sheng di** and **shi hu** nourish *yin*; **bai shao** and **gan cao** combine sour and sweet to generate *yin*, ease spasms and alleviate discomfort.

16.3.2 Liver and Stomach *yin* deficiency, with *qi* stagnation

YI GUAN JIAN 一贯煎
(*Linking Decoction*) modified

This prescription is selected when Stomach *yin* deficiency is complicated by Liver *qi* stagnation, a common situation. Strong *qi* regulating herbs may disperse Stomach *yin*, so a gentle approach is indicated. The aim of treatment is to nourish Stomach *yin* and gently regulate *qi*.

sheng di (Radix Rehmanniae Glutinosae) 生地 15-30g
gou qi zi (Fructus Lycii) 枸杞子 12-15g
sha shen (Radix Adenophorae seu Glehniae) 沙参 12-15g
mai dong (Tuber Ophiopogonis Japonici) 麦冬 12-15g
dang gui (Radix Angelicae Sinensis) 当归 9-12g
chuan lian zi (Fructus Meliae Toosendan) 川楝子 9-12g
bai shao (Radix Paeoniae Lactiflora) 白芍 12-24g
shi hu (Herba Dendrobi) 石斛 12-15g
yu zhu (Rhizoma Polygonati Odorati) 玉竹 9-12g
fo shou (Fructus Citri Sarcodactylis) 佛手 9-12g
mai ya (Fructus Hordei Vulgaris Germinantus) 麦芽 15-30g
gan cao (Radix Glycyrrhizae Uralensis) 甘草 3-6g

Method: Decoction. **Sheng di, gou qi zi, sha shen, mai dong, shi hu** and **yu zhu** moisten and nourish Liver and Stomach *yin* and clear Heat; **dang gui, bai shao** and **gou qi zi** nourish Liver Blood, soften the Liver and ease tension and spasm in the muscles and Stomach; **chuan lian zi** and **fo shou** regulate *qi* and stop pain; **bai shao** and **gan cao** combine sweet and sour to generate *yin* and ease spasms to stop pain; **mai ya** alleviates food stagnation and protects the Stomach. (Source: *Zhong Yi Nei Ke Shou Ce*)

Modifications (where not already included)

- With epigastric pain and distension, gentle non drying *qi* moving herbs may be included. These include **fo shou** (Fructus Citri Sarcodacylis) 佛手 6-9g, **ba yue zha** (Fructus Akebiae) 八月扎 6-9g, **xiang yuan pi** (Pericarpium Citri Medica) 香橼皮 6-9g and **mei gui hua** (Flos Rosae Rugosae) 玫瑰花 6-9g.
- With vomiting or regurgitation of sour fluids, add **huang lian** (Rhizoma Coptidis) 黄连 3-6g and **wu zhu yu** (Fructus Evodiae Rutaecarpae) 吴茱萸 1-2g.

- With dry stools or constipation, add **xuan shen** (Radix Scrophulariae) 玄参 18-24g and **huo ma ren** (Semen Cannabis Sativae) 火麻仁 9-12g.
- With *qi* deficiency, add **zhi huang qi** (honey fried Radix Astragali Membranacei) 炙黄芪 18-30g, **tai zi shen** (Radix Pseudostellariae Heterophyllae) 太子参 15-18g and **shan yao** (Radix Dioscoreae Oppositae) 山药 15-18g.
- With stagnant Blood (intermittent stabbing pain, or a focal area that is painful with pressure), add **dan shen** (Radix Salviae Miltiorrhizae) 丹参 12-18g and **tao ren** (Semen Persicae) 桃仁 9-12g.
- For atrophy of the gastric mucosa, add **dan shen** (Radix Salviae Miltiorrhizae) 丹参 12-18g and **zhi huang qi** (honey fried Radix Astragali Membranacei) 炙黄芪 18-30g.

Variations and additional prescriptions

Post febrile yin deficiency

- If this condition follows a febrile disease it may simply damage Stomach *yin*. This is different to the pattern where Heat congeals fluids to Phlegm Heat (16.1.2, p.605). The features of post febrile *yin* damage are indeterminate gnawing hunger, a lingering, low grade feverishness, restless sleep and a red tongue with little or no coat. The aim of treatment is to clear residual Heat from the *qi* level and nourish Stomach *yin* with **ZHI ZI DOU CHI TANG** (*Gardenia and Prepared Soybean Decoction* 栀子豆豉汤) modified.

  shan zhi zi (Fructus Gardeniae Jasminoidis) 山栀子 9-12g
  dan dou chi (Semen Sojae Preparatum) 淡豆豉 9-12g
  shi gao (Gypsum) 石膏 15g
  mai dong (Tuber Ophiopogonis Japonici) 麦冬 9-12g
  sha shen (Radix Adenophorae seu Glehniae) 沙参 12-15g
  gan cao (Radix Glycyrrhizae Uralensis) 甘草 3-6g

  Method: Decoction. **Shi gao** is decocted for 30 minutes prior to the other herbs. **Shan zhi zi** and **dan dou chi** clear lingering Heat from the *qi* level and alleviate irritability; **shi gao** clears Heat from the Stomach; **mai dong** and **sha shen** nourish Stomach *yin*; **gan cao** protects the Stomach.

Patent medicines

Gu Ben Wan 固本丸 (Gu Ben Wan, Ren Shen Ku Pen Wan)
Sheng Mai San Wan 生脉散丸 (Sheng Mai San Wan)
- *qi* and *yin* deficiency

Acupuncture (select from)

Ren.12 (*zhong wan* +) .... *mu* point of the Stomach, nourishes and supplements Stomach *yin*, regulates the Stomach and directs Stomach *qi* downwards

Liv.13 (*zhang men* +) .... *mu* point of the Spleen and *hui* point of the *zang*, strengthens the Spleen, supplements *yin*, improves digestion and promotes Liver function

Bl.20 (*pi shu* +) .... *shu* points of the Spleen and Stomach, nourish
Bl.21 (*wei shu* +) and supplement *yin* and *qi* and regulate the Spleen and Stomach

St.36 (*zu san li* +) .... *he* sea point of the Stomach, powerfully strengthens the Spleen and Stomach, supplements *qi* and *yin* and stimulates the *qi* mechanism

Ren.4 (*guan yuan* +) .... these points benefit the Stomach and Kidneys
Sp.6 (*san yin jiao* +) and supplement *yin*

Bl.23 (*shen shu* +) .... these points strengthen the source of all
Kid.6 (*zhao hai* +) inherited *yin*, the Kidney, releasing stored *yin* to
Kid.3 (*tai xi* +) support Stomach *yin*

- *Ear points*: stomach, liver, oesophagus, kidney, sympathetic, subcortex, *shen men*

Clinical notes

- Stomach *yin* deficiency type indeterminate gnawing hunger may be diagnosed biomedically as chronic atrophic gastritis or peptic ulcer disease.
- This is a common pattern of indeterminate gnawing hunger and can be quite difficult to treat satisfactorily. Even though systemic *yin* is being replenished, it often takes some time (weeks to months) before the patient gets symptomatic relief, so the discouragement and drop out factor is high. Results will eventually arrive, so diligence and persistence of both patients and practitioner are the key to success.
- The use of slippery elm powder, before meals or bed, can be of assistance in lining the Stomach and easing discomfort.
- For dietary recommendations, see p.876.

胃气虚弱

16.4 STOMACH QI DEFICIENCY

Pathophysiology

- Stomach *qi* deficiency is a less common cause of indeterminate gnawing hunger than the Heat patterns. The mechanism is associated with the relative decline in Stomach function and consequent digestive inefficiency.
- This pattern is frequently complicated by Phlegm Damp and/or food stagnation.

Clinical features

- indeterminate gnawing hunger, worse when the Stomach is empty and temporarily alleviated with small amounts of warm, easily digested food
- dull epigastric pain, worse with raw or cold natured foods or exposure to cold, but relieved by warmth and pressure
- epigastric and abdominal bloating, worse after eating
- decreased sense of taste, loss of appetite
- hypersalivation, drooling
- sour belching, nausea
- waxy pale complexion
- fatigue, weakness, tired limbs
- tendency to loose stools

T pale, may be swollen with tooth marks, thin, white coat
P thready, deficient, weak

Treatment principle

Strengthen the Spleen, harmonise the Stomach

Prescription

SI JUN ZI TANG 四君子汤
(*Four Major Herbs Combination*) modified

dang shen (Radix Codonopsis Pilosulae) 党参 15-24g
chao bai zhu (dry fried Rhizoma Atractylodes Macrocephalae) 炒白术 12-15g
fu ling (Sclerotium Poriae Cocos) 茯苓 12-15g
zhi gan cao (honey fried Radix Glycyrrhizae Uralensis) 炙甘草 6-9g
shan yao (Radix Dioscoreae Oppositae) 山药 15-24g
bian dou (Semen Dolichos Lablab) 扁豆 12-15g

Method: Grind the herbs to a powder and take 9 grams 2-3 times daily with warm water. May also be decocted with the quantities as shown. **Dang shen, chao bai zhu, fu ling, zhi gan cao** and **shan yao** strengthen the Spleen and Stomach and supplement *qi*; **bai zhu** dries Damp; **fu ling** promotes urination and leaches Damp; **shan yao** nourishes Stomach *yin*; **bian dou** strengthens the Spleen.

Modifications

- With Phlegm Damp, nausea or vomiting, add **chen pi** (Pericarpium Citri Reticulatae) 陈皮 9-12g and **ban xia** (Rhizoma Pinelliae Ternatae) 半夏 9-12g.
- With Damp accumulation (thick, greasy tongue coat, heaviness, distension etc.), add **cang zhu** (Rhizoma Atractylodis) 苍术 12-15g and **hou po** (Cortex Magnoliae Officinalis) 厚朴 9-12g.
- With severe *qi* deficiency, add **zhi huang qi** (honey fried Radix Astragali Membranacei) 炙黄芪 18-30g.
- With *qi* stagnation, add **mu xiang** (Radix Aucklandiae Lappae) 木香 6-9g and **sha ren** (Fructus Amomi) 砂仁 6-9g.
- With food stagnation, add **chao shen qu** (dry fried Massa Fermentata) 炒神曲 15g, **chao shan zha** (dry fried Fructus Crataegi) 炒山楂 15g, **chao mai ya** (dry fried Fructus Hordei Vulgaris Germinantus) 炒麦芽 15-30g and **chao lai fu zi** (dry fried Semen Raphani Sativi) 炒莱服子 9-12g.
- With epigastric and abdominal fullness and distension, add **zhi ke** (Fructus Citri Aurantii) 枳壳 9-12g and **chen pi** (Pericarpium Citri Reticulatae) 陈皮 9-12g.
- With cold intolerance and cold extremities, add **gan jiang** (Rhizoma Zingiberis Officinalis) 干姜 6-9g.
- With epigastric pain, add **gao liang jiang** (Rhizoma Alpiniae Officinari) 高良姜 6-9g and **xiang fu** (Rhizoma Cyperi Rotundi) 香附 9-12g.

Variations and Additional Prescriptions

Cold and Deficiency of the Stomach

- In some cases, with Cold complicating the middle *jiao qi* deficiency, the patient wakes during the night or first thing in the morning with indeterminate gnawing hunger, and then vomits. The vomitus is watery and sour and there may be acid reflux. The patient is cold intolerant, with little appetite and a pale tongue. Some suffer migraine type headaches. The aim of treatment is to warm the Liver and Stomach, direct Stomach *qi* downward and stop vomiting with **WU ZHU YU TANG** (*Evodia Combination* 吴茱萸汤).

wu zhu yu (Fructus Evodiae Rutaecarpae) 吴茱萸 6-9g
dang shen (Radix Codonopsis Pilosulae) 党参 15-24g
sheng jiang (Rhizoma Zingiberis Officinalis Recens) 生姜 9-15g
da zao (Fructus Zizyphi Jujubae) 大枣 4pce

Method: Decoction, best taken cool. When warm it can cause vomiting. **Wu zhu yu** warms the Stomach and Liver, directs rebellious *qi* downwards and stops vomiting; **sheng jiang** warms the Stomach and assists **wu zhu yu** in stopping vomiting; **dang shen** strengthens the Spleen and protects Stomach *qi* and *yin* from the effects of severe vomiting; **da zao** moderates the dispersing and drying nature of **wu zhu yu**.

Variations and additional prescriptions

Heart Blood and Spleen qi deficiency

- When the Spleen and Stomach are weak, insufficient Blood will be produced, and *qi* and Blood deficiency will result. Patients with Blood deficiency will experience postural dizziness, palpitations, sleep disturbances with disturbing dreams, poor memory, anxiety, sallow pale complexion, pale lips, nails and conjunctivae, dry skin and hair, a pale tongue and thready pulse. The aim of treatment is to supplement and strengthen the Heart, Spleen, *qi* and Blood with **GUI PI TANG** (*Ginseng and Longan Combination* 归脾汤, p.728).

Patent medicines

Shen Ling Bai Zhu Wan 参苓白术丸 (Shen Ling Bai Zhu Wan)
- *qi* and *yin* deficiency

Gui Pi Wan 归脾丸 (Gui Pi Wan, Angelicae Longana Tea, Kwei Be Wan)
- Heart Blood and Spleen *qi* deficiency

Xiang Sha Yang Wei Wan 香砂养胃丸 (Xiang Sha Yang Wei Wan, Hsiang Sha Yang Wei Wan)
- with *qi* stagnation

Li Zhong Wan 理中丸 (Li Zhong Wan)
- with Cold and *yang* deficiency

Acupuncture (select from)

Ren.12 (*zhong wan* +▲) .. these points warm and strengthen the Stomach
Ren.13 (*shang wan* +▲) and middle *jiao*

St.21 (*liang men* +▲) .... promotes the function of the Spleen and Stomach

St.36 (*zu san li* +▲) .... *he* sea point of the Stomach, powerfully warms and strengthens the Spleen and Stomach, regulates and supplements *qi*

Sp.6 (*san yin jiao*) .... strengthens and regulates the Spleen and supplements *qi*

Bl.20 (*pi shu* +▲) .... *shu* points of the Spleen and Stomach, warm
Bl.21 (*wei shu* +▲) and strengthen middle *jiao qi* function

- with Phlegm Damp, add PC.5 (*jian shi*), St.40 (*feng long* -) and Sp.3 (*tai bai*)
- a moxa box over the epigastrium is useful, especially for *yang* deficiency
- *Ear points*: stomach, spleen, lung, sympathetic, adrenal, *shen men*

Clinical Notes

- Stomach *qi* deficiency indeterminate gnawing hunger may be diagnosed biomedically as chronic gastritis, functional dyspepsia or indigestion.
- Indeterminate gnawing hunger of this type responds reliably to correct TCM treatment, but the greater the deficiency, the longer the course or treatment required.
- For dietary recommendations, see pp.870.

血瘀阻胃

16.5 BLOOD STAGNATION

Pathophysiology

- Blood stagnation is always a chronic pattern of indeterminate gnawing hunger, and represents the culmination of years of other Stomach pathology, typically *qi* stagnation and/or *yin* deficiency. This is not a particularly common presentation, as Stomach Blood stagnation patterns usually present with pain and/or bleeding, but it does occasionally occur in patients taking aspirin or NSAIDs.
- Because of the chronicity and the fact that the patient most likely eats very little, deficiency patterns usually complicate the presentation.

Clinical features

- Chronic and persistent indeterminate gnawing hunger that is worse with eating and at night, with occasional aggravations of focal pain; the epigastric region feels firm or hard, and is focally tender when pressed.
- dark complexion and lips, dark rings around the eyes
- nausea, belching, acid reflux; in severe cases there may be occasional vomiting of a sour, dark or purplish coffee ground-like material, and the stools may be black and tarry
- poor appetite or anorexia, weight loss
- spider naevi across the cheeks, chest, epigastrium and flanks

T dark or purplish body, or with purple or brown stasis spots; dark, distended sublingual veins

P wiry, or thready and choppy

Treatment principle

Invigorate the circulation of *qi* and Blood
Eliminate stagnant Blood and harmonise the Stomach

Prescription

DANG GUI SI NI TANG 当归四逆汤
(*Dang Gui Decoction for Frigid Extremities*) modified

dang gui (Radix Angelicae Sinensis) 当归 9-12g
gui zhi (Ramulus Cinnamomi Cassiae) 桂枝 6-9g
xi xin (Herba cum Radice Asari) 细辛 3-6g
chi shao (Radix Paeoniae Rubrae) 赤芍 12-15g
zhi gan cao (honey fried Radix Glycyrrhizae Uralensis)
炙甘草 6-9g
wu zhu yu (Fructus Evodiae Rutaecarpae) 吴茱萸 3-6g
gan jiang (Rhizoma Zingiberis Officinalis) 干姜 6-9g
dan shen (Radix Salviae Miltiorrhizae) 丹参 12-18g

hong hua (Flos Carthami Tinctorii) 红花 9-12g
sheng pu huang (Pollen Typhae) 生蒲黄 9-12g

Method: Decoction. **Dang gui** nourishes and invigorates Blood; **gui zhi** and **xi xin** are warm, pungent and dispersing, and are used to warm the channels and disperse Cold; **gan jiang** and **wu zhu yu** warm the Stomach and direct *qi* downwards; **chi shao**, **dan shen**, **hong hua** and **sheng pu huang**, invigorate Blood and eliminate stagnant Blood. (Source: *Zhong Yi Nei Ke Shou Ce*)

Modifications

- With Blood deficiency, add **bai shao** (Radix Paeoniae Lactiflora) 白芍 12-18g, **ji xue teng** (Radix et Caulis Jixueteng) 鸡血藤 18-24g and **shu di** (Radix Rehmanniae Glutinosae Conquitae) 熟地 15-18g.
- With *qi* deficiency add **huang qi** (Radix Astragali Membranacei) 黄芪 18-30g, **chao bai zhu** (dry fried Rhizoma Atractylodes Macrocephalae) 炒白术 12-15g and **huang jing** (Rhizoma Polygonati) 黄精 15-18g.
- With *yin* deficiency, add **sheng di** (Radix Rehmanniae Glutinosae) 生地 15-18g and **sha shen** (Radix Adenophorae seu Glehniae) 沙参 12-15g.
- Patients with Blood stagnation in the Stomach will have impaired digestion and may have difficulty processing some Blood moving herbs. In most cases it is useful to add digestion improving herbs, such as **chao shan zha** (dry fried Fructus Crataegi) 炒山楂 15g and **shen qu** (Massa Fermentata) 神曲 15g.

XUE FU ZHU YU TANG 血府逐瘀汤
(*Achyranthes and Persica Combination*) p.83

This, more general, prescription is selected for Blood and *qi* stagnation patterns that follow years of Liver *qi* invading the Stomach.

Patent medicines

Xue Fu Zhu Yu Wan 血府逐瘀丸 (Xue Fu Zhu Yu Wan)
- *qi* and Blood stagnation

Tao Hong Si Wu Wan 桃红四物丸 (Tao Hong Si Wu Wan)
- with Blood deficiency

Tong Jing Wan 痛经丸 (Tong Jing Wan)
- relatively severe Blood stagnation, can be combined with another patent medicine

Fu Ke Wu Jin Wan 妇科乌金丸 (Woo Garm Yuen Medical Pills)
- with Cold and *qi* deficiency

Sheng Tian Qi Pian 生田七片 (Raw Tian Qi Ginseng Tablets)
- for Blood stagnation with bleeding

Acupuncture (select from)

Ren.12 (*zhong wan* -) .... *mu* point of the Stomach, regulates *qi* and Blood in the Stomach
St.21 (*liang men* -) .... regulates Stomach *qi*
St.36 (*zu san li* -) .... *he* sea point of the Stomach, powerfully invigorates movement of *qi* and Blood and regulates the Stomach
Bl.17 (*ge shu* -) .... *hui* point for Blood, eliminates stagnant Blood
Bl.18 (*gan shu* -) .... *shu* point of the Liver, invigorates Liver *qi* and Blood
Bl.21 (*wei shu* -) .... *shu* point of the Stomach, eliminates Stagnant Blood from the Stomach
Sp.10 (*xue hai* -) .... regulates and invigorates Blood
Sp.6 (*san yin jiao*) .... strengthens the Spleen, regulates Liver *qi* and invigorates *qi* and Blood

- with nausea and vomiting, add PC.6 (*nei guan*)
- with Liver *qi* invading the Stomach, add Liv.13 (*zhang men* -)
- with irritability or depression, add Liv.3 (*tai chong*) or Liv.1 (*da dun* ▲)
- *Ear points*: stomach, liver, sympathetic, subcortex, *shen men*

Clinical notes

- Blood stagnation type indeterminate gnawing hunger may be diagnosed biomedically as stomach cancer, chronic atrophic gastritis and peptic ulcer disease.
- This condition can be difficult to treat successfully, but it may respond with prolonged and persistent treatment. When cancer is the western diagnosis, TCM is best as a support to biomedical treatment.
- For dietary recommendations, see p.886.

饮食积滞

16.6 FOOD STAGNATION

Pathophysiology

- Food stagnation is more likely to present in clinic with acid reflux and heartburn, or epigastric and abdominal distension, than as indeterminate gnawing hunger. However, food stagnation can lead to development of the Heat patterns that are most likely to cause indeterminate gnawing hunger.

Clinical features

- indeterminate gnawing hunger
- epigastric and abdominal distension and/or discomfort and/or borborygmus, all of which are relieved following belching or passing gas, and are worse for overeating and pressure
- acid reflux, heartburn
- foul belching, bad breath
- nausea or vomiting
- foul flatulence
- constipation, difficult or irregular stools, occasional diarrhoea, foul stools

T thick, white or yellow, greasy coat
P wiry and slippery or slippery and rapid

Treatment principle

Relieve food stagnation and harmonise the Stomach

Prescription

BAO HE WAN 保和丸
(*Citrus and Crategus Formula*)

This prescription is best for relatively mild food stagnation, with little or no deficiency, Damp or Heat accumulation.

chao shan zha (dry fried Fructus Crataegi) 炒山楂 18-24g
chao shen qu (dry fried Massa Fermentata) 炒神曲 12-15g
chao lai fu zi (dry fried Semen Raphani Sativi)
炒莱服子 9-12g
ban xia (Rhizoma Pinelliae Ternatae) 半夏 9-12g
fu ling (Sclerotium Poriae Cocos) 茯苓 12-15g
chen pi (Pericarpium Citri Reticulatae) 陈皮 6-9g
lian qiao (Fructus Forsythia Suspensae) 连翘 6-9g

Method: Grind herbs to a powder and form into 9-gram pills with water. The dose is one pill 2-3 times daily. May also be decocted with the quantities as shown. **Shan zha**, **shen qu** and **lai fu zi** improve digestion and alleviate food stagnation; **ban xia** and **chen pi** eliminate Phlegm; **lian qiao** disperses accumulation and clears Heat; **fu ling** strengthens the Spleen. (Source: *Shi Yong Zhong Yi Nei Ke Xue*)

Patent medicines

Bao He Wan 保和丸 (Bao He Wan)
Zi Sheng Wan 资生丸 (Zi Sheng Wan, Zi Sheng Stomachic Pills)
Shen Qu Cha 神曲茶 (Shen Chu Cha)
Liu He Bao He Wan 六合保和丸 (Bo Wo Yuen Medical Pills)
Jian Pi Wan 健脾丸 (Jian Pi Wan)
- with Spleen deficiency

Acupuncture (select from)

Ren.12 (*zhong wan* -) .... *mu* point of the Stomach, clears Heat and alleviates food stagnation
St.21 (*liang men* -) .... promotes the function of the Spleen and Stomach
St.36 (*zu san li* -) .... *he* sea point of the Stomach, regulates and strengthens the Stomach, supplements *qi* and stops vomiting
St.40 (*feng long* -) .... *luo* point of the Stomach, transforms Phlegm and clears stagnant food, Heat and Phlegm from the Stomach
LI.11 (*shou san li* -) .... benefits digestion and regulates gastro-intestinal function
St.44 (*nei ting* -) .... *rong* spring and Water point of the Stomach, clears Heat from the Stomach and alleviates food stagnation

- with nausea, add PC.6 (*nei guan* -)
- with Spleen deficiency, add Sp.6 (*san yin jiao*)
- with abdominal pain, add Sp.8 (*di ji* -) and Sp.4 (*gong sun* -)
- with borborygmus, add Sp.5 (*shang qiu* -)
- with constipation, add St.37 (*shang ju xu* -) and SJ.6 (*zhi gou* -)
- *Ear points*: stomach, spleen

Clinical notes

- This is a disorder of gluttony and dietary irregularity. In isolation it needs no treatment other than a sensible approach to diet and eating habits, however if bad habits persist it can become a more serious problem. Herbs and acupuncture can assist in rapidly dispelling the food stagnation and easing the indeterminate gnawing hunger.
- *See also* Clinical Notes, p.354.

SUMMARY OF GUIDING FORMULAE FOR INDETERMINATE GNAWING HUNGER

Stomach and Liver Heat - *Dan Zhi Xiao Yao San* 丹栀逍遥散

Phlegm Heat - *Wen Dan Tang* 温胆汤

Liver *qi* invading the Stomach - *Chai Hu Shu Gan San* 柴胡疏肝散
- with multiple complications - *Yue Ju Wan* 越鞠丸 plus *Zuo Jin Wan* 左金丸
- with Blood deficiency - *Xiao Yao San* 逍遥散 plus *Zuo Jin Wan* 左金丸

Stomach and Liver *yin* deficiency - *Yi Wei Tang* 益胃汤
- with *qi* stagnation - *Yi Guan Jian* 一贯煎
- following a fever - *Zhi Zi Dou Chi Tang* 栀子豆豉汤

Stomach *qi* deficiency - *Si Jun Zi Tang* 四君子汤
- with Cold - *Wu Zhu Yu Tang* 吴茱萸汤
- with Blood deficiency - *Gui Pi Tang* 归脾汤

Blood stagnation - *Dang Gui Si Ni Tang* 当归四逆汤
- with *qi* stagnation - *Xue Fu Zhu Yu Tang* 血府逐瘀汤

Food stagnation - *Bao He Wan* 保和丸

17. Indigestion (Functional Dyspepsia)

Food stagnation
Liver *qi* invading the Spleen
Mixed Cold, Heat and deficiency
Phlegm Damp
Spleen *qi/yang* deficiency

17 INDIGESTION (Functional Dyspepsia)

xiao hua bu liang 消化不良

Indigestion is a term that patients use to describe vague discomfort and dysfunction of the upper digestive tract, especially the stomach. It is a term we shall use to cover a common gastro-intestinal syndrome comprising a number of symptoms, which tend to occur in combination (Box 17.1). In such cases, identifying one main disease symptom for TCM analysis is often difficult or impractical.

This chapter outlines a way to analyse and treat, as a whole, the collection of symptoms called indigestion. TCM texts describe a number of broad acting prescriptions which embrace all aspects of this multifarious and sometimes difficult to define complaint. In practice, mixed patterns are commonly encountered, typically involving the components of the pathological triad described on p.912, complicated with food stagnation. In the early stages of indigestion, the pattern is likely to be caused by an excess accumulation of some kind; such as food stagnation, Phlegm Damp, Heat, Damp Heat, *qi* stagnation, or, commonly, a mixture. As the condition progresses, the deficiency elements will become more and more prominent.

AETIOLOGY

The fundamental mechanisms that generate indigestion are the same as those that produce abdominal bloating, acid reflux and heartburn, and abdominal pain. Disruption to the harmonious functioning of *qi* mechanism (p.xix) is the main factor.

Diet

Probably the most common cause of indigestion in the Western world is simply overeating, that is, overloading the processing capacity of the digestive system with too much food, or with indigestible foods. This behaviour contributes to food stagnation and the various pathologies that can flow on from that, such as accumulation of Heat, Damp Heat and Phlegm (*see also*

BOX 17.1 SYMPTOMS DEFINING INDIGESTION (may not all be present)

- mild nausea
- acid reflux/heartburn/hyperacidity
- upper abdominal discomfort
- epigastric and abdominal bloating, fullness and distension
- flatulence
- belching

p.3).

The western diet contributes significantly to indigestion. A tendency to overconsume sweet foods, icy cold foods, alcohol and rich, oily, deep fried or junk food is common in many communities, directly introducing elements that encourage Dampness, Damp Heat, Phlegm and Spleen deficiency.

Certain habits and foods are renowned for their ability to contribute to indigestion. Eating at irregular times or eating while under stress and pressure causes malfunction and weakness of the Spleen and Stomach, with consequent accumulation of Dampness and the generation of Damp Heat. This specific feature appears to be more and more common, as people's work schedules become more demanding.

Modern medical practice can be a significant contributor to indigestion, in particular the widespread use of cooling drugs, such as antibiotic therapy, which weakens the Spleen and generates Dampness, and NSAIDs which directly damage the stomach.

BOX 17.2 SOME BIOMEDICAL CAUSES OF INDIGESTION

- gastro-oesophageal reflux
- chronic gastritis
- *Giardia lamblia, Helicobacter pylori*
- hiatus hernia
- functional dyspepsia
- peptic ulcer disease
- hepatitis
- biliary dyskinesia
- gall stones
- pancreatitis
- irritable bowel syndrome
- stress
- neoplasms of the oesophagus, stomach or pancreas
- food allergies
- pregnancy
- depression, anxiety

Drugs
- alcohol and tobacco
- NSAIDs, aspirin
- anticholinergics
- corticosteroids
- digitalis
- narcotics
- theophylline
- tricyclic antidepressants
- tetracycline

Emotion

The Spleen and Stomach are very sensitive to the emotional state, and in many people, the course of a gastro-intestinal complaint mirrors stress levels. There is often a constitutional tendency to 'nervous Stomach' problems, and these problems often run in families. The Liver is the main organ system implicated in this type of disorder. It is the Liver's tendency to 'overcontrol' and bully its controlling (*ke* 克) cycle relations, the Spleen and Stomach, when Liver *qi* is constrained that lies at the root of the problem. Stress, frustration, anger, repressed emotion, bitterness and hatred may all conspire to disrupt the Liver's role in controlling the free distribution of *qi* and Blood to the correct location, at the appropriate time.

The function of the Gallbladder is also important, although often as a secondary effect of Liver dysfunction. The Gallbladder is similarly affected by stagnation originating from the Liver's response to stress, and adequate bile may not be released into the Intestines to aid digestion.

TREATMENT

Treatment of indigestion with TCM is usually quite successful, and often provides solutions where other medical therapies fail. There are a large number of prescriptions and variations that can be used to treat indigestion. The prescriptions presented in this chapter are broad enough in their action to cover most elements of a pattern of indigestion. Other chapters may be consulted for prescriptions with a bias towards a particular aspect of indigestion, such as nausea, distension or acid reflux.

饮食积滞

17.1 FOOD STAGNATION

Pathophysiology

- Food stagnation is one of the commonest causes of indigestion and is essentially due to eating too much food, or eating food that is difficult to digest. The undigested food remains in the Stomach and upper Intestine too long, 'fermenting and rotting', disrupting the *qi* mechanism. Food stagnation may occur as an isolated event, following a specific episode of overconsumption, however it is often chronic. Chronic food stagnation occurs when individuals who habitually overconsume adapt to, and become unconscious of, the symptoms of their overindulgence. The acute symptoms of isolated episodes of indigestion are not registered. Instead, a low level of ongoing gastro-intestinal dysfunction and indigestion is seen. In most cases, the food stagnation is complicated by either Heat and/or Dampness and Phlegm and/or Spleen deficiency, often all three.
- Alleviating food stagnation is the treatment of choice in most cases of acute indigestion due to overindulgence, regardless of the underlying pathology.

Clinical features

- Indigestion characterised by upper abdominal and epigastric distension and fullness, relieved following belching or passing gas; worse for pressure, tight clothes and overeating (or eating certain poorly tolerated foods).
- foul belching, halitosis
- acid reflux, heartburn
- nausea or occasional vomiting of undigested food
- foul flatulence
- tendency to constipation, difficult or irregular stools, occasional diarrhoea, foul stools

T thick, white or yellow, greasy coat
P full, wiry and slippery or slippery and rapid

Treatment principle

Alleviate food stagnation and harmonise the Stomach

BAO HE WAN 保和丸
(*Citrus and Crategus Formula*)

This prescription is best for relatively mild food stagnation, with little or no deficiency, Damp or Heat accumulation.

chao shan zha (dry fried Fructus Crataegi) 炒山楂 18-24g
chao shen qu (dry fried Massa Fermentata) 炒神曲 12-15g

chao lai fu zi (dry fried Semen Raphani Sativi)
炒莱服子 9-12g
ban xia (Rhizoma Pinelliae Ternatae) 半夏 9-12g
fu ling (Sclerotium Poriae Cocos) 茯苓 12-15g
chen pi (Pericarpium Citri Reticulatae) 陈皮 6-9g
lian qiao (Fructus Forsythia Suspensae) 连翘 6-9g

Method: Grind herbs to a powder and form into 9-gram pills with water. The dose is one pill 2-3 times daily. May also be decocted with the quantities as shown. **Shan zha** assists in the digestion of greasy, rich and oily food; **shen qu** alleviates the effects of excessive alcohol consumption; **lai fu zi** assists in the digestion of starch and carbohydrates; **ban xia** and **chen pi** regulate *qi* and correct the *qi* mechanism; **fu ling** strengthens the Spleen and leaches out Dampness; **lian qiao** dissipates accumulation and clears Heat. (Source: *Shi Yong Zhong Yi Nei Ke Xue*)

Modifications

- With severe distension and discomfort, add **zhi shi** (Fructus Immaturus Citri Aurantii) 枳实 9-12g and **hou po** (Cortex Magnoliae Officinalis) 厚朴 9-12g.
- In cases of relatively severe food stagnation, with a firm and tender epigastrium, add **san leng** (Rhizoma Sparganii Stoloniferi) 三棱 9-12g and **e zhu** (Rhizoma Curcumae Ezhu) 莪术 9-12g.
- With lots of gas (belching and flatulence) add **sha ren** (Fructus Amomi) 砂仁 6-9g and **mu xiang** (Radix Aucklandiae Lappae) 木香 6-9g.
- With persistent belching, add **dai zhe shi** (Haematitum) 代赭石 15g and **shi di** (Calyx Diospyri Kaki) 柿蒂 9-12g.
- With Phlegm Damp, combine with **PING WEI SAN** (*Magnolia and Ginger Formula* 平胃散, p.153).
- With acid reflux or heartburn, add **huang lian** (Rhizoma Coptidis) 黄连 3-6g and **wu zhu yu** (Fructus Evodiae Rutaecarpae) 吴茱萸 1-2g.
- With some Heat or Damp Heat (irritability, red tongue tip and sides, rapid pulse), add **shan zhi zi** (Fructus Gardeniae Jasminoides) 山栀子 9-12g and **huang lian** (Rhizoma Coptidis) 黄连 3-6g.
- With Cold, add **gan jiang** (Rhizoma Zingiberis Officinalis) 干姜 6-9g.
- With mild Spleen deficiency, add **bai zhu** (Rhizoma Atractylodes Macrocephalae) 白术 12-15g.
- With a degree of *qi* stagnation, add **xiang fu** (Rhizoma Cyperi Rotundi) 香附 9-12g.
- With constipation or difficult stools, add **da huang** (Radix et Rhizoma Rhei) 大黄 6-9g and **bing lang** (Semen Arecae Catechu) 槟榔 9-12g.
- If the indigestion is associated with a protein and oil rich meat diet, increase the dose of **shan zha**.
- If indigestion is associated with starchy foods, such as noodles and grains, increase the dose of **chao lai fu zi**.

- With severe nausea or vomiting, add **zhu ru** (Caulis Bambusae in Taeniis) 竹茹 12-15g and **sheng jiang** (Rhizoma Zingiberis Officinalis Recens) 生姜 9-12g.

Variations and additional prescriptions

With Damp Heat or Phlegm Heat

- Chronic food stagnation type indigestion is often complicated by Heat, Damp Heat or Phlegm Heat, generated in much the same way as rotting compost manufactures heat. The features are relatively severe indigestion, epigastric and abdominal distension and pain (worse for pressure), tendency towards constipation or difficult stools, a thick, greasy, yellow tongue coat and a deep, strong pulse. The aim of treatment is to guide stagnation downward, clear Heat and dispel Damp with **ZHI SHI DAO ZHI WAN** (*Immature Bitter Orange Pill to Guide out Stagnation* 枳实导滞丸, p.181).

With Spleen deficiency

- Chronic indigestion from food stagnation is frequently accompanied by Spleen *qi* deficiency. An elegant and effective approach is to strengthen the Spleen, dry Damp, and correct the *qi* mechanism with the simple **ZHI ZHU WAN** (*Immature Bitter Orange and Atractylodes Macrocephala Pill* 枳术丸).

bai zhu (Rhizoma Atractylodes Macrocephalae)
白术 .... 60 (12-18)g
zhi shi (Fructus Immaturus Citri Aurantii) 枳实 .... 30(6-9)g

Method: Grind the herbs to a fine powder and form into 9-gram pills with water. The dose is one pill 2-3 times daily. May also be decocted with the quantities shown in brackets. **Bai zhu** strengthens the Spleen, encourages correct ascent of Spleen *qi* and dries Dampness; **zhi shi** directs *qi* downwards and alleviates focal accumulation in the epigastrium; together these herbs neatly balance each other, encouraging the correct ascent and descent of middle *jiao qi*, thus facilitating the flow of *qi* through the middle *jiao*.

Patent medicines

Bao He Wan 保和丸 (Bao He Wan)
Mu Xiang Shun Qi Wan 木香顺气丸 (Mu Xiang Shun Qi Wan)
- with sluggish stools
Zi Sheng Wan 资生丸 (Zi Sheng Wan, Zi Sheng Stomachic Pills)
Jian Pi Wan 健脾丸 (Jian Pi Wan)
- with Spleen deficiency
Xiang Sha Yang Wei Wan 香砂养胃丸 (Xiang Sha Yang Wei Wan, Hsiang Sha Yang Wei Wan)
- with *qi* stagnation
Wei Te Ling 胃特灵 (Wei Te Ling Stomach Sedative)

- an antacid formula that can be combined with the appropriate constitutional formula for symptomatic relief of reflux and heartburn

Xiang Lian Wan 香蓮丸 (Xiang Lian Wan)

- this patent medicine can be combined with the appropriate constitutional formula above for symptomatic relief of heartburn

Acupuncture (select from)

Ren.12 (*zhong wan* -) .... *mu* point of the Stomach, reducing method clears Heat and alleviates stagnation

St.25 (*tian shu* -) .... *mu* point of the Large Intestine, regulates Intestinal function and encourages the downward movement of *qi*

Ren.6 (*qi hai* -) .... regulates *qi* and alleviates distension

St.36 (*zu san li* -) .... *he* sea point of the Stomach, regulates and strengthens the Stomach, stops vomiting

St.40 (*feng long* -) .... *luo* point of the Stomach, transforms Phlegm and clears stagnant food, Heatand Phlegm from the Stomach

LI.10 (*shou san li* -) .... benefits digestion and regulates gastro-intestinal function

St.44 (*nei ting* -) .... *rong* spring and Water point of the Stomach, clears Heat from the Stomach and alleviates food stagnation

- with nausea, add PC.6 (*nei guan* -)
- with Spleen deficiency, add Sp.6 (*san yin jiao*)
- with abdominal pain, add Sp.8 (*di ji* -) and Sp.4 (*gong sun* -)
- with borborygmus, add Sp.5 (*shang qiu* -)
- with constipation, add St.37 (*shang ju xu* -) and SJ.6 (*zhi gou* -)
- *Ear points*: stomach, spleen, sympathetic

Clinical notes

- Regulating the diet is the most important element in correcting indigestion due to food stagnation. The use of herbs and acupuncture will relieve symptoms in the meantime.
- Sipping small amounts of certain teas, (in particular green tea), while eating helps assist digestion, especially of fats, and reduces the risk of food stagnation. European cultures use table wine in much the same way, hence 'a little wine for thy stomach's sake'. Similarly, 'bitters', combinations of bitter herbs and alcohol, are a common accompaniment to food, either as a digestive aid following a meal, or as an aperitive. The bitterness of the herbs assists the descent of Stomach *qi* and dries Damp.

肝气犯胃

17.2 LIVER QI INVADING THE STOMACH

Pathophysiology

- Liver invading the Stomach is a common cause of both acute and chronic indigestion. Constrained Liver *qi* invades the Stomach via the controlling (*ke*) cycle and disrupts the *qi* mechanism, causing Stomach *qi* to accumulate and rise.
- Because this is such a common cause and tends to be a long term problem, it is almost invariably complicated by other patterns. The common complications are food stagnation, stagnant Heat, Spleen deficiency and *yin* deficiency.

Clinical features

- recurrent indigestion which is clearly related to the emotional state and stress levels of the patient
- epigastric fullness and discomfort; 'knot' in the stomach when upset
- hypochondriac discomfort, ache or tightness
- belching, frequent sighing
- borborygmus, flatulence
- loss of appetite
- acid reflux, heartburn
- mild or vague nausea, often worse in the morning
- irritability, moodiness, depression
- tendency to loose stools, or alternating constipation and diarrhoea

T thin, white coat, or thicker and greasy coat; may be red edges
P wiry, and/or slippery

Treatment principle

Regulate *qi*, harmonise the Liver and Stomach
Direct Stomach *qi* downwards, alleviate food stagnation
Strengthen the Spleen and Stomach

Prescription

MU XIANG SHUN QI WAN 木香顺气丸
(*Saussurea Pill to Order the Qi*)

This is an excellent prescription for Liver *qi* stagnation complicated with food stagnation.

xiang fu (Rhizoma Cyperi Rotundi) 香附 9-12g
wu yao (Radix Linderae Strychnifoliae) 乌药 6-9g
mu xiang (Radix Aucklandiae Lappae) 木香 6-9g
zhi ke (Fructus Citri Aurantii) 枳壳 6-9g
chen pi (Pericarpium Citri Reticulatae) 陈皮 6-9g

chao shen qu (dry fried Massa Fermentata) 炒神曲 12-15g
chao shan zha (dry fried Fructus Crataegi) 炒山楂 12-15g
chao mai ya (dry fried Fructus Hordei Vulgaris Germinatus) 炒麦芽 15-30g
lai fu zi (Semen Raphani Sativi) 莱服子 9-12g
fu ling (Sclerotium Poria Cocos) 茯苓 12-15g
bing lang (Semen Arecae Catechu) 槟榔 9-12g
qing pi (Pericarpium Citri Reticulatae Viride) 青皮 6-9g
gan cao (Radix Glycyrrhizae Uralensis) 甘草 3-6g

Method: Grind the herbs to a fine powder and form into 6-gram pills with water. The dose is one pill 2-3 times daily. May also be decocted with quantities as shown. **Mu xiang**, **xiang fu** and **wu yao** regulate *qi* and alleviate distension and pain; **zhi ke**, **qing pi** and **bing lang** break up stagnant *qi* and direct *qi* downwards; **chen pi** transforms Phlegm and dries Damp, regulates middle *jiao qi* and corrects the *qi* mechanism; **chao shen qu**, **chao shan zha**, **chao mai ya** and **lai fu zi** improve digestion and alleviate food stagnation; **fu ling** strengthens the Spleen and leaches out Damp; **gan cao** harmonises the Stomach. (Source: *Shi Yong Fang Ji Xue*)

Variations and additional prescriptions

Qi stagnation in the Spleen and Stomach

- If the focus of the pathology is in the epigastrium, with a smaller component of Liver *qi* stagnation, then a more general *qi* moving approach may be useful. The best prescription for this is **YUE JU WAN** (*Escape Restraint Pill* 越鞠丸, p.17), appropriately modified. This is a important and effective prescription for indigestion with numerous complicating features, as it was designed with the 'six stagnations' (food, Damp, Phlegm, Fire, *qi*, Blood) in mind, any and all of which can disrupt and obstruct the *qi* mechanism.

With Phlegm

- *Qi* stagnation is frequently complicated by Phlegm, because the damage inflicted by the Liver on the middle *jiao* weakens digestion, thus creating the potential for accumulation of Dampness. In addition, movement of fluids is retarded, encouraging accumulation and congealing into Phlegm. The aim of treatment is to regulate Liver *qi*, transform Phlegm and stimulate digestion with **JIE GAN JIAN** (*Loosen the Liver Decoction* 解肝煎).

chai hu (Radix Bupleuri) 柴胡 9-12g
zhi shi (Fructus Immaturus Citri Aurantii) 枳实 9-12g
chen pi (Pericarpium Citri Reticulatae) 陈皮 6-9g
ban xia (Rhizoma Pinelliae Ternatae) 半夏 9-12g
hou po (Cortex Magnoliae Officinalis) 厚朴 12-15g
fu ling (Sclerotium Poria Cocos) 茯苓 12-15g

zi su ye (Folium Perillae Frutescentis) 紫苏叶 9-12g
sha ren (Fructus Amomi) 砂仁 6-9g
bai shao (Radix Paeoniae Lactiflora) 白芍 12-18g
sheng jiang (Rhizoma Zingiberis Officinalis Recens) 生姜 9-12g

Method: Decoction. **Sha ren** is added a few minutes before the end of cooking (*hou xia* 后下). **Chai hu** and **bai shao** soften the Liver and regulate Liver *qi*; **zhi shi** and **hou po** direct *qi* downwards; **ban xia** and **chen pi** transform Phlegm Damp and harmonise the Stomach; **fu ling** strengthens the Spleen and leaches out Dampness; **zi su ye** and **sha ren** regulate *qi* and harmonise the Stomach; **sheng jiang** warms and harmonises the Stomach. (Source: *Shi Yong Zhong Yi Nei Ke Xue*)

With stagnant Heat

- Chronic Liver *qi* stagnation is frequently complicated by stagnant Heat. The Heat component will tend to aggravate the rising of Stomach *qi* and make the patient more irritable. The aim of treatment is to move and regulate Liver *qi* and clear stagnant Heat with **DAN ZHI XIAO YAO SAN** (*Bupleurum and Paeonia Formula* 丹栀逍遥散, p.113).

With qi deficiency

- If *qi* stagnation is complicated by *qi* deficiency, strong *qi* regulating and dispersing herbs may aggravate the deficiency. A simple solution is to use a gentle combined regulating and supplementing prescription such as **SI MO TANG** (*Four Milled-Herb Decoction* 四磨汤).

dang shen (Radix Codonopsis Pilosulae) 党参 15-24g
bing lang (Semen Arecae Catechu) 槟榔 9-12g
wu yao (Radix Linderae Strychnifoliae) 乌药 9-12g
chen xiang (Lignum Aquilariae) 沉香 3-6g

Method: Grind the herbs to a fine powder and take as a draft in boiled water. May also be decocted. **Dang shen** strengthens the Spleen and supplements *qi*; **bing lang** and **chen xiang** direct *qi* downwards and promote movement of *qi*; **wu yao** regulates *qi* and stops pain.

Patent medicines

Mu Xiang Shun Qi Wan 木香顺气丸 (Mu Xiang Shun Qi Wan) - with sluggish stools
Chai Hu Shu Gan Wan 柴胡疏肝丸 (Chai Hu Shu Gan Wan)
Xiao Yao Wan 逍遥丸 (Xiao Yao Wan, Hsiao Yao Wan, Bupleurum Sedative Pills) - especially good for women
Jia Wei Xiao Yao Wan 加味逍遥丸 (Jia Wei Xiao Yao Wan, Dan Zhi Xiao Yao Wan) - with stagnant Heat
Chen Xiang Hua Qi Wan 沉香化气丸 (Chen Xiang Hua Qi Wan) - with constipation

Acupuncture (select from)

Ren.12 (*zhong wan* -) .... *mu* point of the Stomach, clears pathogens, directs Stomach *qi* downwards and harmonises the Stomach
Liv.13 (*zhang men*) .... *mu* point of the Spleen, regulates the Liver and Spleen
St.25 (*tian shu* -) .... *mu* point of the Large Intestine, regulates Intestinal function and encourages the downward movement of *qi*
Ren.6 (*qi hai* -) .... regulates *qi* and alleviates distension
PC.6 (*nei guan* -) .... *luo* point of the Pericardium, master point of *yin wei mai*, regulates the middle *jiao* and regulates Liver *qi*

Liv.3 (*tai chong* -) .... together these points regulate Liver *qi*, pacify
GB.34 (*yang ling quan*) the Liver and harmonise the Liver and Stomach

- in most cases, points to calm the *shen* should be added: select one or two points from *yin tang* (M-HN-3), Du.19 (*hou ding*), Du. 24 (*shen ting*)
- with Blood or *yin* deficiency, add Sp.6 (*san yin jiao* +), St.36 (*zu san li* -), Bl.18 (*gan shu* +) and Bl.23 (*shen shu* +)
- with Phlegm or plum stone throat, add PC.5 (*jian shi* -), St.40 (*feng long* -) and Sp.3 (*tai bai*)
- with fat intolerance, pale or pasty stools and right hypochondriac pain or distension, add GB.24 (*ri yue*), GB.40 (*qiu xu* -) and *dan nang xue* (M-LE-23)
- *Ear points*: *shen men*, liver, stomach, spleen, sympathetic

Clinical notes

- The long term solution to Liver invading the Stomach is multifaceted. Herbs and acupuncture are effective, but should be combined with appropriate stress reduction techniques. Long courses of acupuncture are especially good, as the necessary physiological re-learning required to alter the unconscious responses of the individual to the stress triggers, takes time. Stress management, yoga, regular aerobic exercise, meditation and avoidance of triggers are all important factors to consider. Avoidance of tension during meals (for example, not during business meetings or in the office) is important.
- For dietary recommendations, see p.878.

热寒虚都杂

17.3 MIXED COLD, HEAT AND DEFICIENCY IN THE STOMACH AND INTESTINES

Pathophysiology

- This is a common pattern of indigestion and closely reflects the complex pathology many patients in the Western world develop, hence its inclusion here as a separate pattern. Traditionally, the symptoms were thought to be the result of inappropriate treatment for a *shao yang* pathogen–purging rather than harmonising, which weakened the middle *jiao* sufficiently to enable the pathogen to penetrate deeper, and lodge in the Stomach and Intestines.
- Nowadays, it reflects a complex mixture of aetiological features that weaken digestion, disrupt the *qi* mechanism, and enable a mixture of Heat and Cold pathogens to accumulate in the Stomach and Intestines. A poor diet, eating food on the run and a stressful 'on the go' lifestyle, combine to make this a common presentation in Western societies.

Clinical features

- indigestion. characterised by epigastric distension (traditionally the key feature of this pattern), that feels soft and non-tender when palpated
- mild morning nausea, dry retching or vomiting, often first thing in the morning
- loss of appetite
- heartburn
- borborygmus
- tendency to diarrhoea or loose stools; possibly constipation

T thin, greasy, yellow or mixed white and yellow coat
P soft, slippery, slightly wiry and possibly rapid

Treatment principle

Harmonise the Stomach, clear Heat and supplement *qi*
Redirect *qi* downwards and correct the *qi* mechanism

Prescription

BAN XIA XIE XIN TANG 半夏泻心汤
(*Pinellia Combination*)

ban xia (Rhizoma Pinelliae Ternatae) 半夏 6-12g
gan jiang (Rhizoma Zingiberis Officinalis) 干姜 6-9g
huang qin (Radix Scutellariae Baicalensis) 黄芩 6-9g
huang lian (Rhizoma Coptidis) 黄连 3-6g
dang shen (Radix Codonopsis Pilosulae) 党参 12-15g
zhi gan cao (honey fried Radix Glycyrrhizae Uralensis)
炙甘草 3-6g

da zao (Fructus Zizyphi Jujubae) 大枣 4pce

Method: Decoction. **Ban xia** transforms Phlegm, dries Damp, directs rising Stomach *qi* downwards and stops nausea and vomiting; **gan jiang**, pungent and hot, warms Spleen and Stomach *yang* and dispels Cold; **huang qin** and **huang lian**, bitter and cold, clear Heat; **dang shen** and **da zao** strengthen the Spleen, supplement *qi*, and prevent the dispersing action of the principal herbs from injuring the Spleen and Stomach *qi* and *yin*; **zhi gan cao** strengthens the Spleen and harmonises the Stomach.

Modifications

- With significant *qi* stagnation, add **chai hu** (Radix Bupleuri) 柴胡 6-9g and **bai shao** (Radix Paeoniae Lactiflora) 白芍 12-15g.
- With Damp Heat, increase the dose of **huang qin** (Radix Scutellariae Baicalensis) 黄芩 to 12g.
- With significant Spleen deficiency, add **chao bai zhu** (dry fried Rhizoma Atractylodes Macrocephalae) 炒白术 9-12g and increase the dose of **zhi gan cao** to 9g.
- With pathological water in the epigastrium (a splash heard during palpation), dry retching and loud borborygmus, add **sheng jiang** (Rhizoma Zingiberis Officinalis Recens) 生姜9-12g.
- With food stagnation, add **zhi shi** (Fructus Immaturus Citri Aurantii) 枳实 9-12g, **chao shan zha** (dry fried Fructus Crataegi) 炒山楂 15g and **chao shen qu** (dry fried Massa Fermentata) 炒神曲 15g.

Patent medicines

Chen Xiang Hua Qi Wan 沉香化气丸 (Chen Xiang Hua Qi Wan)

Acupuncture (select from)

Ren.12 (*zhong wan* -) .... *mu* point of the Stomach, clears pathogens, regulates and harmonises the Stomach

Liv.13 (*zhang men*) .... *mu* point of the Spleen, regulates the Liver and Spleen, strengthens the Spleen and supplements *qi*

St.25 (*tian shu* -) .... *mu* point of the Large Intestine, regulates Intestinal function, directs Stomach *qi* downward and alleviates distension

Ren.6 (*qi hai* -) .... regulates *qi* and alleviates distension

St.36 (*zu san li* -) .... *he* sea point of the Stomach, regulates and strengthens the Spleen and Stomach and supplements *qi*

St.37 (*shan ju xu* -) .... lower *he* point of the Large Intestine, eliminates stagnation and accumulation from the Stomach and Intestines and clears Damp Heat

PC.6 (*nei guan* -) .... *luo* point of the Pericardium, master point of *yin wei mai*, regulates the middle *jiao* and regulates Liver *qi*

LI.11 (*qu chi* -) .... *he* sea point of the Large Intestine, clears Damp Heat from *yang ming*

- with lots of Heat in the Stomach, add St.44 (*nei ting* -) and LI.4 (*he gu* -)
- with constipation or dry stools, add SJ.6 (*zhi gou* -)
- with Dampness, add Sp.9 (*yin ling quan* -) and Sp.6 (*san yin jiao*)
- with Phlegm or plum stone throat, add PC.5 (*jian shi* -), St.40 (*feng long* -) and Sp.3 (*tai bai*)
- with fat intolerance, pale or pasty stools and right hypochondriac pain or distension, add GB.24 (*ri yue*), GB.40 (*qiu xu* -) and *dan nang xue* (M-LE-23)
- with *shao yang* symptoms, add GB.39 (*xuan zhong* -), SJ.5 (*wai guan* -) and GB.34 (*yang ling quan* -)
- *Ear points*: spleen, stomach, liver, large intestine, small intestine, sympathetic

Clinical notes

- This is a common pattern of chronic indigestion, and will be diagnosed biomedically as functional dyspepsia, peptic ulcer disease, gastric hyperacidity or gastritis.
- The recommended prescription can be used for several months before requiring review. The patient should experience improvement within 2-3 weeks.
- For dietary recommendations, see pp.870, 882.

痰湿阻凝

17.4 PHLEGM DAMP

Pathophysiology

- Phlegm Damp accumulation effectively clogs the *qi* mechanism and blocks the ascent of Spleen *qi* and the descent of Stomach *qi*.
- In practice, Phlegm Damp patterns are frequently complicated by Spleen *qi* deficiency. Patients with Phlegm Damp type indigestion may occasionally have a constitutional component, in which case there usually will be a life long history of gastric disorders.

Clinical features

- indigestion characterised by abdominal and epigastric distension, fullness and discomfort, belching, acid reflux, nausea, poor appetite and loss of taste
- fatigue, lethargy, sluggishness, heaviness in the body and limbs, frequent desire to sleep, after which the patient often feels worse or more sluggish
- poor concentration, heavy or foggy-headedness
- copious salivation
- dizziness, palpitations or headaches that can be triggered by strong smells
- stuffiness in the chest
- may be chronic mucus production from the sinuses and lungs
- greasy skin, musty body odour
- tendency to obesity, pear shape

T thick, greasy, white coat, possible swollen or flabby tongue body
P slippery, wiry, moderate

Treatment principle

Dry Dampness and transform Phlegm
Promote the correct movement of *qi*, harmonise the Stomach

Prescription

PING CHEN TANG 平陈汤
(*Calm the Stomach plus Citrus and Pinellia Decoction*)

This prescription combines **PING WEI SAN** and **ER CHEN TANG** to dry Dampness and transform Phlegm. When the Phlegm Damp is resolving, the emphasis of treatment should shift to strengthening the Spleen to prevent continued creation of Damp and Phlegm. *See* also Spleen deficiency, p.647.

cang zhu (Rhizoma Atractylodis) 苍术 12-15g
hou po (Cortex Magnoliae Officinalis) 厚朴 9-12g
ban xia (Rhizoma Pinelliae Ternatae) 半夏 9-12g

chen pi (Pericarpium Citri Reticulatae) 陈皮 9-12g
fu ling (Sclerotium Poria Cocos) 茯苓 12-15g
gan cao (Radix Glycyrrhizae Uralensis) 甘草 3-6g

Method: Decoction. **Cang zhu** powerfully parches and dries Damp, liberating the Spleen, thus allowing it to function correctly; **hou po** regulates *qi*, transforms Damp and directs *qi* downward; **ban xia** and **chen pi** transform Phlegm and dry Damp, regulate middle *jiao qi* and correct the *qi* mechanism; **fu ling** strengthens the Spleen and leaches out Damp; **gan cao** strengthens the Spleen and harmonises the Stomach.

Modifications

- With food stagnation and constipation, add **lai fu zi** (Semen Raphani Sativi) 莱服子 9-12g, **da fu pi** (Pericarpium Arecae Catechu) 大腹皮 9-12g, **zhi shi** (Fructus Immaturus Citri Aurantii) 枳实 9-12g, **chao mai ya** (dry fried Fructus Hordei Vulgaris Germinantus) 炒麦芽 15-30g and **chao gu ya** (dry fried Fructus Oryzae Sativae Germinatus) 炒谷芽 15-30g.
- With severe Phlegm Damp (nausea, thick, greasy tongue coat, heaviness, distension etc.) add **huo xiang** (Herba Agastaches seu Pogostemi) 藿香 12-15g and **pei lan** (Herba Eupatorii Fortunei) 佩兰 9-12g.
- With foggy-headedness and poor concentration, add **yuan zhi** (Radix Polygalae Tenuifoliae) 远志 6-9g and **shi chang pu** (Rhizoma Acori Graminei) 石菖蒲 6-9g.
- If prolonged stagnation of Dampness generates a degree of Heat, giving rise to a greasy, yellow tongue coat, yellow urine, irritability and a rapid pulse, add **huang qin** (Radix Scutellariae Baicalensis) 黄芩 6-9g, **shan zhi zi** (Fructus Gardeniae Jasminoides) 山栀子 6-9g, **zhu ru** (Caulis Bambusae in Taeniis) 竹茹 9-12g and **yi ren** (Semen Coicis Lachryma-jobi) 苡仁 15-24g.
- With Cold, add **rou gui** (Cortex Cinnamomi Cassiae) 肉桂 3g and **gan jiang** (Rhizoma Zingiberis Officinalis) 干姜 6-9g.

Patent medicines

Ping Wei San 平胃散 (Ping Wei San, Tabellae Pingwei)
Xiang Sha Liu Jun Zi Wan 香砂六君子丸 (Xiang Sha Liu Jun Wan, Aplotaxis-Ammomum Pills, Six Gentlemen Tea Pills)
- with Spleen deficiency
Xiang Sha Yang Wei Wan 香砂养胃丸 (Xiang Sha Yang Wei Wan, Hsiang Sha Yang Wei Wan) - with *qi* and Damp stagnation

Acupuncture (select from)

Ren.12 (*zhong wan* -) .... *mu* point of the Stomach, clears pathogens, directs Stomach *qi* downwards and harmonises the Stomach

St.25 (*tian shu* -) .... *mu* point of the Large Intestine, regulates Intestinal function and encourages the downward movement of *qi*

Sp.15 (*da heng*) .... strengthens the Spleen and resolves Damp

Liv.13 (*zhang men*) .... *mu* point of the Spleen, harmonises the Liver and Spleen, strengthens the Spleen and supplements *qi*

St.40 (*feng long* -) .... *luo* point of the Stomach, transforms Phlegm and clears stagnant food, Heatand Phlegm from the Stomach

Sp.3 (*tai bai*) ....*yuan*, *shu* stream and Earth point of the Spleen, strengthens the Spleen and supplements *qi* to transform Dampness

Sp.5 (*shang qiu* -)...............*jing* river point of the Spleen, transforms Dampness

- with Spleen deficiency, add St.36 (*zu san li* -)
- with fluid retention and oedema, add St.28 (*shui dao* -), Sp.9 (*yin ling quan* -) and Sp.6 (*san yin jiao*)
- with sluggish stools or constipation, add SJ.6 (*zhi gou* -), St.37 (*shang ju xu* -) and St.41 (*jie xi* -)
- with Liver *qi* stagnation, add Liv.3 (*tai chong*) and PC.6 (*nei guan*)
- with plum stone throat, add PC.5 (*jian shi* -)
- with foggy-headedness, add GB.20 (*feng chi*) and Bl.62 (*shen mai*)
- with Wind Phlegm, add GB.40 (*qiu xu* -), St.8 (*tou wei*) and St.41 (*jie xi* -)
- with Cold Phlegm, apply moxa cones to Bl.20 (*pi shu* ▲) and Bl.21 (*wei shu* ▲)
- with muscle aches and heaviness, add Sp.21 (*da bao*)
- with somnolence, add Kid.6 (*zhao hai*) and Bl.62 (*shen mai*)
- *Ear points*: spleen, stomach, sympathetic

Clinical notes

- Phlegm Damp type indigestion responds well to correct treatment as long as the dietary sources are identified and eliminated or substantially reduced. When there is a constitutional tendency to Phlegm Damp, treatment, while still effective for alleviating the symptoms, will need to be ongoing for long term relief. Prolonged herbal therapy is usually required for resolving Phlegm Damp.
- For dietary recommendations, see p.880.

脾气阳虚

17.5 SPLEEN QI/YANG DEFICIENCY

Pathophysiology

- Spleen deficiency is a common cause of chronic indigestion, as the Spleen has such a critical role to play in transforming food into *qi*. This is an energy intensive process, and even mild Spleen weakness can lead to the typical symptoms of indigestion. Spleen deficiency is often at the basis of the other pathologies in this chapter. For example, poor processing and breakdown of food leads to accumulation of undigested materials, and thus food stagnation and Phlegm Damp; a weak Spleen can 'invite' the unwanted attentions of an otherwise passive Liver; deficiency plus accumulation can generate Heat.

Clinical features

- chronic indigestion characterised by loss of appetite, early satiety, loss of sense of taste, epigastric and/or abdominal distension which is worse with eating (especially raw food)
- waxy, pale or lustreless complexion
- shortness of breath, reluctance to speak, low voice
- tiredness, lethargy and fatigue, tired weak limbs
- loose stools
- puffiness around the eyes or in the fingers; quick weight fluctuations
- **With Cold**: cold intolerance, cold extremities, undigested food in the stools, dull abdominal pain

T pale with a white coat; or pale and swollen with tooth marks

P weak, thready or deficient, or big and weak (especially right middle position)

Treatment principle

Supplement, strengthen and warm the Spleen

Regulate *qi* and harmonise the Stomach

Prescription

XIANG SHA LIU JUN ZI TANG 香砂六君子汤
(*Saussurea and Cardamon Combination*)

dang shen (Radix Codonopsis Pilosulae) 党参 15-24g
chao bai zhu (dry fried Rhizoma Atractylodis Macrocephalae) 炒白术 12-15g
fu ling (Sclerotium Poriae Cocos) 茯苓 12-15g
ban xia (Rhizoma Pinelliae Ternatae) 半夏 9-12g
chen pi (Pericarpium Citri Reticulatae) 陈皮 6-9g
sha ren (Fructus Amomi) 砂仁 6-9g
mu xiang (Radix Aucklandiae Lappae) 木香 6-9g

zhi gan cao (honey fried Radix Glycyrrhizae Uralensis)
炙甘草 3-6g

Method: Decoction. **Sha ren** is added towards the end of cooking (*hou xia* 后下). **Dang shen** and **zhi gan cao** supplement *qi* and strengthen the Spleen; **chao bai zhu** strengthens the Spleen and dries Dampness; **fu ling** strengthens the Spleen and leaches out Dampness through the urine; **ban xia** transforms Phlegm, dries Damp, regulates *qi* and directs rising Stomach *qi* downwards; **chen pi** transforms Phlegm and dries Damp, regulates middle *jiao qi* and corrects the *qi* mechanism; **sha ren** and **mu xiang** regulate and mobilise *qi* in the middle *jiao*, alleviate distension and stimulate the appetite.

Modifications

- With severe Dampness (thick, greasy tongue coat, heaviness, distension etc.), add **cang zhu** (Rhizoma Atractylodis) 苍术 12-15g and **hou po** (Cortex Magnoliae Officinalis) 厚朴 9-12g.
- With heartburn, add **wu zhu yu** (Fructus Evodiae Rutaecarpae) 吴茱萸 3-6g.
- With poor muscle tone (and possible hiatus hernia) or diarrhoea, add **huang qi** (Radix Astragali Membranacei) 黄芪 18-30g.
- With food stagnation add **chao mai ya** (dry fried Fructus Hordei Vulgaris Germinantus) 炒麦芽 15-30g and **chao gu ya** (dry fried Fructus Oryzae Sativae Germinatus) 炒谷芽 15-30g.
- With Cold in the Stomach, add **gan jiang** (Rhizoma Zingiberis Officinalis) 干姜 6-12g.
- With fluid retention, puffy eyes or oedema, increase the dose of **fu ling** (Sclerotium Poriae Cocos) 茯苓 to 18g, and add **ze xie** (Rhizoma Alismatis Orientalis) 泽泻 9-12g and **che qian zi** (Semen Plantaginis) 车前子 9-12g, or combine with **WU LING SAN** (*Hoelen Five Formula* 五苓散, p.910).
- With Liver *qi* stagnation, combine with **XIAO YAO SAN** (*Bupleurum and Dang Gui Formula* 逍遥散, p.159) or consider **SI MO TANG** (*Four Milled-Herb Decoction* 四磨汤, p.639) .
- With loss of appetite, add **sha ren** (Fructus Amomi) 砂仁 6-9g and **chao shen qu** (dry fried Massa Fermentata) 炒神曲 15g.
- With suspected parasites, add a small dose of **da huang** (Radix et Rhizoma Rhei) 大黄 1-3g, **bai zhi** (Radix Angelicae Dahuricae) 白芷 9-12g, **zi su ye** (Folium Perillae Frutescentis) 紫苏叶 9-12g and **bo he** (Herba Mentha Haplocalycis) 薄荷 6g.
- With sluggish bowel movements, add **rou cong rong** (Herba Cistanches Deserticolae) 肉苁蓉 18-24g.

Acupuncture (select from)

Ren.12 (*zhong wan* +▲) .. *mu* point of the Stomach, strengthens the Spleen and Stomach

St.36 (*zu san li* +▲) .... *he* sea point of the Stomach, powerfully strengthens the Spleen and Stomach, supplements *qi*, regulates and corrects the *qi* mechanism

Sp.3 (*tai bai*) .... *yuan*, *shu* stream and Earth point of the Spleen, strengthens the Spleen and supplements *qi* to transforms Dampness

Sp.6 (*san yin jiao*) .... strengthens the Spleen, regulates Liver *qi* and benefits the Kidneys

Bl.20 (*pi shu* +▲) .... *shu* point of the Spleen, strengthens the Spleen and supplements *qi*

Bl.21 (*wei shu* +▲) .... *shu* point of the Stomach, strengthens the Stomach and regulates the *qi* mechanism

- with fluid retention and oedema, add St.28 (*shui dao* -) and Sp.9 (*yin ling quan* -)
- with Liver *qi* stagnation, add Liv.3 (*tai chong*) and PC.6 (*nei guan*)
- *Ear points*: spleen, stomach, adrenal, sympathetic

Patent medicines

Xiang Sha Liu Jun Zi Wan 香砂六君子丸 (Xiang Sha Liu Jun Wan, Aplotaxis-Ammomum Pills, Six Gentlemen Tea Pills)

Xiang Sha Yang Wei Wan 香砂养胃丸 (Xiang Sha Yang Wei Wan, Hsiang Sha Yang Wei Wan)
- with *qi* stagnation

Jian Pi Wan 健脾丸 (Jian Pi Wan)
- with food stagnation

Li Zhong Wan 理中丸 (Li Zhong Wan)
- Spleen *yang* deficiency

Fu Zi Li Zhong Wan 附子理中丸 (Carmichaeli Tea Pills, Fu Tzu Li Chung Wan, Li Chung Yuen Medical Pills)
- severe Cold

Clinical notes

- Spleen deficiency patterns may be diagnosed biomedically as functional dyspepsia, chronic gastritis or peptic ulcer disease.
- Spleen *qi* and *yang* deficiency patterns respond well to correct treatment, and the patient will often feel better quite quickly. For lasting results however, treatment usually needs to persist for at least a few months, depending on the length and severity of the initial condition.
- For dietary recommendations, see p.870-873.

SUMMARY OF GUIDING FORMULAE FOR INDIGESTION

Food stagnation - *Bao He Wan* 保和丸
- with Damp Heat - *Zhi Shi Dao Zhi Wan* 枳实导滞丸
- with Spleen deficiency - *Zhi Zhu Wan* 枳术丸

Liver *qi* invading the Stomach - *Mu Xiang Shun Qi Wan* 木香顺气丸
- with primary Stomach *qi* stagnation - *Yue Ju Wan* 越鞠丸
- with Phlegm - *Jie Gan Jian* 解肝煎
- with stagnant Heat - *Dan Zhi Xiao Yao San* 丹栀逍遥散
- with *qi* deficiency - *Si Mo Yin* 四磨饮

Phlegm Damp - *Ping Chen Tang* 平陈汤

Mixed Heat, Cold and deficiency - *Ban Xia Xie Xin Tang* 半夏泻心汤

Spleen and Stomach *qi/yang* deficiency - *Xiang Sha Liu Jun Zi Tang* 香砂六君子汤

18. Intestinal Abscess

Early stage (*qi* and Blood stagnation)
Suppurative stage (Flourishing Heat)
Late stage (Toxic Heat)
Chronic or recurrent abscess

18 INTESTINAL ABSCESS

chang yong 肠痈

In TCM terms an Intestinal abscess (*chang yong*[1]) is an accumulation of focal Damp or Toxic Heat, usually in the left or right iliac fossa. In the acute stage, Intestinal abscess is characterised by excess Heat and stagnation of both *qi* and Blood. In subacute or chronic cases, the pattern is generally one of excess and stagnation, with or without deficiency and Cold.

Acute Intestinal abscess tends to be more common in younger individuals, whose diagnosis is usually quite straight forward. In elderly patients and those with weak *qi*, the manifestations, when there is fairly serious illness, may be subdued, and the diagnosis more obscure.

In the western clinic, chronic or subacute cases are more often seen than acute Intestinal abscesses. Chronic abscesses generally lack the obvious signs of acute Heat, such as fever and chills or rigors, malaise, sweating, nausea and vomiting. The chronic presentation is generally characterised by a fixed lower abdominal pain, and possibly a mass upon palpation. It may be that these cases are associated with a low grade or dormant focus of infection that has been isolated from the rest of the body in such a way as to render it inaccessible to the body's immune system.

In biomedical terms, a TCM defined Intestinal abscess has most commonly been associated with acute appendicitis. As noted in Box 18.1 however, numerous biomedical diseases may fall into the TCM category of Intestinal abscess. Once one of the most common acute abdominal disorders, the incidence of acute appendicitis is decreasing in the developed world, and more chronic disorders, such as diverticulitis and diverticulosis, are becoming more common.

AETIOLOGY

Diet

Various dietary factors can contribute to Intestinal abscess. Overeating, frequently varying the quantity of food consumed and eating irregularly or at odd hours, can all disrupt Spleen and Stomach *qi* and lead to food stagnation. Too much cold natured or raw food weakens Spleen *qi* and *yang*. Overconsumption in general, and excessive consumption of rich and hot natured foods in particular, can lead to the accumulation of food and Damp Heat in the Intestines. Some specific types of foods are thought to be particularly liable to create foci around which stagnation can build, in particular some difficult to digest seeds, pips and nuts.

---

[1]Wiseman's 'Intestinal welling abscess'

Food stagnation can cause of Damp Heat accumulation (*see* p.3) and Intestinal abscess. By habitually overloading the Spleen and Stomach and exceeding their capacities to process the food ingested, the food lingers longer than it should, accumulating and stagnating.. This stagnation can produce Heat which intensifies the process of putrefaction. The Spleen and Stomach are weakened, further inhibiting their abilities to perform their digestive tasks efficiently. The weakened Spleen produces Damp which combines with the Heat to produce Damp Heat, further impeding the descent of Stomach and Large Intestine *qi*. If the stagnation intensifies further it becomes 'Toxic', and an Intestinal abscess is formed.

BOX 18.1 SOME BIOMEDICAL CAUSES OF INTESTINAL ABSCESS

- acute appendicitis
- appendicular abscess
- chronic appendicitis
- diverticulitis, diverticulosis
- peritoneal abscess
- peritonitis
- abscesses in the pelvic basin
- pelvic inflammatory disease, salpingitis
- mesenteric adenitis

Emotion

The gastro-intestinal tract is sensitive to, and easily disturbed by emotion, indeed the gut is perhaps the most common area of the body to store difficult to process emotional patterns. Due to the relationship between the *yin* and *yang* organ systems, the emotions that affect a primary *zang* may be stored in the partner *fu*. In the case of Intestinal abscess, the main emotional patterns are those that affect the Liver, Spleen and Lungs. These include anger, resentment and repressed emotions, grief, separation and loss and sadness.

These emotional elements are generally insufficient in themselves to generate Intestinal abscesses. They can, however, predispose an individual to a variety of complaints involving the Large Intestine, including Intestinal abscess.

Stagnation of Liver *qi* contributes to Intestinal abscess formation by causing a spasm and inefficient peristalsis in the Intestines, leading to focal accumulation. Chronic Liver *qi* stagnation can cause other complications. The prolonged pressure can create Heat, which can combine with any Dampness present to generate Damp Heat. Long term *qi* stagnation can also lead to Blood stagnation.

The emotions experienced following the death or absence of a parent or loved one, a sudden change from a comfortable routine to an unfamiliar one (such as starting school), or physical and social isolation, can cause Lung *qi* to accumulate. The Lung system, which incorporates the Large Intestine, is affected, and *qi* begins to knot.

In addition to the emotional factors that upset the Liver and Lungs, worry, obsessive thinking and prolonged concentration, in combination with a sedentary lifestyle and poor diet, will weaken Spleen *qi*, predisposing it to (or inviting) invasion by Liver *qi*, resulting in further damage.

External pathogenic invasion

External pathogens are a less common than diet and emotions as a cause of Intestinal abscess. However, both Damp Heat and Cold can invade and accumulate in the gastro-intestinal tract. The prolonged presence of a Cold pathogen, from the diet or environment, disrupts the local circulation of *qi* and Blood. Because Cold is such an efficient obstructor, it can easily generate the Heat necessary to damage tissues and create an abscess. Damp Heat is usually a seasonal invader, contributing to diarrhoea or dysenteric disorder. Damp Heat has a tendency to linger and can sometimes be difficult to completely eradicate. Any residual Damp Heat can smoulder at a particular locus in the Large Intestine, promoting the conditions for abscess formation.

Trauma

A trauma to the abdomen and Intestines, either from a previous intestinal illness, surgery, or a penetrating or blunt injury, can cause localised Blood stagnation and the formation of a mass. Once a Blood stagnation mass is present, it will further impede *qi* and Blood circulation, potentially generating the necessary Heat for acute abscess formation.

TCM DIFFERENTIAL DIAGNOSIS

- **Epigastric pain** (*wei tong* 胃痛): epigastric pain is centred in the epigastric region above the umbilicus, bordered laterally by the hypochondria. Pathology that causes epigastric pain usually affects the Stomach and is accompanied by Stomach specific symptoms, such as belching and reflux.
- **Intestinal worms** (*chong tong* 虫痛): Worm infestation tends to primarily affect infants and children, and can mimic Intestinal abscess. Worms can cause periumbilical pain, however the fever and chills and abdominal guarding that are characteristic of acute Intestinal abscess are absent. Chronic Intestinal abscess can be difficult to distinguish from parasites.
- **Painful urination syndrome** (*lin zheng* 淋证): Painful urination syndrome is characterised by central suprapubic fullness and discomfort, along with urinary frequency, urgency and pain. (*See* Volume 1.) Pain from Intestinal abscess tends to be in the lateral abdomen and generally does not disrupt urination.
- ***Shan qi*** (疝气): *Shan qi* patterns are characterised by lower abdominal pain, however the pain tends to be more generalised, may radiate to the external genitals, and is generally not accompanied by the presence of a mass.

- **Gynaecological conditions** (ectopic pregnancy, mittlesmertz, ovarian cysts): may be easily confused with Intestinal abscess, and indeed some gynaecological conditions may fall into the Intestinal abscess disease category (for example, pelvic inflammatory disease and salpingitis). There will usually be vaginal discharge, but sometimes ultrasound is necessary for definitive diagnosis.

TREATMENT

In the acute phase the treatment priority is based on three principles which take priority at different stages:

1. Open the bowels

Pathogens and areas of focal stagnation can be conveniently cleared from the gastro-intestinal system through the bowel (or as the Chinese put it, the 'big exit' *da men* 大门). This method is given priority in the early stages of Intestinal abscess, when stagnation is primary and Heat is beginning to evolve. It is not recommended as a primary method once the Heat is fully evolved. The reason for this is that purgative herbs (specifically **da huang**) stimulate extensive peristalsis in the intestine. Intense peristalsis is not desirable when some locus is severely inflamed and swollen, as the lesion may rupture.

2. Clearing Damp Heat and Toxic Heat

Damp Heat and Toxic Heat clearing is introduced as the primary method when Heat is intense or fully evolved. The main aim at this stage is to quickly clear the Heat, while gently promoting expulsion of the pathogen through the bowel. Strong purgation is avoided for the reasons outlined above.

3. Regulate Blood and eliminate stagnant Blood

Any pathogen or accumulation has the potential to disrupt the circulation of Blood. This is particularly the case when the pathology in question is treated with cooling or cold natured drugs. The method of regulating Blood has two aims:

1. to aid the circulation of *qi* and Blood in the local area during the acute episode
2. to prevent possible Blood stagnation complications following the acute episode, thereby minimising the potential for recurrence

Blood regulation takes third priority in acute cases, but is often the primary method used in chronic cases.

Overall, the treatment of the early and chronic stages of an Intestinal abscess is quite effective. However patients with severe Heat and pain, usually those in the Flourishing Heat or Toxic Heat stages, are critically ill and should be managed in a hospital.

A note on the use of da huang

Da huang (Radix et Rhizoma Rhei) 大黄, known for its purgative and Blood regulating action, is a key herb in all the acute patterns of Intestinal abscess. However it's intended action varies depending on the stage of the disorder. **Da huang** has quite different therapeutic properties, depending on how it is processed and how long it is cooked. The unprocessed root (**sheng da huang** 生大黄) is the most purgative, and its purgative qualities are retained if cooking is kept to a minimum. For the most powerful purge, cook for a few minutes only, or simply steep the root in the hot, strained decoction. Processed **zhi da huang** 制大黄 is less purgative and more Blood moving. The more the root is cooked, the less purgative it becomes, and the more its Blood moving action evolves.

We can harness these differences in action to effect varying outcomes in the treatment of Intestinal abscess. For example, in the early stage of an Intestinal abscess, the primary aim of treatment is to open the bowels with **sheng da huang**, thus providing an outlet for the developing accumulation. In the inflammatory stage, the purgative action of **da huang** is de-emphasised (with long cooking and the use of **zhi da huang**), and the Heat clearing and Blood moving aspect brought to the fore.

气滞血瘀证

18.1 QI AND BLOOD STAGNATION STAGE

Pathophysiology

- The early stage of an acute Intestinal abscess is associated with a focal area of stagnation, either from a lodged food item or locally accumulated Dampness and Heat. The stagnation affects *qi* and Blood movement, but has yet to intensify sufficiently to break down tissue and form much pus.
- At this stage there is generally little internal Heat, although Heat may be developing. The main aim of treatment is therefore to open the bowels and purge the developing accumulation.

Clinical features

- Acute intermittent, spasmodic, lower abdominal pain, usually in the left or right iliac fossa. The pain may be quite severe and is worse with pressure. In some cases there is rebound tenderness (that is, the pain is increased when the pressure is suddenly released). The abdominal muscles over the site of pain may or may not feel tight. The pain may have begun over the navel. If *qi* stagnation predominates, the pain may be unlocalised; with Blood stagnation, the pain is focal.
- abdominal distension
- belching, loss of appetite
- nausea, maybe vomiting
- normal stools or constipation
- may or may not be mild fever, or fever and chills

T unremarkable with a thin, white or thin, yellow coat
P wiry or tight

Treatment principle

Open the bowels to purge the accumulating pathogen
Move *qi* and eliminate Blood stasis, clear Heat

Prescription

DA HUANG MU DAN PI TANG 大黄牡丹皮汤
(*Rhubarb and Moutan Decoction*)

sheng da huang (unprocessed Radix et Rhizoma Rhei) 生大黄 9-18g
dong gua ren (Semen Benincasae Hispidae) 冬瓜仁 18-30g
tao ren (Semen Persicae) 桃仁 12-15g
mu dan pi (Cortex Moutan Radicis) 牡丹皮 9-12g
mang xiao (Mirabilitum) 芒硝 6-9g

Method: Decoction. **Da huang** is added a few minutes before the end of cooking (*hou xia* 后下), **mang xiao** is dissolved in the strained decoction (*yang hua* 冲服).

In acute cases this formula is generally not taken (or needed) for more than 3-4 days. The quantities of all herbs should be reduced by 50%-75% for children. **Da huang** as the main ingredient opens the bowels, purges accumulation, clears Heat and eliminates Blood stagnation; **tao ren** and **dong gua ren** eliminate stagnant Blood and disperse accumulations; the saltiness of **mang xiao** softens hardness to support the purging and Heat clearing action of the **da huang**; **mu dan pi** cools the Blood and eliminates stagnant Blood. (Source: *Shi Yong Zhong Yi Nei Ke Xue*)

Modifications

- The dose of da huang can vary depending on the degree of Heat and constipation, and the robustness of the patient. It is usually best to begin with a conservative dose, then increase it on the second dose. Without constipation, processed **da huang** (*zhi da huang* 制大黄) may be used. Remember that it usually takes about six hours for **da huang** to move the bowels.
- Herbs to enhance the accumulation clearing action of the prescription are often added. The most useful are **hong teng** (Caulis Sargentodoxae Cuneatae) 红藤 30g and **bai jiang cao** (Herba cum Radice Patriniae) 败酱草 30g.
- With predominant *qi* stagnation (distension, non localised pain), add **qing pi** (Pericarpium Citri Reticulatae Viride) 青皮 9-12g and **wu yao** (Radix Linderae Strychnifoliae) 乌药 9-12g.
- With Blood stagnation (focal pain, worse with pressure), add **dan shen** (Radix Salviae Miltiorrhizae) 丹参 18-30g.
- With an obvious palpable mass, add **e zhu** (Rhizoma Curcumae Ezhu) 莪术 9-12 and **san leng** (Rhizoma Sparganii Stoloniferi) 三棱 9-12g.
- With severe abdominal distension, add **zhi shi** (Fructus Immaturus Citri Aurantii) 枳实 9-12g and **gua lou** (Fructus Trichosanthis) 栝楼 18-24g.
- With severe pain, add **yan hu suo** (Rhizoma Corydalis Yanhusuo) 延胡索 9-12g, **chuan lian zi** (Fructus Meliae Toosendan) 川楝子 9-12g and **mu xiang** (Radix Aucklandiae Lappae) 木香 6-9g.
- With exterior signs and symptoms (fever and chills), add **zi su ye** (Folium Perillae Frutescentis) 紫苏叶 9-12g.
- With nausea, add **zhu ru** (Caulis Bambusae in Taeniis) 竹茹 12-15g.
- With developing internal Heat (thirst, halitosis, yellow tongue coat), add **pu gong ying** (Herba Taraxici Mongolici) 蒲公英 15-30g, **lian qiao** (Fructus Forsythia Suspensae) 连翘 9-12g and **jin yin hua** (Flos Lonicera Japonicae) 金银花 15-30g.

Variations and additional prescriptions

Subacute Intestinal abscess in robust patients

- **DA HUANG MU DAN PI TANG** (*Rhubarb and Moutan Decoction* 大黄牡丹皮汤) can also be used for robust patients with chronic or subacute intestinal abscess, (as may be seen in chronic appendicitis and diverticulitis, or mesenteric adenitis in children), with a few modifications. The typical presentation is recurrent, and sometimes vague, abdominal pains, intermittent constipation or bowel disturbance and a focal pain in the iliac fossa when palpated. Because the formula will need to be taken for longer than in acute cases, and constipation may not be an issue, it is better to separate the **da huang** and **mang xiao** and take a smaller dose of these herbs, usually just enough to have 2-3 soft bowel movements daily. The patient should not be purged. For patients with chronic Intestinal abscess and obvious Cold or signs of *qi* and Blood deficiency, see p.670.

Liver qi (Blood) stagnation

- Some patients experience a less acute condition, clearly associated with emotional turmoil. The pain, usually in the left or right iliac fossa, comes and goes or varies in quality, sometimes vague and hard to localise, sometimes sharp and focused. The pain is initiated or aggravated when the patient is stressed or upset. There is a specific tender area and possibly a mass upon palpation. The abdomen is soft and there is no fever. Bowel movements are normal or tend to be sluggish. The pulse during an episode is wiry or tight. The treatment aims to move Liver *qi* and eliminate stagnant Blood with **CHAI HU SHU GAN SAN** (*Bupleurum and Cyperus Formula* 柴胡疏肝散) modified.

chai hu (Radix Bupleuri) 柴胡 9-12g
zhi ke (Fructus Citri Aurantii) 枳壳 9-12g
bai shao (Radix Paeoniae Lactiflora) 白芍 12-18g
chi shao (Radix Paeoniae Rubrae) 赤芍 9-12g
chuan xiong (Radix Ligustici Chuanxiong) 川芎 6-9g
da huang (Radix et Rhizoma Rhei) 大黄 3-9g
tao ren (Semen Persicae) 桃仁 9-12g
mu dan pi (Cortex Moutan Radicis) 牡丹皮 9-12g
mang xiao (Mirabilitum) 芒硝 3-6g
bai jiang cao (Herba cum Radice Patriniae) 败酱草 15-30g

Method: Decoction or as powder. **Chai hu** and **zhi ke** regulate *qi*, **bai shao** softens the Liver; **chuan xiong** invigorates *qi* and Blood; **chi shao** and **mu dan pi** cool the Blood and eliminate stagnant Blood; **tao ren** moistens the Intestines and eliminates stagnant Blood; **da huang** and **mang xiao** open the bowel, purge accumulation and clear Heat; **bai jiang cao** clears Toxic Heat and disperses accumulations. (Source: *Zhong Yi Nei Ke Shou Ce*)

During pregnancy

- An Intestinal abscess during pregnancy presents a clinical conundrum as most of the standard herbs and methods (purgation, Blood moving) are contraindicated. An alternative approach is to clear Heat, gently regulate

Blood and calm the foetus with **QING CHANG YIN** (*Cool the Intestine Decoction* 清肠饮).

jin yin hua (Flos Lonicera Japonicae) 金银花 18-30g
dang gui (Radix Angelicae Sinensis) 当归 9-12g
di yu (Radix Sanguisorbae Officinalis) 地榆 9-12g
mai dong (Tuber Ophiopogonis Japonici) 麦冬 9-12g
xuan shen (Radix Scrophulariae Ningpoensis) 玄参 12-15g
yi ren (Semen Coicis Lachryma-jobi) 苡仁 18-24g
huang qin (Radix Scutellariae Baicalensis) 黄芩 9-12g
gan cao (Radix Glycyrrhizae Uralensis) 甘草 6-9g

Method: Decoction or as powder. **Jin yin hua** clears Toxic Heat; **dang gui** regulates and nourishes Blood; **di yu** cools the Blood; **mai dong** nourishes *yin*; **xuan shen** clears Heat, nourishes *yin*, cools the Blood, softens hardness and dissipates pathological accumulation; **yi ren** clears Damp Heat and promotes discharge of pus; **huang qin** clears Damp Heat and calms a restless foetus; **gan cao** protects the Stomach. (Source: *Shi Yong Zhong Yi Wai Ke Xue*)

Patent medicines

Niu Huang Qing Huo Wan 牛黄清火丸 (Niu Huang Qing Huo Wan)
- with constipation

Huang Lian Jie Du Wan 黄连解毒丸 (Huang Lian Jie Du Wan)
- Damp Heat

Chuan Xin Lian Kang Yan Pian 穿心莲抗炎片 (Chuan Xin Lian Antiphlogistic Tablets)
- can be added to one of the patent medicines above to enhance the Toxic Heat clearing action

Acupuncture (select from)

ah shi points .... If the appendix is affected, *lan wei xue* (M-LE-13), about one cun below St.36 (*zu san li*), will be exquisitely tender; if the focus is in another part of the intestine (usually the left iliac fossa), points on the Stomach channel between St.36 (*zu san li*) and St.37 (*shang ju xu*) will be tender.

St.25 (*tian shu* -) .... *mu* point of the Large Intestine, regulates Intestinal function and eliminates stagnation

St.37 (*shan ju xu* -) .... lower *he* point of the Large Intestine, eliminates stagnation and accumulation from the Stomach and Intestines and clears Damp Heat

Sp.8 (*di ji* -) .... *xi* cleft point of the Spleen, regulates and invigorates Blood

- Electro-acupuncture between St.36 (*zu san li*) and *lan wei xue* (M-LE-13), or other *ah shi* points on the Stomach channel on the same side is useful. Strong treatment with a high frequency dense disperse wave, 20-30 minutes.
- with fever, add LI.11 (*qu chi* -), LI.4 (*he gu* -) and St.44 (*nei ting* -)
- with severe pain, add St.34 (*liang qiu* -), St.43 (*xiang gu* -) and Sp.4 (*gong sun* -)
- with nausea and vomiting, add PC.6 (*nei guan*) and Ren.13 (*shang wan*)
- with abdominal distension, add Ren.6 (*qi hai*) and St.41 (*jie xi* -)
- with constipation, add SJ.6 (*zhi gou* -), Sp.14 (*fu jie*) and GB.34 (*yang ling quan* -)
- with emotional stress/Liver *qi* stagnation, add Liv.3 (*tai chong* -) and Liv.5 (*li gou* -)
- with a history of loss or grief, add Lu.3 (*tian fu*), Lu.7 (*lie que*) and Bl.42 (*po hu*)
- *Ear points*: appendix, large intestine, abdomen, sympathetic, *shen men*

Clinical notes

- *Qi* and Blood stagnation stage Intestinal abscess may be diagnosed biomedically as early stage of acute appendicitis, pelvic inflammatory disease, diverticulitis or grumbling appendix.
- This pattern usually responds quickly and well to early treatment.

蕴热证

18.2 FLOURISHING HEAT STAGE

Pathophysiology

- When the stagnation is prolonged or sufficient to create Heat, the affected tissues are broken down and pus is formed. In addition to the initial stagnation, Damp Heat is generated. Depending on the patient and the aetiology, the mixture of Dampness and Heat may be roughly equal or one may predominate, producing a variable clinical picture.

Clinical features

- Severe and increasing focal pain with guarding and possibly rebound tenderness; the patient may lie with legs flexed at the hip.
- high fever (dominant Heat) or low or afternoon fever (dominant Dampness), possibly with rigors
- sweating
- thirst (may be with little desire to relieve it if Dampness dominates), halitosis
- headache, malaise
- fullness and distension in the chest and abdomen
- constipation (Heat) or foul diarrhoea (Damp)
- concentrated urine
- nausea and vomiting

T normal or red tongue body, thick, greasy, yellow coat
P wiry or slippery and rapid

Treatment principle

Open the bowels to expel and eliminate Damp Heat
Invigorate Blood and eliminate stagnant Blood

Prescription

LAN WEI QING HUA TANG 阑尾清化汤
(*Appendix Cooling and Transforming Decoction*)

jin yin hua (Flos Lonicerae Japonicae) 金银花 30-60g
pu gong ying (Herba Taraxici Mongolici) 蒲公英 18-30g
mu dan pi (Cortex Moutan Radicis) 牡丹皮 12-15g
zhi da huang (processed Radix et Rhizoma Rhei) 制大黄 9-12g
chuan lian zi (Fructus Meliae Toosendan) 川楝子 12-15g
chi shao (Radix Paeoniae Rubrae) 赤芍 12-15g
tao ren (Semen Persicae) 桃仁 12-15g
gan cao (Radix Glycyrrhizae Uralensis) 甘草 6-9g

Method: Decoction. The **da huang** is cooked with the other herbs. **Jin yin hua** and **pu gong ying** clear Damp and Toxic Heat; **mu dan pi** cools the Blood and eliminates stagnant Blood; **da huang** opens the bowels to clears Heat and regulates Blood; **chuan lian zi** regulates *qi* and stops pain; **chi shao** and **tao ren** invigorate Blood and eliminate stagnant Blood; **gan cao** protects the Stomach and clears Heat. (Source: *Shi Yong Zhong Yi Wai Ke Xue*)

Modifications

- With significant Dampness, (thick, greasy tongue coat, low fever, thirst with little desire to drink, diarrhoea, bloating, nausea, slippery pulse), add **huo xiang** (Herba Agastaches seu Pogostemi) 藿香 12-15g, **pei lan** (Herba Eupatorii Fortuneii) 佩兰 9-12g, **dong gua ren** (Semen Benincasae Hispidae) 冬瓜仁 12-15g and **yi ren** (Semen Coicis Lachryma-jobi) 苡仁 18-30g.
- With severe Heat, (high fever, constipation, red tongue, concentrated urine, rapid pulse), add **bai hua she she cao** (Herba Hedyotidis Diffusae) 白花蛇舌草 30g, **huang lian** (Rhizoma Coptidis) 黄连 6-9g and **huang qin** (Radix Scutellariae Baicalensis) 黄芩 9-12g.
- With severe pain, add **yan hu suo** (Rhizoma Corydalis Yanhusuo) 延胡索 9-12g.
- With severe thirst, add **tian hua fen** (Radix Trichosanthes Kirilowii) 天花粉 12-15g.
- With nausea or vomiting, add **zhu ru** (Caulis Bambusae in Taeniis) 竹茹 12-15g.
- With a palpable mass at the site of pain, add **zao jiao ci** (Spina Gleditsiae Sinensis) 皂角刺 9-12g, **hong teng** (Caulis Sargentodoxae Cuneatae) 红藤 30g and **bai jiang cao** (Herba cum Radice Patriniae) 败酱草 30g.

Patent medicines

Niu Huang Qing Huo Wan 牛黄清火丸 (Niu Huang Qing Huo Wan)
- with constipation

Huang Lian Jie Du Wan 黄连解毒丸 (Huang Lian Jie Du Wan)
- Damp and Toxic Heat

Huang Lian Su Pian 黄连素片 (Tabellae Berberini)
- Damp and Toxic Heat

Chuan Xin Lian Kang Yan Pian 穿心莲抗炎片 (Chuan Xin Lian Antiphlogistic Tablets) - can be added to one of the patent medicines above to enhance the Toxic Heat clearing action

Acupuncture (select from)

ah shi points .... If the appendix is affected, *lan wei xue* (M-LE-13) about one cun below St.36 (*zu san li*) will be tender; if the focus is in another part of the intestine (usually the left iliac fossa), points on the Stomach channel between St.36 (*zu san li*) and St.37 (*shang ju xu*) will be tender.

St.25 (*tian shu* -) .... *mu* point of the Large Intestine, regulates Intestinal function and eliminates stagnation

St.37 (*shan ju xu* -) .... lower *he* point of the Large Intestine, eliminates stagnation and accumulation from the Stomach and Intestines and clears Damp Heat

Sp.8 (*di ji* -) .... *xi* cleft point of the Spleen, regulates and invigorates Blood

LI.11 (*qu chi* -) .... *he* sea point of the Large Intestine, clears Heat and Dampness from *yang ming* and regulates *qi* and Blood

St.44 (*nei ting* -) .... *rong* spring and Water point of the Stomach, clears Heat from *yang ming*, the Stomach and Stomach channel

- with a mass and tenderness, surround the focus of the lesion with three or four needles, angled towards the lesion (Fig.18.1)
- Electro-acupuncture between St.36 (*zu san li*) and *lan wei xue* (M-LE-13), or other *ah shi* points on the Stomach channel on the same side is useful. Strong treatment with a high frequency dense disperse wave, 20-30 minutes.
- with nausea and vomiting, add PC.6 (*nei guan*) and Ren.13 (*shang wan*)
- with abdominal distension, add Ren.6 (*qi hai*)
- with constipation, add SJ.6 (*zhi gou* -), Sp.14 (*fu jie*) and GB.34 (*yang ling quan* -)
- with a history of loss or grief, add, Lu.3 (*tian fu*), Lu.7 (*lie que*) and Bl.42 (*po hu*)
- *Ear points*: appendix, large intestine, abdomen, sympathetic, *shen men*

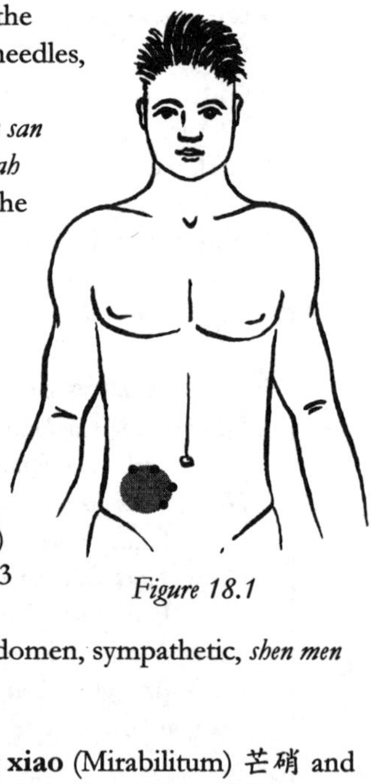

Figure 18.1

Poultice for external application

A poultice made from a mixture of **mang xiao** (Mirabilitum) 芒硝 and mashed garlic can be applied to the affected portion of the abdomen over a layer of vaseline.

Clinical notes

- See p.669.

热毒证

18.3 TOXIC HEAT STAGE

Pathophysiology

- The development of Toxic Heat constitutes a medical emergency, as the patient is very ill at this stage. The abscess has suppurated and may have ruptured.
- The purgative role of **da huang** is de-emphasised (although still utilised) and its Heat clearing and Blood moving action enhanced by longer cooking.

Clinical features

- Severe localised pain, or pain that is spreading to involve the entire abdomen; abdominal rigidity and guarding; any pressure aggravates the pain to the point that the patient cannot bear to be touched.
- epigastric and abdominal hardness and distension
- constipation
- no passing of flatus
- high fever or fever and rigors
- thirst, dryness of the mouth, lips and throat
- red complexion and eyes
- malaise
- headache
- nausea, vomiting, halitosis
- concentrated urine

T deep red or scarlet with a greasy or dry, yellow coat
P flooding and rapid

Treatment principle

Clear Toxic Heat
Invigorate Blood and break up stagnant Blood
Dissipate accumulation and resolve the abscess

Prescription

LAN WEI JIE DU TANG 阑尾解毒汤
(*Detoxify the Appendix Decoction*)

hong teng (Caulis Sargentodoxae Cuneatae) 红藤 30g
bai jiang cao (Herba cum Radice Patriniae) 败酱草 30g
jin yin hua (Flos Lonicerae Japonicae) 金银花 30-60g
pu gong ying (Herba Taraxici Mongolici) 蒲公英 30g
dong gua ren (Semen Benincasae Hispidae) 冬瓜仁 15-18g
chi shao (Radix Paeoniae Rubrae) 赤芍 9-12g
zhi da huang (processed Radix et Rhizoma Rhei)
制大黄 6-9g

mu xiang (Radix Aucklandiae Lappae) 木香 6-9g
huang qin (Radix Scutellariae Baicalensis) 黄芩 9-12g
tao ren (Semen Persicae) 桃仁 9-12g
chuan lian zi (Fructus Meliae Toosendan) 川楝子 9-12g

Method: Decoction. The **da huang** is cooked with the other herbs. **Hong teng, bai jiang cao, jin yin hua** and **pu gong ying** clear Toxic Heat; **hong teng** and **bai jiang cao** also invigorate Blood, aid in the discharge of pus and resolve abscesses; **dong gua ren** clears Heat and promotes the discharge of pus; **huang qin** clears Damp Heat; **chi shao** and **tao ren** invigorate Blood and eliminate stagnant Blood; **mu xiang** and **chuan lian zi** regulate *qi* and stop pain; a small quantity of **da huang** clears Heat through the bowels and breaks up stagnant Blood. (Source: *Shi Yong Fang Ji Xue*)

Modifications

- If vomiting prevents ingestion of the herbs, add **zhu ru** (Caulis Bambusae in Taeniis) 竹茹 12-15g, **ban xia** (Rhizoma Pinelliae Ternatae) 半夏 9-12g and **dai zhe shi** (Haematitum) 代赭石 15g. These herbs can be decocted separately and the decoction can be sipped slowly over a period of time. If the vomiting and nausea are persistent and prevent any ingestion at all, the main prescription can be delivered via a retention enema.
- With high fever and massive thirst, add **shi gao** (Gypsum) 石膏 30g, **zhi mu** (Rhizoma Anemarrhenae Asphodeloides) 知母 15g and **tian hua fen** (Radix Trichosanthes Kirilowii) 天花粉 15g.
- Once the condition begins to settle down, reduce the frequency of ingestion or the quantity of herbs. The effect of the severe Heat and the large quantities of bitter cold herbs may damage *yin*. With signs of *yin* damage, add *yin* nourishing herbs such as **yu zhu** (Rhizoma Polygonati Odorati) 玉竹 12g, **mai dong** (Tuber Ophiopogonis Japonici) 麦冬 12g, **sheng di** (Radix Rehmanniae Glutinosae) 生地 12g and **xuan shen** (Radix Scrophulariae Ningpoensis) 玄参 15g.

Variations and additional prescriptions

With Heat in the ying/Blood

- If the Heat enters the *ying* and/or Blood levels, causing disturbances of consciousness, delirium or febrile rashes, the aim of treatment is to clear Heat from the *ying*/Blood with **QING YING TANG** (*Clear the Ying Decoction* 清营汤) modified.

  shui niu jiao (Cornu Bubali) 水牛角 15-30g
  sheng di (Radix Rehmanniae Glutinosae) 生地 18-30g
  xuan shen (Radix Scrophulariae Ningpoensis) 玄参 18-24g
  mai dong (Tuber Ophiopogonis Japonici) 麦冬 12-15g
  jin yin hua (Flos Lonicera Japonicae) 金银花 30-60g
  lian qiao (Fructus Forsythia Suspensae) 连翘 12-15g

huang lian (Rhizoma Coptidis) 黄连 3-9g
dan shen (Radix Salviae Miltiorrhizae) 丹参 12-18g
dan zhu ye (Herba Lophatheri Gracilis) 淡竹叶 6-12g
pu gong ying (Herba Taraxici Mongolici) 蒲公英 15-30g
zi hua di ding (Herba cum Radice Violae Yedoensitis)
紫花地丁 9-12g
bai hua she she cao (Herba Hedyotidis Diffusae)
白花蛇舌草 30-60g

Method: Decoction. **Shui niu jiao** should be powdered and decocted for 30 minutes before the other herbs are added (*xian jian* 先煎). **Shui niu jiao** is salty and cold, clears Toxic Heat and cools the Blood; **sheng di** and **xuan shen** cool the Blood and nourish *yin*; **mai dong** nourishes *yin* and generates fluids; **jin yin hua**, **lian qiao**, **zi hua di ding** and **bai hua she she cao** clear Toxic Heat; **huang lian** clears Damp Heat and, with **dan zhu ye**, Fire from the Heart; **dan shen** clears Heat and prevents Blood stagnation. (Source: *Shi Yong Zhong Yi Nei Ke Xue*)
NB. Shui niu jiao is an effective substitute for the original ingredient, the horn, **xi jiao** (Cornu Rhinoceri) 犀角, of the endangered rhinoceros.

Residual Spleen and Stomach deficiency

- After recovery, the patient's Spleen and Stomach may be weakened by the purgative and bitter cold herbs. A Spleen strengthening prescription should be employed to bolster and repair the patient's digestive function. Consider prescriptions or patent medicines such as **XIANG SHA LIU JUN ZI TANG** (*Saussurea and Cardamon Combination* 香砂六君子汤, p.149), **SHEN LING BAI ZHU SAN** (*Ginseng and Atractylodes Formula* 参苓白术散, p.243), **LI ZHONG WAN** (*Ginseng and Ginger Formula* 理中丸, p.150) or **BA ZHEN TANG** (*Ginseng and Dang Gui Eight Combination* 八珍汤, p.398).

Residual Blood stagnation

- Blood stagnation is also a common complication of this Toxic Heat pattern. See 18.4 Chronic abscess with Blood stagnation and/or deficiency, p.670.

Damaged yin and qi in the recovery phase

- *Yin*, *qi* and fluids are frequently damaged during the acute phase of this pattern, and it can take some time to recover fully. During recovery, the patient often suffers from persistent fatigue and exhaustion, continuing dryness of the skin and mucous membranes, thirst, scanty urine, nightsweats and restlessness. Convalescence can be accelerated with an appropriate *qi* and *yin* replenishing prescription, such as **YI WEI TANG** (*Benefit the Stomach Decoction* 益胃汤, p.199), **SHENG MAI SAN** (*Generate the Pulse Powder* 生脉散, p.910), **SHA SHEN MAI MEN DONG TANG** (*Adenophora and Ophiopogon Combination* 沙参麦门冬汤,

p.910) or **ZENG YE TANG** (*Increase the Fluids Decoction* 增液汤, p.200).

Patent medicines

Acute phase

Niu Huang Qing Huo Wan 牛黄清火丸 (Niu Huang Qing Huo Wan)
Da Bai Du Jiao Nang 大败毒胶囊 (DBD Capsule)
Wu Wei Xiao Du Wan 五味消毒丸 (Wu Wei Xiao Du Wan)

During convalescence

Xiang Sha Liu Jun Zi Wan 香砂六君子丸 (Xiang Sha Liu Jun Wan, Aplotaxis-Ammomum Pills, Six Gentlemen Tea Pills)
- Spleen deficiency with Damp

Shen Ling Bai Zhu Wan 参苓白术丸 (Shen Ling Bai Zhu Wan)
- *qi* and *yin* deficiency

Li Zhong Wan 理中丸 (Li Zhong Wan)
- Spleen *yang* deficiency

Shi Quan Da Bu Wan 十全大补丸 (Shi Quan Da Bu Wan, Ten Flavour Tea)
- *qi* and Blood deficiency with Cold

Ba Zhen Wan 八珍丸 (Ba Zhen Wan, Women's Precious Pills)
- *qi* and Blood deficiency

Sheng Mai San Wan 生脉散丸 (Sheng Mai San Wan)
- Lung and Stomach *qi* and *yin* deficiency

Gu Ben Wan 固本丸 (Gu Ben Wan, Ren Shen Ku Pen Wan)
- Spleen and Stomach *qi* and *yin* deficiency

Acupuncture (select from)

PC.3 (*qu ze* ↓) .... *he* sea points of the Pericardium and Urinary
Bl.40 (*wei zhong* ↓) Bladder channel respectively, these points cool the Blood when bled

PC.9 (*zhong chong* ↓) ....*jing* well and Wood point of the Pericardium, powerfully clears Heat when bled
LI.11 (*qu chi* -) .... *he* sea point of the Large Intestine, clears Heat and Dampness from *yang ming*
Du.14 (*da zhui* -) .... meeting point of the *yang* channels, excellent for clearing Heat systemically
Du.26 (*ren zhong* -) .... this point has value in situations of possible shock

- with unrelenting fever, add *shi xuan* ↓ (M-UE-1)
- with spasms or convulsions, add Du.12 (*shen zhu* -), LI.4 (*he gu* -) and Liv.3 (*tai chong* -)

- with severe nausea, add PC.6 (*nei guan*)
- with severe pain, add St.34 (*liang qiu* -)
- *Ear points*: appendix, large intestine, abdomen, sympathetic, *shen men*

Clinical notes

- Toxic Heat and flourishing Heat type Intestinal abscess may be diagnosed biomedically as acute appendicitis, suppurative appendicitis, peritonitis, peritoneal abscess, acute pelvic inflammatory disease, suppurative salpingitis or acute diverticulitis.
- This is a potentially dangerous condition and is best managed in hospital. TCM treatment can be applied until IV antibiotic therapy or surgery can be instituted. Once the emergency and Heat is resolved, the various convalescent recovery prescriptions can be applied to good effect.

慢性肠痈

18.4 CHRONIC ABSCESS WITH COLD OR BLOOD STAGNATION AND/OR DEFICIENCY

Pathophysiology

- This pattern reflects either the residue of an incompletely resolved acute episode, or is the result of chronic stagnation of Liver *qi*, and thus Blood. In the aftermath of an acute episode, the free flow of *qi* and Blood can be severely impaired, and the damaged tissues are unable to fully recover health. Similarly, once Heat has been cooled, either by natural transformation or as the result of treatment with bitter cold herbs or medications, the affected tissues and the Spleen/Stomach system may be left in a state of Cold and deficiency, further compromising circulation.
- There are several ways in which a chronic Intestinal abscess can present. Depending on the aetiology of the abscess and the constitution of the patient, other presentations include Cold Damp accumulation, Blood stagnation, *qi* and Blood deficiency, or a mixture of all three.

Clinical features

- Localised lower abdominal mass with or without lower abdominal discomfort and focal tenderness. The mass may feel soft, rubbery and well defined, or firmer and more irregular.
- Discomfort or pain may be intermittent, and may be absent, mild or severe, depending on the pathology. Alternatively, pain may only be evident upon palpation.
- The abdomen may feel taut initially, but with increased palpation and pressure, the tone is lost and the abdomen feels soft or boggy/puffy. The skin tends to be dry and coarse.
- no fever or chills
- bowel movements may be normal, loose or sluggish
- **Cold Damp**: There may be little or no pain and the mass may have been discovered on routine palpation. The tissue overlying the mass may feel cooler then the surrounds. The tongue coat is white and greasy, especially on the root.
- **Blood stagnation**: The focus of pathology is usually quite painful, perhaps sharp or piercing, and worse with palpation. Any palpable mass tends to be firm and tender. Spider naevi or broken vessels may be apparent on the lower extremities. The tongue may be dark or purplish or have brown or purple stagnation spots and distended sublingual vessels, the pulse is wiry or choppy.
- **Qi and Blood deficiency**: There will be mild discomfort, a soft abdomen, tendency to loose stools, fatigue and weakness. The complexion is pale or sallow, the tongue pale and swollen, the pulse weak and thready.

Treatment principle

Reduce swelling, dissipate masses, aid discharge of pus
Warm *yang*, disperse Cold Damp, eliminate Blood stagnation, supplement *qi* and Blood as appropriate.

Prescription

18.4.1 Cold Damp accumulation

YI YI FU ZI BAI JIANG SAN 薏苡附子败酱散
(*Coicis, Prepared Aconite and Patrinia Powder*) modified

chao yi ren (dry fried Semen Coicis Lachryma-jobi) 炒苡仁 30g
bai jiang cao (Herba cum Radice Patriniae) 败酱草 30g
zhi fu zi (Radix Aconiti Carmichaeli Praeparata) 制附子 3-9g
huang qi (Radix Astragali Membranacei) 黄芪 18-30g
dong gua ren (Semen Benincasae Hispidae) 冬瓜仁 18-30g
dang gui (Radix Angelicae Sinensis) 当归 9-12g
mu dan pi (Cortex Moutan Radicis) 牡丹皮 9-12g
bai zhu (Rhizoma Atractylodes Macrocephalae) 白术 12-15g
zao jiao ci (Spina Gleditsiae Sinensis) 皂角刺 9-12g

Method: Decoction. **Zhi fu zi** is decocted for 30 minutes prior to the other herbs (*xian jian* 先煎). **Yi ren, bai jiang cao, dong gua ren** and **zao jiao ci** aid in the discharge of pus; **yi ren** clears Damp and Heat; **bai jiang cao** clears Toxic Heat and invigorates Blood; **zhi fu zi** warms and balances out the cold nature of the cooling herbs, it also disperses Cold and opens up the channels to facilitate the circulation of *qi* and Blood; **huang qi** supplements *qi* and promotes the circulation of *qi* and Blood; **dang gui** regulates and nourishes Blood; **mu dan pi** invigorates Blood; **bai zhu** strengthens the Spleen and dries Damp. (Source: *Zhong Yi Nei Ke Lin Chuang Shou Ce*)

18.4.2 Cold and Blood stagnation

SHAO FU HUA YU TANG 少腹化瘀汤
(*Decoction to Transform Blood Stagnation in the Lower Abdomen*)

hong teng (Caulis Sargentodoxae Cuneatae) 红藤 15-30g
chuan niu xi (Radix Cyathulae Officinalis) 川牛膝 12-15g
tao ren (Semen Persicae) 桃仁 9-12g
hong hua (Flos Carthami Tinctorii) 红花 9-12g
dang gui (Radix Angelicae Sinensis) 当归 9-12g
yan hu suo (Rhizoma Corydalis Yanhusuo) 延胡索 9-12g
pao jiang (quick fried Rhizoma Zingiberis Officinalis) 炮姜 6-9g
chai hu (Radix Bupleuri) 柴胡 6-9g
gui zhi (Ramulus Cinnamomi Cassiae) 桂枝 6-9g

chuan lian zi (Fructus Meliae Toosendan) 川楝子 9-12g
xiao hui xiang (Fructus Foeniculi Vulgaris) 小茴香 9-12g
xiang fu (Rhizoma Cyperi Rotundi) 香附 9-12g

Method: Decoction. **Hong teng** clears Heat, invigorates Blood and aids in discharge of pus; **niu xi, tao ren** and **hong hua** invigorate Blood and eliminate stagnant Blood; **dang gui** regulates and nourishes Blood; **yan hu suo** and **chuan lian zi** stops pain; **pao jiang, gui zhi** and **xiao hui xiang** warm and open the channels and *yang qi* and promote circulation of *qi* and Blood; **chai hu** and **xiang fu** regulate Liver *qi*. (Source: *Zui Xin Fang Ji Shou Ce*)

18.4.3 *Qi* and Blood deficiency

MU DAN PI SAN 牡丹皮散
(*Paeonia Suffruticosa Powder*)

dang shen (Radix Codonopsis Pilosulae) 党参 15-30g
huang qi (Radix Astragali Membranacei) 黄芪 15-30g
dang gui (Radix Angelicae Sinensis) 当归 9-15g
mu dan pi (Cortex Moutan Radicis) 牡丹皮 9-12g
tao ren (Semen Persicae) 桃仁 9-12g
chi shao (Radix Paeoniae Rubrae) 赤芍 9-12g
yi ren (Semen Coicis Lachryma-jobi) 苡仁 18-30g
chuan xiong (Radix Ligustici Chuanxiong) 川芎 6-9g
bai zhi (Radix Angelicae Dahuricae) 白芷 6-9g
mu xiang (Radix Aucklandiae Lappae) 木香 6-9g
gan cao (Radix Glycyrrhizae Uralensis) 甘草 6-9g
rou gui (Cortex Cinnamomi Cassiae) 肉桂 3g

Method: Decoction. **Dang shen, huang qi, dang gui** and **chuan xiong** supplement *qi* and Blood; **rou gui** encourages production and movement of *qi* and Blood; **mu dan pi, tao ren** and **chi shao** invigorate Blood and eliminate stagnant Blood; **bai zhi** and **yi ren** aid in discharge of pus; **gan cao** supplements *qi* and clears Toxin. (Source: *Shi Yong Fang Ji Xue*)

Variations and additional prescriptions

Subacute intestinal abscess in robust patients

- *See* p.658

Patent medicines

Cold Damp

Fu Ke Wu Jin Wan 妇科乌金丸 (Woo Garm Yuen Medical Pills)

Blood stagnation

Xue Fu Zhu Yu Wan 血府逐瘀丸 (Xue Fu Zhu Yu Wan)
- *qi* and Blood stagnation

Gui Zhi Fu Ling Wan 桂枝茯苓丸 (Gui Zhi Fu Ling Wan)

- mild Blood stagnation

Nei Xiao Luo Li Wan 内消瘰疬丸 (Nei Xiao Luo Li Wan)
- Blood and Phlegm stagnation masses

Tao Hong Si Wu Wan 桃红四物丸 (Tao Hong Si Wu Wan)
- with Blood deficiency

Fu Ke Wu Jin Wan 妇科乌金丸 (Woo Garm Yuen Medical Pills)
- with Cold and deficiency

Qi and Blood deficiency

Xiang Sha Liu Jun Zi Wan 香砂六君子丸 (Xiang Sha Liu Jun Wan, Aplotaxis-Ammomum Pills, Six Gentlemen Tea Pills)

Shi Quan Da Bu Wan 十全大补丸 (Shi Quan Da Bu Wan, Ten Flavour Tea)

Ba Zhen Wan 八珍丸 (Ba Zhen Wan, Women's Precious Pills)

Gui Zhi Fu Ling Wan 桂枝茯苓丸 (Gui Zhi Fu Ling Wan)
- this medicine can be added to one of the above patents to gently invigorate Blood

Acupuncture (select from)

ah shi points .... over the site of the lesion and distal points on the corresponding channel, usually the Stomach channel between St.36 (*zu san li*) and St.39 (*xia ju xu*), Spleen, *dai mai* or Kidney channels.

St.25 (*tian shu* -) .... *mu* point of the Large Intestine, regulates Intestinal function and eliminates stagnation from the Intestines

St.36 (*zu san li* +▲) .... *he* sea point of the Stomach, powerfully warms and strengthens the Spleen and Stomach, supplements *qi* and invigorates movement of *qi* and Blood

Sp.6 (*san yin jiao*) .... strengthens the Spleen, regulates Liver *qi*, benefits the Kidneys, invigorates *qi* and Blood and removes obstruction from the *jing luo*

Ren.6 (*qi hai* ▲) .... regulates *qi* in the lower abdomen and dispels Cold Damp

Bl.25 (*da chang shu*) .... *shu* point of the Large Intestine, regulates the Intestines and eliminates stagnation

Bl.17 (*ge shu* -) .... these points may be added when Blood stagnation features
Sp.10 (*xue hai* -)
Sp.8 (*di ji* -)

LI.4 (*he gu* -) .... the 'four gates', both *yuan* points, invigorate *qi*
Liv.3 (*tai chong*) and Blood, powerful sedative and calming action, relieve mental cloudiness and ease muscle spasm

- Non-scarring moxa cones or a moxa box over the *ren mai* points of the lower abdomen are good for warming and invigorating the circulation of *qi* and Blood.
- *Ear points*: appendix, large intestine, distal segment rectum, uterus, abdomen, sympathetic, *shen men*

Retention enema

- For chronic Intestinal abscess, a retention enema may be useful. The herbs are decocted in the normal fashion, strained and cooled to body temperature. 60-150 mls are inserted into the rectum with a commercial enema device. The enema is given once daily for 7-14 days, and can be retained (with the patient lying down) for 30 minutes to 2 hours, or better, overnight, with the patient's hips elevated in bed.

hong teng (Caulis Sargentodoxae Cuneatae) 红藤 30g
bai jiang cao (Herba cum Radice Patriniae) 败酱草 30g
zao jiao ci (Spina Gleditsiae Sinensis) 皂角刺 30g
pu gong ying (Herba Taraxici Mongolici) 蒲公英 30g
xu chang qing (Herba cum Radice Cynanchum Paniculatum) 徐长卿 30g
dan shen (Radix Salviae Miltiorrhizae) 丹参 15g

Method: Decoction. (*Zhong Yi Zhi Liao Yi Nan Za Bing Mi Yao*)

Clinical notes

- Intestinal abscess of a chronic type may be diagnosed biomedically as chronic appendicitis, chronic pelvic inflammatory disease, chronic salpingitis, diverticular disease or chronic colitis.
- Chronic abscesses usually respond well to correct treatment, but will generally take a lengthy period of time.

SUMMARY OF GUIDING FORMULAE FOR INTESTINAL ABSCESS

Qi and Blood stagnation - *Da Huang Mu Dan Pi Tang* 大黄牡丹皮汤
- with Liver *qi* stagnation - *Chai Hu Shu Gan San* 柴胡疏肝散
- during pregnancy - *Qing Chang Yin* 清肠饮

Flourishing Heat - *Lan Wei Qing Hua Tang* 阑尾清化汤

Toxic Heat - *Lan Wei Jie Du Tang* 阑尾解毒汤
- with Heat in the *ying*/Blood - *Qing Ying Tang* 清营汤

Chronic Intestinal abscess
- Cold Damp - *Yi Yi Fu Zi Bai Jiang San* 意苡附子败酱散
- Blood stagnation - *Shao Fu Hua Yu Tang* 少腹化瘀汤
- *qi* and Blood deficiency - *Mu Dan Pi San* 牡丹皮散

19. Lip Wind

Wind Damp Heat (Fire)
Wind Heat (Fire) with Spleen and Stomach Damp Heat
Liver *qi* stagnation with stagnant Heat, Fire
Spleen *qi* deficiency with residual Wind

19 LIP WIND

chun feng 唇风

Lip Wind is a disorder of the lips characterised by redness, swelling, itching, cracking, blistering, and in severe cases, exfoliation. The lips may tremble or quiver. Most commonly the lower lip is affected. Because swelling of the lower lip is a common and prominent feature, Lip Wind is also known as 'Donkey Mouth Wind' (*lü zui feng* 驴嘴风).

In Chinese medicine the lips are considered part of the Spleen organ system. The quality of the Spleen and the Blood is reflected in the lips. The lips may be predisposed to damage when the Spleen organ system is weak, or when Blood is deficient. Once the lips are predisposed to damage, all it takes is the trigger of external exposure, Heating elements in the diet, or stress and *qi* stagnation, to spark an episode. The most common pattern is associated with the combined effects of internally accumulated Heat or Damp Heat affecting the Spleen and Stomach, stirred up by exposure to the elements, repeated Wind invasion, or Liver *qi* stagnation and Liver Fire. The Heat or Damp Heat is lofted upwards through the Spleen and Stomach channels and lodges in the lips, making them red, swollen or blistered.

AETIOLOGY

External Heat/Dryness invasion/exposure

Exposure to a windy, sunny or drying environment is a trigger that mobilises dormant/latent Heat or Damp Heat in the Spleen and Stomach to ooze up through their channels to the lips. Other triggers include local contact with irritant substances such as chillies and chilli oil, raw garlic and cigarette smoke.

Diet

Irregular dietary habits and a diet rich in spicy, heating, drying and/or Damp inducing foods, lays the foundations for Lip Wind. All it then takes is the trigger of a Wind invasion or other irritant to begin the process.

The common dietary causes of this accumulation of Damp Heat are the repeated ingestion of heating and/or Damp inducing substances–chillies, alcohol, sugar and chocolate, spicy food, dairy products, stimulant drugs (including illicit and prescription), coffee and tobacco. Smouldering Damp Heat in the Spleen and Stomach can also be due to overindulgence or irregular dietary habits (eating late at night, midnight snacks, eating while upset, eating too quickly etc.) that weaken the Spleen and Stomach and create food stagnation and stagnant Heat.

Emotion

Emotions also contribute to Lip Wind through the agent of the Liver. When normal Liver function is disrupted by anger, frustration, or stress, the resulting pent up stagnation of *qi* frequently vents sideways, damaging and disrupting Spleen function and creating stagnant Heat, or, in severe cases, Fire. The weakened Spleen may produce Damp. The stagnant Heat and Damp can combine to form Damp Heat. Damp, which accumulates and stagnates, may over time produce its own Heat. In either case, the end result is an accumulation of Damp Heat with a background of *qi* stagnation and Spleen deficiency. Liver Fire can heat the Stomach, creating Stomach Heat or Fire.

BOX 19.1 SOME BIOMEDICAL CORRELATIONS OF LIP WIND

- exfoliative cheilitis
- actinic cheilitis
- herpes simplex

TREATMENT

Treatment involves avoidance of irritants and environmental conditions that aggravate dryness of the lips. Treatment of recurrent cases is often difficult, and prolonged therapy, in association with appropriate dietary modification, is usually necessary to eliminate the lurking Damp Heat. All pathological elements need to be addressed in complex cases, when multiple patterns may coexist.

Figure 19.1 *Aetiology of Lip Wind*

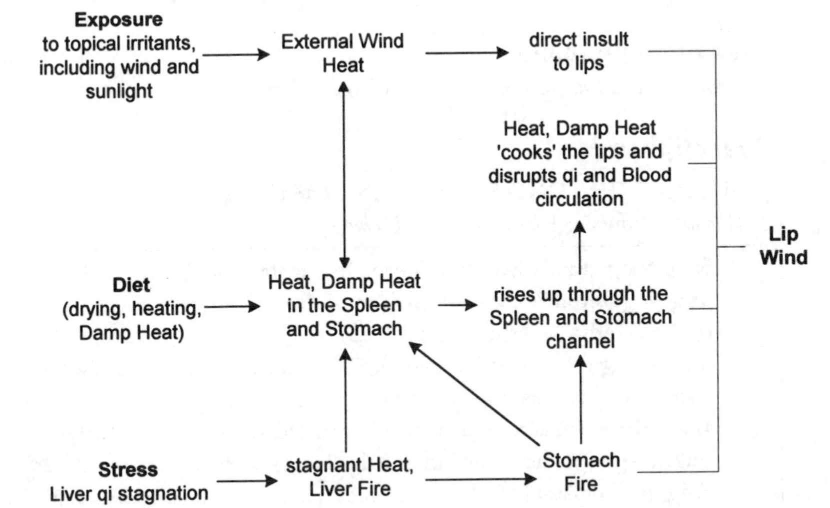

风湿热唇风

19.1 WIND DAMP HEAT (FIRE)

Pathophysiology

- Wind Heat (with Damp) affecting the lips is essentially an external disorder associated with exposure to sun or dry wind. When Heat is sufficiently severe to cause bleeding and significant swelling, erosion and cracking, it is denoted as Wind Fire.
- The manifestations depend to an extent on the relative balance of Wind, Dampness and Heat–when Wind predominates, quivering and itch prevail; when Damp is predominant, swelling, blisters, erosion and a serous exudate occur; when Heat predominates, dryness, cracking, redness and pain occur.

Clinical features

- In the early stages, the lips are itchy or experience a tingling or burning pain; the lips become red and swollen, and over time become blistered or cracked, and exude a serous exudate. The lips may quiver or tremble. There may be bleeding, dryness, erosion, gradual exfoliation and scabbing. A thin yellow membrane may appear over the mucous membrane of the inner lip.
- fever, or fever and chills, or alternating fever and chills
- thirst with desire for cool drinks
- halitosis
- constipation, dry stools
- concentrated urine
- frontal headache

T red or with a red tip and a thin, yellow coat

P floating in the early stage, becoming slippery or wiry and rapid

Treatment principle

Dispel Wind Damp Heat and clear Toxic Heat

Prescription

SHUANG JIE TONG SHENG SAN 双解通圣散
(*Doubly Dispersing Powder to Sagely Unblock*)

fang feng (Radix Ledebouriellae Divaricatae) 防风 9-12g
jing jie (Herba Schizonepetae Tenuifoliae) 荆芥 9-12g
bo he (Herba Mentha Haplocalycis) 薄荷 6-9g
ma huang (Herba Ephedrae) 麻黄 6-9g
lian qiao (Fructus Forsythiae Suspensae) 连翘 12-15g
shan zhi zi (Fructus Gardeniae Jasminoidis) 山栀子 12-15g
huang qin (Radix Scutellariae Baicalensis) 黄芩 9-12g
shi gao (Gypsum) 石膏 30g

jie geng (Radix Platycodi Grandiflori) 桔梗 6-9g
chuan xiong (Radix Ligustici Chuanxiong) 川芎 6-9g
dang gui (Radix Angelicae Sinensis) 当归 12-15g
bai shao (Radix Paeoniae Lactiflorae) 白芍 12-18g
gan cao (Radix Glycyrrhizae Uralensis) 甘草 3-6g
bai zhu (Rhizoma Atractylodes Macrocephalae) 白术 9-12g
hua shi (Talcum) 滑石 30g

Method: Decoction. **Shi gao** is decocted for 30 minutes prior to the other herbs (*xian jian* 先煎); **bo he** is added a few minutes before the end of cooking (*hou xia* 后下). **Fang feng**, **jing jie**, **bo he** and **ma huang** dispel Wind; **lian qiao**, **shan zhi zi** and **huang qin** clear Toxic and Damp Heat; **shi gao** and **jie geng** clear Heat from the *qi* level; **chuan xiong** and **dang gui** regulate and nourish Blood; **bai shao** and **gan cao** combine sweet and sour to generate *yin* and stop pain; **bai zhu** strengthens the Spleen and dries Damp; **hua shi** leaches Damp Heat out through the urine. (Source: *Zhong Yi Er Bi Hou Ke Xue*)

Modifications

- With no fever, delete **shi gao**.
- With no chills, delete **ma huang**.
- With Fire (red or crimson, swollen or bleeding lips, relentless high fever), add **huang lian** (Rhizoma Coptidis) 黄连 6-9g, **ban lan gen** (Radix Isatidis seu Baphicacanthi) 板蓝根 15-30g and **shui niu jiao** (Cornu Bubali) 水牛角 30g.
- With strong exterior signs and symptoms, and dominant Wind, delete **dang gui**, **bai shao** and **bai zhu**, and add **qiang huo** (Rhizoma et Radix Notopterygii) 羌活 9-12g and **niu bang zi** (Fructus Arctii Lappae) 牛蒡子 9-12g.
- With dominant Dampness (vesicular blisters, erosion and exudate), add **yi ren** (Semen Coicis Lachryma-jobi) 苡仁 30g, **ze xie** (Rhizoma Alismatis Orientalis) 泽泻 9-12g and **che qian zi** (Semen Plantaginis) 车前子 9-12g.
- With alternating fever and chills, delete **shi gao** and **ma huang** and add **chai hu** (Radix Bupleuri) 柴胡 9-12g.
- With blistering, add **ban lan gen** (Radix Isatidis seu Baphicacanthi) 板蓝根 15-30g.
- With constipation, add **da huang** (Radix et Rhizoma Rhei) 大黄 3-6g and **mang xiao** (Mirabilitum) 芒硝 3-6g.

Topical therapy

HUANG LIAN GAO (*Coptis Ointment* 黄连膏)

Moistens dryness, clears Heat, stops pain.

huang lian (Rhizoma Coptidis) 黄连 9g
huang bai (Cortex Phellodendri) 黄柏 9g
dang gui (Radix Angelicae Sinensis) 当归 15g

sheng di (Radix Rehmanniae Glutinosae) 生地 30g
jiang huang (Rhizoma Curcumae Longae) 姜黄 9g

Method: Steep the herbs in 360g of sesame oil for a day, then gently heat the oil and herbs for several hours until the herbs are brown and all their goodness has been extracted. Discard the herbs. Mix the oil in with a stabilising wax or setting agent such as lanolin. Apply topically.

Patent medicines

Fang Feng Tong Sheng Wan 防风通圣丸 (Fang Feng Tong Sheng Wan)
- internal and external excess Heat

Huang Lian Shang Qing Pian 牛黄上清片 (Huang Lien Shang Ching Pien)

Niu Huang Jie Du Pian 牛黄解毒片 (Peking Niu Huang Chieh Tu Pien)
- the last two patent medicines for Toxic Heat in the upper body

Xi Gua Shuang 西瓜霜 (Watermelon Frost)
- topically to relieve swelling and pain

Acupuncture (select from)

St.44 (*nei ting* -) .... together these points clear Heat from the
LI.4 (*he gu* -) Stomach channel and *yang ming*, and dispel Wind from the lips

LI.11 (*qu chi* -) .... *he* sea point of the Large Intestine, clears Heat and Dampness from *yang ming* and eliminates Wind

Du.14 (*da zhui* - Ω) .... meeting point of the *yang* channels, clears Heat and pathogens from the exterior

St.36 (*zu san li* -) .... *he* sea point of the Stomach, strengthens and regulates the Spleen and Stomach and clears Damp and Heat

Ren.24 (*cheng jiang*) .... local points for lip disease, select one or two
Du.26 (*ren zhong*)
Du.27 (*dui duan*)
St.4 (*di cang*)

- with constipation, add SJ.6 (*zhi gou* -) and St.25 (*tian shu* -)
- with severe Heat, redness and swelling, add St.45 (*li dui* ↓)
- *Ear points*: mouth, lips, spleen, *shen men*

Clinical notes

- In all cases, patients at risk of exposure should be advised to cover their lips with a soothing emollient such as lanolin, chap stick or sunscreen.
- For dietary recommendations, see p.882.

19.2 WIND HEAT (FIRE) WITH SPLEEN AND STOMACH DAMP HEAT

风火引动脾胃湿热

Pathophysiology

- This pattern describes a Wind Heat (Fire) invasion on top of pre-existing Damp Heat in the Spleen and Stomach. Because of the Spleen's relationship to the lips, this latent Damp Heat makes the lips vulnerable to invasion by external Wind. Damp Heat also contributes to the protracted, recalcitrant and recurrent nature of this disorder. At the same time, the prolonged presence of Damp Heat begins to damage *yin*. Occasionally there is a seasonal component, the disorder recurring during periods of dry or cold weather.

Clinical features

- Chronic or recurrent swelling, redness, dryness, cracking and bleeding, blistering, erosion, scaling, exfoliation, crusting and burning pain of the lips.
- dry mouth, bitter taste, sticky or cloying sensation in the mouth; thirst with little or no desire to drink
- red complexion, greasy skin, possibly strong body odour
- loss of appetite, morning nausea
- fullness and stuffiness in the chest
- restlessness, irritability
- possibly low grade fever or afternoon fever
- heavy sensation in the body, lethargy
- loose stools or a tendency to sluggish stools or constipation; the stools are generally not dry
- concentrated urine

T reddish with a dry or greasy, yellow coat

P slippery or soggy and rapid; or thready and rapid

Treatment principle

Dispel Wind and Heat, clear Damp Heat

Nourish and cool the Blood, moisten *yin* and dryness

Prescription

SI WU XIAO FENG SAN 四物消风散
(*Eliminate Wind Powder with the Four Substances*) modified

dang gui (Radix Angelicae Sinensis) 当归 9-15g
chuan xiong (Radix Ligustici Chuanxiong) 川芎 6-9g
chi shao (Radix Paeoniae Rubrae) 赤芍 9-12g
sheng di (Radix Rehmanniae Glutinosae) 生地 12-18g

jing jie (Herba Schizonepetae Tenuifoliae) 荆芥 12-15g
fang feng (Radix Ledebouriellae Divaricatae) 防风 9-12g
bo he (Herba Mentha Haplocalycis) 薄荷 6-9g
chai hu (Radix Bupleuri) 柴胡 6-9g
chan tui (Periostracum Cicadae) 蝉蜕 9-12g
gan cao (Radix Glycyrrhizae Uralensis) 甘草 3-6g
huang qin (Radix Scutellariae Baicalensis) 黄芩 6-12g
mu dan pi (Cortex Moutan Radicis) 牡丹皮 6-12g
xuan shen (Radix Scrophulariae) 玄参 18-24g
mai dong (Tuber Ophiopogonis Japonici) 麦冬 9-12g
shi hu (Herba Dendrobi) 石斛 12-15g

Method: Decoction. **Bo he** is added towards the end of cooking (*hou xia* 后下). **Dang gui**, **chuan xiong** and **chi shao** regulate and invigorate Blood; **fang feng**, **bo he**, **jing jie**, **chai hu** and **chan tui** dispel Wind and clear Heat; **sheng di** and **gan cao** cool the Blood and clear Toxic Heat; **huang qin** clears Damp Heat; **mu dan pi**, **xuan shen**, **mai dong** and **shi hu** clear Heat and nourish *yin*. (Source: *Zhong Yi Er Bi Hou Ke Xue*)

Modifications

- With prominent blistering and Dampness, add **ban lan gen** (Radix Isatidis seu Baphicacanthi) 板蓝根 15-30g, **yi ren** (Semen Coicis Lachryma-jobi) 苡仁 30g and **che qian zi** (Semen Plantaginis) 车前子 9-12g.
- With prominent Heat, add **jin yin hua** (Flos Lonicerae Japonicae) 金银花 18-30g and **lian qiao** (Fructus Forsythiae Suspensae) 连翘 9-12g.
- With itching, add **bai xian pi** (Cortex Dictamni Dasycarpi Radicis) 白藓皮 9-12g.
- With quivering or spasm of the lips, add **quan xie** (Buthus Martensi) 全蝎 1-3g.

Topical therapy

HUANG LIAN GAO (*Coptis Ointment* 黄连膏, p.681)
ZI DANG YOU (*Lithospermum and Angelica Oil* 紫当油)
Steep 20 grams each of powdered **zi cao** (Radix Arnebiae seu Lithospermi) 紫草 and **dang gui** (Radix Angelicae Sinensis) 当归 in 100mls of hot sesame oil for several hours. Tip off the oil and apply topically to the lips.
Xi Gua Shuang 西瓜霜 (Watermelon Frost)

Patent medicines

Xiao Feng Wan 消风丸 (Xiao Feng Wan) combined with *Si Wu Wan* 四物丸 (Si Wu Wan)

Xi Gua Shuang 西瓜霜 (Watermelon Frost)
- topically to relieve swelling and pain

Acupuncture (select from)

Sp.9 (*yin ling quan*) .... *he* sea point of the Spleen, promotes urination and drains Damp Heat through the urine

LI.11 (*qu chi* -) .... *he* sea point of the Large Intestine, clears Heat and Dampness from *yang ming*, eliminates Wind and regulates *qi* and Blood

LI.4 (*he gu* -) .... *yuan* point of the Large Intestine, clears Wind and Heat, clears Heat from *yang ming*, stops pain, activates the dispersing function of the Lungs and invigorates *qi* and Blood

Ren.12 (*zhong wan* -) .... *mu* point of the Stomach, clears Damp Heat from the Spleen and Stomach

St.36 (*zu san li* -) .... *he* point of the Stomach, regulates and strengthens the Spleen and Stomach and clears Dampness and Heat

Liv.8 (*qu quan* -) .... *he* sea and Water point of the Liver, supplements Liver *yin*, clears Damp Heat and relaxes the muscle channels

Ren.24 (*cheng jiang*) .... local points for lip disease, select one or two
Du.26 (*ren zhong*)
Du.27 (*dui duan*)
St.4 (*di cang*)

- *Ear points*: mouth, lips, spleen, *shen men*

Clinical notes

- In all cases, patients at risk of exposure should be advised to cover their lips with a soothing emollient such as lanolin, chap stick or sunblock.
- For dietary recommendations, see p.882-884.

肝气郁热

19.3 LIVER QI STAGNATION WITH STAGNANT HEAT, LIVER FIRE

Pathophysiology

- Chronic stress, emotional turmoil, a high pressure job or lifestyle, combined with poor diet, smoking, alcohol and sedentary work, can contribute to the generation of Liver *qi* stagnation and stagnant Heat. A sudden increase in stress levels may be sufficient to ignite the stagnant Heat, creating Fire which then affects the Spleen and Stomach. Such an increase in stress may also stir up any pre-existing Heat or Damp Heat in the Spleen and Stomach.

肝火

Clinical features

- Chronic or recurrent blistering, vesicles, swelling, redness, erosion, crusting and burning pain of the lips. Outbreaks are initiated by stress.
- frontal or temporal headaches, shoulder and neck tension, tooth grinding at night
- red eyes, facial flushing
- depression, irritability, moodiness, patient easily angered
- hypochondriac tension or discomfort
- dizziness
- bitter taste in the mouth
- irregular menstruation, premenstrual syndrome and breast tenderness

T unremarkable or dark with a thin white or yellow coat, or with red edges and a thick, yellow coat with Heat or Fire

P wiry and possibly rapid

Treatment principle

Regulate Liver *qi*, clear Heat and Damp
Purge Fire

Prescription

LONG DAN XIE GAN TANG 龙胆泻肝汤
(*Gentiana Combination*) modified

This formula is selected for acute episodes with Heat or Fire.

long dan cao (Radix Gentianae Longdancao) 龙胆草 6-9g
chai hu (Radix Bupleuri) 柴胡 9-12g
huang qin (Radix Scutellariae Baicalensis) 黄芩 9-12g
shan zhi zi (Fructus Gardeniae Jasminoidis) 山栀子 9-12g
sheng di (Radix Rehmanniae Glutinosae) 生地 15-18g
che qian zi (Semen Plantaginis) 车前子 9-12g
gan cao (Radix Glycyrrhizae Uralensis) 甘草 3-6g
ban lan gen (Radix Isatidis seu Baphicacanthi) 板蓝根 15-30g

niu bang zi (Fructus Arctii Lappae) 牛蒡子 9-12g
ye ju hua (Flos Chrysanthemi Indici) 野菊花 9-12g

Method: Decoction. **Long dan cao, huang qin** and **shan zhi zi** cool the Liver and purge Fire; **sheng di** cools the Blood; **chai hu** clears Heat and regulates *qi*; **che qian zi** promotes urination to leach Damp; **gan cao** protects the Stomach; **ban lan gen** and **ye ju hua** clear Toxic Heat; **niu bang zi** clears Wind Heat from the face. (Source: *Shi Yong Zhong Yi Nei Ke Xue*)

Modifications

- With pain, add **yan hu suo** (Rhizoma Corydalis Yanhusuo) 延胡索 9-12g, **chuan lian zi** (Fructus Meliae Toosendan) 川楝子 9-12g and **dan shen** (Radix Salviae Miltiorrhizae) 丹参 15g.
- With constipation or dry stools, add **da huang** (Radix et Rhizoma Rhei) 大黄 6-9g and **zhi shi** (Fructus Citri Aurantii Immaturus) 枳实 9-12g.
- With severe Dampness, add **yi ren** (Semen Coicis Lachryma-jobi) 苡仁 30g and **ze xie** (Rhizoma Alismatis Orientalis) 泽泻 9-12g.

Variations and additional prescriptions

Without stagnant Heat or Fire

- If patients have been subject to repeated episodes over a period of months or years, the Heat aspects during an acute outbreak often become muted, due to the development of underlying deficiency. Without clears signs of Heat, the aim of treatment is to regulate *qi*, strengthen the Spleen, nourish Blood and eliminate pathogens with **XIAO YAO SAN** (*Bupleurum and Dang Gui Formula* 逍遥散) modified.

chai hu (Radix Bupleuri) 柴胡 9-12g
dang gui (Radix Angelicae Sinensis) 当归 9-12g
bai shao (Radix Paeoniae Lactiflora) 白芍 12-15g
bai zhu (Rhizoma Atractylodis Macrocephalae) 白术 9-12g
fu ling (Sclerotium Poriae Cocos) 茯苓 12-15g
bo he (Herba Mentha Haplocalycis) 薄荷 6-9g
zhi gan cao (honey fried Radix Glycyrrhizae Uralensis)
炙甘草 3-6g
wei jiang (roasted Rhizoma Zingiberis Officinalis) 煨姜 ... 3-6g
ban lan gen (Radix Isatidis seu Baphicacanthi) 板蓝根 12-15g
huang lian (Rhizoma Coptidis) 黄连 2-3g

Method: Decoction. **Bo he** is added a few minutes before the end of cooking (*hou xia* 后下). **Chai hu** moves Liver *qi*; **dang gui** and **bai shao** nourish Liver Blood and soften the Liver; **bai zhu** and **fu ling** strengthen the Spleen and dry and leach out Dampness respectively; **zhi gan cao** supplements *qi* and, with **bai shao**, eases muscle spasm; **wei jiang** warms and harmonises the Stomach; **bo he** assists **chai hu** in moving Liver *qi*; the relatively small doses of **ban lan gen** and **huang lian** clear any pathogenic Damp and Heat. (Source: *Zhong Yi Zhi Liao Yi Nan Za Bing Mi Yao*)

In between episodes, to regulate qi

- In between acute episodes, a constitutional prescription to regulate Liver *qi* and eliminate any residual Damp Heat is recommended. Over time, this will reduce the frequency and severity of outbreaks. There are a number of suitable prescriptions, depending on the strength of the patient. Consider **XIAO YAO SAN** (*Bupleurum and Dang Gui Formula* 逍遥散, p.159), **CHAI HU SHU GAN SAN** (*Bupleurum and Cyperus Formula* 柴胡疏肝散, p.356) or **DAN ZHI XIAO YAO SAN** (*Bupleurum and Paeonia Formula* 丹栀逍遥散, p.113).

Topical therapy

HUANG LIAN GAO (*Coptis Ointment* 黄连膏, p.681)
ZI DANG YOU (*Lithospermum and Angelica Oil* 紫当油, p.684)
Xi Gua Shuang 西瓜霜 (Watermelon Frost)

Patent medicines

Jia Wei Xiao Yao Wan 加味逍遥丸 (Jia Wei Xiao Yao Wan)
- Liver *qi* stagnation with stagnant Heat

Long Dan Xie Gan Wan 龙胆泻肝丸 (Long Dan Xie Gan Wan, Lung Tan Xie Gan Wan)
- Liver Fire

Xiao Yao Wan 逍遥丸 (Xiao Yao Wan, Hsiao Yao Wan, Bupleurum Sedative Pills) - Liver *qi* stagnation

Ban Lan Gen Chong Ji 板蓝根冲剂 (Ban Lan Gen Chong Ji)
- Toxic Heat, can be combined with an appropriate constitutional patent medicine above

Bei Jing Niu Huang Jie Du Pian 牛黄解毒片 (Peking Niu Huang Chieh Tu Pien) - Toxic Heat in the upper body, can be combined with an appropriate constitutional patent medicine above

Xi Gua Shuang 西瓜霜 (Watermelon Frost)
- topically to relieve swelling and pain

Acupuncture (select from)

Liv.13 (*zhang men*) .... *mu* point of the Spleen, regulates and harmonises the Liver and Spleen and strengthens the Spleen

GB.34 (*yang ling quan* -) ... *he* sea point of the Gallbladder, regulates *qi* and subdues exuberant Liver *yang*

St.44 (*nei ting* -) .... together these points clear Heat from the
LI.4 (*he gu* -) Stomach and Liver and dispel Wind from the
Liv.2 (*xing jian* -) lips

Liv.3 (*tai chong* -) .... *yuan*, *shu* and Earth point of the Liver, regulates Liver *qi*
St.36 (*zu san li* -) .... *he* sea point of the Stomach, strengthens and regulates the Spleen and Stomach and supplements *qi*
Ren.24 (*cheng jiang*) .... local points for lip disease, select one or two
Du.26 (*ren zhong*)
Du.27 (*dui duan*)
St.4 (*di cang*)

- with Damp, add Sp.9 (*yin ling quan* -)
- with nausea, add PC.6 (*nei guan* -)
- with epigastric pain, add St.21 (*liang men* -) and St.34 (*liang qiu* -)
- *Ear points*: liver, mouth, lips, spleen, *shen men*

Clinical notes

- Acute episodes usually resolve quickly, but preventing recurrence takes time and effort on the part of the patient for a sustained result. Long term results require an appropriate treatment plan which includes lifestyle modification, diet (especially reducing alcohol), relaxation, exercise and stress management.
- For dietary recommendations, see p.878, 882.

脾气虚

19.4 SPLEEN QI DEFICIENCY (WITH RESIDUAL WIND)

Pathophysiology

- The Spleen manifests in the lips and determines their integrity. When the Spleen is weak, *qi* fails to ascend and nourish the lips, making them vulnerable to invasion or retention of pathogens.

Clinical features

- Chronic or recurrent dull redness, swelling, dryness, cracking and bleeding, crusting and tingling of the both lower and upper lips.
- pale or sallow complexion
- loss of appetite
- abdominal distension, early satiety
- weight loss, poor muscle tone
- fatigue, weakness, shortness of breath
- cold intolerance, cold extremities
- tendency to loose stools or diarrhoea

T pale and swollen with tooth marks; thin or thickish coat
P weak, thready, deficient

Treatment principle

Strengthen the Spleen, supplement *qi*

Prescription

SHEN LING BAI ZHU SAN 参苓白术散
(*Ginseng and Atractylodes Formula*) modified

dang shen (Radix Codonopsis Pilosulae) 党参 15-30g
chao bai zhu (dry fried Rhizoma Atractylodes Macrocephalae) 炒白术 12-15g
chao yi ren (dry fried Semen Coicis Lachryma-jobi) 炒苡仁 15-24g
fu ling (Sclerotium Poriae Cocos) 茯苓 12-15g
chao bian dou (dry fried Semen Dolichos Lablab) 炒扁豆 12-18g
chao shan yao (dry fried Radix Dioscoreae Oppositae) 炒山药 12-18g
lian zi (Semen Nelumbinis Nuciferae) 莲子 12-15g
jie geng (Radix Platycodi Grandiflori) 桔梗 6-9g
sha ren (Fructus Amomi) 砂仁 6-9g
zhi gan cao (honey fried Radix Glycyrrhizae Uralensis) 炙甘草 6-9g
huang qi (Radix Astragali Membranacei) 黄芪 18-30g

Method: Grind the herbs to a powder and take 9-grams 2-3 times daily with warm water. May be decocted with quantities as shown, in which case **sha ren** is added a few minutes before the end of cooking (*hou xia* 后下). **Dang shen, chao bai zhu, chao yi ren, fu ling, chao bian dou, chao shan yao, huang qi** and **zhi gan cao** strengthen the Spleen and supplement *qi*; **bai zhu** dries Damp; **yi ren, fu ling** and **chao bian dou** leach out damp by promoting urination; **lian zi** astringes the Intestines and stops diarrhoea; **jie geng** directs *qi* upwards thus alleviating the diarrhoea; **sha ren** transforms Damp and regulates *qi*. (Source: *Zhong Yi Er Bi Hou Ke Xue*)

Modifications

- With *yang* deficiency (cold extremities, undigested food in the stools, abdominal pain which is better for warmth, and a tight, slow or weak pulse), add **zhi fu zi** (Radix Aconiti Carmichaeli Praeparata) 制附子 6-9g (decocted for 30 minutes prior to the other herbs), and **pao jiang** (quick fried Rhizoma Zingiberis Officinalis) 炮姜 6-9g.
- With prominent Dampness, add **cang zhu** (Rhizoma Atractylodis) 苍术 12-15g.
- With food stagnation, add **shan zha** (Fructus Crataegi) 山楂 15g, **chao mai ya** (dry fried Fructus Hordei Vulgaris Germinantus) 炒麦芽 15-30g and **chao shen qu** (dry fried Massa Fermentata) 炒神曲 15g.

Topical therapy

ZI DANG YOU (*Lithospermum and Angelica Oil* 紫当油, p.684)
Xi Gua Shuang 西瓜霜 (Watermelon Frost)

Patent medicines

Shen Ling Bai Zhu Wan 参苓白术丸 (Shen Ling Bai Zhu Wan)
Li Zhong Wan 理中丸 (Li Zhong Wan)
- Spleen *yang* deficiency

Xi Gua Shuang 西瓜霜 (Watermelon Frost)
- topically to relieve swelling and pain

Acupuncture (select from)

Ren.12 (*zhong wan* +▲) .. *mu* point of the Stomach, warms and strengthens the Spleen and Stomach

St.36 (*zu san li* +▲) .... *he* sea point of the Stomach, powerfully warms and strengthens the Spleen and Stomach and supplements *qi*

Sp.6 (*san yi jiao* +▲) .... strengthens the Spleen, regulates Liver *qi*, benefits the Kidneys and regulates *qi* and Blood

LI.11 (*qu chi* +▲) .... *he* sea point of the Large Intestine, regulates *qi* and Blood, warms the *yang ming* channels when moxaed

Ren.24 (*cheng jiang*) .... local points for lip disease, select one or two
Du.26 (*ren zhong*)
Du.27 (*dui duan*)
St.4 (*di cang*)

- a moxa box over the abdomen is useful
- *Ear points*: spleen, mouth, lips, adrenal, *shen men*

Clinical notes

- In all cases, patients at risk of exposure should be advised to cover the lips with a soothing emollient such as lanolin or chap stick.
- For dietary recommendations, see p.870-873.

SUMMARY OF GUIDING FORMULAE FOR LIP WIND

Wind Damp Heat (Fire) - *Shuang Jie Tong Sheng Tang* 双解通圣散

Wind Heat (Fire) Invasion with Spleen and Stomach Damp Heat - *Si Wu Xiao Feng San* 四物消风散

Liver *qi* stagnation with stagnant Heat, Liver Fire - *Long Dan Xie Gan Tang* 龙胆泻肝汤

- With little Heat - *Xiao Yao San* 逍遥散

Spleen *qi* deficiency - *Shen Ling Bai Zhu San* 参苓白术散

20. Mouth Ulcers

Acute ulcers

External pathogenic invasion

Internal excess Heat

Chronic or recurrent ulcers

Yin deficiency

Yang deficiency

Qi and Blood deficiency

20 MOUTH ULCERS

kou chuang 口疮

Mouth ulcers (*kou chuang*[1]) are a common and sometimes distressing oral disorder, characterised by single or multiple ulcerations on the gums, buccal cavity and/or tongue. The ulcerations may be small (<5mm) or large (>1cm). In mild cases, small ulcerations occur singly or in clusters, and typically heal quickly without scarring. In severe cases, however, multiple ulcers may coalesce to form a large ulcerated area that may persist for weeks and leave a scar. Severe types tend to be recurrent or even continuous, often of many years duration, with new lesions appearing before the old ones heal. Severe ulcers can significantly interfere with a patients health, due to reduced food intake, with possible malnutrition and weight loss.

Mouth ulcers are frequently attributed to pathology of the Heart, Spleen and Stomach. The tongue is the 'sprout of the Heart', and Heart pathology can be reflected in both disordered speech, and physical damage to the tongue tissue itself. A branch of the Spleen channel spreads out on the underside of the tongue, and the mouth in general is the sense organ of the Spleen. The Stomach and *yang ming* channels are closely associated with the gums and buccal cavity.

Mild episodes of mouth ulcers are usually self limiting. Acute cases associated with external pathogens usually resolve spontaneously and with no residual damage. They may occur as a one off event, never appearing again. Patients rarely present in the clinic with these ulcers. The chronic recurrent types are more usual in clinic. TCM treatment is usually quite effective for these ulcers.

There are additional factors to be considered when treating chronic ulcerations. Does the patient chew the buccal cavity or tongue, perhaps unconsciously?, or is the tongue 'fidgeting' around in the mouth, perhaps indicating an anxiety or neurotic state. Are there any structures in the mouth, such as plaque buildup, braces or dentures, that may cause pressure areas and consequent ulceration?.

AETIOLOGY

External pathogens

Invasion of external pathogens is a common cause of acute mouth ulcers, the most common being Heat, usually as Wind Heat, Damp Heat, or in severe cases, Toxic Heat. Any pathogen, however, is capable of causing mouth ulcers, if it transforms into Heat.

---

[1]Wisemans 'Mouth Sore'

The Heart and its associated structures are easily affected by Heat. Heat or Fire in the Heart may occur during severe febrile diseases, when external Heat penetrates deep into the body, lodging at the *ying* or Blood level. In this situation, fever is accompanied by disordered consciousness as the Heat disturbs the *shen*.

BOX 20.1 SOME BIOMEDICAL CAUSES OF THE ORAL PATHOLOGY DESCRIBED IN THIS CHAPTER

- denture pressure
- viral (coxsackievirus, herpes simplex)
- oral thrush
- periodontitis mucosa neurotica recurrens
- Crohn's disease
- ulcerative colitis
- coeliac disease
- Beçhet's syndrome
- blood dyscrasia
- Reiter's syndrome
- allergic reaction to, or side effects of, drugs such as antibiotics, Methotrexate and protease inhibitors
- erosive lichen planus
- apthous stomatitis
- anaemia
- post radiotherapy

Stagnant Heat in the Heart & Stomach/Spleen

Stagnant Heat in the Heart and Stomach/Spleen describes the common pathology underlying recurrent episodes of mouth ulcers. The smouldering Heat predisposes the oral cavity to development of repeated mouth ulcers, which may be triggered by some irritant, emotional upset or heating substance. There may be no obvious trigger. There are two factors that contribute to the generation of this internal Heat, diet and emotional stress. The common dietary cause of this stagnant Heat is the repeated ingestion of heating substances such as chillies, alcohol, sugar and chocolate, spicy food, stimulant drugs (including illicit and prescription), coffee and tobacco. Smouldering Heat in the Stomach and Spleen can also be caused by overindulgence or irregular dietary habits (eating late at night, midnight snacks, eating while upset, eating too quickly etc.). Such habits weaken the Spleen and Stomach and create food stagnation and stagnant Heat.

Prolonged worry, anxiety and depression, or a sudden shock, can retard the movement of Heart *qi*. The resulting accumulation of *qi* creates a focus of pressure in the chest, which then generates Heat further affecting the Heart. This type of *qi* accumulation is slightly different to Liver *qi* stagnation in that the focus of Liver *qi* stagnation is usually below the diaphragm (although its effects may be systemic). Smouldering Heat in the Heart and Heart Fire may also develop if Heat is transmitted from the Liver to the Heart. Heart Fire, like Liver Fire, is more likely to occur in those with some pre-existing Heat, whether from diet or congenital factors.

Once stagnant Heat is present, it can easily be triggered by external pathogens, and emotional or dietary changes.

Phlegm Heat

Phlegm and Phlegm Heat, tend to complicate pre-existing pathology, rather than being a primary cause of oral ulcers. The obstruction by Phlegm to *qi* and Blood circulation in the oral mucous membranes, gums or tongue, makes the ulcers persistent and chronic. The Phlegm or Phlegm Heat may:

- represent a constitutional tendency exacerbated by a rich, fatty diet
- be secondary to *yin* deficiency whereby physiological fluids are scant, and deficient Heat thickens these fluids to Phlegm or Phlegm Heat
- be secondary to Liver *qi* stagnation, which contributes to stasis of body fluids and stagnant Heat, thereby causing thickening of physiological fluids to create Phlegm or Phlegm Heat
- result from a failure of fluid metabolism from *qi* or *yang* deficiency affecting Kidney, Spleen or Heart, leading to an accumulation of fluids which, over time, congeal into Phlegm.

Once Phlegm is present, Heat can be generated by the resulting obstruction.

Table 20.1 Characteristics of mouth ulcers

	Excess type ulcers	Deficient type ulcers
Duration	generally acute and of short duration	chronic or recurrent, can persist for a long time and heal very slowly
Appearance of ulcer	can be small or large, obviously inflamed with a raised red margin and red base; maybe with a thickish yellow or white exudate	mostly small, but may be large, with several ulcers coalescing to involve large patches of the buccal cavity, tongue and gums; the margins may or may not be red, and are not particularly raised; the base of the ulcer may be the same colour as the surrounding tissue or may be an ash grey colour
Halitosis	obvious	absent
Pain	quite painful	mild to moderate pain, or only painful with certain foods, such as citrus and salt
Systemic symptoms	excess: fever, fever and chills, muscle aches, dry stools or constipation, insomnia, thirst, red complexion, irritability, etc.	deficiency: hypofunction, fatigue, obvious signs of Spleen and/or Kidney weakness, or dryness and Heat (yin deficiency)

BOX 20.2 KEY DIAGNOSTIC POINTS

- See Box 10.2, p.386

Yin deficiency with Fire

Mouth ulcers, especially of the tongue, are often the result of Heart Fire which arises from deficiency of Heart and Kidney *yin*. The relationship between the Heart and Kidney is one of the fundamental relationships of the body and mind. This relationship functions on both a physical and a mental level. Kidney Water (*yin*) keeps Heart Fire in check, preventing a runaway blaze and overheating. Heart Fire activates Kidney Water, preventing stagnation and accumulation of fluids.

If Kidney *yin* is damaged by overwork, excess sexual activity, insufficient rest and sleep, ageing, etc., there may be a breakdown in the relationship between the Heart and Kidney (via the controlling cycle). Kidney Water no longer keeps Heart Fire in check, and the resultant Heat further consumes *yin*.

Heart *yin* may be damaged directly by stimulant and recreational drugs, including heavy coffee drinking (or caffeine in chocolate), chronic marijuana use, and especially frequent use of speed or cocaine. Heart *yin* may also be depleted by ongoing mental stress and emotional turmoil.

Loss of communication between the Heart and Kidney can also be acute, following a major shock or trauma, such as the sudden death of a loved one, relationship breakdown, or commonly, a motor vehicle accident. This can occur in otherwise robust individuals. The ulceration, and associated insomnia, dream disturbed sleep, flashbacks, anxiety or panic attacks, are accompanied by fewer systemic symptoms since the *yin* of the organs is not damaged. It may also occur in someone with pre-existing *yin* damage, in which case the deficiency is suddenly exacerbated.

Spleen *yang* (*qi*) deficiency

Yang deficiency mouth ulcers are very chronic and slow to heal. In contrast to ulcers involving Heart pathology, there is little or no emotional component in *yang* deficiency ulcers.

These ulcers typically follow years of significant digestive weakness, and are clearly related (at least initially) to what the patient eats or doesn't eat. Typical factors that contribute to Spleen *yang* deficient ulcers include prolonged or serious illness, prolonged starvation or digestive insult, such as occurs in patients with a history of anorexia nervosa or bulimia, or in women following severe morning sickness. Spleen *yang* is also weakened by excessive consumption of cold raw food and irregular eating habits, or by too many cold natured herbs or antibiotics in the treatment of a febrile or other hot disease. Gastric or abdominal surgery can occasionally damage Spleen *yang*.

Heart Blood and Spleen *qi* deficiency

Mouth ulcers of this type are chronic and recurrent, and usually have both a dietary and emotional component. The ulcers arise because *qi* and Blood are unable to adequately perfuse and nourish the tissues of the mouth.

Overwork, physical and mental exhaustion, worry, irregular diet and too much cold, raw or sweet food can damage the Spleen, which then fails to generate sufficient *qi* and Blood. Similarly, any situation that overwhelms the Spleen's ability to replace *qi* and Blood, like a prolonged or severe illness, can lead to *qi* and Blood deficiency. The primary weakness in this pattern is in the Spleen, which is unable to generate enough Blood to nourish the Heart.

Heart Blood and Spleen *qi* weakness can be more acute, following a postpartum haemorrhage or difficult pregnancy and labour. This pattern is common in women who return to work too soon following pregnancy, without fully recovering their investment of *qi* and Blood. It also occurs in those who breast-feed for lengthy periods of time while expending energy working or looking after demanding children. The elderly are another group who frequently suffer from insufficient *qi* and Blood.

Figure 20.1 *Diagnostic strategy for mouth ulcers*

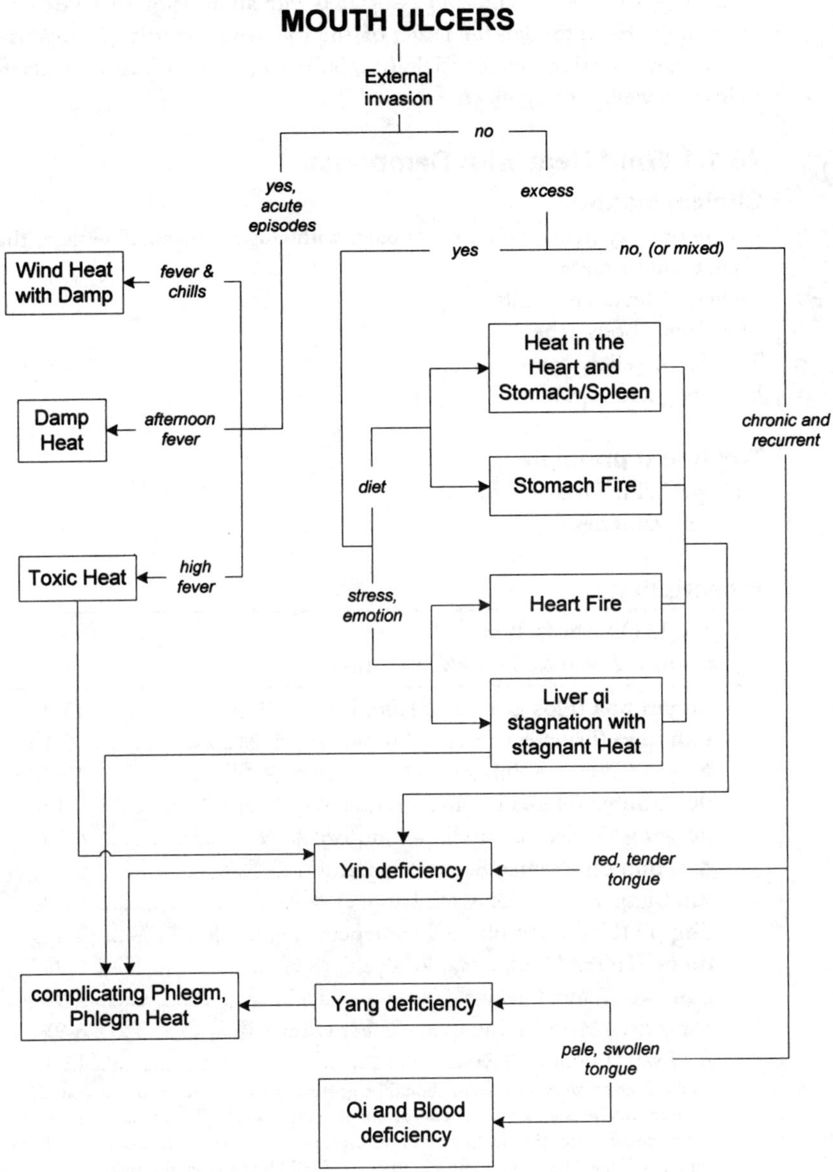

20.1 ACUTE EXTERNAL INVASION

Pathophysiology

- This type of ulcer is acute and associated with an invasion of an external pathogen. Even though the target of the following external pathogens is usually the exterior, Lungs and Spleen/Stomach, the Heat easily affects the Heart as well, causing ulcers.

风热夹湿

20.1.1 Wind Heat with Dampness

Clinical features

- acute oral erythema, redness and pain, with clusters of small vesicles that burst and ulcerate
- fever, or fever and chills
- headache, body aches

T white or yellow coat
P floating and rapid

Treatment principle

Dispel Wind Heat
Drain Dampness

Prescription

YIN QIAO SAN 银翘散
(*Lonicera and Forsythia Formula*) modified

jin yin hua (Flos Lonicerae Japonicae) 金银花 15-30g
lian qiao (Fructus Forsythia Suspensae) 连翘 12-15g
lu gen (Rhizoma Phragmitis Communis) 芦根 15-30g
dan zhu ye (Herba Lophatheri Gracilis) 淡竹叶 9-12g
jie geng (Radix Platycodi Grandiflori) 桔梗 6-9g
dan dou chi (Semen Sojae Preparatum) 淡豆豉 9-12g
niu bang zi (Fructus Arctii Lappae) 牛蒡子 9-12g
jing jie (Herba seu Flos Schizonepetae Tenuifolia) 荆芥 9-12g
bo he (Herba Mentha Haplocalycis) 薄荷 6-9g
gan cao (Radix Glycyrrhizae Uralensis) 甘草 3-9g
tong cao (Medulla Tetrapanacis Papyriferi) 通草 6-9g
hua shi (Talcum) 滑石 12-18g

Method: Decoction. The herbs should be gently simmered for no longer than 20 minutes. **Bo he** is added at the end of cooking (*hou xia* 后下). Take cool or at room temperature. **Jin yin hua** and **lian qiao** clear Heat from the exterior and eliminate Toxic Heat; **niu bang zi** disperses Wind Heat and with **gan cao** and **jie geng**, benefits the throat; **bo he** and **dan dou chi** clear Wind Heat; **jing jie** disperses Wind without drying; **dan zhu ye, lu gen** and **gan cao** generate fluids and stop thirst; **jie geng** promotes the Lungs dispersing function and benefits the throat; **tong cao** and **hua shi** promotes urination to clear Heat through the Urinary Bladder. (Source: *Shi Yong Zhong Yao Xue*)

Modifications

- With predominant Wind (fever and chills, mobile muscle aches, frontal headache), add **fang feng** (Radix Ledebouriellae Divaricatae) 防风 9-12g and **chan tui** (Periostracum Cicadae) 蝉蜕 9-12g.
- With obvious Dampness (heaviness in the head and body, large water or fluid filled vesicles and a thick tongue coat), add **pei lan** (Herba Eupatorii Fortuneii) 佩兰 9-12g, **huo xiang** (Herba Agastaches seu Pogostemi) 藿香 12g-15, **yi ren** (Semen Coicis Lachryma-jobi) 苡仁 18-30g and **che qian zi** (Semen Plantaginis) 车前子 9-12g.
- With strong Heat (high fever, thirst, red tongue), add **huang qin** (Radix Scutellariae Baicalensis) 黄芩 9-12g, **shi gao** (Gypsum) 石膏 15-30g (decocted for 30 minutes prior to the other herbs), and **tian hua fen** (Radix Trichosanthis Kirilowii) 天花粉 12-15g.
- If a viral pathogen is involved, add two or three of the following herbs: **ban lan gen** (Radix Isatidis seu Baphicacanthi) 板蓝根 15-30g, **da qing ye** (Folium Daqingye) 大青叶 15-30g, **hu zhang** (Radix et Rhizoma Polygoni Cuspidati) 虎杖 9-12g, **ye ju hua** (Flos Chrysanthemi Indici) 野菊花 9-12g or **pu gong ying** (Herba Taraxici Mongolici) 蒲公英 15-30g.

Topical therapies

- Decoct **ban lan gen** (Radix Isatidis seu Baphicacanthi) 板蓝根 15g and rinse frequently.
- *Shuang Liao Hou Feng San* 双料喉风散 (Superior Sore Throat Powder) can be applied frequently.
- A strong brew of black tea used to rinse the mouth is soothing. A used teabag can be applied topically.

Patent medicines

Yin Qiao Jie Du Pian 银翘解毒片 (Yin Chiao Chieh Tu Pien, Yinchiao Plus)

Lian Qiao Bai Du Pian 连翘败毒片 (Lien Chiao Pai Tu Pien)

- these two patent medicines are good for the systemic effects of Wind Heat and Toxic Heat

Ban Lan Gen Chong Ji 板蓝根冲剂 (Ban Lan Gen Chong Ji)

Chuan Xin Lian Kang Yan Pian 穿心莲抗炎片 (Chuan Xin Lian Antiphlogistic Tablets)

- these two patent medicines are usually added to enhance the anti-Toxic (specifically antiviral, but also antibacterial) action of the primary prescription

Shuang Liao Hou Feng San 双料喉风散 (Superior Sore Throat Powder)
- topical powder, good when there is infection or suppuration

Acupuncture (select from)

LI.4 (*he gu* -) .... together these points dispel Wind Heat; LI.4
SJ.5 (*wai guan* -) also benefits the mouth and stops pain

LI.11 (*qu chi* -) .... *he* sea point of the Large Intestine, clears Heat and Dampness from *yang ming* and dispels Wind
Lu.11 (*shao shang*) .... *jing* well and Wood point of the Lungs, clears Heat from the Lungs and dispels Wind Heat
Ren.24 (*cheng jiang*) .... local points for oral disease, select one or two
St.6 (*jia che*) closest to the site of the lesion(s)
St.4 (*di cang*)
qian zheng (N-HN-20)
ah shi points .... in the cheeks over the site of the lesion(s)

Du.14 (*da zhui* - Ω) .... meeting point of the *yang* channels, clears Heat and pathogens from the exterior
Bl.12 (*feng men* -Ω) .... dispels Wind and regulates Lung *qi*
Bl.13 (*fei shu* -Ω) .... *shu* point of the Lungs, dispels Wind and regulates Lung *qi*

- with constipation, add SJ.6 (*zhi gou* -) and St.25 (*tian shu* -)
- with cough, add Lu.5 (*chi ze* -)
- *Ear points*: mouth, tongue, lungs, *shen men*

湿热 20.1.2 Damp Heat

Clinical features

- Acute white, porridge like spots or plaques on the tongue, buccal cavity and/or hard palate; if the plaque is scraped off (which may be difficult), an erosion with a red base is revealed. The tongue and mouth are sensitive to certain foods, typically acid, sour or salty foods.
- lethargy, heaviness, muscle aches
- afternoon fever, accompanied by an oozing sweat
- stuffiness and fullness in the chest and abdomen
- poor appetite, thirst with no desire to drink, nausea

T thick and greasy
P slippery and rapid

Treatment principle

Clear Damp Heat, transform and drain Damp

Prescription

GAN LU XIAO DU DAN 甘露消毒丹
(*Sweet Dew Special Pill to Eliminate Toxin*)

yin chen (Herba Artemisiae Yinchenhao) 茵陈 15-24g
hua shi (Talcum) 滑石 15-18g
lian qiao (Fructus Forsythia Suspensae) 连翘 9-12g
huang qin (Radix Scutellariae Baicalensis) 黄芩 9-12g
huo xiang (Herba Agastaches seu Pogostemi) 藿香 12-15g
bai dou kou (Fructus Amomi Kravanh) 白豆蔻 6-9g
she gan (Rhizoma Belamacandae) 射干 9-12g
bo he (Herba Mentha Haplocalycis) 薄荷 6-9g
chuan bei mu (Bulbus Fritillariae Cirrhosae) 川贝母 9-12g
mu tong (Caulis Mutong) 木通 6-9g
shi chang pu (Rhizoma Acori Graminei) 石菖蒲 6-9g

Method: Decoction. The herbs should be gently simmered for no longer than 20 minutes. **Bo he** is added at the end of cooking (*hou xia* 后下). Take cool or at room temperature. **Yin chen**, **mu tong** and **hua shi** clear Damp Heat from the middle and lower body by promoting urination; **huang qin**, **lian qiao** and **bo he** clear Heat from the upper body; **she gan** and **chuan bei mu** clear Heat from the Lungs; **bai kou ren** and **hua xiang** fragrantly transform Dampness; **shi chang pu** clears Dampness from the Head. (Source: *Shi Yong Zhong Yi Nei Ke Xue*)

Topical therapies

- To gently dislodge the spots or plaques, use a piece of sterile gauze dipped in a decoction of **jin yin hua** (Flos Lonicerae Japonicae 金银花), then use a topical powder on the exposed lesions. *Shuang Liao Hou Feng San* 双料喉风散 (Superior Sore Throat Powder) is excellent for this.
- A strong brew of black tea used to rinse the mouth is soothing. A used teabag can be applied topically.

Patent medicines

Huo Xiang Zheng Qi Pian 藿香正气片 (Huo Xiang Zheng Qi Pian)
Xing Jun San 行军散 (Marching Powder, Five Pagodas Brand)
Liu Shen Shui 六神水 (Liu Shen Shui)
Bei Jing Niu Huang Jie Du Pian 北京牛黄解毒片 (Peking Niu Huang Chieh Tu Pien) - This is an excellent remedy for all excess Heat mouth ulcers.
Xi Gua Shuang 西瓜霜 (Watermelon Frost)
- This is an excellent topical remedy for all types of ulcer, both excess and deficient. It stops pain and promotes healing. It comes in two forms, powder and lozenges. The powder can be sprayed directly on the ulcer itself, the lozenges dissolved slowly in the mouth.

Shuang Liao Hou Feng San 双料喉风散 (Superior Sore Throat Powder)
- good when there is infection or suppuration

Acupuncture (select from)

Lu.6 (*kong zui* -) .... together, these points promote the dispersing
LI.4 (*he gu* -) function of the Lungs, clear the exterior and transform Dampness

SJ.6 (*zhi gou* -) .... *jing* river point of the *san jiao*, promotes movement and transformation of *san jiao qi* and aids in clearance of Damp Heat

Sp.9 (*yin ling quan*) .... *he* sea point of the Spleen, promotes urination and drains Dampness through the Urinary Bladder

Ren.24 (*cheng jiang*) .... local points for oral disease, select one or two
St.6 (*jia che*) closest to the site of the lesion(s)
St.4 (*di cang*)
qian zheng (N-HN-20)
ah shi points .... in the cheeks over the site of the lesion(s)

- with high fever, add Du.14 (*da zhui* -)
- with nausea, add PC.6 (*nei guan*)
- with diarrhoea, add *zhi xie* (N-CA-3), Bl.25 (*tian shu*)
- with muscle aches, add Sp.21 (*da bao*)
- with abdominal bloating, add St.36 (*zu san li* -) and St.25 (*tian shu* -)
- *Ear points:* mouth, tongue, spleen, lungs, *shen men*

热毒

20.1.3 Toxic Heat

Clinical features

- Painful, large, hot, yellow or brown scab-like lesions on the buccal cavity and hard palate; the lesions resemble old porridge and the oral cavity is obviously inflamed.
- high fever, or fever with chills or rigors
- constipation
- thirst, with desire for cold drinks
- halitosis

T red with a thick dry yellow coat; the tongue may be swollen
P slippery and rapid, or bounding and rapid

Treatment principle

Clear Toxic Heat, cool the Blood

Prescription

HUANG LIAN JIE DU TANG 黄连解毒汤
(*Coptis and Scute Combination*) modified

huang lian (Rhizoma Coptidis) 黄连 6-9g
huang qin (Radix Scutellariae Baicalensis) 黄芩 9-12g
huang bai (Cortex Phellodendri) 黄柏 9-12g
shan zhi zi (Fructus Gardeniae Jasminoidis) 山栀子 9-12g
xuan shen (Radix Scrophulariae) 玄参 12-24g

Method: Decoction. **Huang lian**, **huang qin** and **huang bai** clear Damp Heat; **huang lian** clears Heat from the Heart and Stomach; **huang qin** clears Heat from the Lungs and upper body; **huang bai** clears Heat from the lower *jiao*; **shan zhi zi** clears Heat from all three *jiao* through the urine; **xuan shen** cools the Blood, nourishes *yin*, softens hardness and disperses Phlegm. (Source: *Shi Yong Zhong Yi Nei Ke Xue*)

Modifications

- With high fever, add **ban lan gen** (Radix Isatidis seu Baphicacanthi) 板蓝根 15-30g and **da qing ye** (Folium Daqingye) 大青叶 15-30g.
- With delirium, disturbances of consciousness or febrile rashes, add **shui niu jiao** (Cornu Bubali) 水牛角 15-30g.
- With severe dryness and thirst, add **shi hu** (Herba Dendrobii) 石斛 12-15g and **tian hua fen** (Radix Trichosanthis Kirilowii) 天花粉 12-15g.
- With constipation, add **da huang** (Radix et Rhizoma Rhei) 大黄 6-9g.

Topical therapies

- Decoct **ban lan gen** (Radix Isatidis seu Baphicacanthi) 板蓝根 15g and rinse frequently.
- A strong brew of black tea used to rinse the mouth is soothing. A used teabag can be applied topically.
- *Shuang Liao Hou Feng San* 双料喉风散 (Superior Sore Throat Powder)

Patent medicines

Bei Jing Niu Huang Jie Du Pian 北京牛黄解毒片 (Peking Niu Huang Chieh Tu Pien) - an excellent remedy for all excess Heat mouth ulcers

Huang Lian Shang Qing Pian 黄连上清片 (Huang Lien Shang Ching Pien)

Huang Lian Jie Du Wan 黄连解毒丸 (Huang Lian Jie Du Wan)

Xi Gua Shuang 西瓜霜 (Watermelon Frost)

- An excellent topical remedy for all types of ulcer, both excess and deficient. It stops pain and promotes healing. It comes in two forms, powder and lozenges. The powder can be sprayed directly on the ulcer itself, the lozenges dissolved slowly in the mouth.

Shuang Liao Hou Feng San 双料喉风散 (Superior Sore Throat Powder)
- especially good when there is infection or suppuration

Acupuncture (select from)

St.44 (*nei ting* -) .... together these points clear Heat from *yang ming*
LI.4 (*he gu* -) and have a special effect on oral pathology

LI.11 (*qu chi* -) .... *he* sea point of the Large Intestine, clears Heat and Damp Heat from *yang ming*
Du.14 (*da zhui* -) .... meeting point of the *yang* channels, excellent for clearing Heat

PC.3 (*qu ze* ↓) .... *he* sea points of the Pericardium and Urinary
Bl.40 (*wei zhong* ↓) Bladder channel respectively, these points cool the Blood and powerfully clear Toxic Heat when bled
PC.9 (*zhong chong* ↓) .... *jing* well and Wood point of the Pericardium, clears Heat

- with unrelenting fever, add *shi xuan* ↓ (M-UE-1)
- with spasms or convulsions, add Du.12 (*shen zhu* -) and Liv.3 (*tai chong* -)
- with severe nausea, add PC.6 (*nei guan*)
- with severe headache, add *tai yang* ↓ (M-HN-9)
- *Ear points:* mouth, tongue, stomach, heart, lungs, *shen men*

Clinical notes

- Excess Heat type mouth ulcers may be diagnosed biomedically as apthous stomatitis, viral stomatitis, acute oral thrush, herpes simplex, hand foot and mouth disease or an acute episode of auto-immune disorder such as Beçhet's syndrome.
- For dietary recommendations, see p.882.

20.2 ACUTE INTERNAL HEAT

心脾积热

The excess Heat patterns are similar in many ways, and in practice are often subtle in their differences and difficult to distinguish clearly. There are, however, different prescriptions depending on the organ system primarily affected. The Heart opens into the tongue and the Spleen into the mouth, so, by extension, non specific ulcerations in the mouth involve these organ systems. Indirectly, the Liver may also be involved via prolonged *qi* stagnation and the generation of stagnant Heat. Stagnant Heat then affects the Heart (via the generating cycle) or the Stomach/Spleen (via the controlling cycle).

Clinical features

Excess Heat in the Heart and Stomach/Spleen

Mouth ulcers which appear with no other systemic signs and symptoms are diagnosed as Heat in the organs which supply the area, the Heart, Spleen and Stomach.

- Single, or more usually, multiple ulcers on the tongue, gums or buccal cavity which, in severe cases, may coalesce into a large ulcerated area. The ulcers are burning and painful, with a yellow or white floor and a red, swollen margin. There may be no clear trigger.

Stomach Heat/Fire

Ulcers related to Stomach Heat will be provoked by overindulgence in heating foods and substances. The appearance of the ulcers is the same as above, with the following additional symptoms:

- the ulcer or ulcers may be concentrated on the gums and buccal cavity
- frequent hunger, halitosis
- tendency to constipation or dry stools
- thirst, dry mouth and lips

T redder in the centre, dry, with a yellow coat

P large in the middle positions, rapid

Heart Fire

Ulcers related to Heart Fire may be provoked by stress or emotional upset.

- the ulcer or ulcers tend to be concentrated on the tongue, particularly towards the anterior
- irritability, restlessness
- insomnia, palpitations
- scanty, concentrated or burning urine

T redder on the tip with a yellow coat

P large in the distal position, especially the left, and rapid

Treatment principle

Clear Heat
Reduce swelling and stop pain

Prescription

20.2.1 With no systemic signs and symptoms

LIANG GE SAN 凉膈散
(*Cool the Diaphragm Powder*) modified

This prescription is selected when the diagnosis is excess Heat in the Heart and Stomach/Spleen

lian qiao (Fructus Forsythia Suspensae) 连翘 12-18g
huang qin (Radix Scutellariae Baicalensis) 黄芩 9-12g
shan zhi zi (Fructus Gardeniae Jasminoidis) 山栀子 9-12g
gan cao (Radix Glycyrrhizae Uralensis) 甘草 6-9g
bo he (Herba Mentha Haplocalycis) 薄荷 6-9g
dan zhu ye (Herba Lophatheri Gracilis) 淡竹叶 9-12g

Method: Decoction. **Bo he** is added near the end of cooking (*hou xia* 后下). **Lian qiao** clears Toxic Heat and cools the Lungs; **huang qin** clears Heat from the upper and middle *jiao*; **shan zhi zi** clears Heat from all three *jiao* through the urine and enters the Heart to relieve irritability; **bo he** clears Heat from the upper body and eases the throat; **dan zhu ye** clears Heat from the Heart and promotes urination. (Source: *Zhong Yi Er Bi Hou Ke Xue*)

Modifications

- With large and very painful ulcers and swelling of the cheeks, add **huang lian** (Rhizoma Coptidis) 黄连 6-9g and **shi chang pu** (Rhizoma Acori Graminei) 石菖蒲 6-9g.
- With obvious Heat, add **huang lian** (Rhizoma Coptidis) 黄连 6-9g and **xuan shen** (Radix Scrophulariae) 玄参 18-24g.
- With constipation, add **da huang** (Radix et Rhizoma Rhei) 大黄 6-9g and **mang xiao** (Mirabilitum) 芒硝 6-9g.
- With pain in the throat and a cough (i.e. Lung and Stomach Heat), add **jie geng** (Radix Platycodi Grandiflori) 桔梗 9-12g, **niu bang zi** (Fructus Arctii Lappae) 牛蒡子 9-12g, **ban lan gen** (Radix Isatidis seu Baphicacanthi) 板蓝根 15-30g and **shan dou gen** (Radix Sophorae Tonkinensis) 山豆根 9-12g.
- With blister-like eruptions that precede the ulcers (i.e. Dampness and Heat), add **yi ren** (Semen Coicis Lachryma-jobi) 苡仁 18-30g, **hua shi** (Talc) 滑石 15-18g and **che qian zi** (Semen Plantaginis) 车前子 9-12g.
- With mild signs of *yin* deficiency, add **sheng di** (Radix Rehmanniae Glutinosae) 生地 12-15g and **mai dong** (Tuber Ophiopogonis Japonici) 麦冬 9-12g.

20.2.2 With mild Stomach/Spleen Heat

XIE HUANG SAN 泻黄散
(*Drain the Yellow Powder*)

This elegant prescription uses both cooling and dispersing herbs to reveal, and then cool and clear, the hidden Heat that afflicts the Stomach/Spleen.

shi gao (Gypsum) 石膏 12-18g
shan zhi zi (Fructus Gardeniae Jasminoidis) 山栀子 9-12g
fang feng (Radix Ledebouriellae Divaricatae) 防风 9-12g
huo xiang (Herba Agastaches seu Pogostemi) 藿香 9-15g
gan cao (Radix Glycyrrhizae Uralensis) 甘草 3-6g

Method: Decoction. **Shi gao** is decocted for 30 minutes prior to the other herbs (*xian jian* 先煎). **Shi gao** clears Heat from the Spleen and Stomach; **shan zhi zi** clears Heat from all three *jiao* through the urine, and enters the Heart to relieve irritability; **fang feng**, being pungent, warm and light in nature, aids in dispersal of smouldering Heat, enabling the cooling herbs to clear the Heat; **huo xiang's** fragrant nature revives the Spleen and invigorates the *qi* mechanism, it also assists **fang feng** in uncovering the Heat so it can be cleared; **gan cao** harmonises and protects the Stomach. (Source: *Zui Xin Fang Ji Shou Ce*)

20.2.3 With vigorous Stomach Heat/Fire

QING WEI TANG 清胃汤
(*Clear the Stomach Decoction*)

This prescription is suitable when there are clear signs of vigorous Stomach Heat without constipation.

shi gao (Gypsum) 石膏 18-30g
huang qin (Radix Scutellariae Baicalensis) 黄芩 9-12g
sheng di (Radix Rehmanniae Glutinosae) 生地 12-15g
mu dan pi (Cortex Moutan Radicis) 牡丹皮 9-12g
huang lian (Rhizoma Coptidis) 黄连 6-9g
sheng ma (Rhizoma Cimicifugae) 升麻 3-6g

Method: Decoction. **Shi gao** is decocted for 30 minutes prior to the other herbs (*xian jian* 先煎). **Shi gao** clears Heat from the Spleen and Stomach; **huang qin** and **huang lian** clear Heat from the Lungs, Heart and Stomach; **sheng di** cools the Blood and nourishes Stomach *yin*; **mu dan pi** cools the Blood; **sheng ma** raises and disperses Heat, and enables the other cooling herbs to more thoroughly access and clear the Heat; the rising nature of **sheng ma** is nicely balanced with the descending nature of the cooling herbs, thus enabling Heat to be cleared and dispersed without causing damage to *qi* or *yin*. (Source: *Zhong Yi Er Bi Hou Ke Xue*)

20.2.4 With vigorous Stomach Heat and constipation

TIAO WEI CHENG QI TANG 调味承气汤
(*Regulate the Stomach and Order the Qi Decoction*)

This prescription is selected when there is Stomach Heat with quite severe constipation. Only use until the bowels move, then use **QING WEI TANG** (above).

da huang (Radix et Rhizoma Rhei) 大黄 6-9g
mang xiao (Mirabilitum) 芒硝 9-12g
gan cao (Radix Glycyrrhizae Uralensis) 甘草 3-6g

Method: Decoction. **Da huang** purges the Intestines and clears Heat; **mang xiao** purges the Intestines, softens hardness and assists **da huang** in moving a hard stool; **gan cao** protects the Stomach. (Source: *Zhong Yi Er Bi Hou Ke Xue*)

20.2.5 Heart Fire

DAO CHI SAN 导赤散
(*Rehmannia and Akebia Formula*)

This prescription clears Fire from the Heart to treat ulcers affecting the tongue.

sheng di (Radix Rehmanniae Glutinosae) 生地 15-30g
dan zhu ye (Herba Lophatheri Gracilis) 淡竹叶 9-12g
mu tong (Caulis Mutong) 木通 3-6g
gan cao shao (tips of Radix Glycyrrhizae Uralensis) 甘草梢 3-6g

Method: Decoction. **Sheng di** cools the Blood and nourishes *yin*; **mu tong** clears Heat from the Heart and promotes urination; **dan zhu ye** clears Heat and promotes urination; **gan cao shao** harmonises the other herbs and alleviates painful urination. (Source: *Zhong Yi Er Bi Hou Ke Xue*)

Modifications (applies to all prescriptions where not already included)

- With severe Heat or Heart Fire, irritability and insomnia, add **huang lian** (Rhizoma Coptidis) 黄连 6g.
- With painful urination, add **chi fu ling** (Sclerotium Poriae Cocos Rubrae) 赤茯苓 9-12g, **zhu ling** (Sclerotium Polypori Umbellati) 猪苓 9-12g and **ze xie** (Rhizoma Alismatis Orientalis) 泽泻 9-12g.
- If the lesions are vesicular or fluid filled, combine with **WU LING SAN** (*Hoelen Five Formula* 五苓散, p.910).
- With mild signs of *yin* deficiency, add **shi hu** (Herba Dendrobii) 石斛 9-12g and **zhi mu** (Rhizoma Anemarrhenae Asphodeloidis) 知母 9-12g.

Variations and additional prescriptions

Liver qi stagnation with stagnant Heat

- In cases with prolonged Liver *qi* stagnation, the stagnant Heat generated may affect the Heart and/or Spleen/Stomach, causing oral ulcers provoked by stress. In addition to the ulcers, the clinical features are irritability, chronic neck and upper back tension, temporal headaches, facial flushing, a tendency to constipation, red edges and tip on the tongue and a wiry, rapid pulse. The aim of treatment is to regulate *qi* and clear stagnant Heat from the Liver and Heart with **DAN ZHI XIAO YAO SAN** (*Bupleurum and Paeonia Formula* 丹栀逍遥散) modified.

chai hu (Radix Bupleuri) 柴胡 9-12g
bai shao (Radix Paeoniae Lactiflora) 白芍 12-18g
fu ling (Sclerotium Poriae Cocos) 茯苓 12-15g
shan zhi zi (Fructus Gardeniae Jasminoidis) 山栀子 9-12g
dang gui (Radix Angelicae Sinensis) 当归 9-12g
bai zhu (Rhizoma Atractylodes Macrocephalae) 白术 9-12g
mu dan pi (Cortex Moutan Radicis) 牡丹皮 9-12g
zhi gan cao (honey fried Radix Glycyrrhizae Uralensis) 炙甘草 3-6g
huang lian (Rhizoma Coptidis) 黄连 3-6g
dan zhu ye (Herba Lophatheri Gracilis) 淡竹叶 9-12g

Method: Decoction. **Chai hu** and **bai shao** regulate and move Liver *qi*; **fu ling**, **bai zhu** and **zhi gan cao** strengthen the Spleen; **fu ling** leaches out Damp and promotes urination; **bai zhu** dries Damp; **dang gui** and **bai shao** nourish Blood and soften the Liver; **shan zhi zi** and **mu dan pi** cool the Liver and Heart and clear stagnant Heat; **huang lian** and **dan zhu ye** clear Heat from the Heart.

Ulcers following radiotherapy

- Mouth ulcers, inflammation, or other oral lesions that occur in the aftermath of radiotherapy for neoplasms of the head or neck, are usually associated with damage to *yin* in combination with localised accumulation of Toxic Heat. Oral dryness, thirst, pain and bleeding are common. The aim of treatment is to nourish *yin*, generate fluids and clear Toxic Heat with **ZI YIN GAN LU YIN** (*Sweet Dew Decoction to Nourish Yin* 滋阴甘露饮) modified.

sheng di (Radix Rehmanniae Glutinosae) 生地 12-18g
shu di (Radix Rehmanniae Glutinosae Conquitae) 熟地 12-18g
xuan shen (Radix Scrophulariae) 玄参 18-24g
mai dong (Tuber Ophiopogonis Japonici) 麦冬 9-15g
tian dong (Tuber Asparagi Cochinchinensis) 天冬 9-15g
shi hu (Herba Dendrobii) 石斛 9-15g
jiu huang qin (wine fried Radix Scutellariae Baicalensis) 酒黄芩 9-12g
zhi ke (Fructus Citri Aurantii) 枳壳 9-12g
gan cao (Radix Glycyrrhizae Uralensis) 甘草 6-9g

zhi mu (Rhizoma Anemarrhenae Asphodeloidis) 知母 9-12g
tian hua fen (Radix Trichosanthis Kirilowii) 天花粉 12-15g
bai mao gen (Rhizoma Imperatae Cylindricae) 白茅根 30g

Method: Decoction. **Sheng di**, **xuan shen** and **mai dong** make up **Zeng Ye Tang** (*Increase the Fluids Decoction* 增液汤) an important prescription for nourishing *yin* and generating fluids; **shu di** nourishes Kidney *yin*; **sheng di** and **xuan shen** cool the Blood; **mai dong**, **tian dong** and **shi hu** nourish Stomach *yin* and clear Heat; **zhi ke** regulates and directs *qi* downwards and harmonises the Stomach; **huang qin** clears Damp Heat; **gan cao** clears Heat and protects the Stomach; **zhi mu** nourishes *yin*, clears Heat and generates fluids; **tian hua fen** clears Heat and generates fluids; **bai mao gen** clears Heat from the Lungs and Stomach and stops bleeding. (Source: *Xiao Hua Ke Zhuan Bing*)

Topical therapies (apply to all internal Heat types)

The main aim of external treatment is to clear Heat and Toxins, reduce swelling, stop pain and promote healing.

Mouth wash

- Decoct **jin yin hua** (Flos Lonicerae Japonicae) 金银花 15g and **bo he** (Herbs Mentha Haplocalycis) 薄荷 9g (added at the end), and rinse several times daily.
- A wet cooled teabag (ordinary english style tea) can be applied directly to the ulcerated area.

Powder

- There are various powders available commercially and others that can be made up, depending on need. Powders are finely ground herbs that are blown directly onto the ulcers with a straw or other appropriate implement. Most practical are the widely available patent powders *Xi Gua Shuang* 西瓜霜 (Water Melon Frost) and *Shuang Liao Hou Feng San* 双料喉风散 (Superior Sore Throat Powder). Powders, such as the following, can also be manufactured from raw materials and stored for lengthy periods without deterioration. In all cases, powders are applied to the ulcers 3-5 times daily.

20.2.6 Mild cases

BING PENG SAN 冰硼散
(*Borneol and Borax Powder*) modified

This formula is good for mild cases, and is suitable for sore throat as well.

bing pian (Borneol) 冰片 1.5g
xuan ming fen (Mirabilitum Purum) 玄明粉 15g
peng sha (Borax) 硼砂 15g

Method: Grind the substances to a powder. Blow a small amount onto affected area 2-3 times daily. (Source: *Zhong Yi Er Bi Hou Ke Xue*)

NB: The original prescription contains the mercury compound **zhu sha** (Cinnabaris) 朱砂 1.8g

20.2.7 Severe cases

ZHU HUANG SAN 珠黄散
(*Mother of Pearl and Cow Gallstone Powder*) modified

This formula is for severe cases. Also used for very sore throats.

huang lian (Rhizoma Coptidis) 黄连 1.5g
qing dai (Indigo Pulverata Levis) 青黛 3g
hai er cha (Pasta Acaciae seu Uncariae) 孩儿茶 3g
xuan ming fen (Mirabilitum Purum) 玄明粉 1.5g
peng sha (Borax) 硼砂 3g
niu huang (Calculus Bovis) 牛黄 1g
bo he (Herbs Mentha Haplocalycis) 薄荷 1.5g
wu mei (Fructus Pruni Mume) 乌梅 1g
zhen zhu (Margarita) 珍珠 1g

Method: Grind the substances to a powder. Blow a small amount onto affected area 2-3 times daily. (Source: *Zhong Yi Er Bi Hou Ke Xue*)

Patent medicines

Bei Jing Niu Huang Jie Du Pian 北京牛黄解毒片 (Peking Niu Huang Chieh Tu Pien) - an excellent remedy for all excess Heat mouth ulcers

Huang Lian Shang Qing Pian 黄连上清片 (Huang Lien Shang Ching Pien)

Qing Fei Yi Huo Pian 清肺抑火片 (Ching Fei Yi Huo Pien)
- Lung and Stomach Heat

Xi Gua Shuang 西瓜霜 (Watermelon Frost)
- This is an excellent topical remedy for all types of ulcer, both excess and deficient. It stops pain and promotes healing. It comes in two forms, powder and lozenges. The powder can be sprayed directly on the ulcer itself, the lozenges dissolved slowly in the mouth.

Shuang Liao Hou Feng San 双料喉风散 (Superior Sore Throat Powder)
- especially when there is infection or suppuration

Acupuncture (select from)

St.44 (*nei ting* -) .... together these points clear Heat from *yang ming*
LI.4 (*he gu* -) and have a special effect on oral pathology

Ren.12 (*zhong wan* -) .... *mu* point of the Stomach, clears Heat from the Stomach

PC.8 (*lao gong* -) .... *rong* spring and Fire point of the Pericardium, drains Heat from the Stomach channel, cools the Blood and clears Heart Fire

St.36 (*zu san li* -) .... *he* sea point of the Stomach, regulates and clears the Spleen and Stomach

Ren.24 (*cheng jiang*) .... local points for oral disease, select one or two
St.6 (*jia che*) closest to the site of the lesion(s)
St.4 (*di cang*)
qian zheng (N-HN-20)
ah shi points .... in the cheeks over the site of the lesion(s)

- with severe Heart Fire, add Ht.9 (*shao chong* ↓) and Ht.7 (*shen men*)
- with severe Stomach Fire, add St.45 (*li dui* ↓)
- with severe oral pain, add St.41 (*jie xi* -)
- with constipation, add SJ.6 (*zhi gou* -) and St.25 (*tian shu* -)
- *Ear points:* mouth, tongue, heart, spleen, stomach, lungs, *shen men*. Select ear points according to the location of the lesions and the organ system relationships. For example for ulcers on the anterior tongue, use heart and lung. For ulcers on the edges of the tongue use liver, on the buccal cavity use spleen, on the gums use stomach.

Clinical notes

- Excess Heat type mouth ulcers may be diagnosed biomedically as apthous stomatitis, viral stomatitis, acute episode of Beçhet's syndrome or Reiter's syndrome, post radiation stomatitis or ulcerative stomatitis.
- For dietary recommendations, see p.882.

陰虛火旺

CHRONIC OR RECURRENT MOUTH ULCERS

20.3 YIN DEFICIENCY

• with Phlegm or Phlegm Heat

Yin deficiency is a common cause of chronic and recurrent mouth ulcers. The ulcers may be of many years standing, or may occur following an acute febrile illness that consumes the *yin*. There are several suitable prescriptions, depending on the balance of involved organ systems, aetiology and accompanying symptoms. *Yin* deficiency mouth ulcers are often complicated by Phlegm or Phlegm Heat.

Heart and Kidney *yin* deficiency

Pathophysiology

- Heart and Kidney *yin* deficiency mouth ulcers are the most common variety of chronic or recurrent ulcerations. The persistent deficiency of Heart *yin* predisposes the oral cavity, in particular the tongue, to damage. The low grade Heat rises and irritates the tissues of the tongue. When sufficiently strong, or triggered by an increase in emotional stress, the Heat scorches and dries the surface of the tongue and tissue sloughs off.

Clinical features

- Recurrent mouth ulcers, which appear in clusters and tend to aggregate on the tongue or tongue tip. The ulcers are painful and hot, with a narrow, slightly swollen, mildly red margin. They frequently recur and persist for up to several weeks before resolving. Often of many years duration, the ulcers tend to be provoked or aggravated when the patient is stressed, anxious or upset.
- nervy, anxious individual
- insomnia, vivid dreaming, panic attacks
- palpitations, forgetfulness, dizziness, tinnitus
- lower back ache
- sensation of heat in the palms and soles ('five Hearts hot')
- dry mouth and throat
- nightsweats

T red with little or no coat, redder at the tip
P thready and rapid

Treatment principle

Nourish Heart and Kidney *yin*
Clear Heat, calm the *shen*

Prescription

20.3.1 Heart and Kidney *yin* deficiency

TIAN WANG BU XIN DAN 天王补心丹
(*Ginseng and Zizyphus Formula*) modified

This is the representative formula for Heart and Kidney *yin* (and *qi*) deficiency patterns and is excellent for patterns characterised by chronic oral ulceration and *shen* disturbance.

sheng di (Radix Rehmanniae Glutinosae) 生地 .... 120 (24)g
xuan shen (Radix Scrophulariae) 玄参 .... 30 (18)g
tian dong (Tuber Asparagi Cochinchinensis) 天冬 .... 30 (12)g
mai dong (Tuber Ophiopogonis Japonici) 麦冬 .... 30 (12)g
suan zao ren (Semen Zizyphi Spinosae) 酸枣仁 .... 30 (12)g
dan shen (Radix Salviae Miltiorrhizae) 丹参 .... 15 (12)g
fu ling (Sclerotium Poriae Cocos) 茯苓 .... 15 (12)g
dang gui (Radix Angelicae Sinensis) 当归 .... 30 (9)g
wu wei zi (Fructus Schizandrae Chinensis) 五味子 .... 30 (9)g
bai zi ren (Semen Biotae Orientalis) 柏子仁 .... 30 (9)g
ren shen (Radix Ginseng) 人参 .... 15 (9)g
jie geng (Radix Platycodi Grandiflori) 桔梗 .... 15 (9)g
yuan zhi (Radix Polygalae Tenuifoliae) 远志 .... 15 (6)g
lian xin (Plumula Nelumbinis Nuciferae) 莲心 .... 15 (6)g

Method: Grind herbs to a powder and form into 9-gram pills with honey. The dose is one pill 2-3 times daily. May also be decocted with the quantities in brackets. **Sheng di** and **xuan shen** nourish Kidney *yin* to restrain Heart Fire, and cool the Blood; **tian dong** and **mai dong** nourish *yin*; **dan shen** and **dang gui** nourish and regulate Blood and prevent the supplementing herbs from causing stasis; **suan zao ren**, **bai zi ren** and **yuan zhi** calm the *shen*; **ren shen** (or **dang shen**) and **fu ling** strengthen the Spleen and supplement *qi*; **wu wei zi** and **lian xin** astringe Heart *qi* and *yin* and calm the *shen*; **jie geng** conducts the action of the other herbs to the upper body; **xuan shen** and **yuan zhi** transform Phlegm.

20.3.2 Kidney *yin* deficiency with deficient Heat

ZHI BAI BA WEI WAN 知柏八味丸
(*Anemarrhena, Phellodendron and Rehmannia Formula*) modified

This prescription is selected when the Kidney *yin* deficiency and deficient Heat is prominent, with signs and symptoms such as facial flushing, heat in the palms and soles, nightsweats and a red peeled tongue.

shu di (Radix Rehmanniae Glutinosae Conquitae) 熟地 18-24g
shan yao (Radix Dioscoreae Oppositae) 山药 12-18g
shan zhu yu (Fructus Corni Officinalis) 山茱萸 12-15g
fu ling (Sclerotium Poria Cocos) 茯苓 12-15g

mu dan pi (Cortex Moutan Radicis) 牡丹皮 9-12g
ze xie (Rhizoma Alismatis Orientalis) 泽泻 9-12g
zhi mu (Rhizoma Anemarrhenae Asphodeloidis) 知母 9-12g
huang bai (Cortex Phellodendri) 黄柏 9-12g
xuan shen (Radix Scrophulariae) 玄参 18-24g

Method: Grind the herbs to powder and form into 9-gram pills with honey. The dose is 2-3 pills daily. May also be decocted with the quantities as shown. **Shu di** and **shan yao** nourish Liver and Kidney *yin*; **shan yao** strengthens the Spleen and nourishes *yin*, **fu ling** strengthens the Spleen and promotes urination, **ze xie** promotes urination; **mu dan pi** cools the Blood and eliminates stagnant Blood. Together these last three herbs moderate the cloying and stagnation inducing tendency of the *yin* supplementing herbs. **Zhi mu** and **huang bai** clear deficient Heat; **xuan shen** cools the Blood, nourishes *yin* and transforms Phlegm. (Source: *Shi Yong Er Bi Hou Ke Xue*)

Variations and additional prescriptions

Ulcers in the aftermath of a febrile illness

- If mouth ulcers appear in the aftermath of a febrile disease that has damaged Heart *yin*, the correct treatment is to clear Fire, nourish *yin*, stop irritability and calm the *shen* with **HUANG LIAN E JIAO TANG** (*Coptis and Ass-Hide Gelatin Decoction* 黄连阿胶汤) modified.

huang lian (Rhizoma Coptidis) 黄连 9-12g
huang qin (Radix Scutellariae Baicalensis) 黄芩 6-12g
e jiao (Gelatinum Corii Asini) 阿胶 9-12g
bai shao (Radix Paeoniae Lactiflora) 白芍 6-15g
ji zi huang (egg yolk) .... 2 yolks
gou qi zi (Fructus Lycii) 枸杞子 12-15g

Method: Decoction. **E jiao** is melted in the hot strained decoction (*yang hua* 烊化). The egg yolks are stirred into the strained decoction. **Huang lian** and **huang qin** clear Heart Fire; **e jiao** nourishes Heart *yin* and Blood; **bai shao** assists **e jiao** in nourishing *yin*; **ji zi huang** assists **e jiao** in nourishing *yin* and Blood and at the same time clears Heat; **gou qi zi** nourishes *yin* and Blood. (Source: *Shi Yong Zhong Yi Nei Ke Xue*)

With Phlegm Heat

- If *yin* deficiency is complicated by Phlegm Heat, ulcers tend to be resistant and more difficult to treat. The presence of the Phlegm may be surmised if:
  1. The mouth ulcers of a patient with an obvious *yin* deficiency pattern fail to respond noticeably to an appropriate *yin* supplementing treatment within 1-2 months.
  2. The ulcers ooze a sticky yellow or white mucus like material.
  3. In between episodes of actual ulceration, the mouth and tongue feel tender and raw. This tenderness is aggravated by spicy, sour and salty foods.

4. The patient appears relatively robust, despite the length of the illness and the obvious presence, albeit intermittently, of *yin* deficiency symptoms. Energy and vitality remain good. The pulse may be thready or otherwise weak, reflecting the deficiency in between episodes of ulceration, and slippery, wiry or otherwise of an excess type during periods of ulceration, reflecting the ascendency of the Phlegm.

- When the presence of Phlegm is suspected as a complication of *yin* deficiency, or another primary pathology, it should be moistened and softened with salty herbs so as to facilitate its dispersal. Usually two or three appropriate Phlegm softening herbs will be added to, (or increased in dosage if already included), the appropriate guiding prescription. Especially suitable herbs include **xuan shen** (Radix Scrophulariae) 玄参, **zhe bei mu** (Bulbus Fritillariae Thunbergii) 浙贝母 and **mu li** (Concha Ostreae) 牡蛎. Together these three herbs form the base Phlegm nodule resolving formula **XIAO LUO WAN** (*Reduce Scrophula Pill* 消瘰丸, p.910).
- Other herbs that may be considered include **gua lou** (Fructus Trichosanthis) 瓜楼 15-24g, **tian hua fen** (Radix Trichosanthis Kirilowii) 天花粉 9-12g, **hai ge ke** (Concha Cyclinae Sinensis) 海蛤壳 9-15g, **hai fu shi** (Pumice) 海浮石 9-12 and **wa leng zi** (Concha Arcae) 瓦楞子 9-15g.

Topical therapies

Powders

see Patent Medicines

Mouth wash

- Steep 10 grams of **rou gui** (Cortex Cinnamomi Cassiae) 肉桂 in one cup of hot water for 10 minutes and gargle with the cooled liquid.

Patent medicines

Tian Wang Bu Xin Dan 天王补心丹 (Emperors Tea, Tien Wang Pu Hsin Tan) - Heart and Kidney *yin* deficiency

Zhi Bai Ba Wei Wan 知柏八味丸 (Zhi Bai Ba Wei Wan, Chih Pai Pa Wei Wan) - Kidney *yin* deficiency with deficient Heat

Xi Gua Shuang 西瓜霜 (Watermelon Frost)

- An excellent topical remedy for all types of ulcer, both excess and deficient. It stops pain and promotes healing. It comes in two forms, powder and lozenges. The powder can sprayed directly on the ulcer itself, the lozenges dissolved slowly in the mouth.

Shuang Liao Hou Feng San 双料喉风散 (Superior Sore Throat Powder)

- especially good when there is lots of heat

Hai Zao Wan 海藻丸 (Hai Zao Wan)
- add to one of the above constitutional patent medicines when there is Phlegm

Wen Dan Wan 温胆丸 (Wen Dan Wan)
- add to one of the above constitutional patent medicines when there is Phlegm Heat

Acupuncture (select from)

Kid.6 (*zhao hai* +) .... together these points open *yin qiao mai* and *ren*
Lu.7 (*lie que* +) *mai*, nourish *yin*, clear Heat and benefit the mouth and throat

Ht.8 (*shao fu* -) .... *rong* spring and Fire point of the Heart, clears Heart Fire and calms the *shen*
LI.4 (*he gu*) .... special point for all oral disorders
St.36 (*zu san li* +) .... *he* sea point of the Stomach, powerfully strengthens the Spleen and Stomach and supplements Stomach *qi* and *yin*
Sp.6 (*san yin jiao* +) .... with Ren.4, nourishes *yin* of the whole body
Kid.3 (*tai xi* +) .... *yuan* point to nourish Kidney *yin*
Ren.4 (*guan yuan* +) .... meeting point of the *yin* channels, nourishes *yin* of whole body, especially with Sp.6
Bl.15 (*xin shu* +) .... *shu* point of the Heart, nourishes Heart *yin* and clears Heat from the Heart
Bl.20 (*pi shu* +) .... *shu* point of the Spleen, nourishes Spleen and Stomach *qi* and *yin*
Bl.23 (*shen shu* +) .... *shu* point of the Kidney, nourishes Kidney *yin*

Ren.24 (*cheng jiang*) .... local points for oral disease, select one or two
St.6 (*jia che*) closest to the site of the lesion(s)
St.4 (*di cang*)
qian zheng (N-HN-20)
ah shi points .... in the cheeks over the site of the lesion(s)

- if the ulceration is predominantly on the tongue, add *jin jin* ↓ (M-HN-20) and *yu ye* ↓ (M-NH-20)
- with Phlegm, add St.40 (*feng long* -) and PC.5 (*jian shi* -)
- with Phlegm Heat, add PC.8 (*lao gong* -), Lu.6 (*kong zui* -) and Liv.2 (*xing jian* -)
- **wu zhu yu** (Fructus Evodiae Rutaecarpae) 吴茱萸 5g can be powdered and mixed with vinegar to form a paste and applied bilaterally to Kid.1 (*yong quan*). Tape the paste in place with a sticking plaster or bandage and keep dry. Best applied at night and left on

until morning. This treatment redirects the errant Fire back to its source (the Kidneys).

- *Ear points:* mouth, tongue, *shen men*; lungs, heart, liver, kidney, spleen, stomach. Select ear points according to the location of the lesions and the organ system relationships. For example for ulcers on the anterior tongue, use heart and lung. For ulcers on the edges of the tongue use liver, on the buccal cavity use spleen, on the gums use stomach.

Clinical notes

- *Yin* deficiency type mouth ulcers may be diagnosed biomedically as chronic apthous stomatitis, ulcerative stomatitis, auto-immune disorders such as Reiter's syndrome and Beçhet's syndrome, ulcerative colitis, Crohn's disease or periodontitis mucosa neurotica recurrens.
- These ulcers can be difficult to treat, especially when complicated by Phlegm, but do eventually respond to correct treatment. In most cases, of 3-9 months of therapy will be required for satisfactory long term results.
- For dietary recommendations, see p.876.

阳虚口疮

20.4 YANG DEFICIENCY

Pathophysiology

- *Yang* deficient mouth ulcers occur because *yang* circulation is unable to adequately repair any breach in the mucous membrane of the mouth. In contrast to *yin* deficiency, where a degree of Heat scorches and dries the mucous membranes, here the mucous membranes are soggy and flaccid, and *yang* simply cannot infiltrate all areas of the mouth.
- Most frequently, the deficiency affects the Spleen; the Kidney will usually be involved to some degree, mostly as a secondary effect of Spleen *yang* deficiency draining Kidney *yang*.

Clinical features

- Chronic, recurrent and often extensive ulceration of the gums and buccal cavity, less often the tongue. The ulcerations are not particularly painful, but are sensitive to certain foods, particularly fruit and salt. The colour of the floor of the ulcerated area is much the same as the surrounding mucous membrane, or appears ash grey. The margins are narrow and not raised. New areas of ulceration often begin before the old ulcers have healed.
- swollen tissues of the buccal cavity, so the inner cheeks press upon the teeth, and leave a ridge like elevation of tissue along the bite line
- severe abdominal bloating; abdomen may feel cool when palpated
- poor appetite; often a restricted diet because of avoidance of aggravating foods, and subsequent weight loss
- diarrhoea with undigested food in the stools
- cold extremities, cold intolerance
- puffy eyes and fingers
- fatigue, weakness, depression
- **with weak Kidney *yang*:** lower back ache, frequent urination and nocturia, or scanty urination and oedema in the lower body, loss of hearing, tinnitus

T swollen, pale with tooth marks and a thin, white coat
P deep, weak

Treatment principle

Warm and supplement Spleen and Kidney *yang*

Prescription

20.4.1 Spleen *yang* deficiency

FU ZI LI ZHONG WAN 附子理中丸
(*Aconite, Ginseng and Ginger Formula*)

zhi fu zi (Radix Aconiti Carmichaeli Praeparata) 制附子 9-15g
gan jiang (Rhizoma Zingiberis Officinalis) 干姜 9-12g

dang shen (Radix Codonopsis Pilosulae) 党参 15-24g
chao bai zhu (dry fried Rhizoma Atractylodis Macrocephalae) 炒白术 12-15g
zhi gan cao (honey fried Radix Glycyrrhizae Uralensis) 炙甘草 6-9g

Method: Grind herbs into powder and form into 3-gram pills with honey. The dose is one pill 2-3 times daily on an empty stomach. May also be prepared as a decoction, in which case **zhi fu zi** is cooked for 30 minutes prior to the other herbs (*xian jian* 先煎). **Zhi fu zi** powerfully warms Spleen and Stomach *yang*, dispels Cold and invigorates the circulation of *qi* and Blood; **gan jiang** warms Spleen and Stomach *yang* and dispels Cold; **dang shen** supplements *qi* and strengthens the Spleen; **chao bai zhu** strengthens the Spleen and dries Dampness; **zhi gan cao** supplements *qi* and harmonises the Stomach.

20.4.2 Kidney *yang* deficiency

JIN KUI SHEN QI WAN 金匮肾气丸
(*Rehmannia Eight Formula*)

This prescription can be selected as the primary prescription, or can be combined with the previous prescription (without doubling of common ingredients), when there are elements of Kidney *yang* deficiency. It can also be introduced after a period of Spleen *yang* strengthening treatment.

shu di (Radix Rehmanniae Glutinosae Conquitae) 熟地...... 15-24g
shan yao (Radix Dioscoreae Oppositae) 山药 15-18g
shan zhu yu (Fructus Corni Officinalis) 山茱萸 12-15g
fu ling (Sclerotium Poria Cocos) 茯苓 12-15g
ze xie (Rhizoma Alismatis Orientalis) 泽泻 9-12g
mu dan pi (Cortex Moutan Radicis) 牡丹皮 6-9g
zhi fu zi (Radix Aconiti Carmichaeli Praeparata) 制附子 6-12g
rou gui (Cortex Cinnamomi Cassiae) 肉桂 3-6g

Method: Grind the herbs to powder and form into 9-gram pills with honey. The dose is 2-3 pills daily. May also be decocted with quantities as shown. When decocted, **zhi fu zi** is cooked for 30 minutes before the other herbs are added (*xian jian* 先煎), **rou gui** is added towards the end of cooking (*hou xia* 后下). **Shu di** and **shan zhu yu** nourish Liver and Kidney; **shan yao** strengthens the Spleen and nourishes *qi* and *yin*; **fu ling**, **ze xie** and **mu dan pi** regulate the Spleen, Kidneys and Liver and moderate the cloying tendency of the supplementing herbs; **zhi fu zi** and **rou gui** warm *yang*, dispel Cold, unblock the channels, promote the transformation of *qi* and improve fluid metabolism. (Source: *Shi Yong Zhong Yi Nei Ke Xue*)

Variations and additional prescriptions

Difficult or resistant ulcerations

- In resistant cases, with the possibility of Phlegm accumulation, consider **YANG HE TANG** (*Yang-Heartening Decoction* 阳和汤). This formula can be used topically, as a mouthwash, and taken internally. If the formula is modified, the relative proportions of **shu di** to **ma huang** must be maintained. After the ulcers have resolved, one of the above formulae may be given.

shu di (Radix Rehmanniae Glutinosae Conquitae) 熟地 30g
lu jiao jiao (Colla Cornu Cervi) 鹿角胶 9g
rou gui (Cortex Cinnamomi Cassiae) 肉桂 3g
bai jie zi (Semen Sinapsis Albae) 白芥子 6g
pao jiang (quick fried Rhizoma Zingiberis Officinalis)
炮姜 1.5g
ma huang (Herba Ephedrae) 麻黄 1.5g
gan cao (Radix Glycyrrhizae Uralensis) 甘草 3g

Method: Decoction. **Lu jiao jiao** can melted in the hot strained decoction (*yang hua* 烊化), or powdered and taken separately; **rou gui** is added towards the end of cooking (*hou xia* 后下). **Shu di** supplements the Kidneys and nourishes Blood; **lu jiao jiao** supplements Blood and Kidney *yang* and opens up the channels; **rou gui** and **pao jiang** warm and invigorate *yang*, dispel Cold and unblock areas of stagnation; **bai jie zi** disperses Cold Phlegm; **ma huang** in small doses opens up the channels, dispels Cold and promotes movement of *qi*; **gan cao** harmonises the other herbs and protects the Stomach. (Source: *Shi Yong Zhong Yi Nei Ke Xue*)

Jing deficiency

- In severe cases with evidence of both *yang*, *yin* and *jing* deficiency, consider prescriptions that have a stronger *jing* nourishing effect, such as **YOU GUI WAN** (*Eucommia and Rehmannia Formula* 右归丸, p.333).

Topical therapies

Mouthwash

- **YANG HE TANG** (Yang-*Heartening Decoction* 阳和汤, see above)
- Steep 10 grams of **rou gui** (Cortex Cinnamomi Cassiae) 肉桂 in one cup of hot water for 10 minutes and hold the cooled liquid in the mouth.

Lozenges

- *Xi Gua Shuang Pian* 西瓜霜片 (Watermelon Frost Lozenges) can be sucked to relieve discomfort and sensitivity of *yang* deficiency ulcers. They are less cooling than the Watermelon Frost powder.

Patent medicines

Fu Zi Li Zhong Wan 附子理中丸 (Fu Tzu Li Chung Wan, Carmichaeli Tea Pills, Li Chung Yuen Medical Pills)
- Spleen *yang* deficiency with severe Cold

Li Zhong Wan 理中丸 (Li Zhong Wan)
- Spleen *yang* deficiency

Jin Kui Shen Qi Wan 金匮肾气丸 (Fu Gui Ba Wei Wan, Sexoton Pills, Golden Book Tea)
- Kidney *yang* deficiency

Lu Rong Jiao 鹿茸胶 (Lu Rong Jiao)
- *Jing* and Blood deficiency, can be added as powder to a primary prescription to enhance the result.

Xi Gua Shuang Pian 西瓜霜片 (Watermelon Frost Lozenges)

Acupuncture (select from)

Ren.12 (*zhong wan* +▲) .. *mu* point of the Stomach, warms and strengthens the Spleen and Stomach
Ren.6 (*qi hai* +▲) .... regulates *qi*, strengthens the Kidneys, warms and supplements *yang*
St.36 (*zu san li* +▲) .... *he* sea point of the Stomach, powerfully warms and strengthens the Spleen and Stomach and supplements *qi*
Sp.6 (*san yi jiao* +▲)........ strengthens the Spleen, regulates Liver *qi*, benefits the Kidneys and regulates *qi* and Blood
LI.11 (*qu chi* +▲) .... *he* sea point of the Large Intestine, regulates *qi* and Blood and warms the *yang ming* channels when moxaed
LI.4 (*he gu*) ....*yuan* point of the Large Intestine, invigorates *qi* and Blood, a special point for oral pathology
Bl.20 (*pi shu* +▲) .... *shu* point of the Spleen, warms and strengthens the Spleen and supplements *qi*

Ren.24 (*cheng jiang* ▲) ..... local points for oral disease, select one or two
St.6 (*jia che* ▲) closest to the site of the lesion(s)
St.4 (*di cang* ▲)
qian zheng ▲ (N-HN-20)
ah shi points .... over the lesion(s)

- a moxa box over the abdomen is useful; also strong moxa on Ren.8 (*shen que*), usually on salt. Place a piece of thin cloth over the navel and fill it with salt. Burn large cones of moxa on the salt. The cloth enables quick removal of the salt and prevents excessive burning.
- with Kidney *yang* deficiency, add Bl.23 (*shen shu* +▲), Du.4 (*ming men* +▲) and Ren.4 (*guan yuan* +▲)
- *Ear points:* mouth, tongue, *shen men*; lungs, heart, liver, kidney, spleen, stomach. Select ear points according to the location of the lesions and the organ system relationships. For example, for ulcers on the anterior tongue, use heart and lung. For ulcers on the edges of the

tongue use liver, on the buccal cavity use spleen, on the gums use stomach.

Clinical notes

- *Yang* deficiency mouth ulcers may be diagnosed biomedically as chronic apthous stomatitis, ulcerative stomatitis, malnutrition, malabsorption syndrome, coeliac disease, erosive lichen planus or periodontitis mucosa neurotica recurrens.
- Symptoms of *yang* deficiency generally respond well to correct treatment, although profound or long term deficiency always needs long term therapy. Treatment may need to persist for 9-12 months for a satisfactory result.
- For dietary recommendations, see p.873.

气血虚弱

20.5 QI AND BLOOD DEFICIENCY

Pathophysiology

• *Qi* and Blood deficiency ulcers are chronic and recurrent. There are several variations on the basic theme of *qi* and Blood deficiency depending on the aetiological factors involved. However, by definition the Spleen and Heart must be involved. Both the Spleen and Heart influence the tongue, and weakness of these organ systems can lead to a general failure of *qi* and Blood nourishment in the tissues of the mouth.

Clinical features

• Chronic, recurrent ulceration of the tongue, and to a lesser extent the gums and buccal cavity. The ulcer margins are narrow, slightly red and slightly raised. The buccal cavity may be slightly swollen, so the inner cheeks press upon the teeth, and leave a ridgelike elevation of tissue along the bite line. The ulcers are provoked or initiated when the patient is run down, fatigued and anxious, or following a menstrual period.
• postural dizziness, light-headedness, blurred vision
• pale, sallow complexion, pale nails and conjunctivae
• fatigue, lethargy, weakness
• shortness of breath with exertion, low weak voice
• spontaneous sweating

T pale, with a thin white coat
P thready and weak

Treatment principle

Supplement *qi* and Blood, strengthen the Spleen

Prescription

20.5.1 Heart Blood and Spleen *qi* deficiency

GUI PI TANG 归脾汤
(*Ginseng and Longan Combination*)

This formula is selected when there are clear signs of Spleen *qi* and Heart Blood deficiency–*shen* disturbance, insomnia, anxiety and palpitations. The ulcers, which tend to be concentrated on the tongue, may be provoked or aggravated when the patient is anxious.

zhi huang qi (honey fried Radix Astragali Membranacei) 炙黄芪 18-30g
dang shen (Radix Codonopsis Pilosulae) 党参 15-24g
fu ling (Sclerotium Poria Cocos) 茯苓 12-15g
chao bai zhu (dry fried Rhizoma Atractylodes Macrocephalae) 炒白术 12-15g

dang gui (Radix Angelicae Sinensis) 当归 9-12g
long yan rou (Arillus Euphoriae Longanae) 龙眼肉 9-12g
suan zao ren (Semen Zizyphi Spinosae) 酸枣仁 12-15g
yuan zhi (Radix Polygalae Tenuifoliae) 远志 6-9g
mu xiang (Radix Aucklandiae Lappae) 木香 6-9g
zhi gan cao (honey fried Radix Glycyrrhizae Uralensis)
炙甘草 6-9g

Method: Decoction. **Zhi huang qi, dang shen, bai zhu** and **zhi gan cao** strengthen the Spleen and supplement *qi*; **dang gui** and **zhi huang qi** together have a special effect on building Blood; **suan zao ren, long yan rou** and **yuan zhi** nourish the Heart and calm the *shen*; **fu ling** benefits the Spleen and calms the *shen*; **mu xiang** regulates *qi* and aids the Spleen in digesting the Blood supplementing herbs; **zhi gan cao** supplements *qi* and harmonises the Stomach. (Source: *Shi Yong Er Bi Hou Ke Xue*)

Modifications

- With stagnant Heat generated by Liver *qi* stagnation, add **shan zhi zi** (Fructus Gardeniae Jasminoidis) 山栀子 9-12g and **mu dan pi** (Cortex Moutan Radicis) 牡丹皮 9-12g.

20.5.1 *Qi* and Blood deficiency with Cold

SHI QUAN DA BU TANG 十全大补汤
(*Ginseng and Dang Gui Ten Combination*)

This prescription is selected when the symptoms of *qi* and Blood deficiency are less organ system specific, with general Blood deficiency features such as postural dizziness, shortness of breath, fatigue and weakness, weak limbs, a thready pulse and general pallor.

shu di (Radix Rehmanniae Glutinosae Conquitae) 熟地 15-24g
zhi huang qi (honey fried Radix Astragali Membranacei)
炙黄芪 18-30g
dang shen (Radix Codonopsis Pilosulae) 党参 15-24g
chao bai zhu (dry fried Rhizoma Atractylodes
Macrocephalae) 炒白术 12-15g
fu ling (Sclerotium Poria Cocos) 茯苓 12-15g
chao bai shao (dry fried Radix Paeoniae Lactiflorae)
炒白芍 12-18g
dang gui (Radix Angelicae Sinensis) 当归 9-12g
chuan xiong (Radix Ligustici Chuanxiong) 川芎 6-9g
rou gui (Cortex Cinnamomi Cassiae) 肉桂 3g
gan cao (Radix Glycyrrhizae Uralensis) 甘草 3-6g

Method: Decoction. **Shu di, chao bai shao** and **dang gui** nourish Blood; **zhi huang qi, dang shen, chao bai zhu, fu ling** and **gan cao** supplement *qi* and strengthen the Spleen; **chuan xiong** invigorates *qi* and Blood; **rou gui** warms *yang* and encourages the production of Blood. (Source: *Shi Yong Zhong Yi Nei Ke Xue*)

20.5.3 Blood deficiency with Heat

SI WU TANG 四物汤
(*Dang Gui Four Combination*) modified

This prescription is used when Blood deficiency generates a degree of Heat, a relatively common pattern following childbirth or heavy menstruation. In addition to the ulcers, which are often concentrated on the tongue and may be quite painful, the features are those of Blood deficiency (pale tongue, lips, conjunctivae, complexion and nails, postural dizziness, fatigue, thready pulse) and deficient Heat (flushed cheeks, feeling hot and restless at night, heat intolerance, short menstrual cycle). The aim of treatment is to nourish Blood and gently clear away Heat.

shu di (Radix Rehmanniae Glutinosae Conquitae) 熟地...... 9-15g
dang gui (Radix Angelicae Sinensis) 当归 9-12
bai shao (Radix Paeoniae Lactiflorae) 白芍 9-12g
chuan xiong (Radix Ligustici Chuanxiong) 川芎 6-9g
zhi mu (Rhizoma Anemarrhenae Asphodeloidis) 知母 6-9g
huang bai (Cortex Phellodendri) 黄柏 6-9g
mu dan pi (Cortex Moutan Radicis) 牡丹皮 6-9g

Method: Decoction. **Shu di**, **dang gui** and **bai shao** nourish Blood; **chuan xiong** invigorates *qi* and Blood; **zhi mu** clears Heat and generates fluids; **huang bai** clears Heat; **mu dan pi** cools the Blood and invigorates Blood. (Source: *Shi Yong Er Bi Hou Ke Xue*)

Topical therapies

Mouthwash

- **YANG HE TANG** (Yang-*Heartening Decoction* 阳和汤, *see* p.724)
- Steep 10 grams of **rou gui** (Cortex Cinnamomi Cassiae) 肉桂 in one cup of hot water for 10 minutes and hold the cooled liquid in the mouth.

Lozenges

- *Xi Gua Shuang Pian* 西瓜霜片 (Watermelon Frost Lozenges) are best for *qi* and Blood deficiency ulcers, as they are less cooling than the powder. *See* p.725.

Patent medicines

Gui Pi Wan 归脾丸 (Gui Pi Wan, Angelicae Longana Tea, Kwei Be Wan) - Heart and Spleen deficiency
Shi Quan Da Bu Wan 十全大补丸 (Shi Quan Da Bu Wan, Ten Flavour Tea) - *qi* and Blood deficiency with Cold
Wu Ji Bai Feng Wan 乌鸡白凤丸 (Wu Chi Pai Feng Wan)

- *qi* and Blood supplement with black skinned chicken

Dang Gui Ji Jing 当归鸡精 (Chicken Essence with Tang Kuei)
- a popular *qi* and Blood supplement in liquid form, especially good postpartum

Xi Gua Shuang Pian 西瓜霜片 (Watermelon Frost Lozenges)

Acupuncture (select from)

Ren.12 (*zhong wan* +▲) .. *mu* point of the Stomach, warms and strengthens the Spleen and Stomach

St.36 (*zu san li* +▲) .... *he* sea point of the Stomach, powerfully warms and strengthens the Spleen and Stomach and supplements *qi* and Blood

Sp.6 (*san yi jiao* +▲) .... strengthens the Spleen, regulates Liver *qi*, benefits the Kidneys and regulates *qi* and Blood

LI.11 (*qu chi* +▲) .... *he* sea point of the Large Intestine, regulates *qi* and Blood and warms the *yang ming* channels when moxaed

Ht.5 (*tong li*) .... *luo* point of the Heart, regulates Heart and tongue *qi* and calms the *shen*

Ht.7 (*shen men*) ....*yuan* and *shu* stream point of the Heart, supplements and regulates Heart *qi* and Blood

Bl.20 (*pi shu* +▲) .... *shu* point of the Spleen, warms and strengthens the Spleen and supplements *qi* and Blood

Ren.24 (*cheng jiang* ▲) ..... local points for oral disease, select one or two
St.6 (*jia che* ▲) closest to the site of the lesion; gentle and
St.4 (*di cang* ▲) shallow needling or moxa
qian zheng ▲ (N-HN-20)

- a moxa box over the abdomen is useful
- with bruising or heavy periods add Sp.10 (*xue hai*) and Sp.1 (*yin bai* ▲)
- with dizziness add Du.20 (*bai hui* ▲)
- *Ear points:* mouth, tongue, *shen men*; lungs, heart, liver, kidney, spleen, stomach. Select ear points according to the location of the lesions and the organ system relationships. For example for ulcers on the anterior tongue, use heart and lung. For ulcers on the edges of the tongue use liver, on the buccal cavity use spleen, on the gums use stomach.

Clinical notes

- Heart and Spleen deficiency patterns respond well to treatment, which should continue until it is clear the Spleen is strong enough to make sufficient Blood. Careful diet and eating patterns will enhance the result. Blood supplementing, iron rich foods are useful after each menstrual period. Iron supplements are also useful. For other dietary recommendations, see pp.870, 874.
- Ulcers of this type may be found in patients with anaemia.
- Acupuncture can be effective at supplementing Spleen *qi*, but if the patient is already Blood deficient, herbs will usually be necessary as well.

SUMMARY OF GUIDING FORMULAE FOR MOUTH ULCERS

Acute patterns

External Heat

Wind Heat with Dampness - *Yin Qiao San* 银翘散

Damp Heat - *Gan Lu Xiao Du Dan* 甘露消毒丹

Toxic Heat - *Huang Lian Jie Du Tang* 黄连解毒汤

Internal Heat

Stagnant Heat in the Heart and Spleen - *Liang Ge San* 凉膈散

Heart Fire - *Dao Chi San* 导赤散

Stomach Heat/Fire - *Qing Wei Tang* 清胃汤
- with constipation - *Tiao Wei Cheng Qi Tang* 调味承气汤

Liver *qi* stagnation with stagnant Heat - *Dan Zhi Xiao Yao San* 丹栀逍遥散

Chronic or recurrent patterns

Yin deficiency
- Heart and Kidney *yin* deficiency - *Tian Wang Bu Xin Dan* 天王补心丹
- Kidney *yin* deficiency with Heat - *Zhi Bai Ba Wei Wan* 知柏八味丸
- Following a febrile illness - *Huang Lian E Jiao Tang* 黄连阿胶汤
- with Phlegm - *Xiao Luo Wan* 消瘰丸 (as an addition)

Yang deficiency - *Fu Zi Li Zhong Wan* 附子理中丸
- Kidney *yang* deficiency - *Jin Kui Shen Qi Wan* 金匮肾气丸
- with Phlegm - *Yang He Tang* 阳和汤

Qi and Blood deficiency - *Gui Pi Tang* 归脾汤
- generalised - *Shi Quan Da Bu Tang* 十全大补汤
- with Heat - *Si Wu Tang* 四物汤

21. Nausea, Vomiting

Excess patterns

External pathogens invading the Stomach
Food stagnation
Phlegm Damp
Liver *qi* invading the Stomach

Deficient patterns

Spleen and Stomach (*qi* or *yang*) deficiency
Stomach *yin* deficiency

21 NAUSEA, VOMITING

e xin 恶心, *ou tu* 呕吐

Nausea and vomiting are symptoms of rising Stomach *qi*. Normally, Stomach *qi* descends, taking the waste products of digestion to the Intestines. However, Stomach *qi* can be blocked by a pathogen, or it can simply be too weak to descend. In either case, rising Stomach *qi* is a form of 'rebellious' *qi*.

In adults, nausea and vomiting can be caused by dysfunction of almost any organ system, reflecting a large range of different disorders, ranging from simple acute viral infections to emotional stress to cancer.

In children, vomiting may be the first sign of an infection. All children with vomiting accompanied by fever, should, in addition to the obvious gastrointestinal infection, be checked for middle ear, urinary tract, upper respiratory tract or central nervous system infection.

AETIOLOGY

External pathogens

Invasion by external pathogens into the Stomach is a common cause of both nausea and vomiting, and is typically associated with a seasonal pathogen, or with eating spoiled food. The most frequent cause is Dampness, either alone or in combination with another pathogen. Nausea and vomiting of this type most commonly occur during the humid months of Summer and Autumn, but may occur at any time of the year. External invasion usually cause acute, self limiting illnesses. However, in some cases, the illness can drag on and become entrenched. Chemotherapy for cancer, a frequent cause of nausea and vomiting, often resembles an external pathogen, and may be treated as such.

Diet

The type of food consumed, and the way it is consumed, are important aetiological factors in the generation of nausea and vomiting. Eating spoiled or contaminated food can produce acute vomiting, which, in TCM terms, may resemble the invasion of an external pathogen, such as Summerheat or Summerdamp.

Too much cold natured or raw food can introduce Cold into the Stomach and weaken Spleen *qi* and *yang*. Overconsumption in general, and excessive consumption of rich heating or supplementing foods in particular, can lead to the accumulation of food (*see* p.3), and Heat or Damp Heat in the Stomach and Intestines. An excess of heating foods can create Stomach Heat or damage Stomach *yin*. Sugar, dairy products and some medications, such as antibiotics, create Dampness and Phlegm. All these pathogens can obstruct the *qi* mechanism and cause Stomach *qi* to rise.

The way food is eaten is as important as the type of food that is consumed. Irregular eating times, eating late at night, or while stressed, or in excessive quantities can all tax the capacity of the Stomach and Spleen to digest and distribute food. These habits can contribute to excess, deficiency and mixed pathologies.

In addition, the manipulations of modern agri-business have added a raft of new and potentially disruptive substances to many of our foods. Pesticides, fertilisers, hormones and antibiotics find their way into our daily foods as residues of the production process. Artificial colouring and flavouring agents, preservatives and stabilisers are added to enhance shelf life and palatability. It seems that some people are unable to metabolise these compounds adequately; they become sensitised and ingestion of the offending agent produces symptoms of nausea, vomiting, abdominal distension, flatulence and pain.

BOX 21.1 SOME BIOMEDICAL CAUSES OF NAUSEA AND VOMITING

Infection, inflammation
- appendicitis, meningitis, hepatitis, pyelonephritis, peritonitis, cholecystitis, pancreatitis, malaria, food poisoning, gastroenteritis

Gastro-intestinal
- postoperative
- peptic ulcers
- gastritis
- food intolerance
- stomach cancer

Mechanical (vomiting)
- bowel obstruction
- volvulus
- pyloric stenosis

Trauma (vomiting)
- following head injury (concussion)

Renal
- uraemia, chronic renal failure

Cerebral, neurological
- tumours (sudden vomiting without preceding nausea)
- Meniere's disease, labyrinthine disturbance

Physiological
- pregnancy
- motion sickness

Psychogenic
- stress, anxiety

Medication, poisons
- chemotherapy
- alcohol intoxication
- NSAIDs

Emotion

Frustration, anger, resentment, prolonged emotional turmoil, repressed emotions and stress disrupt the circulation of Liver *qi*. These emotions cause a low grade spasm and tension in the smooth muscle of the digestive tract. Nausea or vomiting associated with Liver *qi* stagnation is generally intermittent and related to the patient's emotional state.

When the smooth movement of Liver *qi* is impeded, it finds alternative pathways. In this case, the stagnant *qi* is discharged sideways, overcontrolling

BOX 21.2 KEY DIAGNOSTIC POINTS

Accompanying signs and symptoms
- acute with cramping abdominal pain - external pathogen, Liver *qi* stagnation
- with epigastric distension, belching and bad breath - food stagnation
- with an emotional component - *qi* stagnation
- with headache and fever - external pathogen

Aggravation
- with strong odours - Phlegm or Dampness
- with emotion - Liver *qi* stagnation

Type of vomitus
- sour and foul smelling - Heat
- with undigested food - food stagnation, *yang* deficiency
- dry retching - *yin* deficiency
- watery and inoffensive - deficient and Cold or Phlegm Fluids

the Stomach through the controlling cycle), disrupting the descent of Stomach *qi* and causing nausea and vomiting.

There are several consequences of Liver *qi* invading the Stomach. When *qi* stagnates for any length of time, the resulting pressure can generate Heat. Chronic Heat in the Stomach will eventually consume Stomach *yin*. Stagnant *qi* can disrupt the Spleen, weakening it and contributing to the development of Dampness and Phlegm, which block the descent of Stomach *qi*.

Liver *qi* invading the Stomach can be a long term, or even lifetime disorder, and may have a constitutional component. Liver *qi* stagnation can run in families, with several members prone to emotional gastro-intestinal upsets.

Phlegm Damp

Phlegm Damp is generated by overindulgence in Phlegm or Damp producing foods and by eating habits that weaken Spleen *qi*. Repeated courses of antibiotics can damage Spleen *qi*, allowing the generation and accumulation of Dampness. Foods that can weaken the Spleen if consumed to excess include dairy products, fatty, rich, sweet or raw foods, and alcohol. Once the Spleen is weak, inefficient digestion allows accumulation of Dampness, which over time congeals into Phlegm. In the presence of Heat, Damp may be condensed to form Phlegm in a shorter time.

Poor fluid metabolism, due to Spleen, Lung or Kidney dysfunction, may cause accumulation and thickening of physiological fluids into Phlegm. In addition, prolonged Liver *qi* stagnation can contribute to the condition by weakening the Spleen and by retarding the movement of fluids, which gradually condense into Phlegm.

Phlegm may also arise following a serious acute febrile illness. The pathogenic Heat cooks and congeals fluid into Phlegm Heat. Once present, Phlegm or Phlegm Heat blocks the *qi* mechanism and the descent of Stomach *qi*, provoking nausea and vomiting.

Spleen and Stomach deficiency

This refers to *qi*, *yang* or *yin* deficiency. The most common cause of Spleen *yang qi* deficiency nausea or vomiting is prolonged or excessive consumption of cold raw food and irregular eating habits, or the inappropriate use of cold natured herbs or antibiotics in the treatment of a febrile disease. Prolonged insult to the Stomach or severely limited food intake, such as occurs in patients with bulimia and anorexia nervosa, can seriously damage Spleen and Stomach *yang qi*. Excessive mental strain or prolonged concentration may deplete Spleen *qi*. The damage is aggravated when an irregular diet is combined with sustained mental activity and too much sitting. The Spleen and Stomach can also be weakened following an acute invasion of Cold and/or Dampness. Gastric surgery can deplete Spleen *yang* and cause Blood stagnation. When Stomach *qi* is weakened, it can become too feeble to descend properly. The *qi* mechanism is disordered, *qi* accumulates and eventually rises causing nausea and vomiting.

Stomach *yin* deficiency may follow a febrile disease, long term consumption of spicy heating foods, or excessive consumption of drugs such as steroids, illicit stimulants and *yang* supplementing substances. It also may result from prolonged or excessive vomiting from an excess pathogen, or another chronic Stomach pathology, especially one characterised by Heat or dryness.

Spleen and Stomach deficiency may also be constitutional, and in patients with a component of inherited weakness, there will often be a history of recurrent nausea or vomiting since childhood.

TCM DIFFERENTIAL DIAGNOSIS

- **Regurgitation** (*fan wei* 反胃): Regurgitation is a type of vomiting. In regurgitation, the vomiting occurs some time after eating, usually at least 12 hours later. The vomitus is generally composed of undigested or partially digested food. In addition, there is significant epigastric distension and weakness. Regurgitation is usually a chronic disorder.
- **Dysphagia** (*yi ge* 壹膈): Dysphagia is difficulty swallowing, a situation that may result in immediate regurgitation of the ingested material. In mild cases the patient can swallow, although there may be discomfort, and the amount of food that can be ingested at one time is reduced. In severe cases, even swallowing water may be difficult.

- **Sudden Turmoil Disorder** (*huo luan* 霍乱): Sudden turmoil is characterised by sudden onset of vomiting, diarrhoea and abdominal pain. It is due to invasion by seasonal, usually epidemic, pathogens, and overlaps with some varieties of vomiting discussed in this chapter. Biomedically, Sudden Turmoil Disorder corresponds to conditions such as food poisoning, acute gastroenteritis or cholera.

TREATMENT

In general, both excess and deficient patterns of nausea and vomiting respond well to acupuncture and herbs. Due to the nature of the problem, however, and the fact that patients may not be able to tolerate or hold down medicine, acupuncture is often the treatment of choice, at least in the early stages.

Delivery of medicine to patients with nausea and vomiting, especially Chinese herb decoctions, presents a clinical challenge. There are several methods that may assist. Decoctions may be drunk cool or cold, sipped in tiny amounts through a straw placed at the back of the tongue, or in extremis, delivered per rectum as an enema. Acupuncture is effective in quickly alleviating nausea, even temporarily, and allowing the ingestion of medicine. A useful technique involves strong needling or finger pressure on PC.6 (*nei guan*) prior to ingestion of the herbs. Gently patting the spine around T7-T12 may also help some patients.

Vomiting, depending on the cause, can often be relieved quite quickly. Nausea also responds quite well, but may on occasion prove persistent. Depending on the underlying cause, treatment will often need to persist beyond alleviation of the symptoms, so as to rebuild *yin* or *yang*, completely eliminate Damp, etc., so as to prevent a recurrence of the problem.

Figure 21.1 *Diagnostic strategy for nausea and vomiting*

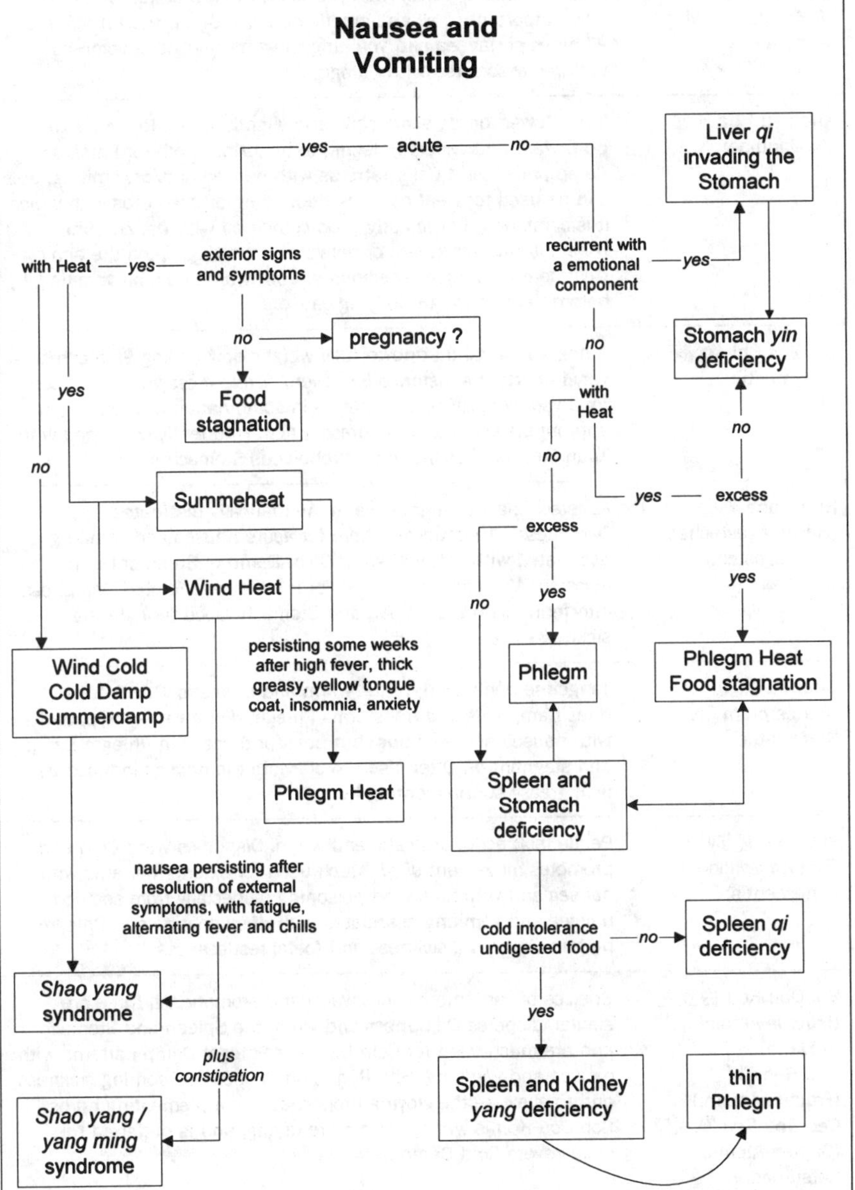

Table 21.1 *Herbs with anti-emetic properties*

Ban Xia 半夏 (Rhizoma Pinelliae Ternatae)	Pinellia rhizome; acrid, warm, toxic (in the raw state). One of the most important of all anti-emetic herbs, with a powerful effect on all types of nausea and vomiting. Best for nausea or vomiting patterns associated with Phlegm Damp.
Xuan Fu Hua 旋复花 (Flos Inulae)	Inula flower; bitter, acrid, salty and slightly warm. Redirects *qi* downward and expels Phlegm. An important herb for Phlegm Damp or deficient Cold patterns with nausea and/or vomiting, but can be used for Heat patterns depending on the herbs with which it is combined. Particularly good combined with Dai Zhe Shi (Haematitum) for severe or persistent vomiting, when the aim of treatment is to drive rebellious *qi* downward and stop vomiting, before treating the underlying cause.
Dai Zhe Shi 代赭石 (Haematitie)	A heavy mineral that powerfully weighs down rising Stomach *qi*. A very important substance for severe or relentless vomiting. Used for a variety of different patterns in combination with an appropriate constitutional prescription. Frequently combined with Xuan Fu Hua (Flos Inulae) for rebellious Stomach *qi*.
Huo Xiang 藿香 (Herba Agastaches seu Pogostemi)	Agastache; acrid, slightly warm. Aromatically dissipates Dampness. An important herb for acute nausea and vomiting associated with external Wind Cold, Damp or Summer Damp invasion. Also commonly used for internally generated Dampness interfering with the Spleen and Stomach. Good for morning sickness.
Chen Pi 陈皮 (Pericarpium Citri Reticulatae)	Tangerine peel; acrid, bitter, warm and aromatic. Regulates *qi*, dries Dampness and transforms Phlegm. For a variety of patterns with nausea and vomiting, but best for those with Phlegm Damp and stagnant *qi*. Often used to alleviate the nausea induced by rich, greasy supplementing herbs.
Zi Su Ye 紫苏叶 (Folium Perillae Frutescentis)	Perilla leaf; acrid, aromatic and warm. Disperses Wind Cold and promotes movement of *qi*. Much used for exterior patterns with nausea and vomiting, food poisoning (especially from seafood), nausea and vomiting associated with *qi* stagnation and Phlegm patterns, morning sickness and foetal restlessness.
Bai Dou Kou 白豆蔻 (Fructus Amomi Kravanh) Sha Ren 砂仁 (Fructus Amomi) Cao Dou Kou 草豆蔻 (Semen Alpiniae Katsumadai)	Species of cardamon; acrid, warm and aromatic. All three are similar, disperse Dampness and warm the Spleen and Stomach and are much used for Cold Damp or Phlegm Damp patterns with nausea and vomiting. Sha Ren is often used for morning sickness and to alleviate the cloying properties of supplementing herbs. Cao Dou Kou is warmer and more drying, and is preferred for more severe Cold Damp patterns.

Table 21.1 *Herbs with anti-emetic properties (cont.)*

Wu Zhu Yu 吴茱萸 (Fructus Evoidae Rutaecarpae)	Evodia fruit; acrid, bitter, hot, slightly toxic. Disperses Cold and redirects *qi* downwards. For nausea and vomiting associated with interior Cold patterns, particularly those with acid reflux, hypersalivation and migraine or vertex headaches.
Gan Jiang 干姜 (Rhizoma Zingiberis Officinalis)	Dry ginger rhizome; acrid and hot. Warms the Spleen and Stomach and expels internal Cold. For nausea and vomiting associated with excess or deficient Cold patterns affecting the Spleen or Stomach, and Phlegm and fluid accumulation.
Sheng Jiang 生姜 (Rhizoma Zingiberis Officinalis)	Fresh ginger rhizome; acrid and warm. Disperses Wind Cold and warms the Spleen and Stomach. For a variety of patterns presenting with nausea and vomiting, especially those associated with Cold or exterior pathogens. Can be used for Heat patterns when combined with other cooling herbs. Much used as a simple remedy for morning and motion sickness.
Pi Pa Ye 枇杷叶 (Folium Eriobotryae Japonicae)	Loquat leaf; bitter and cool. For Stomach Heat patterns causing nausea and vomiting.
Lu Gen 芦根 (Rhizoma Phragmitis Communis)	Phragmites rhizome; sweet and cool. For Stomach Heat patterns causing nausea and vomiting.
Zhu Ru 竹茹 (Caulis Bambusae in Taeniis)	Bamboo shavings; sweet and cool. For Phlegm Heat, Damp Heat or Stomach Heat patterns with nausea and vomiting. Particularly good when associated with symptoms of *shen* disturbance. Can be used for deficiency patterns when combined with the appropriate herbs.
Zhang Nao 樟脑 (Camphora)	Camphor; acrid and hot. Extremely aromatic substance that appears in some patent medicines, notably *Xing Jun San* (Marching Powder). Used for acute vomiting and diarrhoea due to pestilential or seasonal pathogens. Powerfully disperses turbid Dampness or Cold Damp clogging the Spleen and Stomach.

外邪犯胃

21.1 EXTERNAL PATHOGENS INVADING THE STOMACH

Pathophysiology

- Nausea and vomiting, caused by external pathogens invading the Stomach, is usually a seasonal disorder, appearing at various times of the year, most typically Summer and Autumn. It may also be caused by ingestion of pathogens in spoiled food.
- Regardless of the origin of the pathogen, it blocks the descent of Stomach *qi* which then rebels upwards, often with force.
- With simultaneous vomiting and diarrhoea, see Sudden Turmoil Disorder, p.826.

Clinical features

- The nausea and vomiting is acute, and accompanied by variable signs and symptoms, depending on the type of pathogen involved (*See* Table 21.2).

Treatment principle

Expel the pathogen, harmonise the Stomach
Redirect Stomach *qi* downwards, stop nausea and vomiting

Prescription

21.1.1 Wind Cold, Summerdamp

HUO XIANG ZHENG QI SAN 藿香正气散
(*Agastache Formula*)

huo xiang (Herba Agastaches seu Pogostemi) 藿香 12-15g
fu ling (Sclerotium Poriae Cocos) 茯苓 12-15g
bai zhu (Rhizoma Atractylodes Macrocephalae) 白术 9-12g
zi su ye (Folium Perillae Frutescentis) 紫苏叶 9-12g
ban xia (Rhizoma Pinelliae Ternatae) 半夏 9-12g
da fu pi (Pericarpium Arecae Catechu) 大服皮 9-12g
chen pi (Pericarpium Citri Reticulatae) 陈皮 9-12g
bai zhi (Radix Angelicae Dahuricae) 白芷 9-12g
hou po (Cortex Magnoliae Officinalis) 厚朴 9-12g
jie geng (Radix Playcodi Grandiflori) 桔梗 6-9g
gan cao (Radix Glycyrrhizae Uralensis) 甘草 3-6g
sheng jiang (Rhizoma Zingiberis Officinalis Recens)
生姜 6-9g
da zao (Fructus Zizyphi Jujubae) 大枣 2pce

Method: Decoction. The herbs should be simmered for no longer than 20 minutes in a pot with a close fitting lid. **Huo xiang** fragrantly disperses Damp turbidity, harmonises the Stomach and stops vomiting; **zi su ye** and **bai zhi** dispel Wind Cold and transform Dampness; **hou po** regulates *qi*, directs *qi* downwards, transforms Phlegm Damp and alleviates fullness; **chen pi** regulates *qi*, corrects the *qi* mechanism, transforms Phlegm Damp and harmonises the Stomach; **ban xia** transforms Phlegm Damp and stops vomiting; **da fu pi** directs *qi* and Dampness downwards and alleviates fullness; **bai zhu** and **fu ling** strengthen the Spleen, dry Dampness and promote urination; **jie geng** assists the dispersing function of the Lungs; **gan cao, sheng jiang** and **da zao** harmonise the other herbs and regulate the Stomach. (Source: *Shi Yong Zhong Yi Nei Ke Xue*).

Modifications

- When the exterior symptoms are severe, increase the dose of **zi su ye** to 12-15g, and add **jing jie** (Herba seu Flos Schizonepetae Tenuifolia) 荆芥 12-15g and **fang feng** (Radix Ledebouriellae Divaricatae) 防风 9-12g. *See also* Variations and additional prescriptions below.
- With food stagnation (vomiting of undigested food, severe epigastric bloating), delete **bai zhu, gan cao** and **da zao**, and add **shen qu** (Massa Fermentata) 神曲 15g, **mai ya** (Fructus Hordei Vulgaris Germinantus) 麦芽 15-30g and **ji nei jin** (Endothelium Corneum Gigeriae Galli) 鸡内金 12g.

Table 21.2 *Comparison of externally generated vomiting patterns*

Wind Cold	acute nausea and vomiting, simultaneous fever and chills, the chills are often more prominent than the fever, no sweating, occipital headache, muscle aches, neck stiffness, nasal obstruction, or runny nose with thin watery mucus, sneezing, cough or wheezing with thin watery mucus, thin, white tongue coat, floating and tight pulse
Wind Heat	acute nausea and vomiting, fever with little or no chills, sore, dry or scratchy throat, mild sweating, headache (usually frontal), thirst, cough with thick or sticky, yellow sputum, nasal obstruction, or a nasal discharge which is thick and yellow or green, thin, yellow tongue coat, floating and rapid pulse
Summerdamp	acute nausea and vomiting, diarrhoea, muscle aches, heaviness in the limbs, foggy-headedness, lethargy and tiredness, loss of appetite, thick white, greasy tongue coat, floating, soft pulse
Summerheat	acute nausea and vomiting, relatively high fever which is unrelieved by sweating, heaviness in the body, diarrhoea, foggy-headedness, fatigue and lethargy, thirst, irritability and restlessness, concentrated urine, greasy, white or yellow tongue coat, soft, soggy, possibly rapid pulse
Shao yang syndrome	nausea and vomiting, anorexia, alternating fever and chills, dry throat, dizziness, bitter taste in the mouth, fullness in the chest and hypochondrium, heartburn and a wiry pulse
Shao yang Yang ming syndrome	continuous nausea and vomiting, burning diarrhoea or constipation, alternating fever and chills, bitter taste in the mouth, fullness or pain in the epigastrium, a yellow tongue coat and a strong, wiry pulse

- With severe Dampness (severe vomiting, thick, greasy tongue coat), delete **bai zhu** and add **cang zhu** (Rhizoma Atractylodis) 苍术 12-15g and **pei lan** (Herba Eupatorii Fortuneii) 佩兰 9-12g.
- With *qi* stagnation, add **mu xiang** (Radix Aucklandiae Lappae) 木香 6-9g and **zhi ke** (Fructus Citri Aurantii) 枳壳 9-12g.
- With scanty urine, add **mu tong** (Caulis Mutong) 木通 6-9g and **ze xie** (Rhizoma Alismatis Orientalis) 泽泻 9-12g.

Variations and additional prescriptions

With severe Wind Cold

- If the exterior Wind Cold signs are severe (acute nausea or vomiting, strong chills, no sweating, occipital headache, severe tightness or stiffness in the upper back and neck), a more powerful exterior clearing formula such as **GE GEN JIA BAN XIA TANG** (*Kudzu Decoction plus Pinellia* 葛根加半夏汤) may be appropriate.

  ge gen (Radix Puerariae) 葛根 12-15g
  ma huang (Herba Ephedra) 麻黄 6-9g
  ban xia (Rhizoma Pinelliae Ternatae) 半夏 9-12g
  gui zhi (Ramulus Cinnamomi Cassiae) 桂枝 6-9g
  bai shao (Radix Paeoniae Lactiflora) 白芍 6-9g
  zhi gan cao (honey fried Radix Glycyrrhizae Uralensis) 炙甘草 3-6g
  sheng jiang (Rhizoma Zingiberis Officinalis Recens) 生姜 9-12g
  da zao (Fructus Zizyphi Jujubae) 大枣 2pce

  Method: Decoction. **Ge gen** eases the muscles and clears the exterior; **ma huang** and **gui zhi** are a strong diaphoretic combination to disperse Wind Cold and induce sweating; **ban xia** transforms Phlegm Damp and stops vomiting; **gui zhi** and **bai shao** work synergistically to regulate the *ying* and *wei qi* and disperse pathogens, while preventing excessive diaphoresis; **gan cao**, **sheng jiang** and **da zao** harmonise the other herbs and regulate the Stomach. (Source: *Formulas and Strategies*)

21.1.2 Wind Heat

YIN QIAO SAN 银翘散
(*Lonicera and Forsythia Formula*) modified

This prescription is selected for Wind Heat patterns.

jin yin hua (Flos Lonicerae Japonicae) 金银花 15-24g
lian qiao (Fructus Forsythia Suspensae) 连翘 12-15g
lu gen (Rhizoma Phragmitis Communis) 芦根 15-30g
dan zhu ye (Herba Lophatheri Gracilis) 淡竹叶 9-12g
dan dou chi (Semen Sojae Preparatum) 淡豆豉 9-12g
niu bang zi (Fructus Arctii Lappae) 牛蒡子 9-12g

jing jie (Herba seu Flos Schizonepetae Tenuifolia) 荆芥 9-12g
bo he (Herbs Mentha Haplocalycis) 薄荷 6-9g
gan cao (Radix Glycyrrhizae Uralensis) 甘草 3-6g
zhu ru (Caulis Bambusae in Taeniis) 竹茹 9-12g
chen pi (Pericarpium Citri Reticulatae) 陈皮 6-9g

Method: Decoction. The herbs should be gently simmered for no longer than 20 minutes. **Bo he** is added at the end of cooking (*hou xia* 后下). Take cool or at room temperature. **Jin yin hua** and **lian qiao** clear Heat from the exterior and eliminate Toxic Heat; **niu bang zi** disperses Wind Heat and with **gan cao**, benefits the throat; **bo he** and **dan dou chi** clear Wind Heat; **jing jie** disperses Wind without drying; **dan zhu ye, lu gen** clear Heat, and, with **gan cao**, generate fluids and stop thirst; **zhu ru** and **chen pi** harmonise the Stomach and stop nausea and vomiting. (Source: *Shi Yong Zhong Yi Nei Ke Xue*)

21.1.3 Summerheat

XIN JIA XIANG RU YIN 新加香薷饮
(*Newly Augmented Elsholtzia Decoction*)

This prescription is selected for Summerheat patterns, or exterior patterns with obvious Heat and digestive symptoms.

xiang ru (Herba Elsholtzia seu Moslae) 香薷 9-12g
jin yin hua (Flos Lonicerae Japonicae) 金银花 15-24g
lian qiao (Fructus Forsythia Suspensae) 连翘 9-12g
bian dou (Semen Dolichos Lablab) 扁豆 12-15g
hou po (Cortex Magnoliae Officinalis) 厚朴 9-12g

Method: Decoction. The herbs should be gently simmered for no longer than 20 minutes. This formula should be taken cool as **xiang ru** can aggravate vomiting when taken hot. **Xiang ru** clears the exterior, harmonises the *qi* mechanism and disperses Summerheat; **bian dou** and **hou po** harmonise the Stomach and transform Dampness to alleviate fullness and stop vomiting; **jin yin hua** and **lian qiao** clear Heat from the exterior and eliminate Toxic Heat. (Source: *Shi Yong Zhong Yi Nei Ke Xue*)

Variations and additional prescriptions

Very severe vomiting

- In severe cases with extreme and persistent vomiting, 1-2 grams of **YU SHU DAN** (*Jade Pivot Special Pill* 玉枢丹) modified, can be given first to suppress the urge to vomit. This formula uses toxic and cathartic herbs to forcefully drive *qi* downward, and is reserved for severe cases of relentless vomiting caused by pestilential pathogenic invasion, food poisoning or chemical poisoning. It is available as a patent medicine.

shan ci gu (Pseudobulbus Shancigu) 山慈菇 9g
wu bei zi (Galla Rhois Chinensis) 五倍子 9g
da ji (Radix Euphorbiae seu Knoxiae) 大戟 4.5g
qian jin zi (Semen Euphorbiae Lathyridis) 千金子 3g

xiong huang (Realgar) 雄黄 3g
zhu sha (Cinnabaris) 朱砂 3g

Method: Grind the herbs and substances to fine powder, mix and store in an airtight container. The dose is 0.5-1 grams in a little water two or three times as needed, until the patient can ingest the primary prescription. **Shan ci gu, xiong huang, zhu sha** and **wu bei zi** disperse pestilential Toxins; **qian jin zi** and **da ji** drive pestilential Toxins down and out through the bladder and bowels. (Source: *Shi Yong Zhong Yi Nei Ke Xue*)

NB. The original prescription contained a gram of **she xiang** (Secretio Moschus) 麝香, a product derived from the musk deer, an endangered animal.

Shao yang syndrome

- If pathogens penetrate further into the body, they can lodge in the *shao yang* level. This happens in people who are run down, or who don't rest properly during an acute infection. It can also happen if the pathogen is strong. The symptoms occur some days after the initial episode, often described as 'a cold that never really went away'. The features are nausea, occasional vomiting, loss of appetite, alternating fever and chills, dry throat, dizziness, bitter taste in the mouth, fullness in the chest and hypochondrium, heartburn and a wiry pulse. The tongue coat is usually not thick. The aim of treatment is to harmonise *shao yang* and clear any residual pathogen with **XIAO CHAI HU TANG** (*Minor Bupleurum Combination* 小柴胡汤).

chai hu (Radix Bupleuri) 柴胡 9-12g
ban xia (Rhizoma Pinelliae Ternatae) 半夏 9-12g
huang qin (Radix Scutellariae Baicalensis) 黄芩 9-12g
sheng jiang (Rhizoma Zingiberis Officinalis Recens)
生姜 6-9g
dang shen (Radix Codonopsis Pilosulae) 党参 12-15g
zhi gan cao (honey fried Radix Glycyrrhizae Uralensis)
炙甘草 6-9g
da zao (Fructus Zizyphi Jujubae) 大枣 4pce

Method: Decoction. **Chai hu** harmonises and closes off the *shao yang* level to lurking pathogens, clears Heat and regulates *qi*; **huang qin** clears Heat from the Liver, Gallbladder and the *shao yang* level. Together these two herbs are the main synergistic pair for dispersing pathogens from *shao yang*. **Ban xia** and **sheng jiang** harmonise the Stomach and stop vomiting; **dang shen** and **gan cao** support *zheng qi* and assist in preventing the pathogen from penetrating further; **sheng jiang** and **da zao** support **ban xia** in harmonising the Stomach and stopping nausea and vomiting.

Shao yang / yang ming syndrome

- A variation of the *shao yang* syndrome above that can cause serious nausea and vomiting, is the simultaneous overlap of the pathogen into *yang ming*. This is generally more intense than the simple *shao yang* pattern, and is characterised by continuous vomiting and nausea, burning diarrhoea or constipation, strong alternating fever and chills, fullness or pain in the epigastrium and a strong wiry pulse. The aim of treatment is to harmonise *shao yang* and purge Heat from the Stomach and Intestines with **DA CHAI HU TANG** (*Major Bupleurum Combination* 大柴胡汤) modified.

chai hu (Radix Bupleuri) 柴胡 12-15g
ban xia (Rhizoma Pinelliae Ternatae) 半夏 12-15g
huang qin (Radix Scutellariae Baicalensis) 黄芩 9-12g
zhi shi (Fructus Immaturus Citri Aurantii) 枳实 9-12g
bai shao (Radix Paeoniae Lactiflorae) 白芍 12-15g
da huang (Radix et Rhizoma Rhei) 大黄 6-9g
sheng jiang (Rhizoma Zingiberis Officinalis Recens) 生姜 6-9g
da zao (Fructus Zizyphi Jujubae) 大枣 4pce
huang lian (Rhizoma Coptidis) 黄连 6-9g
wu zhu yu (Fructus Evodiae Rutaecarpae) 吴茱萸 2-3g

Method: Decoction. **Chai hu** harmonises and closes off the *shao yang* level to lurking pathogens, clears Heat and regulates *qi*; **huang qin** clears Heat from the Liver, Gallbladder and the *shao yang* level; **ban xia** and **sheng jiang** harmonise the Stomach and stop vomiting; **zhi shi** regulates *qi*, breaks up accumulated *qi*, directs *qi* downwards, alleviates distension and assists **da huang** in draining the accumulated Heat downwards; **da huang** purges accumulated Heat from *yang ming* and opens the bowels; **bai shao** softens the Liver, alleviates spasms and pain and assists **da zao** in preventing damage to *yin* by the harsh purgative action of **da huang**; **sheng jiang** and **da zao** support **ban xia** in harmonising the Stomach and stopping nausea and vomiting. (Source: Formulas and Strategies)

Lingering Damp Heat

- Following an unresolved, or incompletely resolved, acute invasion of Damp Heat that causes vomiting and diarrhoea (classified as Sudden Turmoil Disorder), some patients are left with lingering Damp Heat accumulation in the Spleen and Stomach. The symptoms include persistent nausea with occasional vomiting, loss of appetite, muscle aches, heaviness, afternoon fever, abdominal distension and fatigue. The tongue coat is thick, white and/or yellow, and greasy. The aim of treatment is to Clear smouldering Damp Heat from the middle *jiao* with **LIAN PO YIN** (*Coptis and Magnolia Bark Decoction* 连朴饮, p.27).

Residual Phlegm Heat

- Continuous nausea and vomiting that persists for some weeks after a severe febrile illness can be due to Phlegm Heat. The Phlegm Heat results from the congealing of body fluids by the intense Heat of the fever. In addition to the nausea there is insomnia and anxiety, a thick, greasy yellow tongue coat and a slippery, rapid pulse. The correct treatment is to resolve Phlegm Heat and stop vomiting with **WEN DAN TANG** 温胆汤 (*Bamboo and Hoelen Combination*, p.758).

Mixed Heat and Cold

- Incorrect treatment at the *shao yang* stage, specifically giving a purge rather than harmonising, can deplete Stomach *qi* and enable the pathogen to penetrate further into the Stomach and Intestines. The resulting pattern is characterised by a mix of excess and deficiency, Heat and Cold signs and symptoms. The main features are nausea and/or vomiting, or dry retching, epigastric discomfort and distension, acid reflux, indigestion, loss of appetite, tendency to loose stools and a greasy, yellowish tongue coat. The aim of treatment is to harmonise the Stomach and redirect rebellious *qi* downward with **BAN XIA XIE XIN TANG** (*Pinellia Combination* 半夏泻心汤, p.32).

Patent medicines

In general, the dose of all the following patent medicines can be increased by 50%-100% over the recommended dose for a quick result.

Huo Xiang Zheng Qi Pian 藿香正气片 (Huo Xiang Zheng Qi Pian)
Liu Shen Shui 六神水 (Liu Shen Shui)
Xing Jun San 行军散 (Marching Powder, Five Pagodas Brand)
- The three formulae above are for acute vomiting due to external pathogens of any type, but are best when Heat signs are not severe.

Yin Qiao Jie Du Pian 银翘解毒片 (Yin Chiao Chieh Tu Pien, Yin Chiao Plus) - add for Wind Heat

Kang Ning Wan 康宁丸 (Pill Curing)
- Wind Cold

Bao Ji Wan 保济丸 (Po Chai Pills)
- Summerheat

Xiao Chai Hu Wan 小柴胡丸 (Xiao Chai Hu Wan)
- *shao yang* syndrome

Acupuncture (select from)

Du.14 (*da zhui* - Ω) .... meeting point of the *yang* channels, clears pathogens from the exterior

SJ.5 (*wai guan*) ....
PC.6 (*nei guan*) these two points can be joined by deep needling to stop vomiting and dispel Wind from the exterior

St.44 (*nei ting* -) .... together these points clear Heat from *yang*
LI.4 (*he gu* -) *ming*

Ren.12 (*zhong wan* -) .... *mu* point of the Stomach, harmonises Stomach *qi* and directs *qi* downwards

- in severe cases, bleed PC.3 (*qu ze* ↓) and Bl.40 (*wei zhong* ↓)
- with dry retching apply 7 cones of moxa to PC.5 (*jian shi* ▲)
- with epigastric pain, add Sp.4 (*gong sun* -)
- with Phlegm or severe Damp, add St.40 (*feng long* -) and Sp.3 (*tai bai*)
- with dizziness add GB.20 (*feng chi* -)
- with alternating fever and chills add SJ.5 (*wai guan* -) and GB.39 (*xuan zhong* -)
- vomiting bile, add GB.40 (*qiu xu* -), GB.24 (*ri yue*)
- with jaundice add Du.9 (*zhi yang* -)
- *Ear points*: lungs, stomach, liver, subcortex, sympathetic, *shen men*

Clinical notes

- Nausea and vomiting of this type may be diagnosed biomedically as stomach flu, acute viral gastroenteritis, giardia or food poisoning.
- In severe cases, some patients may be unable to tolerate ingesting medicine. Sipping tiny doses through a straw placed at the back of the tongue may help. Keeping a slice of root ginger on the tongue may also be useful.
- These acute patterns are usually self limiting. However, in severe or improperly treated cases, the pathogen can get locked in and linger for lengthy periods. This can cause periodic episodes of the same symptoms, or *shao yang* symptoms. In cases with a Damp pathogen, treatment should persist for a few days after the patient feels well again, to ensure complete expulsion of the Dampness.

饮食停积

21.2 FOOD STAGNATION

Pathophysiology

- Food stagnation is mostly related to overindulgence or unrestrained dietary habits. In the developed world, where people consistently overeat and are often sedentary, the pattern combines with weakness of Spleen and Stomach *qi*, creating a chronic condition. Clinically, this pattern is mixed excess and deficiency. As the pattern progresses the deficiency will become more and more prominent.
- In recurrent cases, there can be several complications depending on the patient and the type of food consumed. Typical complications include Damp or Phlegm Heat, *qi* stagnation, Cold or deficiency.

Clinical features

- Acute or recurrent nausea or vomiting of sour material with undigested food. The patient feels much better after vomiting. Acute episodes will usually be clearly related to an episode of overindulgence; recurrent cases may not be related to a particular event.
- epigastric and abdominal fullness and distension, foul belching, aversion to food and abdominal pain, all symptoms relieved by vomiting
- halitosis, flatulence
- constipation or foul diarrhoea

T thick, greasy coat
P slippery

Treatment principle

Relieve food stagnation and harmonise the Stomach
Redirect Stomach *qi* downward

Prescription

BAO HE WAN 保和丸
(*Citrus and Crategus Formula*)

chao shan zha (dry fried Fructus Crataegi) 炒山楂 18-24g
chao shen qu (dry fried Massa Fermentata) 炒神曲 12-15g
chao lai fu zi (dry fried Semen Raphani Sativi)
炒莱服子 9-12g
ban xia (Rhizoma Pinelliae Ternatae) 半夏 9-12g
fu ling (Sclerotium Poriae Cocos) 茯苓 12-15g
chen pi (Pericarpium Citri Reticulatae) 陈皮 6-9g
lian qiao (Fructus Forsythia Suspensae) 连翘 6-9g

Method: Grind herbs to a powder and form into 9-gram pills with water. The dose is one pill 2-3 times daily. May also be decocted. **Chao shan zha, chao shen qu** and **chao lai fu zi** improve digestion and alleviate food stagnation; **chao lai fu**

zi also directs *qi* downwards; **ban xia** and **chen pi** harmonise the Stomach, resolve Phlegm and promote the movement of *qi*; **fu ling** strengthens the Spleen and leaches out Damp; **lian qiao** dissipates accumulations and clears Heat. (Source: *Shi Yong Zhong Yi Nei Ke Xue*)

Modifications

- In severe cases, add one or two of the following herbs: **huo xiang** (Herba Agastaches seu Pogostemi) 藿香 12-15g, **pei lan** (Herba Eupatorii Fortunei) 佩兰 9-12g, **xuan fu hua** (Flos Inulae) 旋复花 12-15g or **sheng jiang** (Rhizoma Zingiberis Officinalis) 生姜 9-12g.
- With Heat in the Stomach, add **lu gen** (Rhizoma Phragmitis Communis) 芦根 15-30g and **huang lian** (Rhizoma Coptidis) 黄连 6-9g.
- With Cold in the Stomach, delete **lian qiao**, and add **gan jiang** (Rhizoma Zingiberis Officinalis) 干姜 9-12g and **sha ren** (Fructus Amomi) 砂仁 6-9g.
- With Liver *qi* stagnation, add **fo shou** (Fructus Citri Sarcodactylis) 佛手 9-12g, and **mei gui hua** (Flos Rosae Rugosae) 玫瑰花 6-9g.
- With Spleen deficiency, add **chao bai zhu** (dry fried Rhizoma Atractylodes Macrocephalae) 炒白术 12-15g.
- With constipation, add **da huang** (Radix et Rhizoma Rhei) 大黄 6-9g and **bing lang** (Semen Arecae Catechu) 槟榔 9-12g.
- If the stagnation is associated with consumption of excessive meat, increase the dose of **shan zha** (Fructus Crataegi) 山楂 to 30g.
- If the food stagnation is associated with an excessive consumption of starchy foods such as noodles or grains, increase the dose of **lai fu zi** to 15g.
- With severe abdominal distension, add **zhi shi** (Fructus Immaturus Citri Aurantii) 枳实 9-12g.
- In some acute cases, the patient may feel nauseous and bloated but is unable to vomit to relieve the stagnation. In these cases, a dose of warm salty water may help induce vomiting.

Variations and additional prescriptions

Resistant cases

- In resistant cases, a few doses of a mild purge, like **TIAO WEI CHENG QI TANG** (*Regulate the Stomach and Order the Qi Decoction* 调胃承气汤, p.468) may be useful to powerfully redirect *qi* downwards and clear the stagnation through the bowels.

Chronic or recurrent food stagnation with Damp Heat

- For more chronic cases, with significant digestive disruption and the generation of Damp Heat, the aim of treatment is to thoroughly clear the stagnation downwards and out of the Intestines, clear Heat and dispel Damp with **ZHI SHI DAO ZHI WAN** (*Immature Bitter Orange Pill to Guide out Stagnation* 枳实导滞丸, p.181).

Patent medicines

Bao He Wan 保和丸 (Bao He Wan)
Liu He Bao He Wan 六合保和丸 (Bo Wo Yuen Medical Pills)
Jian Pi Wan 健脾丸 (Jian Pi Wan)
- with Spleen deficiency

Acupuncture (select from)

Ren.12 (*zhong wan* -) .... *mu* point of the Stomach, clears Heat and alleviates food stagnation
PC.6 (*nei guan* -) .... *luo* point of the Pericardium, regulates the middle *jiao* and stops vomiting
St.36 (*zu san li* -) .... *he* sea point of the Stomach, regulates and strengthens the Stomach and stops vomiting
St.44 (*nei ting* -) .... *rong* spring and Water point of the Stomach, clears Heat from the Stomach and alleviates food stagnation
St.40 (*feng long* -) .... *luo* point of the Stomach, transforms Phlegm and clears Heat, food stagnation and Phlegm from the Stomach
LI.10 (*shou san li* -) .... benefits digestion and regulates gastro-intestinal function

- with constipation, add SJ.6 (*zhi gou* -), Sp.15 (*da heng* -) and St.25 (*tian shu* -)
- with Spleen deficiency, add Sp.4 (*gong sun*) and Bl.20 (*pi shu* +)
- with severe abdominal distension add St.25 (*tian shu* -) and Ren.6 (*qi hai*)
- *Ear points*: spleen, stomach, small intestine, liver, abdomen

Clinical notes

- Because this is largely a disorder of overindulgence and irregular dietary habits, the patient should be counselled accordingly, and generally the resultant changes alone are enough to cure the problem.
- The Chinese have long known the benefits of sipping small amounts of certain teas while eating. The action of such teas helps assist digestion, especially of fats, and reduces the risk of food stagnation. European cultures use table wine in much the same way, hence 'a little wine for thy stomach's sake'. Similarly, 'bitters', combinations of bitter herbs and alcohol, are a common accompaniment to food, either as a digestive aid following a meal, or as an aperitive. The bitterness of the herbs assists the descent of Stomach *qi* and dries Damp.

痰湿阻胃

21.3 PHLEGM DAMP

Pathophysiology

- The Phlegm patterns are common causes of nausea and vomiting. The presence of Phlegm in the Stomach obstructs the *qi* mechanism and the descent of Stomach *qi*, and retards distribution of *qi* and fluids. Clinical presentation depends on the duration of the disorder, any accompanying pathogens and the degree of deficiency beneath the excess.
- Phlegm may be the primary pathogen, that is, the result of overconsumption of food in general, and Phlegm producing foods such as dairy and ice cream in particular, in which case there may be little underlying deficiency. More commonly, however, Phlegm is the product of poor fluid metabolism and Spleen weakness, or the retardation of fluids by stagnant Liver *qi*. If Phlegm accumulation is the product of an underlying Spleen *yang* deficiency, the Phlegm may initially manifest as thin watery fluids congesting the Spleen and Stomach. Successful treatment ultimately depends on determining the relative degree of deficiency and excess, and prescribing the correct balance of herbs and points to resolve Phlegm and strengthen Spleen *qi*.
- Phlegm can generate Heat through it's capacity to cause obstruction. Phlegm Heat patterns can also follow an acute febrile disorder that has congealed fluids.

Clinical features

- Nausea and/or vomiting, which may be worse first thing in the morning, or when the patient is assailed by strong odours such as perfume or petrol. The vomitus may contain a mucus-like material.
- epigastric and abdominal fullness, distension and stuffiness
- loss of appetite, decreased sense of taste, borborygmus, belching, acid reflux
- sticky sensation in the mouth, or dry mouth with no desire to drink
- fatigue, lethargy, tiredness (may be worse in the morning), increased desire to sleep, heaviness in the body, heavy tired limbs
- dizziness or vertigo, foggy-headedness
- may be chronic mucus production from the sinuses and lungs
- greasy skin, musty body odour
- tendency to obesity, pear shape

T thick, greasy, white coat; the tongue body may be flabby

P slippery or wiry or moderate

Treatment principle

Warm, dry and transform Phlegm and fluids
Strengthen the Spleen and harmonise the Stomach
Stop nausea and vomiting

Prescription

ER CHEN TANG 二陈汤
(*Citrus and Pinellia Combination*)

This is the basic formula for all Phlegm Damp patterns, and serves as the foundation on which to build the majority of Phlegm treatments.

jiang ban xia (ginger fried Rhizoma Pinelliae Ternatae) 姜半夏 9-12g
chen pi (Pericarpium Citri Reticulatae) 陈皮 9-12g
fu ling (Sclerotium Poria Cocos) 茯苓 12-15g
zhi gan cao (honey fried Radix Glycyrrhizae Uralensis) 炙甘草 3-6g

Method: Decoction. **Jiang ban xia** transforms Phlegm, dries Dampness, directs rising Stomach *qi* downwards and stops nausea and vomiting; **chen pi** transforms Phlegm and dries Dampness, regulates middle *jiao qi* and corrects the *qi* mechanism; **fu ling** strengthens the Spleen and leaches out Dampness; **zhi gan cao** strengthens the Spleen and harmonises the Stomach. (Source: *Shi Yong Zhong Yi Nei Ke Xue*)

Modifications

As noted above **ER CHEN TANG** forms the basis of most other Phlegm prescriptions, some of which are listed in the additional prescriptions section below. Some of the modifications listed here are replicated in the additional prescriptions section, which contains commercially prepared powdered or patent formulae.

- With Cold in the Stomach, add **gan jiang** (Rhizoma Zingiberis Officinalis) 干姜 9-12g and **sha ren** (Fructus Amomi) 砂仁 6-9g.
- With Heat, add **huang lian** (Rhizoma Coptidis) 黄连 3-6g, **huo xiang** (Herba Agastaches seu Pogostemi) 藿香 12-15g and **yi ren** (Semen Coicis Lachryma-jobi) 苡仁 15-24g.
- With heartburn or acid reflux, add **huang lian** (Rhizoma Coptidis) 黄连 3-6g and **wu zhu yu** (Fructus Evodiae Rutaecarpae) 吴茱萸 1-2g.
- With vomiting of bile (green, sour or bitter vomitus), add **huang lian** (Rhizoma Coptidis) 黄连 3-6g, **huang qin** (Radix Scutellariae Baicalensis) 黄芩 9-12g, **sheng jiang** (Rhizoma Zingiberis Officinalis) 生姜 9-12g, **yin chen** (Herba Artemisiae Yinchenhao) 茵陈 12-15g and **yu jin** (Tuber Curcumae) 郁金 9-12g.
- For morning sickness (of a Phlegm type), add **zi su ye** (Folium Perillae Frutescentis) 紫苏叶 6-9g, **huang qin** (Radix Scutellariae Baicalensis) 黄芩 3g and **zhu ru** (Caulis Bambusae in Taeniis) 竹茹 6-9g.
- For vomiting of thin, watery, mucus-like material, add **cang zhu** (Rhizoma Atractylodis) 苍术 9-12g and **bai zhu** (Rhizoma Atractylodes Macrocephalae) 白术 9-12g.
- In severe or resistant cases, add **xuan fu hua** (Flos Inulae) 旋复花 9-

15g and **huo xiang** (Herba Agastaches seu Pogostemi) 藿香 12-15g.

- With food stagnation, add **shen qu** (Massa Fermentata) 神曲 15g, **chao mai ya** (dry fried Fructus Hordei Vulgaris Germinantus) 炒麦芽 15-30g, **zhi shi** (Fructus Immaturus Citri Aurantii) 枳实 9-12g and **xiang fu** (Rhizoma Cyperi Rotundi) 香附 9-12g.
- For nausea or vomiting due to excess alcohol consumption, add **zhu ling** (Sclerotium Polypori Umbellati) 猪苓 9-12g and **ge hua** (Flos Puerariae) 葛花 12-18g.
- With constipation or sluggish stools, add **da huang** (Radix et Rhizoma Rhei) 大黄 3-9g, **hou po** (Cortex Magnoliae Officinalis) 厚朴 9-12g and **zhi shi** (Fructus Immaturus Citri Aurantii) 枳实 9-12g.
- If Cold Dampness accumulates in the Stomach as a result of overconsumption of raw or cold natured foods, with nausea and vomiting, belching, acid reflux, epigastric and abdominal distension, heaviness in the limbs, loose stools and an increased desire to sleep, combine with **PING WEI SAN** (*Magnolia and Ginger Formula* 平胃散, p.153).

Variations and additional prescriptions

Chronic Phlegm with Spleen qi deficiency

- When Spleen deficiency is the source of the Phlegm (chronic morning nausea, food sensitivities, abdominal distension, reflux, pale tongue, fatigue), the aim of treatment is to strengthen the Spleen to resolve Phlegm with **XIANG SHA LIU JUN ZI TANG** (*Saussurea and Cardamon Combination* 香砂六君子汤).

dang shen (Radix Codonopsis Pilosulae) 党参 12-15g
chao bai zhu (dry fried Rhizoma Atractylodes Macrocephalae) 炒白术 12-15g
fu ling (Sclerotium Poria Cocos) 茯苓 12-18g
ban xia (Rhizoma Pinelliae Ternatae) 半夏 9-12g
chen pi (Pericarpium Citri Reticulatae) 陈皮 9-12g
gan cao (Radix Glycyrrhizae Uralensis) 甘草 3-6g
sha ren (Fructus Amomi) 砂仁 6-9g
mu xiang (Radix Aucklandiae Lappae) 木香 6-9g

Method: Decoction. **Dang shen, bai zhu, fu ling** and **gan cao** constitute **SI JUN ZI TANG**, the basic prescription for Spleen *qi* deficiency; **dang shen** supplements *qi* and strengthens the Spleen; **chao bai zhu** strengthens the Spleen and dries Dampness; **fu ling** strengthens the Spleen and leaches out Dampness; **gan cao** supplements *qi*; **ban xia** and **chen pi** transform Phlegm, dry Dampness, direct rising Stomach *qi* downwards and stop nausea and vomiting; **sha ren** and **mu xiang** regulate *qi* in the middle *jiao*.

Thin Phlegm and Spleen yang deficiency

- An underlying tendency to Spleen *yang* deficiency can give rise to accumulation of thin fluids in the epigastrium, and consequent chronic nausea and vomiting of watery fluids. In addition, the patient may experience dizziness, fullness in the chest and epigastrium, palpitations, shortness of breath, a productive cough, a pale, swollen tongue and a slippery or soggy pulse. The aim of treatment is to warm and transform Phlegm and fluids, and strengthen the Spleen with **LING GUI ZHU GAN TANG** (*Atractylodes and Hoelen Combination* 苓桂术甘汤) modified. Follow with a lengthy course of an appropriate Spleen supplementing prescription.

fu ling (Sclerotium Poria Cocos) 茯苓 12-18g
bai zhu (Rhizoma Atractylodes Macrocephalae) 白术 12-15g
gui zhi (Ramulus Cinnamomi Cassiae) 桂枝 9-12g
zhi gan cao (honey fried Radix Glycyrrhizae Uralensis)
炙甘草 3-6g
gan jiang (Rhizoma Zingiberis Officinalis) 干姜 9-12g
ban xia (Rhizoma Pinelliae Ternatae) 半夏 9-12g

Method: Decoction. **Fu ling** strengthens the Spleen and leaches out Dampness; **gui zhi** warms *yang* and supports metabolism and transformation of fluids; **bai zhu** strengthens the Spleen and dries Dampness; **zhi gan cao** strengthens the Spleen and harmonises the Stomach; **gan jiang** warms the Spleen and Stomach and stops vomiting, **ban xia** transforms Phlegm, dries Dampness, directs rising Stomach *qi* downwards and stops nausea and vomiting. (Source: *Shi Yong Zhong Yi Nei Ke Xue*)

Phlegm Heat

- With Phlegm Heat (frequent nausea or vomiting, flushing with vomiting, indeterminate gnawing hunger, insomnia, anxiety, greasy, yellow tongue coat and a slippery, rapid pulse) the aim of treatment is to resolve Phlegm Heat and stop vomiting with **WEN DAN TANG** 温胆汤 (*Bamboo and Hoelen Combination*). This pattern may also occur in the recovery phase of an acute febrile illness, in which case it typically persists for up to six weeks after the fever has abated. This prescription is also suitable for Liver and Stomach Heat type vomiting.

zhu ru (Caulis Bambusae in Taeniis) 竹茹 9-12g
zhi shi (Fructus Immaturus Citri Aurantii) 枳实 9-12g
ban xia (Rhizoma Pinelliae Ternatae) 半夏 9-12g
chen pi (Pericarpium Citri Reticulatae) 陈皮 6-9g
fu ling (Sclerotium Poria Cocos) 茯苓 12-15g
gan cao (Radix Glycyrrhizae Uralensis) 甘草 3-6g
sheng jiang (Rhizoma Zingiberis Officinalis Recens)
生姜 6-9g

Method: Decoction. **Zhu ru** clears Phlegm Heat from the Stomach and Gallbladder, directs Stomach *qi* downwards and stops vomiting; **zhi shi** breaks up stagnant *qi*, directs *qi* downwards and alleviates distension; **ban xia** transforms Phlegm, dries Dampness, directs rising Stomach *qi* downwards and stops nausea and vomiting; **chen pi** transforms Phlegm and dries Dampness, regulates middle *jiao qi* and corrects the *qi* mechanism; **fu ling** strengthens the Spleen and leaches out Dampness; **gan cao** strengthens the Spleen and harmonises the Stomach; **sheng jiang** assists the other herbs in stopping nausea and vomiting. (Source: *Shi Yong Zhong Yi Nei Ke Xue*)

Wind Phlegm

- The obstructive nature of Phlegm can generate sufficient pressure to create Wind, and thus Wind Phlegm, in some patients. The Wind manifests itself when it suddenly carries Phlegm up to the head, causing severe nausea and vomiting, accompanied by dizziness or vertigo (in severe cases bed spins) and tinnitus. The aim of treatment is to eliminate Wind and transform Phlegm with a formula such as **BAN XIA BAI ZHU TIAN MA TANG** (*Pinellia and Gastrodia Combination* 半夏白术天麻汤). *See also* Dizziness, Vol.1.

ban xia (Rhizoma Pinelliae Ternatae) 半夏 9-12g
bai zhu (Rhizoma Atractylodes Macrocephalae) 白术 12-15g
tian ma (Rhizoma Gastrodiae Elatae) 天麻 9-12g
chen pi (Pericarpium Citri Reticulatae) 陈皮 6-9g
fu ling (Sclerotium Poria Cocos) 茯苓 9-15g
gan cao (Radix Glycyrrhizae Uralensis) 甘草 3-6g
sheng jiang (Rhizoma Zingiberis Officinalis Recens)
生姜 6-12g
da zao (Fructus Zizyphi Jujubae) 大枣 3pce

Method: Decoction. **Ban xia** transforms Phlegm, dries Dampness, directs rising Stomach *qi* downwards and stops nausea and vomiting, **tian ma** calms the Liver and extinguishes Wind, together these herbs effectively treat Wind Phlegm; **bai zhu** and **fu ling** strengthen the Spleen, and dry and leach out Dampness respectively, as well as treating the root cause of the Phlegm; **chen pi** transforms Phlegm and dries Dampness, regulates middle *jiao qi* and corrects the *qi* mechanism; **sheng jiang** transforms Phlegm and assists the other herbs in stopping nausea and vomiting; **da zao** and **gan cao** strengthen the Spleen and harmonise the Stomach.

Morning sickness

- Phlegm type morning sickness is characterised by morning nausea, vomiting of a mucus like material, aversion to strong smells, fullness and discomfort in the chest, palpitations, a thick, greasy tongue coat and a slippery pulse. The aim of treatment is to gently strengthen the Spleen to transform Phlegm, leach out Damp and stop vomiting with **XIAO BAN XIA FU LING TANG** (*Minor Pinellia and Hoelen Combination* 小半夏茯苓汤).

jiang ban xia (ginger fried Rhizoma Pinelliae Ternatae)
姜半夏 9-12g

fu ling (Sclerotium Poria Cocos) 茯苓 30g
sheng jiang (Rhizoma Zingiberis Officinalis Recens) 生姜 6-9g

Method: Decoction. **Jiang ban xia** transforms Phlegm, dries Dampness, directs rising Stomach *qi* downwards and stops nausea and vomiting; **fu ling** strengthens the Spleen and leaches out Dampness; **sheng jiang** assists the other herbs in stopping nausea and vomiting.

With some Heat in the Stomach, add **huang qin** (Radix Scutellariae Baicalensis) 黄芩 3g and **zhu ru** (Caulis Bambusae in Taeniis) 竹茹 6-9g. (Source: *Shi Yong Zhong Yi Fu Ke Xue*)

Phlegm with rebellious Stomach qi

- In severe or unresponsive cases, the treatment priority is altered to forcefully direct rising Stomach *qi* downwards, transform Phlegm and harmonise the Stomach with **XUAN FU DAI ZHE TANG** (*Inula and Haematite Decoction* 旋复代赭汤, p.772).

Patent medicines

Er Chen Wan 二陈丸 (Er Chen Wan, Pinellia-Pachyma Compound Pills)
Xiang Sha Liu Jun Zi Wan 香砂六君子丸 (Xiang Sha Liu Jun Wan, Aplotaxis-Ammomum Pills, Six Gentlemen Tea Pills)
- with Spleen *qi* deficiency

Wen Dan Wan 温胆丸 (Wen Dan Wan)
- Phlegm Heat

Fu Zi Li Zhong Wan 附子理中丸 (Fu-Tzu Li-Chung Wan)
- Spleen *yang* deficiency with thin Phlegm

Xiang Sha Yang Wei Wan 香砂养胃丸 (Xiang Sha Yang Wei Wan, Hsiang Sha Yang Wei Wan)
- with *qi* stagnation

Acupuncture (select from)

PC.6 (*nei guan* -) .... *luo* point of the Pericardium, master point of *yin wei mai*, regulates the middle *jiao*, stops vomiting and calms the Heart and *shen*
PC.5 (*jian shi* -) .... *jing* river point of the Pericardium, transforms Phlegm and harmonises the Stomach
Ren.12 (*zhong wan* -) .... *mu* point of the Stomach, clears pathogens, directs Stomach *qi* downwards and harmonises the Stomach
St.40 (*feng long* -) .... *luo* point of the Stomach, transforms Phlegm and clears Heat and Phlegm from the Stomach
Sp.3 (*tai bai*) .... *yuan*, *shu* stream and Earth point of the Spleen, supplements the Spleen and transforms Dampness

- with Spleen deficiency, add St.36 (*zu san li* +) and Liv.13 (*zhang men* +)
- with Liver *qi* stagnation, add GB.34 (*yang ling quan* -) and Liv.3 (*tai chong* -)
- with vomiting of bile, add GB.34 (*yang ling quan* -), GB.24 (*ri yue*) and *dan nang xue* (M-LE-23)
- with foggy-headedness, add GB.20 (*feng chi*) and Bl.62 (*shen mai*)
- with Wind Phlegm, add GB.40 (*qiu xu* -), St.8 (*tou wei*) and St.41 (*jie xi* -)
- with Cold Phlegm, apply moxa cones to Bl.20 (*pi shu* ▲) and Bl.21 (*wei shu* ▲)
- with muscle aches and heaviness, add Sp.21 (*da bao*)
- with fluid retention and oedema, add Sp.9 (*yin ling quan* -) and Sp.6 (*san yin jiao*)
- with somnolence, add Kid.6 (*zhao hai*) and Bl.62 (*shen mai*)
- with severe abdominal distension, add St.25 (*tian shu* -) and Sp.15 (*da heng* -)
- *Ear points*: stomach, spleen, liver, subcortex, sympathetic, *shen men*

Clinical notes

- Nausea and vomiting of a Phlegm accumulation type may be diagnosed biomedically as chronic gastritis, indigestion, Meniere's disease, neurogenic vomiting and morning sickness.
- Phlegm disorders usually respond quite well to correct treatment, however they can be persistent, especially when chronic or constitutional. Prolonged treatment and dietary modification is necessary to disperse the Phlegm and prevent recurrence.
- For dietary recommendations, see p.880.

肝气犯胃

21.4 LIVER QI INVADING THE STOMACH

Pathophysiology

- Liver *qi* invades the Stomach in response to stress or emotional upset. This type of nausea and vomiting may be an acute episode (after sudden or severe emotional aggravation), never to be repeated and with few if any constitutional indicators of *qi* stagnation. It is, however, much more likely to be a chronic and recurrent pattern, a learned and deeply ingrained response to stress.
- Because this is such a common cause of nausea and vomiting, and in general tends to be a long term problem, *qi* stagnation is almost invariably complicated by other patterns. The common complications are stagnant Heat, Blood stagnation, food stagnation, Spleen deficiency and Phlegm accumulation.

Clinical features

- Recurrent or chronic nausea, vomiting, sour belching and acid reflux, all aggravated or initiated by stress, anxiety and emotional turmoil, and relieved by belching and when calm and relaxed.
- loss of appetite, indigestion, heartburn, acid reflux
- fullness, tightness or discomfort in the chest, epigastrium and hypochondrium
- irritability, anger, frustration, anxiety, moodiness, depression
- may be a sensation of something lodged in the throat (plum-stone throat)
- premenstrual syndrome, irregular menstruation

T normal or darkish or with slightly red edges with a thin, possibly greasy coat; in chronic cases with underlying deficiency, the tongue may be pale or pale on the edges

P wiry, or wiry and slippery

Treatment principle

Harmonise the Liver and Stomach and regulate *qi*
Redirect Stomach *qi* downwards, stop nausea and vomiting

Prescription

21.4.1 *Qi* stagnation predominantly in the Stomach

YUE JU WAN 越鞠丸
(*Escape Restraint Pill*) modified

This prescription is selected when the predominant site of the *qi* stagnation is in the Stomach, and Liver symptoms are secondary. This is a broad acting prescription, designed to take into account the common repercussions of *qi* stagnation, such as accumulation of Damp, Phlegm, Blood,

Heat and food. The key features are nausea, poor appetite, indigestion, epigastric fullness and distension, acid reflux, belching, depression and occasional fatigue.

xiang fu (Rhizoma Cyperi Rotundi) 香附 12-15g
cang zhu (Rhizoma Atractylodis) 苍术 9-12g
chuan xiong (Radix Ligustici Chuanxiong) 川芎 6-9g
shan zhi zi (Fructus Gardeniae Jasminoides) 山栀子 6-12g
shen qu (Massa Fermentata) 神曲 9-12g
ban xia (Rhizoma Pinelliae Ternatae) 半夏 9-12g

Method: Decoction. **Xiang fu** is the main herb and disperses stagnant Liver *qi*; **cang zhu** dries Dampness and Phlegm, and works with **xiang fu** to improve Spleen and Stomach function; **chuan xiong** invigorates *qi* and Blood and reinforces the *qi* moving function of **xiang fu**; **shan zhi zi** clears Heat from all three *jiao*; **shen qu** alleviates food stagnation, aids digestion and harmonises the Stomach; **ban xia** transforms Phlegm, dries Damp, directs rising Stomach *qi* downwards and stops nausea and vomiting.

21.4.2 Predominant Liver *qi* stagnation with Heat

SI NI SAN 四逆散
(*Bupleurum and Zhi Shi Formula*) modified

This prescription is selected when Liver *qi* stagnation has generated Heat, and there is significant sour vomiting and acid regurgitation. The Heat has lodged in the Stomach. The associated features that point to this prescription are persistently cold extremities, (especially the fingers and toes) in a generally robust patient with a short temper and irritability, belching, indigestion, bitter taste in the mouth, red edges on the tongue, a yellow coat and a wiry pulse.

chai hu (Radix Bupleuri) 柴胡 9-12g
zhi shi (Fructus Immaturus Citri Aurantii) 枳实 9-12g
bai shao (Radix Paeoniae Lactiflora) 白芍 12-15g
zhi gan cao (honey fried Radix Glycyrrhizae Uralensis)
炙甘草 3-6g
huang lian (Rhizoma Coptidis) 黄连 6-9g
wu zhu yu (Fructus Evodiae Rutaecarpae) 吴茱萸 2-3g

Method: Decoction. **Chai hu** regulates and invigorates Liver *qi* and clears Heat; **zhi shi** breaks up stagnant *qi*, directs *qi* downwards and alleviates distension, it's descending action neatly balances the ascending nature of **chai hu** thus facilitating the correct functioning of the *qi* mechanism; **bai shao** softens the Liver and nourishes *yin* and Blood, thus preventing excessive dispersal of, and damage to, *qi* and Liver *yin* by **chai hu**; **gan cao** harmonises the Stomach and strengthens the Spleen, and with **bai shao** eases spasms thereby alleviating cramping pain; **huang lian** clears Heat from the Liver and Stomach; **wu zhu yu** is pungent and warm and promotes movement of *qi*, together these last two herbs clear Heat and direct Stomach *qi* downward. (Source: *Shi Yong Zhong Yi Nei Ke Xue*)

21.4.3 *Qi* stagnation with Phlegm

BAN XIA HOU PO TANG 半夏厚朴汤
(*Pinellia and Magnolia Combination*)

This prescription is selected in cases of Phlegm and *qi* stagnation, characterised by nausea or vomiting that is provoked by anxiety or stress, and accompanied by sadness, plum-stone throat, tightness in the chest, a greasy tongue coat and a wiry, slippery pulse.

ban xia (Rhizoma Pinelliae Ternatae) 半夏 9-12g
hou po (Cortex Magnoliae Officinalis) 厚朴 9-12g
fu ling (Sclerotium Poriae Cocos) 茯苓 12-15g
sheng jiang (Rhizoma Zingiberis Officinalis Recens) 生姜 6-9g
zi su ye (Folium Perillae Frutescentis) 紫苏叶 6-9g

Method: Decoction. **Ban xia** transforms Phlegm, dries Damp, directs rising Stomach *qi* downwards and stops nausea and vomiting; **hou po** promotes movement of *qi*, transforms Phlegm and Dampness, and directs *qi* downwards; **fu ling** strengthens the Spleen and leaches out Damp; **sheng jiang** warms the Stomach and stops vomiting, **zi su ye** promotes movement of *qi* and settles the Stomach. (Source: *Shi Yong Zhong Yi Nei Ke Xue*)

Modifications (apply to all three prescriptions where not already included)

- With severe nausea or vomiting, add **xuan fu hua** (Flos Inulae) 旋复花 12-15g and **dai zhe shi** (Haematitum) 代赭石 15g.
- For vomiting of bile (greenish, sour vomitus), add **zhi ke** (Fructus Citri Aurantii) 枳壳 9-12g, **yu jin** (Tuber Curcumae) 郁金 9-12g and **jin qian cao** (Herba Lysimachiae) 金钱草 18g.
- With constipation add **da huang** (Radix et Rhizoma Rhei) 大黄 3-9g and **zhi shi** (Fructus Immaturus Citri Aurantii) 枳实 9-12g.
- With food stagnation add **shan zha** (Fructus Crataegi) 山楂 15g, **mai ya** (Fructus Hordei Vulgaris Germinantus) 麦芽 15-30g and **ji nei jin** (Endothelium Corneum Gigeriae Galli) 鸡内金 12g.
- With stagnant Heat and acid reflux, add **huang lian** (Rhizoma Coptidis) 黄连 6-9g and **wu zhu yu** (Fructus Evodiae Rutaecarpae) 吴茱萸 2-3g.
- In chronic cases with damaged *yin* (dry mouth, burning epigastrium, little coat in the centre of the tongue), decrease the dose of the dispersing and drying herbs (**ban xia, chai hu, sheng jiang, zi su ye** etc.), and add **sha shen** (Radix Adenophorae seu Glehniae) 沙参 12-15g and **shi hu** (Herba Dendrobii) 石斛 12-15g.

Variations and additional prescriptions

Chronic nausea associated with Liver and Gallbladder qi stagnation and Damp Heat

- Chronic Liver *qi* stagnation, in combination with a rich diet, can disrupt the smooth flow of bile, which over time may contribute to Gallbladder irritation and the development of gallstones. Patients with this tendency, often women, will often have a long history of low grade digestive symptoms, food intolerances and sensitivity. The typical features are frequent nausea, fat intolerance, distension, a tendency to sluggish and sticky stools, temporal headaches, a thick tongue coat and a soggy or slippery pulse. The treatment is to clear the Gallbladder, regulate *qi*, harmonise the Stomach and transform Phlegm. (*See also* Hypochondriac pain and Gallstones, Volume 1). A reasonable base prescription is **XIAO CHAI HU TANG** (*Minor Bupleurum Combination* 小柴胡汤, p.748). If there is constipation or sluggish stools, **DA CHAI HU TANG** (*Major Bupleurum Combination* 大柴胡汤, p.363) is suitable. With lurking Damp Heat (yellow tongue coat, thirst with no desire to drink, slippery or soggy pulse) **HAO QIN QING DAN TANG** (*Artemisia Annua and Scutellaria Decoction to Clear the Gallbladder* 蒿芩清胆汤) modified, may be suitable.

qing hao (Herba Artemesiae Annuae) 青蒿 12-18g
huang qin (Radix Scutellariae Baicalensis) 黄芩 9-12g
zhu ru (Caulis Bambusae in Taeniis) 竹茹 9-12g
ban xia (Rhizoma Pinelliae Ternatae) 半夏 9-12g
chi fu ling (Sclerotium Poriae Cocos Rubrae) 赤茯苓 12-15g
chen pi (Pericarpium Citri Reticulatae) 陈皮 6-9g
zhi ke (Fructus Citri Aurantii) 枳壳 6-9g
gan cao (Radix Glycyrrhizae Uralensis) 甘草 3-6g
yu jin (Tuber Curcumae) 郁金 9-12g
pu gong ying (Herba Taraxaci Mongolici) 蒲公英 15-30g

Method: Decoction or powder. **Qing hao** and **huang qin** vent *shao yang* and clear Damp Heat from the Liver and Gallbladder; **zhu ru** clears Phlegm Heat from the Stomach and Gallbladder, directs Stomach *qi* downwards and stops vomiting; **ban xia** transforms Phlegm, dries Dampness, directs rising Stomach *qi* downwards and stops nausea and vomiting; **chen pi** transforms Phlegm and dries Dampness, regulates middle *jiao qi* and corrects the *qi* mechanism; **zhi ke** assists the previous two herbs in regulating *qi*, transforming Dampness and harmonising the Stomach; **chi fu ling** leaches out Damp Heat through the urine; **gan cao** assists in clearing Heat; **yu jin** invigorates *qi* and Blood and benefits and cools the Heart and Gallbladder; **pu gong ying** cools and benefits the Liver and Gallbladder.

Persistent or severe vomiting

- For patients who suffer from persistent or severe vomiting associated with anxiety, stress or emotional tension, a useful formula for acute or difficult to control episodes is **XUAN FU DAI ZHE TANG** (*Inula and Haematite Decoction* 旋复代赭汤, p.772). This formula drives down rebellious *qi* to control the vomiting in the short term.

Morning sickness (Heat in the Liver and chong mai)

- Morning sickness or vomiting during pregnancy, associated with Heat in the Liver and Stomach (via the *chong mai*), is characterised by nausea with sour regurgitation or vomiting of sour material, hypochondriac discomfort, belching and sighing, dizziness, moodiness, depression, concentrated urine, a tendency to constipation and a yellow tongue coat. The treatment is to clear Liver and Stomach Heat, redirect *qi* downwards and stop vomiting with **SU YE HUANG LIAN TANG** (*Perilla Leaf and Coptis Decoction* 苏叶黄连汤) modified.

zi su ye (Folium Perillae Frutescentis) 紫苏叶 6-9g
huang lian (Rhizoma Coptidis) 黄连 2-3g
ban xia (Rhizoma Pinelliae Ternatae) 半夏 6-9g
zhu ru (Caulis Bambusae in Taeniis) 竹茹 6-9g
pi pa ye (Folium Eriobotryae Japonicae) 枇杷叶 6-9g
chen pi (Pericarpium Citri Reticulatae) 陈皮 6-9g

Method: Decoction. **Zi su ye** calms a restless foetus, promotes movement of *qi* and settles the Stomach; **huang lian**, **zhu ru** and **pi pa ye** clear Heat from the Liver and Stomach and direct Stomach *qi* downwards; **ban xia** and **chen pi** transform Phlegm, dry Dampness, direct rising Stomach *qi* downwards and stop nausea and vomiting.

With dryness, dry retching or fluid damage, delete **ban xia** and add **mai dong** (Tuber Ophiopogonis Japonici) 麦冬 9g; with severe dizziness, add **ju hua** (Flos Chrysanthemi Morifolii) 菊花 9g and **gou teng** (Ramulus Uncariae cum Uncis) 钩藤 9g. (Source: *Shi Yong Zhong Yi Fu Ke Xue*)

Maintenance treatment to regulate qi

- Once the nausea and vomiting have resolved, other *qi* regulating formulae (for example, **XIAO YAO SAN** (*Bupleurum and Dang Gui Formula* 逍遥散, p.159), **CHAI HU SHU GAN SAN** (*Bupleurum and Cyperus Formula* 柴胡疏肝散, p.356) or **BAN XIA HOU PO TANG** (*Pinellia and Magnolia Combination* 半夏厚朴汤, p.764) should be selected for the long term constitutional treatment of the patient's tendency to Liver *qi* stagnation.

Patent medicines

Shu Gan Wan 舒肝丸 (Shu Gan Wan, Shu Kan Wan)
- with pain

Chai Hu Shu Gan Wan 柴胡疏肝丸 (Chai Hu Shu Gan Wan)
- Liver invading the Stomach, good for robust patients

Chen Xiang Hua Qi Wan 沉香化气丸 (Chen Xiang Hua Qi Wan)
- with constipation

Xiao Yao Wan 逍遥丸 (Xiao Yao Wan, Hsiao Yao Wan, Bupleurum Sedative Pills) - best for constitutional treatment of Liver *qi* stagnation in women and patient's with Spleen and Blood deficiency

Jia Wei Xiao Yao Wan 加味逍遥丸 (Jia Wei Xiao Yao Wan, Dan Zhi Xiao Yao Wan) - Liver *qi* stagnation with stagnant Heat

Li Dan Pian 利胆片 (Lidan Tablets)
- with Damp Heat and Gallbladder involvement

Xiao Chai Hu Wan 小柴胡丸 (Xiao Chai Hu Wan)
- *shao yang* syndrome

Xiang Sha Yang Wei Wan 香砂养胃丸 (Xiang Sha Yang Wei Wan)
- with Spleen and Stomach deficiency

Long Dan Xie Gan Wan 龙胆泻肝丸 (Long Dan Xie Gan Wan, Lung Tan Xie Gan Wan)
- Liver and Gallbladder Fire

Huang Lian Jie Du Wan 黄连解毒丸 (Huang Lian Jie Du Wan)
- severe Stomach Damp Heat, Fire

Acupuncture (select from)

PC.6 (*nei guan* -) .... *luo* point of the Pericardium, master point of *yin wei mai*, spreads Liver *qi*, regulates the middle *jiao*, stops vomiting and calms the Heart and *shen*

Sp.4 (*gong sun*) .... *luo* point of the Spleen, master point of *chong mai*, regulates the Spleen and Stomach

Liv.13 (*zhang men*) .... *mu* point of the Spleen, regulates the Liver and Spleen and strengthens the Spleen

Ren.12 (*zhong wan* -) .... *mu* point of the Stomach, regulates the Stomach and directs Stomach *qi* downwards

Liv.3 (*tai chong* -) .... together these points regulate Liver *qi*,
GB.34 (*yang ling quan* -) pacify the Liver and harmonise the Liver and Stomach

- with severe vomiting, add GB.40 (*qiu xi* -)
- with Gallbladder involvement or vomiting bile, add GB.24 (*ri yue*), GB.40 (*qiu xu* -) and *dan nang xue* (M-LE-23)
- with Spleen deficiency, add St.36 (*zu san li* +) and Bl.20 (*pi shu* +)
- with Phlegm or plum stone throat, add PC.5 (*jian shi* -), St.40 (*feng long* -) and Sp.3 (*tai bai*)
- with alternating fever and chills add SJ.5 (*wai guan* -) and GB.39 (*xuan zhong* -)
- with dizziness, add GB.20 (*feng chi* -)
- In most cases, points to calm the *shen* should be added: select one or two points from Ht.7 (*shen men*), *yin tang* (M-HN-3), Du.19 (*hou ding*), Du. 24 (*shen ting*)
- *Ear points*: liver, stomach, spleen, subcortex, sympathetic, *shen men*

Clinical notes

- Nausea or vomiting of a Liver *qi* invading the Stomach type may be diagnosed biomedically as chronic gastritis, peptic ulcer disease, nervous stomach, indigestion, chronic cholecystitis, chronic hepatitis, inner ear disorders, Meniere's disease or morning sickness.
- Liver *qi* stagnation type nausea and vomiting usually has a good prognosis, particularly if the source of external stress can be resolved. Acupuncture and herbs are certainly among the best and most reliable treatments. Treatment often needs to be prolonged (3 months+) and must be combined with appropriate relaxation and stress management techniques, or other forms of *qi* mobilising activity. Particularly useful is walking, swimming, yoga or *tai ji chuan*, although all exercise is beneficial. Gentle and regular massage, particularly of the abdomen, neck and mid thoracic region is also useful.
- For dietary recommendations, see p.878.

脾胃虛弱

21.5 SPLEEN AND STOMACH QI/YANG DEFICIENCY

Pathophysiology

- Spleen and Stomach deficiency can give rise to nausea and vomiting in two ways. Digestive *qi* can accumulate in the middle *jiao* because of a weakness of correct *qi* movement. The *qi* mechanism is disordered, and Spleen *qi* does not ascend and/or Stomach *qi* does not descend. This accumulated *qi* can back up, giving a feeling of discomfort and mild nausea. Because there is little digestive power, food stagnation and/or Phlegm may complicate the deficiency. Both these pathogens can further disrupt the *qi* mechanism.
- In contrast to the Phlegm patterns which it may resemble, this pattern is predominantly deficient. There are several variations depending on the degree of deficiency and how much excess complication there is.

Clinical features

- Chronic, intermittent nausea or vomiting after eating; food remains undigested for too long after eating. The nausea may be better for warming, easily digestible foods, and worse with raw, or hard to digest, foods and dairy products. It may also be worse in the morning.
- waxy, pale or lustreless complexion
- tiredness, lethargy and fatigue, tired weak limbs
- poor appetite, sweet cravings (that increase the nausea when indulged)
- epigastric and abdominal distension
- loose stools or diarrhoea
- oedema, particularly in the eyelids and fingers
- if *yang* is deficient: cold extremities, cold intolerance, undigested food in the stools, abdominal pain which is better for warmth

T pale and swollen with toothmarks; the coat will vary from thin (in pure deficiency) to thick and greasy (with accumulated Damp)

P weak and thready

Treatment principle

Warm and strengthen the Spleen and Stomach, supplement *qi*
Harmonise the Stomach and redirect *qi* downward
Transform Phlegm and Damp as necessary

Prescription

21.5.1 Spleen *qi* deficiency

LIU JUN ZI TANG 六君子汤
(*Six Major Herbs Combination*)

This prescription is selected for Spleen *qi* deficiency. There may be a degree of accumulated Dampness or Phlegm.

dang shen (Radix Codonopsis Pilosulae) 党参 15-24g
chao bai zhu (dry fried Rhizoma Atractylodes Macrocephalae) 炒白术 12-15g
ban xia (Rhizoma Pinelliae Ternatae) 半夏 9-12g
fu ling (Sclerotium Poriae Cocos) 茯苓 12-15g
chen pi (Pericarpium Citri Reticulatae) 陈皮 6-9g
zhi gan cao (honey fried Radix Glycyrrhizae Uralensis) 炙甘草 3-6g

Method: Decoction. **Dang shen** supplements *qi* and strengthens the Spleen; **chao bai zhu** strengthens the Spleen and dries Dampness; **fu ling** strengthens the Spleen and leaches out Dampness through the urine; **ban xia** transforms Phlegm, dries Dampness, directs rising Stomach *qi* downwards and stops nausea and vomiting; **chen pi** transforms Phlegm and dries Dampness, regulates middle *jiao qi* and corrects the *qi* mechanism; **zhi gan cao** strengthens the Spleen and harmonises the Stomach. (Source: *Shi Yong Zhong Yi Nei Ke Xue*)

21.5.2 Spleen *yang* deficiency

LI ZHONG WAN 理中丸
(*Ginseng and Ginger Formula*)

This prescription is selected for Spleen and Stomach *yang* deficiency.

gan jiang (Rhizoma Zingiberis Officinalis) 干姜 9-12g
dang shen (Radix Codonopsis Pilosulae) 党参 15-24g
chao bai zhu (dry fried Rhizoma Atractylodes Macrocephalae) 炒白术 12-15g
zhi gan cao (honey fried Radix Glycyrrhizae Uralensis) 炙甘草 3-6g

Method: Decoction. **Gan jiang**, the main herb, warms Spleen and Stomach *yang* and dispels Cold; **dang shen** supplements *qi* and strengthens the Spleen; **chao bai zhu** strengthens the Spleen and dries Dampness; **zhi gan cao** supplements *qi* and harmonises the Stomach.

Modifications

- With vomiting of thin, watery or frothy mucus, add **gui zhi** (Ramulus Cinnamomi Cassiae) 桂枝 6-9g and **wu zhu yu** (Fructus Evodiae Rutaecarpae) 吴茱萸 3-6g.
- With morning sickness, use the lower end of the dosage range, and add **huo xiang** (Herba Agastaches seu Pogostemi) 藿香 6-9g and **zhu ru** (Caulis Bambusae in Taeniis) 竹茹 6-9g.
- With abdominal bloating, add **mu xiang** (Radix Aucklandiae Lappae) 木香 6-9g and **sha ren** (Fructus Amomi) 砂仁 6-9g.
- With cold extremities and cold intolerance, add **zhi fu zi** (Radix Aconiti Carmichaeli Praeparata) 制附子 6-9g (decocted for 30 minutes prior to the other herbs), and **rou gui** (Cortex Cinnamomi Cassiae) 肉桂 3g.
- With food stagnation, add **chao shan zha** (dry fried Fructus Crataegi)

炒山楂 15g and **chao shen qu** (dry fried Massa Fermentata) 炒神曲 15g.

- With heartburn or acid reflux, add **huang lian** (Rhizoma Coptidis) 黄连 3g and **wu zhu yu** (Fructus Evodiae Rutaecarpae) 吴茱萸 1.5g.
- With foggy or woolly-headedness or sleepiness, add **shi chang pu** (Rhizoma Acori Graminei) 石菖蒲 6-9g and **yuan zhi** (Radix Polygalae Tenuifoliae) 远志 6-9g.
- With copious Dampness (muscle aches, heaviness, thick, greasy tongue coat), add **huo xiang** (Herba Agastaches seu Pogostemi) 藿香 12g and **pei lan** (Herba Eupatorii Fortunei) 佩兰 9g.

Variations and additional prescriptions

Cold in the Liver and Stomach channels

- An interesting variation involves Cold and deficiency affecting the Liver and Stomach. This pattern typically involves nausea and vomiting, or vomiting immediately after eating, dry retching, acid reflux and cold extremities associated with headache. The tongue is pale with a greasy, white coat. The headache is typically at the vertex or temples. This occurs in some types of migraine. The aim of treatment is to warm the Liver and Stomach, redirect rebellious *qi* downward and stop vomiting with **WU ZHU YU TANG** (*Evodia Combination* 吴茱萸汤).

wu zhu yu (Fructus Evodiae Rutaecarpae) 吴茱萸 9-12g
dang shen (Radix Codonopsis Pilosulae) 党参 12-15g
sheng jiang (Rhizoma Zingiberis Officinalis Recens)
生姜 9-12g
da zao (Fructus Zizyphi Jujubae) 大枣 4pce

Method: Decoction, best taken cool. **Wu zhu yu** warms the Stomach and Liver, directs rebellious *qi* downwards and stops vomiting; **sheng jiang** warms the Stomach and assists the **wu zhu yu** in stopping vomiting; **dang shen** strengthens the Spleen and protects Stomach *qi* and *yin* from the effects of severe vomiting; **da zao** moderates the dispersing and drying nature of **wu zhu yu**.

As the symptoms improve (should be no more than 3-7 days), the dose of **wu zhu yu** should be reduced to 3-6 grams for maintenance.

Complex of Heat, Cold and deficiency

- A common, yet somewhat more complex situation, is one in which Heat and Cold clump in the middle *jiao* against a background of Spleen and Stomach deficiency. The key features are morning nausea, vomiting or dry retching and a sensation of blockage, distension, fullness and discomfort in the epigastrium, which, when palpated, feels soft and without pain. In addition, there may be borborygmus with diarrhoea, poor appetite, a thin, greasy, yellow tongue coat and a soft, slippery, slightly wiry and possibly rapid pulse. The aim of treatment is to harmonise the Stomach, redirect *qi* downwards and disperse accumulation with **BAN XIA XIE XIN TANG** (*Pinellia Combination* 半夏泻心汤) modified.

ban xia (Rhizoma Pinelliae Ternatae) 半夏 9-12g
gan jiang (Rhizoma Zingiberis Officinalis) 干姜 6-9g
huang qin (Radix Scutellariae Baicalensis) 黄芩 6-12g
huang lian (Rhizoma Coptidis) 黄连 3-6g
dang shen (Radix Codonopsis Pilosulae) 党参 12-15g
zhi gan cao (honey fried Radix Glycyrrhizae Uralensis) 炙甘草 3-6g
da zao (Fructus Zizyphi Jujubae) 大枣 4pce
wu zhu yu (Fructus Evodiae Rutaecarpae) 吴茱萸 2-3g

Method: Decoction. **Ban xia** transforms Phlegm, dries Damp, directs rising Stomach *qi* downwards and stops nausea and vomiting; **gan jiang**, pungent and hot, warms Spleen and Stomach *yang* and dispels Cold; **huang qin** and **huang lian**, bitter and cold, clear Heat; **dang shen** and **da zao** strengthen the Spleen, supplement *qi* and prevent the dispersing action of the principal herbs from injuring the Spleen and Stomach *qi* and *yin*; **zhi gan cao** strengthens the Spleen and harmonises the Stomach; **wu zhu yu** warms the Stomach and Liver, and with **huang lian**, forms **ZUO JIN WAN** to reinforce the anti-emetic action.

Persistent nausea and vomiting

- Some patients with Stomach *qi* or *yang* deficiency, complicated by Phlegm obstructing the descent of Stomach *qi*, suffer unrelenting or unresponsive vomiting or nausea. The associated features are a firm and distended epigastrium, regurgitation, vomiting soon after eating, a thick, greasy, white tongue coat and a wiry, deficient pulse. In such cases, the primary aim of treatment is to first stop vomiting by powerfully weighing down the rebellious Stomach *qi*, and transforming Phlegm, and second to supplement *qi* and harmonise the Stomach. The prescription selected is **XUAN FU DAI ZHE TANG** (*Inula and Haematite Decoction* 旋复代赭汤) modified.

xuan fu hua (Flos Inulae) 旋复花 12-15g
dai zhe shi (Haematitum) 代赭石 15g
ban xia (Rhizoma Pinelliae Ternatae) 半夏 9-12g
sheng jiang (Rhizoma Zingiberis Officinalis) 生姜 9-12g
dang shen (Radix Codonopsis Pilosulae) 党参 9-12g
gan cao (Radix Glycyrrhizae Uralensis) 甘草 3-6g
da zao (Fructus Zizyphi Jujubae) 大枣 2pce
chen pi (Pericarpium Citri Reticulatae) 陈皮 6-9g
fu ling (Sclerotium Poria Cocos) 茯苓 12-15g

Method: Decoction. **Xuan fu hua** and **dai zhe shi** are the main substances and are a synergistic pair that forcefully drive down rising Stomach *qi*; **xuan fu hua** also transforms Phlegm, **dai zhe shi** heavily weighs down rising Stomach *qi*; **ban**

xia transforms Phlegm, dries Damp, directs rising Stomach *qi* downwards and stops nausea and vomiting; **sheng jiang** harmonises the Stomach and stops vomiting; **dang shen, da zao, fu ling** and **gan cao** supplement *qi* and strengthen the Spleen; **chen pi** transforms Phlegm and dries Damp, regulates middle *jiao qi* and corrects the *qi* mechanism. (Source: *Shi Yong Zhong Yi Nei Ke Xue*)

Morning sickness and motion sickness

- A simple recipe for Cold in the Stomach type vomiting, particularly useful during pregnancy, and for motion sickness, is 60 grams of **bai dou kou** (Fructus Amomi Kravanh) 白豆蔻, ground into powder and formed into small pills with ginger juice. The dose is 1-3 grams with warm water two or three times daily.

Patent medicines

Xiang Sha Liu Jun Zi Wan 香砂六君子丸 (Xiang Sha Liu Jun Wan, Aplotaxis-Ammomum Pills, Six Gentlemen Tea Pills)
- *qi* deficiency with Phlegm Damp

Xiang Sha Yang Wei Wan 香砂养胃丸 (Xiang Sha Yang Wei Wan, Hsiang Sha Yang Wei Wan)
- *qi* deficiency with *qi* stagnation

Fu Zi Li Zhong Wan 附子理中丸 (Fu Tzu Li Chung Wan, Carmichaeli Tea Pills, Li Chung Yuen Medical Pills)
- Spleen *yang* deficiency with severe Cold

Li Zhong Wan 理中丸 (Li Zhong Wan)
- Spleen *yang* deficiency

Jian Pi Wan 健脾丸 (Jian Pi Wan)
- Spleen deficiency with food stagnation

Acupuncture (select from)

Ren.12 (*zhong wan* +▲) .. *mu* point of the Stomach, warms and regulates the Stomach and directs Stomach *qi* downwards

PC.6 (*nei guan*) .... *luo* point of the Pericardium, master point of *yin wei mai*, regulates the middle *jiao* and stops vomiting

St.36 (*zu san li* +▲) .... *he* sea point of the Stomach, powerfully warms and strengthens the Spleen and Stomach, supplements *qi* and stops vomiting

Sp.4 (*gong sun*) .... *luo* point of the Spleen, master point of *chong mai*, regulates the Spleen and Stomach

Bl.20 (*pi shu* +▲) .... *shu* point of the Spleen, warms and strengthens the Spleen and supplements *qi* and *yang*

- a moxa box over the upper abdomen is useful
- with Dampness, add Sp.3 (*tai bai* -)
- with Liver *qi* stagnation, add Sp.6 (*san yin jiao*)
- with indigestion, add LI.10 (*shou san li*)
- with abdominal distension, add Sp.3 (*tai bai*), St.25 (*tian shu*) and Sp.15 (*da heng*)

Ear points: spleen, stomach, adrenal, sympathetic, *shen men*

Clinical notes

- Spleen and Stomach deficiency type nausea and vomiting may be diagnosed biomedically as chronic gastritis, peptic ulcer disease, chronic indigestion, dyspepsia, food intolerance and allergy, and morning sickness.
- *Qi* deficiency nausea and vomiting respond reliably and quickly to correct treatment. *Yang* deficiency also responds well, but will take somewhat longer for satisfactory and sustained results.
- For dietary recommendations, see pp.870-873

胃阴不足

21.6 STOMACH YIN DEFICIENCY

Pathophysiology

- Stomach *yin* deficiency is usually a complication of some other long standing pathology, most commonly Liver *qi* invading the Stomach, or chronic Stomach Heat patterns. It can, however, be more acute, and follow sudden damage to Stomach *yin* following a febrile illness, typically *yang ming* syndrome.
- The nausea and vomiting of this pattern are associated with the general weakness of the Stomach. This leads to a failure of Stomach *qi* to descend, and the potential development of deficient Heat, which can rise taking Stomach *qi* with it. Stomach *yin* is a superficial aspect of the body's *yin*, more closely associated with fluids than the deeper *yin* of the Kidneys. When Stomach *yin* is deficient, it may not produce *yin* deficiency Heat symptoms. The main feature may be dryness rather than Heat, although in severe cases, there may be significant Heat. Depending on the degree of deficiency and the length of the problem, Kidney *yin* may eventually be drained, provoking the onset of deeper Heat symptoms such as night sweats or bone steaming.
- Chronic Stomach *yin* deficiency is often associated with atrophy of the gastric mucosa.

Clinical features

- Chronic, recurrent, persistent mild nausea, with occasional vomiting or dry retching. The patient may wake in the early hours of the morning with vague epigastric discomfort and nausea that is relieved on arising and eating.
- vague dull or burning epigastric pain, which may feel better for pressure
- dry mouth and throat
- poor appetite, indeterminate gnawing hunger
- constipation or dry stools

T slightly red and dry with little or no coat, or peeled in the centre. In severe cases the tongue may be red and so denuded of papillae as to resemble a piece of liver (mirror tongue), or have numerous surface cracks.

P thready and rapid

Treatment principle

Nourish and supplement Stomach *yin*, and moisten dryness
Redirect Stomach *qi* downward, stop vomiting

Prescription

MAI MEN DONG TANG 麦门冬汤
(*Ophiopogon Combination*)

mai dong (Tuber Ophiopogonis Japonici) 麦冬 12-15g
dang shen (Radix Codonopsis Pilosulae) 党参 12-18g
ban xia (Rhizoma Pinelliae Ternatae) 半夏 6-9g
jing mi (Nonglutinous rice) 粳米 15g
da zao (Fructus Zizyphi Jujubae) 大枣 4pce
gan cao (Radix Glycyrrhizae Uralensis) 甘草 3-6g

Method: Decoction. **Mai dong** nourishes Stomach fluids and *yin* and clears Heat; **dang shen, gan cao, da zao** and **jing mi** benefit Stomach *qi* and generate fluids; **ban xia** directs Stomach *qi* downwards and stops nausea and vomiting. (Source: *Shi Yong Zhong Yi Nei Ke Xue*)

Modifications

- Even though the dose is relatively small, **ban xia** may be excessively drying, and must be monitored carefully, and reduced where necessary. For severe *yin* deficiency, add **shi hu** (Herba Dendrobii) 石斛 12-15g, **sha shen** (Radix Adenophorae seu Glehniae) 沙参 12-15g and **tian hua fen** (Radix Trichosanthis Kirilowii) 天花粉 9-15g.
- If vomiting is frequent, add **zhu ru** (Caulis Bambusae in Taeniis) 竹茹 9-12g, **chen pi** (Pericarpium Citri Reticulatae) 陈皮 6-9g and **pi pa ye** (Folium Eriobotryae Japonicae) 枇杷叶 9-12g.
- If there are dry stools or constipation, add **xuan shen** (Radix Scrophulariae) 玄参 15-24g, **huo ma ren** (Semen Cannabis Sativae) 火麻仁 9-12g and **feng mi** (honey) 蜂蜜.
- With mild deficient Heat symptoms (tidal fever, flushing), add **hu huang lian** (Rhizoma Picrorhixae) 胡黄连 9-12g and **di gu pi** (Cortex Lycii Chinensis) 地骨皮 9-12g.
- With epigastric pain, add **bai shao** (Radix Paeoniae Lactiflora) 白芍 12-24g and increase the dose of **gan cao** to 9g.
- With acid reflux and heartburn, add **hai piao xiao** (Os Sepiae seu Sepiellae) 海螵蛸 15g (or 3g as a powder washed down with the decoction).
- With hypo-acidity, add **wu mei** (Fructus Pruni Mume) 乌梅 9-12g, **shi hu** (Herba Dendrobi) 石斛 12-15g and **shan zha** (Fructus Crataegi) 山楂 15g.
- For atrophy of the gastric mucosa, add **dan shen** (Radix Salviae Miltiorrhizae) 丹参 12-18g and **huang qi** (Radix Astragali Membranacei) 黄芪 18-30g.
- With *Helicobacter pylori*, add **pu gong ying** (Herba Taraxaci Mongolici) 蒲公英 15-30g.

- With stagnant *qi*, add **mei gui hua** (Flos Rosae Rugosae) 玫瑰花 6-9g and **fo shou** (Fructus Citri Sarcodacylis) 佛手 9-12g, or consider **YI GUAN JIAN** (*Linking Decoction* 一贯煎, p.615) as guiding formula.
- If Kidney and/or Liver *yin* is also weakened (lower back ache, flushing, nightsweats and tinnitus) combine with **LIU WEI DI HUANG WAN** (*Rehmannia Six Formula* 六味地黄丸). Patent pills are usually sufficient.

Patent medicines

Gu Ben Wan 固本丸 (Gu Ben Wan, Ren Shen Ku Pen Wan)

Sheng Mai San Wan 生脉散丸 (Sheng Mai San Wan)
- *qi* and *yin* deficiency

Shen Ling Bai Zhu Wan 参苓白术丸 (Shen Ling Bai Zhu Wan)
- good for mild *yin* and *qi* deficiency

Liu Wei Di Huang Wan 六味地黄丸 (Liu Wei Di Huang Wan, Six Flavour Tea)

Mai Wei Di Huang Wan 麦味地黄丸 (Mai Wei Di Huang Wan, Ba Xian Chang Shou Wan)
- A small dose of one of the last two patent medicines may be combined with the principal patent selected when there is Kidney *yin* deficiency. Take care not to allow the cloying, *yin* supplementing herbs to aggravate the nausea in the early stages of treatment.

Acupuncture (select from)

Ren.12 (*zhong wan* +) .... *mu* point of the Stomach, nourishes Stomach *yin*, regulates the Stomach and directs Stomach *qi* downwards

PC.6 (*nei guan*) .... *luo* point of the Pericardium, master point of *yin wei mai*, regulates the middle *jiao* and stops vomiting

St.36 (*zu san li* +) .... *he* sea point of the Stomach, powerfully strengthens the Spleen and Stomach, supplements *qi* and *yin* and stops vomiting

Sp.4 (*gong sun*) .... *luo* point of the Spleen, master point of *chong mai*, regulates the Spleen and Stomach

Bl.20 (*pi shu* +) .... *shu* point of the Spleen, strengthens the Spleen and supplements *qi* and *yin*

Bl.21 (*wei shu* +) .... *shu* point of the Stomach, benefits Stomach *qi* and *yin* and directs Stomach *qi* downwards

Kid.9 (*zhu bin* +) .... *xi* point of *yin wei mai*, with PC.6 (*nei guan*) can direct weak Stomach *qi* downwards

- with deficient Heat, add St.43 (*xian gu* -) and Kid.2 (*ran gu*)
- with Kidney *yin* deficiency, add Bl.23 (*shen shu* +) and Kid.3 (*tai xi* +)

Ear points: spleen, stomach, kidney, endocrine, sympathetic, *shen men*

Clinical notes

- Vomiting or nausea of a Stomach *yin* deficiency type may be diagnosed biomedically as chronic atrophic gastritis, peptic ulcer disease, oesophageal reflux, convalescence from febrile disease or diabetes mellitus.
- Stomach *yin* deficiency is a relatively common cause of chronic vague nausea and can be difficult to treat. Depending on the longevity of the condition, it will often take some weeks before adequate symptomatic relief is obtained with herbs and acupuncture alone. Because Stomach *yin* deficiency may be associated with physical atrophy of the gastric mucosa, the underlying pattern may require 6-9 months of treatment for satisfactory results. Long term results usually require the ingestion of a *yin* building prescription and diet to replenish the depleted *yin*. Mucilaginous substance that put a lining on the oesophageal and gastric wall, such as slippery elm powder, are also useful.
- For dietary recommendations, see p.876.

SUMMARY OF GUIDING FORMULAE FOR NAUSEA AND VOMITING

External invasion
- Wind Cold with Damp, Summerdamp - *Huo Xiang Zheng Qi San* 藿香正气散
- Wind Heat - *Yin Qiao San* 银翘散
- Summerheat - *Xin Jia Xiang Ru Yin* 新加香薷饮
- pestilential and violent - *Yu Shu Dan* 玉枢丹
- *Shao yang* syndrome - *Xiao Chai Hu Tang* 小柴胡汤
- *Shao yang / yang ming* syndrome - *Da Chai Hu Tang* 大柴胡汤
- residual Phlegm Heat after - *Wen Dan Tang* 温胆汤
- mixed Heat and Cold - *Ban Xia Xie Xin Tang* 半夏泻心汤

Food stagnation - *Bao He Wan* 保和丸
- with Damp Heat - *Zhi Shi Dao Zhi Wan* 枳实导滞丸

Phlegm Damp - *Er Chen Tang* 二陈汤
- Phlegm Heat - *Wen Dan Tang* 温胆汤
- persistent vomiting - *Xuan Fu Dai Zhe Tang* 旋复代赭汤
- thin Phlegm - *Ling Gui Zhu Gan Tang* 苓桂术甘汤
- Wind Phlegm - *Ban Xia Bai Zhu Tian Ma Tang* 半夏白术天麻汤
- plus Spleen deficiency - *Xiang Sha Liu Jun Zi Tang* 香砂六君子汤

Liver *qi* invading the Stomach
- with depression - *Yue Ju Wan* 月鞠丸
- with Heat - *Si Ni San* 四逆散
- plum stone throat - *Ban Xia Hou Po Tang* 半夏厚朴汤

Spleen and Stomach deficiency
- *qi* deficiency - *Liu Jun Zi Tang* 六君子汤
- *yang* deficiency - *Li Zhong Wan* 理中丸

Yin deficiency - *Mai Men Dong Tang* 麦门冬汤

Table 21.3 *Differential diagnosis of nausea and vomiting*

Pattern	Duration	Aggravated by	Ameliorated by	Nature of vomit or nausea	Nature of patient	Pulse and tongue
External pathogens invade the Stomach	acute	usually hot humid weather or changes of season		may be frequent and violent vomiting, and associated with cramping abdominal pain and diarrhoea	all ages	T: thin or greasy coat P: floating
Food stagnation	chronic with acute exacerbations	eating	belching, vomiting, fasting	churning in the Stomach, foul vomit with partly digested material	may tend to be overweight	T: thick, greasy coat P: slippery, full
Phlegm Damp	chronic	dairy, cold raw food, sweet food, strong or volatile odours	fasting, avoidance of aggravating foods	nausea may be worse in the morning, mucus like material in the vomit	all ages, may tend to be overweight	T: thick, greasy coat P: slippery, wiry
Liver qi invading the Stomach	chronic and recurrent	anxiety, emotion and stress	relaxation, expulsion of gas	nausea tends to be worse in the morning and when anxious	tense, uptight, nervy, most common 20-50 yrs F>M	T: normal, or dark, or with red edges P: wiry

Spleen and Stomach qi deficiency	chronic	fatigue, cold natured, hard to digest or excessively sweet foods	bland, light, well cooked food, small meals; application of warmth and pressure	mild continuous nausea	pale, fatigued, puffy eyes, low vitality	T: pale, with tooth marks P: weak, deficient
Spleen yang deficiency	chronic	fatigue, cold natured, hard to digest, or excessively sweet, foods	bland, light, well cooked food, small meals; application of warmth and pressure	watery, inoffensive, thin mucus like material	pale, cold intolerant, emaciated	T: pale and swollen P: deep, slow, weak
Stomach yin deficiency	chronic (but may follow an acute febrile disease)	with an empty stomach and at night	bland or liquid diet	vague nausea worse at night, dry retching	older patients, thin, flushed, heat intolerant	T: peeled in the centre or red and peeled P: thready, rapid

22. Rectal Prolapse

Spleen and Lung *qi* deficiency
Spleen and Kidney *yang* deficiency
Damp Heat

22 RECTAL PROLAPSE

tuo gang 脱肛

Rectal prolapse is a protrusion of the rectum through the anus. Rectal bleeding may occur, and faecal incontinence is frequent, while pain is typically absent in the common deficiency patterns. In mild cases, protrusion occurs only when straining during bowel movements and spontaneously retracts, or is easily manually reduced. As the condition deteriorates, protrusion occurs frequently and may occur while walking or standing. Manual replacement becomes more difficult and in severe cases the prolapsed bowel may become irreducible and ischaemic.

In Chinese medicine, there are two types of rectal prolapse, deficiency and excess. The deficiency patterns are characterised by long duration and painlessness, and by typical signs and symptoms of deficiency, such as weakness, pallor, fatigue, a pale tongue and weak pulse.

The excess pattern is characterised by rectal inflammation, with symptoms such as pain, redness, itch, in combination with signs of systemic Heat, a red tongue with a yellow coat and a rapid pulse. The deficiency patterns are more common than the excess pattern.

Rectal prolapse is most common in middle aged women with children, but also affects children and the elderly of both sexes. Transient minor prolapse of the rectal mucosa often occurs in otherwise normal infants, as Spleen and Lung *qi* in infants is delicate and unstable.

AETIOLOGY

Spleen and Lung *qi* deficiency

Spleen and Lung *qi* deficiency type prolapse is associated with loss of tissue tone, and failure of the Spleen to hold the tissues of the lower Intestine in place against the force of gravity. Spleen and Lung *qi* deficiency may be caused by overwork, excessive worry or mental activity, insufficient physical activity, irregular dietary habits, prolonged illness and age. Lung and Spleen *qi* can be seriously depleted by a long or difficult labour, which not only consumes *qi* but causes mechanical trauma to the tissues of the rectum and anus.

Prolonged or excessive consumption of cold natured or uncooked food weakens Spleen *qi* and *yang*. Rectal prolapse is a common sequelae to Spleen deficiency type diarrhoea or chronic dysentery. It can also be provoked by the chronic cough which develops from Lung *qi* deficiency.

Chronic retention of Dampness following an unresolved external invasion, or arising from a damp environment, will eventually drain Spleen *qi* and cause deficiency. Patterns that are initially associated with an excess of Cold Damp often result in Spleen deficiency in susceptible patients. Damp Heat patterns that are treated too enthusiastically with bitter cold herbs and/ or antibiotics, can also transform into Spleen deficiency patterns.

Spleen and Kidney *yang* deficiency

Spleen and Kidney *yang* deficiency prolapse is essentially a deterioration of Spleen and Lung *qi* deficiency patterns, with the added complication of Kidney weakness. The Kidney controls the two lower *yin*, the anus and urethra, and assists the Spleen in the maintenance of tone in these structures. Loss of strength of the anal sphincter compounds the already poor tone of the intestinal smooth muscle.

Another contributing factor is the disordered fluid metabolism that may accompany Spleen and Kidney *yang* deficiency. If fluids are not being adequately processed and metabolised, but are being lost through the urine as excessive or frequent urination, an imbalance in fluid distribution may occur, causing dryness in the Intestine. This can lead to dry stools or constipation, with a consequent increase in the downwards pressure on the already strained rectal mucosa. In men, prostate swelling, from fluid accumulation as a result of *yang* deficiency, may also contribute to increasing the pressure on the rectal mucosa.

Spleen *yang* is weakened by excessive consumption of cold raw food and irregular eating habits, or by ingestion of too many cold natured herbs or antibiotics in the treatment of a febrile or other hot disease. It may represent the deterioration of Spleen *qi* deficiency. Additional factors are prolonged or serious illness, prolonged starvation or digestive insult, such as occurs in famine conditions and in patients with a history of anorexia nervosa or bulimia.

Kidney *yang* deficiency may develop as a result of age, chronic illness, overexertion, overexposure to cold conditions, excessive lifting or standing In women, Kidney *yang* and *jing* are depleted by having many pregnancies. Multiple pregnancies can also stretch and traumatise the tissues of the rectum and anus. Spleen and Kidney *yang* and *qi* deficiency prolapse patterns are most common in middle aged, elderly and multiparous women.

Damp Heat

Damp Heat rectal prolapse is associated with a diet rich in Damp producing and heating foods, or an invasion of external Damp Heat that lodges in the Intestine, causing severe or chronic diarrhoea or dysenteric disorder. External Damp Heat patterns easily complicate the deficiency patterns as the *qi* is often too weak to repel a pathogenic invasion.

TCM DIFFERENTIAL DIAGNOSIS

- **Haemorrhoids** (*zhi chuang* 痔疮): Haemorrhoids are due to a weakness or pouching of the rectal veins. From a pathological point of view they share some aetiological and pathological characteristics with rectal prolapse. Rectal prolapse differs by involving the full thickness of rectal mucosa, and in the later stages at least, being more difficult to treat satisfactorily with TCM alone.

TREATMENT

Prolapse often occurs as the result of some other pathology, for example, chronic diarrhoea or dysentery, chronic cough, or straining from chronic constipation. Any pre-existing condition must be treated at the same time as the prolapse. Mild prolapses usually respond well to TCM treatment. Taping the buttocks together with surgical tape between bowel movements is useful, and assists the local tissues in recovery of tissue tone. For resistant or repeated prolapse, surgery may be the best option. If surgery is required, TCM treatment still offers valuable assistance in rebuilding *qi* and *yang*, or clearing Damp Heat. For other measures see Box 13.2, p.488.

脾肺气虚下陷

22.1 SPLEEN AND LUNG QI DEFICIENCY, SINKING QI

Pathophysiology

- When Spleen *qi* is weak tissue tone tends to be poor. The walls of the rectum become lax and stretched, and the rectum itself is not held firmly in its correct position in the pelvis.
- Deficient Lung *qi*, in combination with Spleen *qi* deficiency, predisposes patients to upper respiratory tract infection and the development of chronic cough. The resulting increase in intra-abdominal pressure can, over time, contribute to prolapse of the rectum. In the case of constitutional Lung weakness, the Large Intestine, the *yang* partner to the Lungs, will also be weak.
- Children, who by nature have immature Lung and Spleen *qi*, are vulnerable to rectal prolapse after chronic diarrhoea or upper respiratory tract infection.

Clinical features

- Variable degrees of rectal prolapse that usually appear whenever downward abdominal pressure is increased, such as during a bowel movement, coughing or sneezing, walking or prolonged standing. The protruding rectal mucosa appears pale red. There may be occasional bleeding or mucus in the stools. Women may experience prolapse of the uterus concurrently.
- abdominal fullness and distension, worse for eating
- poor appetite, early satiety
- frequent bowel movements, chronic loose stools or diarrhoea
- waxy pale complexion
- weakness and fatigue
- shortness of breath, low voice, reluctance to speak
- spontaneous sweating, maybe a chronic weak cough

T pale and swollen with toothmarks
P weak, thready, deficient, moderate

Treatment principle

Strengthen the Spleen and Lungs, supplement *qi*
Promote the elevation of *yang qi*

Prescription

BU ZHONG YI QI TANG 补中益气汤
(*Ginseng and Astragalus Combination*)

zhi huang qi (honey fried Radix Astragali Membranacei)
炙黄芪 30-60g
dang shen (Radix Codonopsis Pilosulae) 党参 15-24g

chao bai zhu (dry fried Rhizoma Atractylodes Macrocephalae) 炒白术 12-15g
dang gui (Radix Angelicae Sinensis) 当归 9-12g
chen pi (Pericarpium Citri Reticulatae) 陈皮 6-9g
zhi gan cao (honey fried Radix Glycyrrhizae Uralensis) 炙甘草 6-9g
sheng ma (Rhizoma Cimicifugae) 升麻 9-12g
chai hu (Radix Bupleuri) 柴胡 6-9g

Method: Decoction. The large quantity of **zhi huang qi** is important here to elevate *yang qi*, lift the prolapse and improve the tone of the rectal mucosa; **dang shen, chao bai zhu, zhi huang qi** and **zhi gan cao** strengthen the Spleen and supplement *qi*; **dang gui** supplements and regulates Blood; **chai hu** and a relatively large quantity of **sheng ma** assist **zhi huang qi** in lifting *yang qi*; **chen pi** regulates *qi*. (Source: *Shi Yong Zhong Yi Nei Ke Xue*)

Modifications

- In chronic or severe cases, astringent herbs may be added to strengthen the tissue toning effect, such as **wu bei zi** (Galla Rhois Chinensis) 五倍子 6g, **wu mei** (Fructus Pruni Mume) 乌梅 9-12g and **jin ying zi** (Fructus Rosae Laevigatae) 金樱子 9-12g.
- With *yang* weakness, cold intolerance and cold extremities, add **zhi fu zi** (Radix Aconiti Carmichaeli Praeparata) 制附子 6-12g (decocted for 30 minutes prior to the other herbs), and **gan jiang** (Rhizoma Zingiberis Officinalis) 干姜 6-9g.
- With bleeding, add **xian he cao** (Herba Agrimoniae Pilosae) 仙鹤草 15-30g.
- With severe abdominal distension and poor appetite, add two or three of the following herbs: **chao shan yao** (dry fried Radix Dioscoreae Oppositae) 炒山药 15g, **ji nei jin** (Endothelium Corneum Gigeriae Galli) 鸡内金 12g, **sha ren** (Fructus Amomi) 砂仁 6-9g, **chao shan zha** (dry fried Fructus Crataegi) 炒山楂 15g, **chao shen qu** (dry fried Massa Fermentata) 炒神曲 15g, **chao gu ya** (dry fried Fructus Oryzae Sativae) 炒谷芽 15-30g or **chao mai ya** (dry fried Fructus Hordei Vulgaris Germinantus) 炒麦芽 15-30g.
- With *qi* stagnation, add **mu xiang** (Radix Aucklandiae Lappae) 木香 6-9g.
- With Blood deficiency, add **chao bai shao** (dry fried Radix Paeoniae Lactiflorae) 炒白芍 9-15g.
- With a degree of Heat in the Intestines, add **huang qin** (Radix Scutellariae Baicalensis) 黄芩 3-6g, **bai shao** (Radix Paeoniae Lactiflorae) 白芍 9-15g and **huai hua** (Flos Sophora Japonicae Immaturus) 槐花 9-12g.
- With anal distension, fullness and discomfort, add **zhi ke** (Fructus Citri

Aurantii) 枳壳 9-12g and **mu xiang** (Radix Aucklandiae Lappae) 木香 6-9g.

- In some patients, constipation or sluggish stools is a feature, as *qi* may be insufficient to propel stools. Add **huo ma ren** (Semen Cannabis Sativae) 火麻仁 9-12g, **hu tao ren** (Semen Juglandis Regiae) 胡桃仁 12-15g and **feng mi** (honey) 蜂蜜.

External wash

- An astringent wash can be used to tone the rectal tissue directly in cases that do not respond, or that respond only slowly. Decoct **shi liu pi** (Pericarpium Punicae Granati) 石榴皮 30g for 30 minutes and add **ming fan** (Alumen) 明矾 15g to the strained decoction. Bathe the rectum in a sitzbath as often as practical.
- A simple astringent wash suitable for mild *qi* deficiency prolapse is a decoction of the white parts of **cong bai** (Bulbus Allii Fistulosi) 葱白 [shallots/scallions].

Patent medicines

Bu Zhong Yi Qi Wan 补中益气丸 (Bu Zhong Yi Qi Wan, Central Qi Pills) - a larger than normal dose (2-3 times) is usually required

Acupuncture (select from)

Du.20 (*bai hui* ▲) .... raises *yang qi*

Ren.12 (*zhong wan* +▲) .. *mu* point of the Stomach, warms and strengthens the Spleen and Stomach

Ren.6 (*qi hai*) .... needle obliquely downwards with a 3-inch needle from Ren.6 (*qi hai*) towards Ren.3 (*zhong ji*). The needle is twirled to anchor it, then raised towards the sternum creating a lifting sensation in the lower abdomen. It can be taped in its lifted position in place for the duration of the treatment.

St.25 (*tian shu* +▲) .... *mu* point of the Large Intestine, warms and regulates Intestinal function

St.36 (*zu san li* +▲) .... *he* sea point of the Stomach, powerfully warms and strengthens the Spleen and Stomach and supplements *qi*

Du.1 (*chang qiang*) .... an important point for all rectal disorders

Bl.57 (*cheng shan*) .... special point for rectal disorders (especially in combination with Du.1), regulates the lower Intestine and rectum, stops bleeding and pain

Bl.20 (*pi shu* +▲) .... *shu* point of the Spleen, warms and strengthens the Spleen and supplements *qi*
Bl.25 (*da chang shu* +▲) .. *shu* point of Large Intestine, regulates Intestinal function
Bl.30 (*bai huan shu* +) ...... special point for anal disorders

- a moxa box over the lower abdomen is useful
- with bleeding, add Sp.1 (*yin bai* ▲) and Sp.3 (*tai bai* +)
- with Lung *qi* deficiency, add Lu.9 (*tai yuan* +) and Lu.1 (*zhong fu* +)
- with chronic or incessant diarrhoea, add *zhi xie* +▲ (N-CA-3) and Ren.8 (*shen que* ▲)
- For patients who can cope with it, the dermal hammer can be gently applied to the tissue around the anus. This rather uncomfortable method is quite good for toning and strengthening the rectal mucosa by encouraging the circulation of *qi* and Blood.
- *Ear points*: prolapse, haemorrhoids, spleen, large intestine, distal segment rectum, adrenal, *shen men*

Clinical notes

- Prolapses of a *qi* deficient type usually respond quite well to correct treatment, although the greater the degree of prolapse the more treatment required. In general, at least 2-3 months of treatment, or several courses of acupuncture will be necessary for satisfactory results.
- For dietary recommendations, see p.870.

脾肾阳虚

22.2 SPLEEN AND KIDNEY YANG DEFICIENCY

Pathophysiology

- Spleen and Kidney *yang* deficiency is essentially a worsening of the Spleen *qi* deficiency pattern. The involvement of the Kidney here implies a weakness of the 'lower *yin*', here the anus, in addition to the sinking *qi* and Spleen deficiency. The weakness of the anal sphincter, combined with the sinking *qi*, produces a more significant prolapse. In addition, excessive loss of fluids through the urine can lead to an imbalance in fluid distribution in the Large Intestine, causing dryness of the stools and consequent straining at stool. This further aggravates the rectal weakness and the frequency and severity of the prolapse.
- Most common in the elderly or debilitated patients.

Clinical features

- relatively severe rectal prolapse that may be continuous or irreducible; dragging, heavy sensation in the anus; possible faecal incontinence
- lower back, knees and legs cold, weak and sore
- dizziness, tinnitus, loss of hearing acuity
- frequent urination, incontinence of urine, nocturia
- cold extremities, cold intolerance
- fatigue, weakness, exhaustion
- breathlessness with exertion
- possible chronic diarrhoea or dysenteric disorder, or cock crow diarrhoea, or a tendency to constipation, straining at stool, possibly with dry stools

T pale and swollen, with toothmarks
P deep, thready, weak

Treatment principle

Warm and supplement Spleen and Kidney *yang*
Promote the elevation of *yang qi*

Prescription

DA BU YUAN JIAN 大补元煎
(*Great Tonify the Basal Decoction*) modified

dang shen (Radix Codonopsis Pilosulae) 党参 15-24g
shan yao (Radix Dioscoreae Oppositae) 山药 12-18g
shu di (Radix Rehmanniae Glutinosae Conquitae)
熟地 15-24g
du zhong (Cortex Eucommiae Ulmoidis) 杜仲 9-15g
dang gui (Radix Angelicae Sinensis) 当归 9-12g
gou qi zi (Fructus Lycii) 枸杞子 9-12g

shan zhu yu (Fructus Corni Officinalis) 山茱萸 9-12g
zhi gan cao (honey fried Radix Glycyrrhizae Uralensis) 炙甘草 6-9g
zhi huang qi (honey fried Radix Astragali Membranacei) 炙黄芪 30-60g
tu si zi (Semen Cuscutae Chinensis) 菟丝子 12-15g
rou cong rong (Herba Cistanches Deserticolae) 肉苁蓉 12-18g
wu wei zi (Fructus Schizandrae Chinensis) 五味子 6-9g

Method: Decoction. **Dang shen, shan yao, huang qi** and **zhi gan cao** strengthen the Spleen and reinforce *qi*; **shu di, shan zhu yu, gou qi zi, du zhong** and **tu si zi** nourish and strengthen the Kidney and benefit *jing*, **dang gui** nourishes Blood and moistens dryness; a large quantity of **zhi huang qi** elevates *yang qi*; **tu si zi, rou cong rong** and **wu wei zi** warm *yang*, and astringe and tone the tissues of the lower *jiao*. (Source: *Shi Yong Zhong Yi Nei Ke Xue*)

Modifications

- To assist in lifting collapsing Spleen *qi*, **chai hu** (Radix Bupleuri) 柴胡 6-9g and **sheng ma** (Rhizoma Cimicifugae) 升麻 9-12g may be added.
- With constipation or dry stools, add **huo ma ren** (Semen Cannabis Sativae) 火麻仁 9-12g, **hu tao ren** (Semen Juglandis Regiae) 胡桃仁 12-15g and **feng mi** 蜂蜜 (honey).
- With chronic diarrhoea, delete **rou cong rong**, and add **bu gu zhi** (Fructus Psoraleae Corylifoliae) 补骨脂 12-15g and **rou dou kou** (Semen Myristicae Fragrantis) 肉豆蔻 6-9g. *See also* Table 7.2, p.301.
- In severe or resistent cases of prolapse, more astringent herbs may be added to strengthen the tissue toning effect, such as **wu bei zi** (Galla Rhois Chinensis) 五倍子 6g, **wu mei** (Fructus Pruni Mume) 乌梅 9-12g and **jin ying zi** (Fructus Rosae Laevigatae) 金樱子 9-12g.
- With severe cold intolerance and cold extremities, add **zhi fu zi** (Radix Aconiti Carmichaeli Praeparata) 制附子 6-12g and **gan jiang** (Rhizoma Zingiberis Officinalis) 干姜 6-9g.
- With a degree of Blood stagnation, delete **shan zhu yu** and add **chuan xiong** (Radix Ligustici Chuanxiong) 川芎 6-9g.
- For elderly or debilitated patients with *jing* and Blood deficiency, add **lu rong** (Cornu Cervi Parvum) 鹿茸 3g daily (taken separately in capsules).

Variations and additional prescriptions

With fluid metabolism problems

- In cases with problems of fluid metabolism and distribution (relatively severe frequency and nocturia), the tendency to prolapse may be complicated by sluggish bowels or even dryish stools, as disproportionately large volumes of fluids are diverted from the Intestines to the Urinary Bladder. The treatment aims to warm, invigorate and elevate *yang* and promote transformation of fluids with **JIN KUI SHEN QI WAN** (*Rehmannia Eight Formula* 金匮肾气丸) modified.

shu di (Radix Rehmanniae Glutinosae Conquitae) 熟地 15-24g
shan yao (Radix Dioscoreae Oppositae) 山药 15-18g
shan zhu yu (Fructus Corni Officinalis) 山茱萸 12-15g
fu ling (Sclerotium Poria Cocos) 茯苓 12-15g
zhi fu zi (Radix Aconiti Carmichaeli Praeparata) 制附子 6-12g
rou gui (Cortex Cinnamomi Cassiae) 肉桂 3-6g
wu wei zi (Fructus Schizandrae Chinensis) 五味子 6-9g
zhi huang qi (honey fried Radix Astragali Membranacei) 炙黄芪 30-60g
sheng ma (Rhizoma Cimicifugae) 升麻 9-12g

Method: Decoction. **Zhi fu zi** is cooked for 30 minutes before the other herbs are added (*xian jian* 先煎), **rou gui** is added towards the end of cooking (*hou xia* 后下). **Shu di, shan yao** and **shan zhu yu** reinforce the Kidney, Spleen and Liver; **fu ling** strengthens the Spleen, leaches out Dampness and prevents digestive upset from the rich supplementing herbs; **zhi fu zi** and **rou gui** warm and mobilise *yang qi* and stimulate the transformation of *qi* and fluid metabolism; **zhi huang qi** strengthens the Spleen and with **sheng ma**, powerfully elevates *yang qi*. (Source: *Zhong Yi Nei Ke Shou Ce*)

Chronic diarrhoea or dysenteric disorder

- For patients with prolapse associated with Spleen and Kidney deficiency and chronic unremitting diarrhoea, or dysenteric disorder to the point of faecal incontinence, the focus of treatment should be towards astringing the Intestines and stopping diarrhoea, while warming and supplementing the middle *jiao*. In addition to the prolapse and diarrhoea, these patients are usually quite severely depleted, with anorexia, exhaustion, lower back and leg weakness and aching, a pale swollen tongue and a weak or imperceptible pulse. The most suitable prescription is **ZHEN REN YANG ZANG TANG** (*True Man's Decoction to Nourish the Organs* 真人养脏汤) modified.

zhi ying su ke (honey fried Pericarpium Papaveris Somniferi) 炙罂粟壳 9-12g
wei he zi (roasted Fructus Terminaliae Chebulae) 煨诃子 9-15g
rou dou kou (Semen Myristicae Fragrantis) 肉豆蔻 9-15g
chao bai zhu (dry fried Rhizoma Atractylodes Macrocephalae) 炒白术 12-15g
dang shen (Radix Codonopsis Pilosulae) 党参 15-24g
chao bai shao (dry fried Radix Paeoniae Lactiflorae) 炒白芍 12-18g

dang gui (Radix Angelicae Sinensis) 当归 6-12g
mu xiang (Radix Aucklandiae Lappae) 木香 6-9g
rou gui (Cortex Cinnamomi Cassiae) 肉桂 3g
zhi gan cao (honey fried Radix Glycyrrhizae Uralensis)
炙甘草 3-6g
zhi huang qi (honey fried Radix Astragali Membranacei)
黄芪 30-60g
sheng ma (Rhizoma Cimicifugae) 升麻 9-12g

Method: Decoction. **Rou gui** is added towards the end of cooking (*hou xia* 后下). **Dang shen**, **chao bai zhu**, **zhi gan cao** and **zhi huang qi** strengthen the Spleen and supplement *qi*; **rou gui** and **rou dou kou** warm the middle *jiao* and Kidney *yang* and disperse Cold; **mu xiang** regulates *qi* and alleviates tenesmus; **dang gui** and **chao bai shao** harmonise the Blood and stop pain; **wei he zi** and **chao ying su ke** astringe the Intestines and stop diarrhoea; **zhi huang qi** and **sheng ma** powerfully elevate *yang qi*. (Source: *Shi Yong Zhong Yi Nei Ke Xue*)

Patent medicines

Bu Zhong Yi Qi Wan 补中益气丸 (Bu Zhong Yi Qi Wan, Central Qi Pills) plus one of the following–

Jin Kui Shen Qi Wan 金匮肾气丸 (Fu Gui Ba Wei Wan, Sexoton Pills, Golden Book Tea)
- Kidney *yang* deficiency

Fu Zi Li Zhong Wan 附子理中丸 (Fu Tzu Li Chung Wan, Carmichaeli Tea Pills, Li Chung Yuen Medical Pills)
- Spleen *yang* deficiency

Li Zhong Wan 理中丸 (Li Zhong Wan)
- Spleen *yang* deficiency

Cong Rong Bu Shen Wan 苁蓉补肾丸 (Cong Rong Bu Shen Wan)
- with sluggish stools

Ba Ji Yin Yang Wan 巴戟阴阳丸 (Ba Ji Yin Yang Wan)
- with urinary frequency.

External wash

- An astringent wash can be used to tone the rectal tissue directly in cases that do not respond, or that respond only slowly. Decoct **shi liu pi** (Pericarpium Punicae Granati) 石榴皮 30g for 30 minutes and add **ming fan** (Alumen) 明矾 15g to the strained decoction. Bathe the rectum in a sitzbath as often as practical.

Acupuncture (select from)

Du.20 (*bai hui* ▲) .... raises *yang qi*
Ren.6 (*qi hai*) .... Needle obliquely downwards with a 3-inch needle from Ren.6 (*qi hai*) towards Ren.3 (*zhong ji*). The needle is twirled to anchor it, then

raised towards the sternum creating a lifting sensation in the lower abdomen. It can be taped in its lifted position in place for the duration of the treatment.

Ren.8 (*shen que* ▲) .... Strong moxa on salt; place a piece of thin cloth over the navel and fill it with salt; burn large cones of moxa on the salt. The cloth enables quick removal of the salt and prevents excessive burning. Powerfully warms *yang* and elevates *yang*.

Du.1 (*chang qiang*) .... an important point for all rectal disorders

Bl.30 (*bai huan shu* +) ...... special point for anal disorders and a milder, but reasonable, alternative to Du.1

Bl.57 (*cheng shan*) .... point for rectal disorders (especially in combination with Du.1), regulates the lower Intestine and rectum, stops bleeding and pain

Bl.23 (*shen shu* +▲)......... *shu* point of the Kidney, warms and stimulates Kidney *yang*

Du.4 (*ming men* +▲) .... warms *yang*

Ren.12 (*zhong wan* +▲) .. *mu* point of the Stomach, warms and strengthens the Spleen and Stomach

St.25 (*tian shu* +▲) .... *mu* point of the Large Intestine, warms and regulates Intestinal function

St.36 (*zu san li* +▲) .... *he* sea point of the Stomach, powerfully warms and strengthens the Spleen and Stomach and supplements *qi*

Bl.20 (*pi shu* +▲) .... *shu* point of the Spleen, warms and strengthens the Spleen and supplements *qi*

Bl.25 (*da chang shu* +▲) .. *shu* point of Large Intestine, regulates Intestinal function

- a moxa box over the lower abdomen or low back is useful
- *Ear points*: spleen, large intestine, prolapse, haemorrhoids, kidney, adrenal, *shen men*

Clinical notes

- This pattern of prolapse can be difficult, especially when there has been significant mechanical trauma to the rectal tissues. It will usually require long treatment to resolve, 6-12 months is not unreasonable. If surgical repair is required, TCM treatment should still proceed to rebuild Spleen and Kidney *yang*.
- For dietary recommendations, see p.873.

湿热下坠

22.3 DAMP HEAT

Pathophysiology

- This type of prolapse is usually associated with chronic Damp Heat type diarrhoea or dysenteric disorder. The relentless downwards pressure of the diarrhoea, in combination with the persistent smouldering Heat, weakens and irritates the local tissues forcing them to protrude. If the Heat aspect is dominant, the stools may tend to be dry, causing constipation and pressure on the rectum.

Clinical features

- Rectal prolapse with a distended feeling, tenesmus and/or a burning sensation in the anus. The rectal mucosa appears dark, purple or deep red, feels firm and may be eroded or ulcerated. There may be bleeding.
- red complexion
- fever, afternoon fever
- dry mouth, thirst, halitosis
- fullness and discomfort in the chest and abdomen
- chronic diarrhoea or dysenteric disorder (with dominant Damp), or a tendency to difficult or dry stools, constipation or incomplete bowel movements (with dominant Heat)
- concentrated urine

T red with a greasy or dry, yellow coat
P soft or slippery and rapid

Treatment principle

Clear Damp Heat from the Intestines

Prescription

LIANG GE QING CHANG SAN 凉膈清肠散
(*Cool the Diaphragm, Clear the Intestine Powder*)

sheng di (Radix Rehmanniae Glutinosae) 生地 15-24g
bai shao (Radix Paeoniae Lactiflora) 白芍 12-18g
chi shao (Radix Paeoniae Rubrae) 赤芍 9-12g
dang gui (Radix Angelicae Sinensis) 当归 9-15g
chuan xiong (Radix Ligustici Chuanxiong) 川芎 6-9g
huang qin (Radix Scutellariae Baicalensis) 黄芩 9-12g
huang lian (Rhizoma Coptidis) 黄连 6-9g
sheng ma (Rhizoma Cimicifugae) 升麻 6-9g
xiang fu (Rhizoma Cyperi Rotundi) 香附 9-12g
gan cao (Radix Glycyrrhizae Uralensis) 甘草 6-9g

Method: Grind the herbs to a fine powder and form into 9-gram pills. The dose is one pill twice daily. May also be decocted with the quantities as shown. **Sheng di** and **chi shao** cool the Blood; **bai shao** cools and softens the Liver and nourishes Blood; **huang qin** and **huang lian** clear Damp Heat; **chi shao, dang gui, xiang fu** and **chuan xiong** regulate *qi* and Blood; **chi shao** and **chuan xiong** eliminate stagnant Blood; **sheng ma** elevates *yang qi*, and clears Toxic Heat; **gan cao** clears Heat and protects the Stomach. (Source: *Shi Yong Zhong Yi Nei Ke Xue*)

Modifications

- With swelling, burning, pain and itching in and around the rectum and anus, add **jin yin hua** (Flos Lonicerae Japonicae) 金银花 18-30g, **huang bai** (Cortex Phellodendri) 黄柏 9-12g, **huai hua** (Flos Sophora Japonicae Immaturus) 槐花 9-12g and **shan zhi zi** (Fructus Gardeniae Jasminoidis) 山栀子 9-12g.
- With difficult, dry or sluggish bowel movements, add **jue ming zi** (Semen Cassiae) 决明子 12g and **da huang** (Radix et Rhizoma Rhei) 大黄 6-9g.
- With concentrated urine, add **hua shi** (Talcum) 滑石 12-15g and **che qian zi** (Semen Plantaginis) 车前子 9-12g.
- If the patient drinks a lot of alcohol, and it is a contributing factor to the pathology, add **ge hua** (Flos Puerariae) 葛花 12-18g.
- With bleeding and rectal pain or discomfort, add **jing jie sui** (Herba seu Flos Schizonepetae Tenuifoliae) 荆芥穗 9-12g and **fang feng** (Radix Ledebouriellae Divaricatae) 防风 9-12g.

External wash

A decoction of **zhu ma gen** (*Boehmeria nivea*) 苎麻根 may be used to wash the rectal area.

Patent medicines

Yi Zi Tang 乙字汤 (Cimicifuga Combination)
- with a tendency to sluggish stools or constipation

Zhong Guo Zhi Gen Duan 中国痔根断 (Chinese Zhi Gen Duan)
- specific for bleeding haemorrhoids, but also useful to clear Damp Heat

Huang Lian Jie Du Wan 黄连解毒丸 (Huang Lian Jie Du Wan)
- Damp Heat

Chuan Xin Lian Kang Yan Pian 穿心莲抗炎片 (Chuan Xin Lian Antiphlogistic Tablets)
- severe Heat

Acupuncture (select from)

Du.20 (*bai hui* ▲) .... raises *yang qi*

Du.1 (*chang qiang*) .... local point for rectal diseases, and excellent with Bl.57 for excess patterns of the rectum

Bl.30 (*bai huan shu* -) .... special point for anal disorders and a milder, but reasonable alternative to Du.1
Bl.57 (*cheng shan* -) .... special point for diseases of the rectum, regulates the lower Intestine and rectum, dispels Wind and stops bleeding
Bl.25 (*da chang shu* -) .... *shu* point of the Large Intestine, clears Damp Heat and regulates the Intestines
Bl.31-34 (*ba liao* -) .... clear Damp Heat from the lower *jiao* and the rectal area; select the most tender
St.37 (*shang ju xu* -) .... lower *he* point of the Large Intestine, clears Damp Heat and regulates the Intestines
LI.11 (*qu chi* -) .... *he* sea point of the Large Intestine, clears Damp Heat from the intestines
Sp.9 (*yin ling quan*) .... *he* sea point of the Spleen, promotes urination and drains Damp

- with swelling and pain add Bl.58 (*fei yang* -) and Bl.54 (*zhi bian* -)
- with Heat in the Liver, add Liv.2 (*xing jian* -)
- magnets can be applied to Du.2 (*yao shu*)
- *Ear points*: large intestine, spleen, prolapse, haemorrhoids, *shen men*

Clinical notes

- Damp Heat rectal prolapse usually responds well to correct treatment, although in chronic cases, 2-3 months treatment will usually be necessary. Attention to diet and alcohol intake is essential.
- For dietary recommendations, see p.884.

SUMMARY OF GUIDING FORMULAE FOR RECTAL PROLAPSE

Spleen *qi* deficiency with sinking *qi* - *Bu Zhong Yi Qi Tang* 补中益气汤

Spleen and Kidney *yang* deficiency - *Da Bu Yuan Jian* 大补元煎
- with fluid metabolism disorder - *Jin Kui Shen Qi Wan* 金匮肾气丸
- with chronic diarrhoea or dysenteric disorder - *Zhen Ren Yang Zang Tang* 真人养脏汤

Damp Heat - *Liang Ge Qing Chang Tang* 凉膈清肠汤

23. Regurgitation

Liver *qi* invading the Stomach
Spleen and Stomach *qi/yang* deficiency
Stomach Heat
Phlegm obstructing the Stomach
Blood stagnation

23 REGURGITATION

fan wei 反胃

Regurgitation (*fan wei* [1]) is a disorder characterised by intermittent vomiting of partially digested food 12 hours or more following the previous meal. The most common presentation is vomiting of the evening meal the next morning. Other symptoms include epigastric fullness, nausea, early satiety, indigestion and loss of appetite. Vomiting may be infrequent if the patient has learned to adapt to a liquid or semiliquid diet.

Regurgitation of ingested material occurs if there is some obstruction to the Stomach *qi* and its natural descent, or if weakness of the Stomach organ is such that it is unable to break down food and pass it on to the Intestines. The undigested food remains in the Stomach until it is regurgitated.

Gastric content has a bitter taste, while regurgitated oesophageal content does not.

Regurgitation may occur as a single episode, especially when associated with an acute emotional upset. More commonly in the TCM clinic however, it appears as a chronic or recurrent event.

AETIOLOGY

Diet

Diet contributes to this disorder if it weakens Spleen and Stomach function, if it encourages Phlegm, or if it creates Heat in the Stomach.

Too much cold natured or raw food can weaken Spleen *qi* and *yang*. Missing meals or eating at odd hours throws the Stomach out of balance, gradually depleting *qi* and *yang*. Restrictive diets and eating disorders can severely damage Spleen and Stomach *yang*.

Overconsumption of too much food in general, and excessive consumption of rich, spicy and heating foods and alcohol in particular, can lead to the accumulation of food, and Heat or Damp Heat in the Stomach. High consumption of alcohol is a common factor in generating Stomach Heat and regurgitation. Sugar and dairy products create Dampness and Phlegm.

Emotion

The Liver is the most commonly implicated organ system when emotional factors lead to regurgitation. The relationship between the Liver, Stomach and Spleen is very close, and errant Liver *qi* will easily invade and disrupt the normal functioning of the Spleen and Stomach, and the *qi* mechanism.

[1] Wiseman's Stomach reflux

Liver *qi* stagnation is the result of chronic stress or emotional turmoil, and contributes to regurgitation directly by disrupting the *qi* mechanism. If the Liver invades the Spleen, the Spleen is weakened and may produce Dampness as a by-product of inefficient digestion. If the Liver invades the Stomach, Stomach *qi* can ascend carrying the acid contents up through the oesophagus. Prolonged *qi* stagnation often generates Heat, which intensifies the rising tendency of the already disordered Stomach *qi*. The Heat plus the increased acid reflux damages Stomach *yin*, drying and tightening the Stomach, oesophagus and associated structures.

BOX 23.1 SOME BIOMEDICAL CAUSES OF REGURGITATION

Gastro-intestinal
- gastric and duodenal ulcers
- acute and chronic gastritis
- gastric and oesophageal diverticulum
- gastric tumours, carcinoma of the antrum
- pyloric stenosis
- scleroderma
- systemic lupus erythematosus
- dermatomyositis
- post gastric surgery

Metabolic
- diabetes
- hypothyroidism

Drugs
- narcotics
- cimetidine
- salbutamol
- anticholinergics

In addition, stagnant *qi* slows and retards fluids which may congeal into Phlegm. Any Heat that has developed may combine with pre-existing Dampness forming Phlegm or Phlegm Heat. Once Phlegm or Phlegm Heat is formed, the nature of the obstruction is more substantial, and physical changes take place in the tissues of the Stomach and oesophagus.

Prolonged accumulation of *qi* and Phlegm, and perhaps Heat and *yin* deficiency, will gradually slow and obstruct the circulation of Blood, and more serious regurgitation develops.

Liver *qi* stagnation is also a common cause of acute or one off episodes of regurgitation, whereby anger or an emotional upset around the dinner table leads to acute Liver invasion of the Stomach and Spleen. When the emotional trigger is intense enough, the Stomach and Spleen can fail to proceed with digestion, and the *qi* mechanism is suddenly shut down. Eventually *qi* rebels and ejects the unprocessed meal.

Trauma

Trauma which may lead to regurgitation includes surgery of the upper abdomen or an injury such as the bruising and Blood stagnation that may occur following a motor vehicle accident in which the lower chest/upper abdomen is damaged.

TCM DIFFERENTIAL DIAGNOSIS

- **Vomiting** (*ou tu* 呕吐): Regurgitation differs from vomiting in that the regurgitated material consists of mostly undigested food. Vomiting which is not regurgitation is usually of sour digested or partially digested food.
- **Dysphagia** (*yi ge* 噎膈): Dysphagia is difficulty swallowing. The ingested material may be ejected if it cannot be swallowed, but if so this will usually occur immediately. In regurgitation there is usually no difficulty swallowing.
- **Acid reflux and Heartburn** (*tu suan* 吐酸): Acid reflux and heartburn is sour gastric acid that can be detected in the mouth, throat or retrosternally. Heartburn specifically refers to a sensation of retrosternal burning that spreads upwards to the throat. In general nothing is ejected from the mouth.

TREATMENT

From a biomedical point of view, one of the most common causes of regurgitation is pathology of the pyloric or cardiac sphincter. This pathology may be functional or structural, involving oedema, inflammation, spasm or stenosis. A knowledge of the mechanism is useful in the selection of herbs and in assessing the prognosis.

In general, the treatment of regurgitation is difficult, and the results with TCM are poor when there is a significant structural component. TCM treatment of regurgitation may be effective for the functional varieties, pyloric spasm, oedema and inflammation. The most responsive patterns are Liver *qi* stagnation, *qi*/*yang* deficiency and Stomach Heat. Blood stagnation and Phlegm accumulation may represent a physical lesion such as pyloric stenosis, oesophageal diverticulum or tumour, and results with TCM treatment are generally variable to poor. Phlegm patterns can sometimes respond to persistent treatment. Patients with Blood stagnation and non-responding Phlegm patterns are best referred to a surgeon.

肝气犯胃

23.1 LIVER QI INVADING THE STOMACH

Pathophysiology

- Liver *qi* invades the Stomach in response to stress or emotional upset. This type of regurgitation is often an acute episode that typically follows an emotional episode while eating. In such cases, it may be a single event never be repeated. Regurgitation associated with *qi* stagnation may also be chronic and recurrent, a learned and deeply ingrained response to stress.
- In long term cases, the *qi* stagnation will eventually be complicated by other pathology, most commonly Spleen deficiency, Phlegm accumulation, stagnant Heat and eventually, Blood stagnation.

Clinical features

- Episodes of recurrent or chronic regurgitation, aggravated or initiated during periods of stress and emotional turmoil, and alleviated when the patient is calm and relaxed.
- loss of appetite, indigestion, heartburn, acid reflux
- fullness, tightness or discomfort in the chest, epigastrium and hypochondrium
- irritability, anger, frustration, anxiety, moodiness, depression
- may be a sensation of something lodged in the throat (plum-stone throat)
- premenstrual syndrome, irregular menstruation

T normal or darkish or with slightly red edges with a thin, possibly greasy coat; in chronic cases with underlying deficiency, the tongue may be pale or pale on the edges

P wiry, or wiry and slippery

Treatment principle

Harmonise the Liver and Stomach and regulate *qi*
Redirect Stomach *qi* downwards

Prescription

CHAI HU SHU GAN SAN 柴胡疏肝散
(*Bupleurum and Cyperus Formula*)

This prescription is suitable for both acute and recurrent episodes of regurgitation.

chai hu (Radix Bupleuri) 柴胡 9-12g
cu bai shao (vinegar fried Radix Paeoniae Lactiflora)
醋白芍 12-18g
xiang fu (Rhizoma Cyperi Rotundi) 香附 9-12g
zhi shi (Fructus Immaturus Citri Aurantii) 枳实 6-9g

chuan xiong (Radix Ligustici Chuanxiong) 川芎 6-9g
gan cao (Radix Glycyrrhizae Uralensis) 甘草 3-6g

Method: Decoction, or ground to a fine powder and taken in 9-gram doses as a draft with hot water. **Chai hu** regulates and invigorates Liver *qi* and clears Heat; **cu bai shao** softens the Liver and nourishes *yin* and Blood, thus preventing excessive dispersal of, and damage to, *qi* and Liver *yin* by **chai hu; xiang fu** regulates *qi* and disperses stagnant Liver *qi*; **zhi shi** breaks up stagnant *qi*, directs *qi* downwards, it's descending action neatly balancing the ascending nature of **chai hu** thus facilitating the correct functioning of the *qi* mechanism; **chuan xiong** invigorates *qi* and Blood and reinforces the *qi* moving function of **xiang fu; gan cao** harmonises the Stomach and strengthens the Spleen, and with **bai shao** eases spasms in the Stomach and oesophagus.

Modifications (apply to all three prescriptions where not already included)

- With severe regurgitation, add **xuan fu hua** (Flos Inulae) 旋复花 12-15g and **dai zhe shi** (Haematitum) 代赭石 15g.
- With regurgitation of bile, **yu jin** (Tuber Curcumae) 郁金 9-12g and **jin qian cao** (Herba Lysimachiae) 金钱草 18g.
- With a tendency to constipation add **da huang** (Radix et Rhizoma Rhei) 大黄 3-9g.
- With food stagnation add **shan zha** (Fructus Crataegi) 山楂 15g, **mai ya** (Fructus Hordei Vulgaris Germinantus) 麦芽 15-30g and **ji nei jin** (Endothelium Corneum Gigeriae Galli) 鸡内金 12g.
- With stagnant Heat and acid reflux, add **huang lian** (Rhizoma Coptidis) 黄连 6-9g and **wu zhu yu** (Fructus Evodiae Rutaecarpae) 吴茱萸 2-3g.

Variations and additional prescriptions

With Phlegm

- Liver *qi* stagnation type regurgitation may be associated with accumulation of Phlegm. The patient experiences regurgitation during times of anxiety or stress, accompanied by a sensation of something lodged in the throat ('plum-stone throat'), tightness in the chest, a greasy tongue coat and a wiry, slippery pulse. The aim of treatment is to regulate *qi* and transform Phlegm with **BAN XIA HOU PO TANG** (*Pinellia and Magnolia Combination* 半夏厚朴汤, p.764).

Maintenance treatment to regulate qi

- In between episodes of regurgitation, *qi* regulating patent medicines (*see* below) may be prescribed on the basis of the patients constitution and accompanying features to prevent recurrence.

Patent medicines

Chai Hu Shu Gan Wan 柴胡疏肝丸 (Chai Hu Shu Gan Wan)
- Liver invading the Stomach, good for robust patients

Chen Xiang Hua Qi Wan 沉香化气丸 (Chen Xiang Hua Qi Wan) - with constipation

Xiao Yao Wan 逍遥丸 (Xiao Yao Wan, Hsiao Yao Wan, Bupleurum Sedative Pills) - best for constitutional treatment of Liver *qi* stagnation in women and patient's with Spleen and Blood deficiency

Jia Wei Xiao Yao Wan 加味逍遥丸 (Jia Wei Xiao Yao Wan, Dan Zhi Xiao Yao Wan) - Liver *qi* stagnation with stagnant Heat

Xiang Sha Yang Wei Wan 香砂养胃丸 (Xiang Sha Yang Wei Wan) - with Spleen and Stomach deficiency

Acupuncture (select from)

Ren.22 (*tian tu*) .... these points regulate *qi* in the chest
Ren.17 (*shan zhong*) and oesophagus, direct *qi* downwards, correct
Ren.14 (*ju que*) the *qi* mechanism in the chest and relax the diaphragm

PC.6 (*nei guan* -) .... *luo* point of the Pericardium, master point of *yin wei mai*, spreads Liver *qi*, regulates the middle *jiao*, stops vomiting and calms the Heart and *shen*

Sp.4 (*gong sun*) .... *luo* point of the Spleen, master point of *chong mai*, regulates the Spleen and Stomach

Liv.13 (*zhang men*) .... *mu* point of the Spleen, regulates the Liver and Spleen and strengthens the Spleen

Ren.12 (*zhong wan* -) .... *mu* point of the Stomach, regulates the Stomach and directs Stomach *qi* downwards

Kid.4 (*da zhong* -) .... *luo* point of the Kidney, a special point for stricture in the oesophagus

Liv.3 (*tai chong* -) .... together these points regulate Liver *qi*,
GB.34 (*yang ling quan* -) pacify the Liver and harmonise the Liver and Stomach

- with Gallbladder involvement or regurgitation of bile, add GB.24 (*ri yue*), GB.40 (*qiu xu* -) and *dan nang xue* (M-LE-23)
- with Spleen deficiency, add St.36 (*zu san li* +) and Bl.20 (*pi shu* +)
- with Phlegm or plum stone throat, add PC.5 (*jian shi* -), St.40 (*feng long* -) and Sp.3 (*tai bai*)
- In most cases, points to calm the *shen* should be added: select one or two points from Ht.7 (*shen men*), *yin tang* (M-HN-3), Du.19 (*hou ding*), Du. 24 (*shen ting*)
- *Ear points*: liver, stomach, spleen, pylorus, oesophagus, subcortex, sympathetic, *shen men*

Clinical notes

- Regurgitation of a Liver *qi* invading the Stomach type may be diagnosed biomedically as oesophageal spasm, gastric spasm, chronic gastritis, peptic ulcer disease, nervous stomach, indigestion, chronic cholecystitis or chronic hepatitis.
- When uncomplicated, Liver *qi* stagnation type regurgitation usually has a good prognosis, particularly if the source of external stress can be resolved. Acupuncture and herbs are certainly among the best and most reliable treatments. Treatment often needs to be prolonged (3 months+) and must be combined with appropriate relaxation and stress management techniques, or other forms of *qi* mobilising activity. Particularly useful is walking, swimming, yoga or *tai ji chuan*, although all exercise is beneficial. Gentle and regular massage, particularly of the abdomen, neck and mid thoracic region is also useful.
- For dietary recommendations, see p.878.

脾胃虚寒

23.2 SPLEEN AND STOMACH QI/YANG DEFICIENCY

Pathophysiology

- When Spleen and Stomach *qi* and *yang* are weak, there is little digestive fire and motive force available to process and move the ingested food. The partially digested or undigested mass remains in the Stomach, further obstructing the descent of Stomach *qi*. Eventually sufficient *qi* backs up behind the food mass and forces the accumulated *qi to* rebel upwards, taking the food with it. A complicating feature of Spleen deficiency patterns is the potential presence of oedema or pathological fluids, here affecting the Stomach and oesophagus, and thus further impeding descent of food.
- This is usually a chronic pattern, in which case malnourishment may become significant.
- Occasionally, regurgitation of this type follows abdominal surgery, if there is direct damage to Spleen and Stomach *yang* by the external Cold of the operating theatre.

Clinical features

- intermittent epigastric and abdominal distension and fullness after eating, followed around 12 hours later by vomiting of the partially digested or undigested previous meal, relieving the discomfort
- the vomitus is relatively inoffensive, with clearly identifiable food items and possibly a watery mucus-like material
- waxy, pale complexion
- loss of appetite, anorexia, weight loss, emaciation
- loose stools, diarrhoea
- fatigue, weakness, listlessness, increased desire to sleep
- cold extremities and abdomen, cold intolerance

T pale and swollen with a white coat
P thready, weak, deep

Treatment principle

Warm and strengthen the Spleen and Stomach
Harmonise the Stomach and redirect *qi* downwards

Prescription

DING KOU LI ZHONG WAN 丁蔻理中丸
(*Regulate the Middle Pills with Clove and Cardamon*) modified

dang shen (Radix Codonopsis Pilosulae) 党参 15-24g
chao bai zhu (dry fried Rhizoma Atractylodis Macrocephalae) 炒白术 12-15g
gan jiang (Rhizoma Zingiberis Officinalis) 干姜 9-12g

zhi gan cao (honey fried Radix Glycyrrhizae Uralensis) 炙甘草 6-9g
ding xiang (Flos Caryophylli) 丁香 3-6g
bai dou kou (Fructus Amomi Kravanh) 白豆蔻 6-9g

Method: Decoction. **Bai dou kou** can be taken separately as a powder or added at the end of cooking (*hou xia* 后下). **Dang shen** supplements *qi* and strengthens the Spleen; **chao bai zhu** strengthens the Spleen and dries Dampness; **gan jiang** warms and invigorates Spleen *yang*; **zhi gan cao** supplements *qi* and harmonises the Stomach; **ding xiang** warms and regulates *qi* and directs *qi* downwards; **bai dou kou** fragrantly warms the Stomach and promotes the movement of *qi*. (*Shi Yong Zhong Yi Nei Ke Xue*)

Modifications

- Depending on the relative degree of deficiency and Cold, the proportion of the herbs can be varied. For example if the *qi* deficiency is primary (that is, there are few Cold symptoms), then the upper dose range of **dang shen** and **chao bai zhu** can be used, and **fu ling** (Sclerotium Poria Cocos) 茯苓 12-15g added. If the Cold aspects are primary, the quantity of **gan jiang** should be 12g, and **wu zhu yu** (Fructus Evodiae Rutaecarpae) 吴茱萸 6g added.
- With severe regurgitation, add **ban xia** (Rhizoma Pinelliae Ternatae) 半夏 9-12g and **xuan fu hua** (Flos Inulae) 旋复花 12-15g.
- With oedema or fluid retention, add **ze xie** (Rhizoma Alismatis Orientalis) 泽泻 9-12g **fu ling** (Sclerotium Poriae Cocos) 茯苓 12-15g and **che qian zi** (Semen Plantaginis) 车前子 9-12g.
- With severe distension and fullness, add **hou po** (Cortex Magnoliae Officinalis) 厚朴 9-12g and **zhi ke** (Fructus Citri Aurantii) 枳壳 9-12g.

Variations and additional prescriptions

With qi stagnation

- When *qi* deficiency is complicated by *qi* stagnation, episodes of regurgitation are initiated or aggravated by changes in the emotional state of the patient. When *qi* stagnation is significant, the aim of treatment is to strengthen the Spleen and regulate the Liver, harmonise the Stomach, alleviate food stagnation and redirect *qi* downwards with **DING XIANG TOU GE SAN** (*Clove Powder to Penetrate the Diaphragm* 丁香透膈散).

ding xiang (Flos Caryophylli) 丁香 3-6g
dang shen (Radix Codonopsis Pilosulae) 党参 12-15g
chao bai zhu (dry fried Rhizoma Atractylodis Macrocephalae) 炒白术 9-12g
xiang fu (Rhizoma Cyperi Rotundi) 香附 9-12g
mu xiang (Radix Aucklandiae Lappae) 木香 6-9g
sha ren (Fructus Amomi) 砂仁 9-12g

bai dou kou (Fructus Amomi Kravanh) 白豆蔻 6-9g
chao mai ya (dry fried Fructus Hordei Vulgaris Germinantus) 炒麦芽 15-30g
shen qu (Massa Fermentata) 神曲 9-15g
zhi gan cao (honey fried Radix Glycyrrhizae Uralensis) 炙甘草 3-6g

Method: Decoction. **Sha ren**, **bai dou kou** and **mu xiang** are added towards the end of cooking (*hou xia* 后下). **Ding xiang** warms and regulates *qi* and directs *qi* downwards; **dang shen**, **chao bai zhu** and **zhi gan cao** support the Spleen and supplement *qi*; **xiang fu** and **mu xiang** regulate *qi* and open up *qi* flow; **sha ren** and **bai dou kou** fragrantly dispel Damp and move *qi*; **chao mai ya** and **shen qu** improve digestion and alleviate food stagnation. (Source: *Shi Yong Zhong Yi Nei Ke Xue*)

With Kidney yang deficiency

- In persistent cases, Kidney *yang* will be drained off to support the weak Spleen. The result is a combined Spleen and Kidney *yang* deficiency. The features are the same as those of the primary pattern, with the addition of Kidney specific signs and symptoms, such as nocturia and urinary frequency, tinnitus and loss of hearing, lower back ache, sore knees and deep, weak pulse at the proximal positions. The treatment aims to strengthen Spleen and Kidney *yang*, harmonise the Stomach and redirect *qi* downwards with **FU ZI LI ZHONG WAN** (*Aconite, Ginseng and Ginger Formula* 附子理中丸) modified.

zhi fu zi (Radix Aconiti Carmichaeli Praeparata) 制附子 9-12g
gan jiang (Rhizoma Zingiberis Officinalis) 干姜 9-12g
fu ling (Sclerotium Poria Cocos) 茯苓 12-15g
rou gui (Cortex Cinnamomi Cassiae) 肉桂 3-6g
bu gu zhi (Fructus Psoraleae Corylifoliae) 补骨脂 12-15g
yi zhi ren (Fructus Alpiniae Oxyphyllae) 益智仁 12-15g
xian ling pi (Herba Epimedii) 仙灵脾 12-15g
chen xiang (Lignum Aquilariae) 沉香 2-3g
chen pi (Pericarpium Citri Reticulatae) 陈皮 6-9g
niu xi (Radix Achyranthis Bidentatae) 牛膝 6-9g
shen qu (Massa Fermentata) 神曲 9-12g

Method: Decoction. **Zhi fu zi** is cooked for 30 minutes before the other herbs (*xian jian* 先煎), **chen xiang** is added towards the end of cooking (*hou xia* 后下). **Zhi fu zi** and **gan jiang** warm Spleen *yang*; **rou gui** and **zhi fu zi** warm the Kidneys and aid in the transformation of *qi*; **bu gu zhi**, **yi zhi ren** and **xian ling pi** supplement and warm Kidney *yang*; **fu ling** strengthens the Spleen and leaches out Dampness; **chen xiang** and **chen pi** regulate *qi*; **niu xi** regulates Blood, directs Blood downwards and strengthens the Kidneys; **shen qu** aids digestion and alleviates food stagnation. (Source: *Zhong Yi Nei Ke Shou Ce*)

Severe, resistant or unresponsive cases with Phlegm accumulation

- In cases of severe regurgitation, often with a degree of accumulated stubborn Phlegm, the principle of treatment may be altered to heavily weigh down the rising Stomach *qi* and transform Phlegm, before strengthening the middle *jiao*. **XUAN FU DAI ZHE TANG** (*Inula and Haematite Decoction* 旋复代赭汤, p.772) is employed to do this.

Patent medicines

Fu Zi Li Zhong Wan 附子理中丸 (Fu Tzu Li Chung Wan, Carmichaeli Tea Pills, Li Chung Yuen Medical Pills)
- Spleen *yang* deficiency with Cold

Li Zhong Wan 理中丸 (Li Zhong Wan)
- Spleen *yang* deficiency

Xiang Sha Liu Jun Zi Wan 香砂六君子丸 (Xiang Sha Liu Jun Wan, Aplotaxis-Ammomum Pills, Six Gentlemen Tea Pills)
- Spleen *qi* deficiency with Phlegm Damp

Jin Kui Shen Qi Wan 金匮肾气丸 (Fu Gui Ba Wei Wan, Sexoton Pills, Golden Book Tea)
- combine with one of the above formulae for Kidney *yang* deficiency

Acupuncture (select from)

Bl.21 (*wei shu* +▲) .... *shu* points of the Stomach and Spleen
Bl.20 (*pi shu* +▲) respectively, warm and strengthen *middle jiao yang qi*

Ren.12 (*zhong wan* +▲) .. *mu* point of the Stomach, warms and strengthens the Spleen and Stomach

Ren.17 (*shan zhong*) .... these points direct rebellious *qi* downward,
Ren.14 (*ju que*) regulates movement of *qi* in the chest and lower oesophagus

Liv.13 (*zhang men* +▲) .... *mu* point of the Spleen and *hui* point of the *zang*, strengthens the Spleen and supplements *qi*

Ren.9 (*shui fen* ▲) .... strong moxibustion, either direct or stick, to mobilise fluids and relieve oedema

St.36 (*zu san li* +▲) .... *he* sea point of the Stomach, warms and strengthens the Spleen and Stomach, and supplements *qi*

- with *qi* stagnation, add Liv.3 (*tai chong*) and PC.6 (*nei guan*)

- with Kidney *yang* deficiency, add Bl.23 (*shen shu* +▲), Du.4 (*ming men* +▲), Ren.4 (*guan yuan* +▲), Kid.3 (*tai xi* +)
- with gastroptosis, add Du.20 (*bai hui* +▲)
- a moxa box over the upper abdomen is useful
- *Ear points*: oesophagus, pylorus, spleen, stomach, kidney, adrenal, sympathetic, *shen men*

Clinical notes

- Regurgitation associated with *qi* and/or *yang* deficiency may be diagnosed biomedically as chronic gastritis, gastroptosis, scleroderma, prolapse of the gastric mucosa, hypo-acidity, gastric diverticulum, post-gastrectomy syndrome and hypothyroidism.
- If the regurgitation results from a functional weakness, the prognosis is generally good, and with persistent treatment (6-12 months), Spleen *yang* will be restored. When structural, referral to a surgeon may be appropriate. Even if surgery is required, TCM treatment is valuable for restoring *yang* and improving the patient's overall health.
- In long term cases, with malnourishment, diet is an especially important part of treatment, not just in addressing the aetiology of the disorder, but in building strength and aiding recovery. Small meals of easily absorbable food, such as broths and soups are most appropriate. For further dietary recommendations, see p.870-873.

胃中积热

23.3 STOMACH HEAT

Pathophysiology

- Stomach Heat subverts the normal descent of Stomach *qi* by causing *qi* and food to rise upwards. This pattern is typically due to ingestion of excessive amounts of heating substances, in particular alcohol.
- Prolonged Stomach Heat will eventually damage Stomach *yin*, or cook and congeal fluids into Phlegm Damp or Phlegm Heat.

Clinical features

- intermittent epigastric and abdominal distension and fullness after eating, followed around 12 hours later by vomiting of the partially digested meal, relieving the discomfort
- the vomitus may be sour and offensive
- irritability, restlessness
- red complexion and lips
- halitosis
- thirst, dry mouth and lips
- tendency to constipation; rarely, diarrhoea
- concentrated urine

T red and dry with a thick, yellow or thick, greasy yellow coat
P slippery and rapid

Treatment principle

Clear Heat from the Stomach
Harmonise the Stomach and redirect *qi* downwards

Prescription

ZHU RU TANG 竹茹汤
(*Bamboo Shavings Decoction*)

zhu ru (Caulis Bambusae in Taeniis) 竹茹 9-12g
shan zhi zi (Fructus Gardeniae Jasminoides) 山栀子 9-12g
ban xia (Rhizoma Pinelliae Ternatae) 半夏 9-12g
chen pi (Pericarpium Citri Reticulatae) 陈皮 9-12g
pi pa ye (Folium Eriobotryae Japonicae) 枇杷叶 12-15g
sheng jiang (Rhizoma Zingiberis Officinalis Recens) 生姜 6-9g
da zao (Fructus Zizyphi Jujubae) 大枣 4pce
gan cao (Radix Glycyrrhizae Uralensis) 甘草 3-6g

Method: Decoction. **Zhu ru** and **shan zhi zi** clear Heat from the Stomach and direct Stomach *qi* downwards; **ban xia, chen pi, pi pa ye** and **zhu ru** harmonise the Stomach and transform Phlegm; **gan cao** clears Heat and with **sheng jiang** and **da zao**, protects the Stomach. (Source: *Shi Yong Zhong Yi Nei Ke Xue*)

Modifications

- With severe Heat, add **huang qin** (Radix Scutellariae Baicalensis) 黄芩 9-12g and **huang lian** (Rhizoma Coptidis) 黄连 3-6g.
- With constipation, add **da huang** (Radix et Rhizoma Rhei) 大黄 6-9g, **zhi shi** (Fructus Immaturus Citri Aurantii) 枳实 9-12g and **hou po** (Cortex Magnoliae Officinalis) 厚朴 9-12g.
- With significant Dampness (a thick tongue coat), add **bing lang** (Semen Arecae Catechu) 槟榔 9-12g and **bai dou kou** (Fructus Amomi Kravanh) 白豆蔻 6-9g.
- With *yin* deficiency (peeled centre of the tongue), add **mai dong** (Tuber Ophiopogonis Japonici) 麦冬 9-12g and **shi hu** (Herba Dendrobii) 石斛 12-15g.

Variations and additional prescriptions

Damage to qi and yin

- In chronic cases, Stomach *yin* and *qi* are consumed, resulting in regurgitation accompanied by dry mouth and lips, constipation, a dry, pink, slightly red or peeled tongue and a thready pulse. The aim of treatment is to benefit *qi*, replenish *yin* fluids, harmonise the Stomach and direct *qi* downwards with **DA BAN XIA TANG** (*Major Pinellia Decoction 大半夏汤*).

  jiang ban xia (ginger fried Rhizoma Pinelliae Ternatae) 姜半夏 9-12g
  dang shen (Radix Codonopsis Pilosulae) 党参 15-24g
  mai dong (Tuber Ophiopogonis Japonici) 麦冬 9-12g
  shi hu (Herba Dendrobii) 石斛 9-12g
  feng mi (honey) 蜂蜜 30g

  Method: Decoction. **Jiang ban xia** stops vomiting; **dang shen** supplements *qi* and generates fluids; **feng mi** prevents the **ban xia** from excessive drying, supplements *qi* and moistens dryness; **mai dong** and **shi hu** nourish Stomach *yin*.

Alcohol as significant aetiological feature, Damp Heat

- If overconsumption of alcohol is a significant contributing factor, then, in addition to moderating alcohol intake, a formula that can decrease desire for alcohol and clear Heat and Damp may be useful. **GE HUA JIE CHENG TANG** (*Pueraria Flower Decoction to Alleviate Hangover* 葛花解酲汤) is selected.

  ge hua (Flos Puerariae) 葛花 15-18g
  sha ren (Fructus Amomi) 砂仁 6-9g
  bai dou kou (Fructus Amomi Kravanh) 白豆蔻 6-9g
  mu xiang (Radix Aucklandiae Lappae) 木香 6-9g
  qing pi (Pericarpium Citri Reticulatae Viridae) 青皮 6-9g
  chen pi (Pericarpium Citri Reticulatae) 陈皮 6-9g

dang shen (Radix Codonopsis Pilosulae) 党参 15-24g
zhu ling (Sclerotium Polypori Umbellati) 猪苓 9-12g
fu ling (Sclerotium Poria Cocos) 茯苓 12-15g
shen qu (Massa Fermentata) 神曲 12-15g
ze xie (Rhizoma Alismatis Orientalis) 泽泻 9-12g
gan jiang (Rhizoma Zingiberis Officinalis) 干姜 6-9g
bai zhu (Rhizoma Atractylodis Macrocephalae) 白术 12-15g

Method: Decoction. **Ge hua** alleviates the effects of excessive alcohol consumption; **sha ren** and **bai dou kou** fragrantly disperse Dampness and invigorate the Spleen; **mu xiang**, **qing pi** and **chen pi** regulate and break up accumulated *qi*; **dang shen** strengthens the Spleen and supplements *qi*; **zhu ling**, **fu ling** and **ze xie** promote urination to provide an outlet for the Dampness; **shen qu** improves digestion; **gan jiang** warms Spleen *yang*; **bai zhu** strengthens the Spleen and dries Damp. (Source: *Shi Yong Zhong Yi Nei Ke Xue*)

Complex mixture of Heat, Cold and deficiency

- In chronic cases, Heat and Cold may coexist, clumping together in the middle *jiao* against a background of Spleen and Stomach deficiency. This is usually associated with poor dietary habits and the effect of stress on the upper gastro-intestinal system. It may also be the result of repeated self induced emesis (bulimia). In addition to the regurgitation, there is a sensation of blockage, distension, fullness and discomfort in the epigastrium, which, when palpated, feels soft and without pain. The patient may also experience nausea, vomiting or dry retching, borborygmus with diarrhoea, poor appetite, a thin, greasy, yellow tongue coat and a soft, slippery, slightly wiry, and possibly rapid, pulse. The treatment is to harmonise the Stomach, redirect *qi* downwards and disperse accumulation with **BAN XIA XIE XIN TANG** (*Pinellia Combination* 半夏泻心汤, p.32).

Patent medicines

Huang Lian Jie Du Wan 黄连解毒丸 (Huang Lian Jie Du Wan)
- Stomach Heat and Damp Heat

Wen Dan Wan 温胆丸 (Wen Dan Wan)
- Phlegm Heat

Niu Huang Qing Huo Wan 牛黄清火丸 (Niu Huang Qing Huo Wan)
- with constipation

Acupuncture (select from)

Ren.17 (*shan zhong*) .... these points direct rebellious *qi* downward,
Ren.14 (*ju que*) regulates movement of *qi* in the chest and lower oesophagus

Ren.12 (*zhong wan* -) .... *mu* point of the Stomach, clears Heat from the Stomach and directs Stomach *qi* downwards

PC.6 (*nei guan*) .... *luo* point of the Pericardium, master point of *yin wei mai*, regulates the middle *jiao* and stops vomiting

PC.8 (*lao gong* -) .... *rong* spring and Fire point of the Pericardium, drains Heat from the Stomach and Stomach channel

St.36 (*zu san li* -) .... *he* sea point of the Stomach, regulates the Spleen and Stomach and corrects the *qi* mechanism

St.44 (*nei ting* -) .... *rong* spring and Water point of the Stomach, clears Heat from *yang ming*, the Stomach and Stomach channel

- with severe Heat, add LI.4 (*he gu* -) and LI.11 (*qu chi* -) or St.45 (*li dui* ↓) and SJ.2 (*ye men* -)
- with constipation, add SJ.6 (*zhi gou* -) and St.25 (*tian shu* -)
- with Phlegm Heat, add St.40 (*feng long* -) and PC.5 (*jian shi*)
- *Ear points*: oesophagus, pylorus, stomach, duodenum, spleen, sympathetic, *shen men*

Clinical notes

- Stomach Heat type regurgitation may be diagnosed biomedically as inflammation of the cardiac or pyloric sphincter caused by acute or chronic gastritis or gastro-oesophageal reflux, alcoholism, bulimia, scleroderma or systemic lupus erythematosus.
- Depending on the longevity and intensity of the pattern, and the degree of structural change, Stomach Heat regurgitation may respond reasonably well to treatment. With scarring or sclerosis of the oesophagus or sphincters, TCM treatment is less effective.
- For dietary recommendations, see p.882.

痰浊阻胃

23.4 PHLEGM OBSTRUCTING THE STOMACH

Pathophysiology

- Phlegm is a pathogen that easily obstructs the correct movement of *qi* and disrupts the *qi* mechanism. In cases of regurgitation, the presence of Phlegm in the Stomach system obstructs the descent of Stomach *qi* and retards distribution of *qi* and fluids. Phlegm may form substantial knots and a degree of structural change in the tissues of the Stomach and oesophagus. Phlegm easily generates Heat, becoming Phlegm Heat.

Clinical features

- frequent epigastric and abdominal distension and fullness, worse after eating, followed by vomiting of the partially digested meal around 12 hours later, relieving the discomfort
- the vomitus may have clearly identifiable undigested food residue, and possibly a thick or thin, frothy mucus, saliva or egg-white-like material
- possible epigastric masses and/or epigastric splash with palpation
- copious salivation
- dizziness, palpitations
- stuffiness in the chest

T greasy, white coat
P slippery or wiry

Treatment principle

Transform and eliminate Phlegm
Harmonise the Stomach and redirect *qi* downward

Prescription

DAO TAN TANG 导痰汤
(*Guide Out Phlegm Decoction*)

ban xia (Rhizoma Pinelliae Ternatae) 半夏 9-12g
chen pi (Pericarpium Citri Reticulatae) 陈皮 9-12g
fu ling (Sclerotium Poriae Cocos) 茯苓 12-15g
zhi shi (Fructus Immaturus Citri Aurantii) 枳实 12-15g
tian nan xing (Rhizoma Arisaematis) 天南星 6-9g
gan cao (Radix Glycyrrhizae Uralensis) 甘草 3-6g

Method: Decoction. **Ban xia** and **tian nan xing** dry Damp and transform Phlegm; **chen pi** and **zhi shi** harmonise the Stomach and direct *qi* downwards; **fu ling** strengthens the Spleen, promotes urination and leaches out Dampness; **gan cao** supplements *qi* and protects the Stomach. (Source: *Shi Yong Zhong Yi Nei Ke Xue*)

Modifications

- With Heat, substitute **dan nan xing** (Pulvis Arisaemae cum Felle Bovis) 胆南星 for **tian nan xing**, and add **huang lian** (Rhizoma Coptidis) 黄连 6g and **zhu ru** (Caulis Bambusae in Taeniis) 竹茹 9-12g.
- With signs of Cold accumulation, add **gan jiang** (Rhizoma Zingiberis Officinalis) 干姜 6-9g and **xi xin** (Herba cum Radice Asari) 细辛 3-6g.
- With frequent regurgitation and cold extremities, add **wu zhu yu** (Fructus Evodiae Rutaecarpae) 吴茱萸 3-6g.
- With an epigastric splash upon palpation, copious salivation or thin watery, white mucus or egg-white-like material in the vomit, add **dang shen** (Radix Codonopsis Pilosulae) 党参 12-15g and **yi zhi ren** (Fructus Alpiniae Oxyphyllae) 益智仁 9-12g.
- With Phlegm masses, combine with **XIAO LUO WAN** (*Reduce Scrophula Pill* 消瘰丸, p.910), or add **hai ge ke** (Concha Cyclinae Sinensis) 海蛤壳 9-15g, **hai fu shi** (Pumice) 海浮石 9-12 and **wa leng zi** (Concha Arcae) 瓦楞子 9-15g.
- With firm masses, add **e zhu** (Rhizoma Curcumae Ezhu) 莪术 9-12g and **san leng** (Rhizoma Sparganii Stoloniferi) 三棱 9-12g.

Variations and additional prescriptions

Robust patients with copious Phlegm and Heat

- In severe cases, with stubborn Phlegm, continuous palpitations, vertigo, tinnitus, a thick, yellow tongue coat and constipation, the aim of treatment is to powerfully drive out Phlegm through the bowel with **GUN TAN WAN** (*Vaporize Phlegm Pill* 滚痰丸). This is suitable for strong or robust patients.

  duan meng shi (calcined Lapis Micae seu Chloriti) 煅礞石 30g
  jiu da huang (wine fried Radix et Rhizoma Rhei) 酒大黄 .. 240g
  huang qin (Radix Scutellariae Baicalensis) 黄芩 240g
  chen xiang (Linum Aquilariae) 沉香 15g

  Method: Grind all substances to a powder and form into small pills with water. The dose is 6-9 grams once or twice daily, with ginger tea. **Meng shi** unearths and drives out stubborn accumulations of Phlegm and directs *qi* downward; **jiu da huang** purges the Intestines, clears Heat, invigorates *qi* and Blood and provides an outlet for the Phlegm; **huang qin** clears Heat from the upper *jiao*; **chen xiang** regulates *qi* and directs *qi* downward. (Source: *Shi Yong Zhong Yi Nei Ke Xue*)

Difficult or persistent regurgitation

- Unrelenting or unresponsive regurgitation may be assisted with a heavy prescription to weigh down the rebellious Stomach *qi* and transform Phlegm, and supplement *qi* and harmonise the Stomach. The formula selected is **XUAN FU DAI ZHE TANG** (*Inula and Haematite Decoction* 旋复代赭汤, p.772).

Patent medicines

Er Chen Wan 二陈丸 (Er Chen Wan, Pinellia-Pachyma Compound Pills)
- base formula for Phlegm disorders

Su Zi Jiang Qi Wan 苏子降气丸 (Su Zi Jiang Qi Wan)
- with thin Phlegm

Wen Dan Wan 温胆丸 (Wen Dan Wan)
- Phlegm Heat

Nei Xiao Luo Li Wan 内消瘰疬丸 (Nei Xiao Luo Li Wan)
- with Blood stagnation

Hai Zao Wan 海藻丸 (Hai Zao Wan)
- a general formula to soften Phlegm

Acupuncture (select from)

St.40 (*feng long* -) .... *luo* point of the Stomach, transforms Phlegm and clears Heat and Phlegm from the Stomach

Ren.12 (*zhong wan* -) .... *mu* point of the Stomach, clears Phlegm from the Stomach and directs Stomach *qi* downwards

Ren.17 (*shan zhong*) ....
Ren.14 (*ju que*) these points direct rebellious *qi* downward, regulates movement of *qi* in the chest and lower oesophagus

PC.6 (*nei guan*) .... *luo* point of the Pericardium, master point of *yin wei mai*, regulates the middle *jiao* and stops regurgitation

Bl.21 (*wei shu* -) ....
Bl.20 (*pi shu* -) *shu* points of the Stomach and Spleen respectively, strengthen the *middle jiao*, transform Phlegm and correct the *qi* mechanism

- with Phlegm Fluids or an epigastric splash, add Lu.7 (*lie que*) and Ren.9 (*shui fen* ▲) and moxa to points on the trunk
- with Phlegm Heat add PC.8 (*lao gong* -), Lu.6 (*kong zui* -) and Liv.2 (*xing jian* -)
- with epigastric masses, add Sp.4 (*gong sun* -) and Liv.13 (*zhang men* -)
- *Ear points*: oesophagus, pylorus, stomach, spleen, sympathetic, *shen men*

Clinical notes

- Phlegm obstructing the Stomach type regurgitation may be diagnosed biomedically as pyloric spasm or oedema, or tumours of the stomach or oesophagus. If the biomedical cause is not structural, Phlegm often responds quite well to persistent TCM treatment, in combination with dietary modification.
- For dietary recommendations, see p.880.

23.5 BLOOD STAGNATION

血瘀反胃

Pathophysiology

- Blood stagnation type regurgitation is likely to be caused by a mass or physical lesion that prevents the passage of food. The accumulated food builds up to the point where it rebels upwards and is regurgitated.

Clinical features

- frequent or constant epigastric and abdominal distension and fullness, worse after eating, followed around 12 hours later by vomiting of the partially digested or undigested meal, relieving the discomfort
- localised or stabbing epigastric pain or firm immobile epigastric masses, which are painful when palpated
- the vomitus has clearly identifiable undigested food residue, possibly with a brown or blood streaked mucus like material
- the stools may be tarry and black, or there may be streaks of blood in the stools
- broken vessels or spider naevi on the face, trunk, inner knee and ankle
- purplish lips, sclera, conjunctiva and nails, dark rings around the eyes
- irritability, short temper, depression, mood swings; dizziness and forgetfulness; dry scaly skin, hair loss on the head and body

T dark or red purple with brown or purple stasis spots; sublingual veins are distended and dark

P thready and choppy or wiry

Treatment principle

Invigorate Blood and eliminate stagnant Blood
Harmonise the Stomach and redirect Stomach *qi* downwards

Prescription

GE XIA ZHU YU TANG 膈下逐瘀汤
(Drive Out Blood Stasis Below the Diaphragm Decoction)

chao wu ling zhi (dry fried Excrementum Trogopteri seu Pteromi) 炒五灵脂 9-12g
dang gui (Radix Angelicae Sinensis) 当归 9-12g
tao ren (Semen Persicae) 桃仁 9-12g
hong hua (Flos Carthami Tinctorii) 红花 9-12g
chi shao (Radix Paeoniae Rubrae) 赤芍 9-12g
xiang fu (Rhizoma Cyperi Rotundi) 香附 9-12g
wu yao (Radix Linderae Strychnifoliae) 乌药 9-12g
gan cao (Radix Glycyrrhizae Uralensis) 甘草 6-9g
chuan xiong (Radix Ligustici Chuanxiong) 川芎 6-9g

mu dan pi (Cortex Moutan Radicis) 牡丹皮 6-9g
zhi ke (Fructus Citri Aurantii) 枳壳 6-9g
cu yan hu suo (vinegar fried Rhizoma Corydalis Yanhusuo) 醋延胡索 6-9g

Method: Decoction. **Wu ling zhi, dang gui, chuan xiong, chi shao, tao ren** and **hong hua** invigorate Blood and disperse stagnant Blood; **xiang fu, wu yao, zhi ke** and **cu yan hu suo** regulate *qi* and stop pain; **gan cao** protects and harmonises the Stomach. (Source: *Shi Yong Zhong Yi Nei Ke Xue*)

Modifications

- If nausea and vomiting are severe, add **ban xia** (Rhizoma Pinelliae Ternatae) 半夏 9-12g and **zhu ru** (Caulis Bambusae in Taeniis) 竹茹 9-12g.
- With epigastric pain, add **ru xiang** (Gummi Olibanum) 乳香 6-9g and **mo yao** (Myrrha) 没药 6-9g.
- With blood in the vomitus or stools, or tarry black stools, add **jiang xiang** (Lignum Dalbergiae Odoriferae) 降香 6-9g and **san qi fen** (powdered Radix Notoginseng) 三七粉 3-6g.
- With clearly palpable, firm masses in the epigastrium, add **mu li** (Concha Ostrae) 牡蛎 15g, **san leng** (Rhizoma Sparganii Stoloniferi) 三棱 9-12g and **e zhu** (Rhizoma Curcumae Ezhu) 莪术 9-12g.

Patent medicines

Tong Jing Wan 痛经丸 (Tong Jing Wan)
- severe Blood stagnation with masses

Xue Fu Zhu Yu Wan 血府逐瘀丸 (Xue Fu Zhu Yu Wan)
- *qi* and Blood stagnation

Shi Xiao Wan 失笑丸 (Shi Xiao Wan)
- to enhance analgesic action

Fu Ke Wu Jin Wan 妇科乌金丸 (Woo Garm Yuen Medical Pills)
- good for Blood stagnation with a degree of deficiency (mostly *yang* or *qi* deficiency).

Sheng Tian Qi Pian 生田七片 (Sheng Tien Qi Pien)
- good when there is mild bleeding.

Tao Hong Si Wu Wan 桃红四物丸 (Tao Hong Si Wu Wan)
- with Blood deficiency

Acupuncture (select from)

Ren.12 (*zhong wan* -) .... *mu* point of the Stomach, clears stagnant Blood from the Stomach and directs Stomach *qi* downwards

Ren.17 (*shan zhong*) .... these points direct rebellious *qi* downward,
Ren.14 (*ju que*) regulates movement of *qi* in the chest and

	lower oesophagus
Bl.17 (*ge shu* -)	*shu* point of the diaphragm, *hui* point for Blood, transforms stagnant Blood and regulates diaphragm function
Bl.18 (*gan shu* -)	*shu* point of the Liver, invigorates Liver *qi* and Blood
St.36 (*zu san li* -)	*he* sea point of the Stomach, regulates the Spleen and Stomach and corrects the *qi* mechanism
Sp.6 (*san yin jiao*)	invigorates *qi* and Blood, removes obstruction from the *jing luo*
Sp.8 (*di ji* -)	*xi* cleft point of the Spleen, regulates and invigorates Blood
Sp.10 (*xue hai* -)	cools the Blood to stop bleeding, regulates and invigorates Blood
a shi points	over the epigastrium, along the Stomach channel between St.36 (*zu san li*) and St.39 (*xia ju xu*), and along the Urinary Bladder channel between Bl.17 (*ge shu*) and Bl.21 (*wei shu*)

- congested spider vessels on the legs (especially around the medial knee and ankle) can be bled with a lancet
- *Ear points*: oesophagus, pylorus, stomach, spleen, liver, sympathetic, *shen men*

Clinical notes

- Blood stagnation type regurgitation may be diagnosed biomedically as pyloric stricture, stomach cancer, oesophageal varices, or scleroderma.
- The prognosis is likely to be poor, and TCM treatment may only be supportive.
- For dietary recommendations, see p.886.

SUMMARY OF GUIDING FORMULAE FOR REGURGITATION

Liver *qi* invading the Stomach - *Chai Hu Shu Gan San* 柴胡疏肝散
- with Phlegm - *Ban Xia Hou Po Tang* 半夏厚朴汤

Spleen and Stomach *qi/yang* deficiency - *Ding Kou Li Zhong Wan* 丁蔻理中丸
- with *qi* stagnation - *Ding Xiang Tou Ge San* 丁香透膈散
- with Spleen and Kidney *yang* deficiency - *Fu Zi Li Zhong Wan* 附子理中丸
- severe cases - *Xuan Fu Dai Zhe Tang* 旋复代赭汤

Stomach Heat - *Zhu Ru Tang* 竹茹汤
- with damage to *qi* and *yin* - *Da Ban Xia Tang* 大半夏汤
- with alcohol as significant aetiological feature - *Ge Hua Jie Cheng Tang* 葛花解酲汤
- with a mixture of Heat, Cold and deficiency - *Ban Xia Xie Xin Tang* 半夏泻心汤

Phlegm obstructing the Stomach - *Dao Tan Tang* 导痰汤
- in robust patients with copious Phlegm - *Gun Tan Wan* 滚痰丸
- severe cases - *Xuan Fu Dai Zhe Tang* 旋复代赭汤

Blood stagnation - *Ge Xia Zhu Yu Tang* 膈下逐瘀汤

24. Sudden Turmoil Disorder

Cold Damp
Damp Heat
Dryness

24 SUDDEN TURMOIL DISORDER

huo luan 霍乱

Sudden Turmoil Disorder (*huo luan*[1]) represents a group of conditions characterised by acute and usually violent simultaneous vomiting and diarrhoea. There may or may not be abdominal pain. The most common cause is an acute invasion of a strong, epidemic or pestilential pathogen that disrupts the *qi* mechanism. As the pressure builds up due to the severe obstruction in the middle *jiao*, the conglomerate of turbid untransformed materials and pathogen is forcefully ejected upwards and downwards.

Even though the pathogenic influence is usually quite strong, patients with Sudden Turmoil Disorder can present with varying degrees of disharmony, from mild to severe. The common types in the Western clinic are generally relatively mild and self limiting, but should always be treated to fully clear the offending pathogen, and thereby preventing recurrence. Severe cases, especially when in children, may require hospital attention.

AETIOLOGY

External pathogens

Invasion by powerful or epidemic external pathogens is the most common cause of Sudden Turmoil Disorder. These pathogens typically occur seasonally, most frequently during periods of hot and humid weather in late Summer and early Autumn, but may occur at any time of the year. Damp Heat, Cold Damp or Summerheat pathogens are the most common.

Diet

Eating spoiled or contaminated food produces Sudden Turmoil Disorder, which in TCM terms may resemble an attack of Damp or Toxic Heat, or Cold Damp. Excessive consumption of certain Damp Heat generating foods can create a Sudden Turmoil Disorder situation, the most familiar being a concentrated alcohol binge.

Constitution

Constitutional factors may be influential in the development of particular types of Sudden Turmoil Disorder. Patients with a tendency to *yang* deficiency, or Spleen deficiency, or those who habitually consume large quantities of raw foods and fruits may tend to develop the Cold patterns of Sudden Turmoil Disorder. Conversely, those with a Hot or *yang* excess constitu-

[1] Wiseman gives *huo luan* as cholera, although he notes that it may be associated with acute gastroenteritis and food poisoning, as well as infection by *Vibrio cholerae*.

tion, or a rich and heating diet, may tend to develop Hot type Sudden Turmoil Disorder.

BOX 24.1 BIOMEDICAL CAUSES OF SUDDEN TURMOIL DISORDER

- acute gastroenteritis associated with infection by numerous bacterial, viral or parasitic agents, most commonly *Campylobacter*, *Salmonella*, *Shigella*, *Giardia* and *Cryptosporidium*
- gastric 'flu'
- food poisoning
- cholera

TREATMENT

In many cases of Sudden Turmoil Disorder, spontaneous resolution occurs anywhere from 24-72 hours after onset. In these cases, the patient is often well or recovering before treatment is sought. For patients prone to repeated episodes, keeping a suitable patent medicine handy is a good solution. TCM treatment can be used to strengthen patients prone to recurrent episodes and to aid recovery from a debilitating episode.

Violent vomiting and diarrhoea can swiftly lead to dehydration and, especially in infants and children, shock and death. Maintenance of body fluids, with fluid replacement, is essential. If positive response to treatment is not quick, referral for specialist or hospital care may be required.

Astringent herbs and pharmaceutical anti-emetics and antidiarrhoeal agents (Stemetil, Lomotil, Imodium, etc.) should be avoided, as they can lock pathogens into the body. A pathogen with no escape route will tend to intensify and cause even greater problems.

寒湿霍乱

24.1 COLD DAMP

Pathophysiology

- In Cold Damp type Sudden Turmoil Disorder there are usually factors, such as the type of diet (raw, cold, Damp), or a constitutional tendency to *yang* deficiency, that facilitate the invasion or accumulation of Cold Damp. A constitutional tendency to Dampness is an additional feature. The Cold Damp obstructs the *qi* mechanism and depletes *yang*; Spleen *qi* is unable to ascend and turbid *qi* to descend, instead mixing in the middle *jiao*. The Cold freezes and constricts all movement in the abdomen, but at some point of pressure, the turbid *qi* is forced out as violent diarrhoea and vomiting.
- Depending on the strength of the pathogen and the strength of the individual's *zheng qi*, symptoms may be mild or severe. The mild type is a common pattern in clinic, often occurring in waves and sweeping through offices or schools. The severe type is a dangerous condition, especially so in infants and children who can dehydrate quickly.

Clinical features

- Acute nausea, vomiting and diarrhoea. The diarrhoea is urgent, and progresses over hours to an opaque, watery discharge. The diarrhoea is largely inoffensive.
- cramping or colicky abdominal pain that may come in waves
- chills, possible mild fever
- no sweating
- generalised muscle aches, dull occipital or general headache
- fullness and discomfort in the chest and abdomen
- lethargy, malaise, heaviness in the head and body, foggy-headedness
- In severe cases the patient evacuates and vomits frequently, appears ashen or grey and dehydrated, is severely cold intolerant with icy cold extremities, physically and mentally exhausted, with sunken eyes, a hoarse voice, muscle spasms or cramps, and copious sweating.

T greasy, white coat

P floating, soggy, soft, slippery, possibly tight; in severe cases deep, thready, imperceptible

Treatment principle

Warm the middle *jiao*, Dispel Cold, transform and eliminate Dampness

Support *zheng qi*

Prescription

24.1.1 Mild Cold Damp

HUO XIANG ZHENG QI SAN 藿香正气散
(*Agastache Formula*)

huo xiang (Herba Agastaches seu Pogostemi) 藿香 12-15g
fu ling (Sclerotium Poriae Cocos) 茯苓 12-15g
bai zhu (Rhizoma Atractylodes Macrocephalae) 白术 9-12g
zi su ye (Folium Perillae Frutescentis) 紫苏叶 9-12g
ban xia (Rhizoma Pinelliae Ternatae) 半夏 9-12g
da fu pi (Pericarpium Arecae Catechu) 大腹皮 9-12g
chen pi (Pericarpium Citri Reticulatae) 陈皮 6-9g
bai zhi (Radix Angelicae Dahuricae) 白芷 6-9g
hou po (Cortex Magnoliae Officinalis) 厚朴 6-9g
jie geng (Radix Platycodi Grandiflori) 桔梗 3-6g
zhi gan cao (honey fried Radix Glycyrrhizae Uralensis)
炙甘草 6-9g
sheng jiang (Rhizoma Zingiberis Officinalis Recens)
生姜 6-9g
da zao (Fructus Zizyphi Jujubae) 大枣 2pce

Method: Decoction. The herbs should be simmered for no longer than 20 minutes in a pot with a close fitting lid. **Huo xiang** fragrantly disperses Wind Cold Damp turbidity, harmonises the Stomach, revives the Spleen and stops vomiting; **zi su ye** and **bai zhi** dispel Wind Cold and transform Dampness; **hou po** regulates and directs *qi* downward, transforms Phlegm Damp and alleviates fullness; **chen pi** regulates and directs *qi* downwards, transforms Phlegm Damp and harmonises the Stomach; **ban xia** warms the Stomach, transforms Phlegm Damp and stops vomiting; **da fu pi** directs *qi* and Dampness downwards and alleviates fullness; **bai zhu** and **fu ling** strengthen the Spleen, dry Dampness and promote urination; **jie geng** assists the dispersing function of the Lungs; **gan cao, sheng jiang** and **da zao** harmonise the other herbs and regulate the Stomach. (Source: *Shi Yong Zhong Yi Nei Ke Xue*).

24.1.1 Severe Cold

LI ZHONG WAN 理中丸
(*Ginseng and Ginger Formula*)

This prescription is suitable for more severe cases with strong Cold signs, such as cold intolerance, cold extremities, waves of severe cramping abdominal pain that are alleviated by warmth, frequent vomiting and watery diarrhoea.

gan jiang (Rhizoma Zingiberis Officinalis) 干姜 9-15g
dang shen (Radix Codonopsis Pilosulae) 党参 15-24g
chao bai zhu (dry fried Rhizoma Atractylodes
Macrocephalae) 炒白术 12-15g

zhi gan cao (honey fried Radix Glycyrrhizae Uralensis) 炙甘草 6-9g

Method: Decoction. **Gan jiang**, the main herb, warms Spleen and Stomach *yang* and dispels Cold; **dang shen** supplements *qi* and strengthens the Spleen; **chao bai zhu** strengthens the Spleen and dries Dampness; **zhi gan cao** supplements *qi* and harmonises the Stomach. (Source: *Shi Yong Zhong Yi Nei Ke Xue*)

Modifications (Li Zhong Wan)

- With severe vomiting, add **ding xiang** (Flos Caryophylli) 丁香 3-6g and **wu zhu yu** (Fructus Evodiae Rutaecarpae) 吴茱萸 3-6g.
- With severe Cold and fading *yang* (copious sweating especially on the head and upper body, ashen complexion, icy extremities), add **zhi fu zi** (Radix Aconiti Carmichaeli Praeparata) 制附子 6-12g.

Variations and additional prescriptions

Copious watery diarrhoea, scanty urine and oedema

- When the patient experiences less nausea and vomiting, but frequent watery diarrhoea, one method of correcting the fluid imbalance is to drain Dampness through the promotion of diuresis. A suitable prescription is **WEI LING TANG** (*Magnolia and Hoelen Combination* 胃苓汤). Even though much fluid is being lost through the bowel, the patient may also have oedema and/or scanty urination.

fu ling (Sclerotium Poria Cocos) 茯苓 15-24g
ze xie (Rhizoma Alismatis Orientalis) 泽泻 12-15g
zhu ling (Sclerotium Polypori Umbellati) 猪苓 12-15g
bai zhu (Rhizoma Atractylodes Macrocephalae) 白术 12-15g
cang zhu (Rhizoma Atractylodis) 苍术 9-15g
chen pi (Pericarpium Citri Reticulatae) 陈皮 6-9g
hou po (Cortex Magnoliae Officinalis) 厚朴 9-12g
gui zhi (Ramulus Cinnamomi Cassiae) 桂枝 6-9g
gan cao (Radix Glycyrrhizae Uralensis) 甘草 3-9g

Method: Decoction. **Fu ling**, **zhu ling** and **ze xie** promote urination to drain Dampness; **bai zhu** and **fu ling** strengthen the Spleen and its fluid metabolism function; **cang zhu** and **bai zhu** dry Dampness and liberate the Spleen; **chen pi** and **hou po** regulate *qi* and transform Phlegm Dampness; **hou po** directs *qi* downwards; **gui zhi** stimulates the transformation of *qi* and fluid metabolism; **gan cao** protects and strengthens the Spleen and Stomach and harmonises the prescription.

Yang collapse

- In severe cases the patient may deteriorate rapidly to the point of *yang* collapse. The patient is ashen or grey with blue lips, sweating copiously, has icy extremities and an imperceptible pulse. *Yin* and *yang* are about to separate. Swift administration of **SI NI JIA REN SHEN TANG** (*Frigid Extremities Decoction plus Ginseng* 四逆加人参汤) may save the patient from collapse. The patient should lie flat with legs elevated. Variations of this prescription are given by intramuscular injection in China.

zhi fu zi (Radix Aconiti Carmichaeli Praeparata) 制附子 9-15g
gan jiang (Rhizoma Zingiberis Officinalis) 干姜 9-12g
ren shen (Radix Ginseng) 人参 9-12g
zhi gan cao (honey fried Radix Glycyrrhizae Uralensis)
炙甘草 6-9g

Method: Decoction. The relatively large quantity of **zhi fu zi** powerfully warms and stimulates *yang* to circulate throughout the body; **gan jiang** warms Spleen and Stomach *yang* and dispels Cold; these are the main herbs and together they can prevent the imminent collapse of *yang qi*; **ren shen** and **zhi gan cao** reinforce *qi* and strengthen the Spleen; **zhi gan cao** alleviates the harsh drying and dispersing nature of the principal herbs. (Source: *Shi Yong Zhong Yi Nei Ke Xue*)

Patent medicines

Huo Xiang Zheng Qi Pian 藿香正气片 (Huo Xiang Zheng Qi Pian, Huo Hsiang Cheng Chi Pien)
- mild type

Xing Jun San 行军散 (Marching Powder, Five Pagodas Brand)
- mild type

Li Zhong Wan 理中丸 (Li Zhong Wan)
- with Cold

Fu Zi Li Zhong Wan 附子理中丸 (Fu Tzu Li Chung Wan, Carmichaeli Tea Pills, Li Chung Yuen Medical Pills)
- severe Cold

Acupuncture (select from)

Ren.12 (*zhong wan* -▲) .... *mu* point of the Stomach, warms and regulates the Stomach, dispels Cold and directs Stomach *qi* downwards

St.25 (*tian shu* -▲) .... *mu* point of the Large Intestine, warms and regulates Intestinal function and dispels Cold

Ren.6 (*qi hai* ▲) .... dispels Cold, warms the abdomen

Sp.4 (*gong sun*) .... *luo* point of the Spleen, master point of *chong mai*, regulates the Spleen and Stomach and stops vomiting and diarrhoea

PC.6 (*nei guan*) .... *luo* point of the Pericardium, master point of *yin wei mai*, regulates the middle *jiao* and stops vomiting

St.36 (*zu san li* ▲) .... *he* sea point of the Stomach, powerfully warms and strengthens the Spleen and Stomach and supplements *qi*

Sp.6 (*san yin jiao*) .... strengthens the Spleen, elevates Spleen *qi* and encourages turbid *qi* to descend

- ginger moxa (best) or a moxa box can be applied to the abdominal points
- with abdominal pain and cramping, add St.34 (*liang qiu* -)
- with leg or calf cramps, add Bl.57 (*cheng shan* -)
- in cases of severe Cold with possible shock or collapse, moxa can be burnt over Ren.8 (*shen que*). Spread a thin cloth over the navel and fill it with salt. Burn large moxa cones over the salt until consciousness is restored. The cloth enables swift removal of the salt and moxa if necessary.
- *Ear points*: lungs, large intestine, small intestine, spleen, abdomen, sympathetic

Other therapies

- A hot ginger compress on the abdomen may be useful. This can be made by simmering a large root of grated ginger wrapped in a muslin cloth in 1-2 litres of water until the water turns slightly milky. A clean cloth or towel is dipped into the simmering water, wrapped in a dry towel and placed on the abdomen. Take care not to burn the patient. If the compress is too hot, place another towel between the compress and the abdomen.
- A paste of powdered **wu zhu yu** (Fructus Evodiae Rutaecarpae) 吴茱萸, or fresh mashed garlic and salt can be applied to the palms of the hands and soles of the feet until redness and heat are felt.

Clinical notes

- Cold Sudden Turmoil Disorder may be diagnosed biomedically as Summer flu, stomach flu, acute gastroenteritis, food poisoning or cholera.
- Because vomiting can inhibit the ingestion of oral decoctions, a useful technique involves strong needling or finger pressure on PC.6 (*nei guan*), prior to ingestion of the herbs. Gently patting the spine around T7-T12 may also help some patients. The herbs should be taken in tiny sips as frequently as possible. Sipping through a straw may help.
- Fluid replacement is an essential feature of treatment. In severe cases, dehydration is a critical factor. Oral isotonic fluid replacement solution should be administered in small amounts frequently. Isotonic solution can be made by adding 3.5 grams of household salt (NaCl), 2.5 grams of sodium bicarbonate, 1.5 grams of potassium chloride (KCl) and 20 grams of sugar to one litre of water. Isotonic drinks are commercially available. Alternatively use lemonade with a teaspoon of salt.

热湿霍乱

24.2 DAMP HEAT

Pathophysiology

- In Damp Heat type Sudden Turmoil Disorder, there are usually factors such as diet (spicy, rich and heating), or a constitutional tendency to *yang* excess or internal Heat, that predisposes towards invasion or development of Damp Heat. Heat and Damp lodge in the middle *jiao*, disrupting the *qi* mechanism. The balance of Heat and Damp can vary considerably, altering the clinical picture and the treatment strategy.
- Depending on the strength of the pathogen and the strength of the individual's *zheng qi*, the symptoms can be mild or severe. The mild type is a common pattern in clinic, tending to occur during the late Summer and early Autumn months, particularly in hot and humid climates.
- The severe type is a dangerous condition, especially so in infants and children who can dehydrate quickly.

Clinical features

- acute and often violent vomiting and diarrhoea; the vomitus and diarrhoea are sour and offensive
- cramping abdominal pain
- severe headache
- fever, afternoon fever, unrelieved by sweating
- sweating that comes in waves and is worse in the afternoon
- thirst, dry mouth and lips
- irritability, restlessness
- sensation of heat in the chest
- scanty, concentrated urine
- heaviness, lethargy
- In severe cases the patient has pain, spasms and cramps in the limbs, sweats copiously, the body feels hot but the limbs are cold, the patient has a bluish tinge to the face, lips and nails and an imperceptible pulse.

T greasy, yellow coat

P soft or slippery and rapid

Treatment principle

Clear Heat and transform Dampness
Promote the correct ascent and descent of *qi*
Harmonise the middle *jiao*

Prescription

24.2.1 Damp greater than Heat

RAN ZHAO TANG 燃照汤
(*Illuminating Decoction*) modified

This prescription is selected for mild cases where Dampness is dominant.

dan dou chi (Semen Sojae Preparatum) 淡豆豉 9-12g
shan zhi zi (Fructus Gardeniae Jasminoidis) 山栀子 9-12g
huang qin (Radix Scutellariae Baicalensis) 黄芩 9-12g
ban xia (Rhizoma Pinelliae Ternatae) 半夏 9-12g
pei lan (Herba Eupatorii Fortuneii) 佩兰 9-12g
hou po (Cortex Magnoliae Officinalis) 厚朴 9-12g
bai dou kou (Fructus Amomi Kravanh) 白豆蔻 6-9g
hua shi (Talcum) 滑石 12-15g

Method: Decoction. The herbs should be gently simmered for no longer than 20 minutes. **Dan dou chi** and **shan zhi zi** clear Heat from the *qi* level and alleviate irritability; **huang qin** clears Damp Heat; **ban xia** and **hou po** transform Dampness and correct the *qi* mechanism; **ban xia** stops vomiting; **pei lan** and **bai dou kou** fragrantly transform Dampness, regulate *qi* and stop vomiting; **hua shi** leads Damp Heat out through the urine. (Source: *Zhong Yi Nei Ke Ji Zheng Zheng Zhi*)

24.2.2 Heat greater than Damp

LIAN PO YIN 连朴饮
(*Coptis and Magnolia Bark Decoction*)

This prescription is selected for mild cases when Heat is dominant. The main features are acute vomiting and diarrhoea, fullness in the chest and epigastrium, afternoon fever unrelieved by sweating, irritability and restlessness, greasy, yellow, tongue coat and dark urine. There may also be small, itchy, fluid filled vesicular eruptions on the neck and trunk (miliaria crystallina).

huang lian (Rhizoma Coptidis) 黄连 3-6g
hou po (Cortex Magnoliae Officinalis) 厚朴 6-9g
shan zhi zi (Fructus Gardeniae Jasminoidis) 山栀子 9-12g
dan dou chi (Semen Sojae Preparatum) 淡豆豉 9-12g
shi chang pu (Rhizoma Acori Graminei) 石菖蒲 6-9g
ban xia (Rhizoma Pinelliae Ternatae) 半夏 6-9g
lu gen (Rhizoma Phragmitis Communis) 芦根 30-60g

Method: Decoction. **Huang lian** and **shan zhi zi** clear Damp Heat and, being bitter and descending, combine well with the pungent warmth of **ban xia** and the descending nature of **hou po** to correct the *qi* mechanism; **ban xia** transforms Dampness and stops vomiting; **dan dou chi** and **shan zhi zi** clear Heat from the *qi* level and alleviate irritability; **shi chang pu** revives the Spleen and transforms Dampness; **lu gen** clears Heat from the Stomach and stops vomiting. (Source: *Shi Yong Fang Ji Xue*)

Modifications

- With abdominal or muscular spasms and cramps, add **can sha** (Excrementum Bombycis Mori) 蚕砂 9g and **mu gua** (Fructus Chaenomelis) 木瓜 9g. *See also* Variations and additional prescriptions.

Variations and additional prescriptions

With severe Heat

- With relatively severe Heat and moderate Dampness (high unrelenting fever, headache, severe dryness and thirst, explosive, foul, burning diarrhoea, scanty, concentrated urine, a rapid pulse and dry, yellow tongue coat), the aim of treatment is to expel Heat, drain Dampness and aid transformation of *qi* with **GUI LING GAN LU YIN** (*Cinnamon and Poria Sweet Dew Decoction* 桂苓甘露饮).

hua shi (Talcum) 滑石 15-30g
shi gao (Gypsum) 石膏 15-30g
han shui shi (Calcitum) 寒水石 15-30g
fu ling (Sclerotium Poria Cocos) 茯苓 9-15g
ze xie (Rhizoma Alismatis Orientalis) 泽泻 9-15g
zhu ling (Sclerotium Polypori Umbellati) 猪苓 9-15g
bai zhu (Rhizoma Atractylodes Macrocephalae) 白术 9-12g
gan cao (Radix Glycyrrhizae Uralensis) 甘草 3-9g
rou gui (Cortex Cinnamomi Cassiae) 肉桂 1-3g

Method: Decoction. **Shi gao** is decocted for 30 minutes prior to the other herbs (*xian jian* 先煎). **Hua shi** leads Damp Heat out through the urine; **shi gao** and **han shui shi** are sweet and cold, and the large dose powerfully clears Heat from the *qi* level without damaging fluids; **fu ling, ze xie, zhu ling, bai zhu** and **rou gui** make up **WU LING SAN**, and serve to promote diuresis and encourage transformation of *qi* and fluids to clear Dampness; the heat of **rou gui** also moderates the cold nature of the mineral substances; **bai zhu, fu ling** and **gan cao** strengthen the Spleen; **gan cao** clears Heat and protects the Stomach, and with **hua shi** makes up **LIU YI SAN**, an important formula for Dampness and Summerheat patterns. (Source: *Shi Yong Zhong Yi Nei Ke Xue*)

Persistent vomiting, diarrhoea and fever

- In some cases the fever, vomiting and diarrhoea can linger or recur after the severe acute phase has passed. Residual Heat remains lodged in the chest and diaphragm (the *qi* level) and the *qi* and *yin* have been damaged. The patient is restless and irritable yet fatigued, nauseous with occasional vomiting and possible diarrhoea. The patient suffers from insomnia characterised by extreme restlessness, and fitful broken sleep. The patient also experiences dryness of the throat, lips and mouth and a stifling sensation in the chest. The tongue is red and dry. This sometimes occurs following incorrect use of antibiotics for viral gastroenteritis. The antibiotics are cooling, but do not adequately disperse the Heat pathogen. The treatment aims to clear residual Heat, generate fluids, supplement *qi* and harmonise the Stomach with **ZHU YE SHI GAO TANG** (*Lophatherus and Gypsum Decoction* 竹叶石膏汤).

dan zhu ye (Herba Lophatheri Gracilis) 淡竹叶 12-15g
shi gao (Gypsum) 石膏 15-30g
dang shen (Radix Codonopsis Pilosulae) 党参 15-30g
mai dong (Tuber Ophiopogonis Japonici) 麦冬 9-12g
ban xia (Rhizoma Pinelliae Ternatae) 半夏 9-12g
jing mi (Semen Oryzae) 粳米 15g
gan cao (Radix Glycyrrhizae Uralensis) 甘草 3-9g

Method: Decoction. **Shi gao** is decocted for 30 minutes prior to the other herbs (*xian jian* 先煎). **Dan zhu ye** and **shi gao** clear Heat from the *qi* level; **dang shen** and **mai dong** generate fluids and protect *yin*; **ban xia** directs Stomach *qi* downward, stops vomiting and prevents cloying by the *yin* nourishing herbs; **gan cao, jing mi** assist in strengthening the Spleen, and protect the Stomach. (Source: *Shi Yong Zhong Yao Xue*)

Muscle spasms and cramps

- Muscle spasms and cramps are a common complication of the rapid fluid and electrolyte loss that accompanies severe diarrhoea and vomiting. From a TCM perspective, smouldering Heat or Damp Heat causes loss of *yin* fluids; the Tendons begin to dry, losing nourishment and lubrication. In mild cases, simple abdominal cramping and skeletal muscle spasms may occur; in more advanced cases, full cramps and severe pain may occur. When cramps are a significant feature, the aim of treatment (in addition to maintaining fluids and electrolytes) is to clear Damp Heat, ease and moisten the tendons and open the channels with **CAN SHI TANG** (*Arrow Like Decoction of Silkworm* 蚕矢汤).

can sha (Excrementum Bombycis Mori) 蚕砂 9-12g
mu gua (Fructus Chaenomelis) 木瓜 9-12g
yi ren (Semen Coicis Lachryma-jobi) 苡仁 15-24g
dou juan (Semen Glycines Germinatum) 豆卷 24g
shan zhi zi (Fructus Gardeniae Jasminoidis) 山栀子 6-12g
huang qin (Radix Scutellariae Baicalensis) 黄芩 6-9g
huang lian (Rhizoma Coptidis) 黄连 3-6g
ban xia (Rhizoma Pinelliae Ternatae) 半夏 6-9g
tong cao (Medulla Tetrapanacis Papyrifera) 通草 3-6g
wu zhu yu (Fructus Evodiae Rutaecarpae) 吴茱萸 2-6g

Method: Decoction. **Can sha** and **mu gua** harmonise the Stomach, transform turbid Dampness and relax the Tendons; **yi ren** clears Damp Heat and promotes urination; **dou juan** clears Summerheat and Damp Heat; **shan zhi zi, huang qin** and **huang lian** clear Damp Heat; **ban xia** and **wu zhu yu** being pungent, warm and dispersing, balance the descending nature of the bitter cold herbs, facilitating dispersal and clearance of the obstructing Heat and Dampness, and correction of the *qi* mechanism; **tong cao** promotes urination to provide an outlet for the Heat and Dampness; **wu zhu yu** and **ban xia** stop vomiting. (Source: *Shi Yong Zhong Yi Nei Ke Xue*)

With severe Heat, delirium, imminent collapse

- In severe cases where the patient is near collapse, with deep internal Heat and cold extremities, a mixture of **BAI HU TANG** (*Anemarrhena and Gypsum Combination* 白虎汤, the prescription below) and the emergency patent medicine **ZI XUE DAN** (*Purple Snow Special Pill* 紫雪丹) may be used to quickly and powerfully clear Heat.
  - **shi gao** (Gypsum) 石膏 30-60g
  - **zhi mu** (Rhizoma Anemarrhenae Asphodeloides) 知母 9-15g
  - **jing mi** (Semen Oryzae) 粳米 15g
  - **gan cao** (Radix Glycyrrhizae Uralensis) 甘草 3-9g

  Method: Decoction. **Shi gao** and **zhi mu** clear Heat from the *qi* level; **zhi gan cao** and **jing mi** protect the Stomach.

Damaged yin and qi in the recovery phase

- *Yin*, *qi* and fluids are invariably damaged during the acute phase of this pattern, and can take some time to recover fully. During recovery, the patient often suffers from fatigue and exhaustion, continuing dryness of the skin and mucous membranes, thirst, scanty urine, nightsweats and restlessness. Convalescence can be accelerated with an appropriate *qi* and *yin* replenishing prescription, such as **YI WEI TANG** (*Benefit the Stomach Decoction* 益胃汤, p.199), **SHENG MAI SAN** (*Generate the Pulse Powder* 脉散, p.910), **ZHI GAN CAO TANG** (*Baked Licorice Combination* 炙甘草汤, p.911) or **ZENG YE TANG** (*Increase the Fluids Decoction* 增液汤, p.200)

Acupuncture (select from)

Ren.12 (*zhong wan* -) .... *mu* point of the Stomach, clears Heat and Dampness

St.25 (*tian shu* -) .... *mu* point of the Large Intestine, regulates Intestinal function and clears Heat and Dampness

PC.3 (*qu ze* ↓) ....
Bl.40 (*wei zhong* ↓) *he* sea points of the Pericardium and Urinary Bladder channel respectively, these points clear Heat, cool the Blood, and stop acute vomiting and diarrhoea when bled

St.36 (*zu san li* -) .... *he* sea point of the Stomach, regulates the *qi* mechanism, strengthens the Stomach and clears Dampness

- with muscular spasms and cramps, add Bl.57 (*cheng shan*) and burn 7 cones of moxa on the tip of the external malleolus.
- with high fever, add Du.14 (*da zhui* -) and LI.11 (*qu chi* -)
- with disturbances of consciousness, needle Du.26 (*ren zhong*) and bleed the finger tips (*shi xuan* ↓ M-UE-1)

Patent medicines

Xing Jun San 行军散 (Marching Powder, Five Pagodas Brand)
Bao Ji Wan 保济丸 (Po Chai Pills)

Clinical notes

- Damp Heat type Sudden Turmoil Disorder may be diagnosed biomedically as Summer flu, stomach flu, acute gastroenteritis, viral illness, food poisoning or cholera.
- Maintenance of fluid and electrolytes is an essential feature of treatment. See p.832.

干霍乱

24.3 DRY

Pathophysiology

- This is the most serious type of Sudden Turmoil Disorder. The pathogen has so disrupted the *qi* mechanism and blocked up the abdomen that, even though the patient feels the need and urge to expel the pathogen, he or she is unable to do so. Like the other Sudden Turmoil patterns, this patterns is in fact associated with Dampness, but the Dampness is locked in the interior and not clearly expressed. There is no external manifestation of the Dampness, hence the description 'Dry'.

Clinical features

- violent cramping abdominal pain accompanied by nausea and a desire to vomit and defecate, but an inability to do so
- severe restlessness, mental confusion bordering on delirium
- In severe cases: bluish green complexion and lips, icy cold extremities, copious sweating from the head, deep and hidden, imperceptible pulse

Treatment principle

Expel turbidity, eliminate Toxins
Regulate and dissipate congested *qi*, correct the movement of *qi*

Prescription

The first approach is to try one of the previous prescriptions described for Heat or Cold Sudden Turmoil, as appropriate. If this does not work a more vigorous approach (below) can be tried.

XING JUN SAN 行军散
(*Marching Powder*) modified

This powerful prescription contains toxic substances to 'fight Toxin with Toxin'. It is used in small doses for severe cases of epidemic Toxin locked in the middle *jiao*. Generally not used for more than a few days.
Note: Although the name is the same, this prescription is different in composition from the frequently mentioned patent medicine.

niu huang (Calculus Bovis) 牛黄 15g
zhen zhu (Margarita) 珍珠 15g
bing pian (Borneol) 冰片 15g
peng sha (Borax) 硼砂 15g
xiong huang (Realgar) 雄黄 24g
huo xiao (Niter) 火硝 1g

Method: Grind all substances to fine powder, mix and store in an airtight container. The dose is 0.3 grams in a little water or blown into the nose. **Niu huang** vaporises Phlegm and eliminates Toxin; **bing pian** dissipates turbidity and

opens the orifices; **zhen zhu** calms the *shen*; **peng sha** eliminates Toxic Heat; **xiong huang** eliminates Toxin and dries Dampness; **huo xiao** clears Heat and dissipates accumulation. (Source: *Shi Yong Zhong Yi Nei Ke Xue*)
NB. This prescription originally included 15 grams of musk (**she xiang** [Secretio Moschus] 麝香), an ingredient derived from the endangered musk deer. No substitution is made, as no substance (save synthetic muscone), is an adequate replacement for real musk, in emergency situations.

Variations and additional prescriptions

Emesis as a way of eliminating pathogens

- An emetic prescription may be used to promote vomiting and the expulsion of the pathogen. The first thing to try is warm salty water. Mix 1 tablespoon of salt to 1 cup of warm water and drink.

  If that fails, try **GUA DI SAN** (*Melon Pedicle Powder* 瓜蒂散). This approach must be used with caution and is reserved for severe cases.

  gua di (Pedicellus Cucumeris) 瓜蒂 3g
  chi xiao dou (Semen Phaseoli Calcarati) 赤小豆 3g
  dan dou chi (Semen Sojae Preparatum) 淡豆豉 10g

  Method: Decoction. Cook for no longer than 5-10 minutes. **Gua di** is a powerful emetic; **chi xiao dou** moderates the harsh nature of the **gua di** to prevent excessive emesis; **dan dou chi** alleviates stagnation in the chest and moderates the harshness of **gua di**. (Source: *Shi Yong Zhong Yi Nei Ke Xue*)

With disturbances of consciousness

- In severe cases, with disturbances of consciousness and icy cold extremities, the treatment is to aromatically warm and open the orifices, transform turbidity and restore consciousness with an emergency medicine such as the patent formula *Su He Xiang Wan* (*Liquid Styrax Pill* 苏合香丸). The pill can be crushed and blown into the nose, or liquid extract can be forced into the mouth, or given via a nasogastric tube until consciousness is restored.

Acupuncture (select from)

Acupuncture treatment depends on whether Heat or Cold dominates.

Heat

PC.3 (*qu ze* ↓) .... *he* sea points of the Pericardium and Urinary
Bl.40 (*wei zhong* ↓) Bladder channel respectively, these points clear Toxic Heat and cool the Blood

shi xuan ↓ (M-UE-1) .... for severe heat and disturbances of consciousness

LI.4 (*he gu* -) .... the 'four gates', both *yuan* points, invigorate *qi*
Liv.3 (*tai chong* -) and Blood, powerfully sedate and calm, relieve mental cloudiness and ease muscle spasm

Cold

Ren.8 (*shen que* ▲) .... for Cold with possible shock or collapse, spread a thin cloth over the navel and fill it with salt. Burn large moxa cones over the salt until consciousness is restored. The cloth enables swift removal of the salt and moxa if necessary.

Ren.12 (*zhong wan* -▲) .... *mu* point of the Stomach, warms and regulates the Stomach, dispels Cold and directs Stomach *qi* downwards

St.25 (*tian shu* -▲) .... *mu* point of the Large Intestine, warms and regulates Intestinal function and dispels Cold

Ren.6 (*qi hai* ▲) .... dispels Cold, warms the abdomen

Sp.4 (*gong sun* -) .... *luo* point of the Pericardium, master point of *chong mai*, regulates the Spleen and Stomach and stops vomiting and diarrhoea

St.36 (*zu san li* -) .... *he* sea point of the Stomach, regulates the *qi* mechanism and strengthens the Spleen and Stomach and supplements *qi*

- with muscular spasms and cramps, add Bl.57 (*cheng shan*) and burn 7 cones of moxa on the tip of the external malleolus.
- with high fever, add Du.14 (*da zhui* -) and LI.11 (*qu chi* -)
- with disturbances of consciousness, needle Du.26 (*ren zhong*) and bleed the finger tips (*shi xuan* ↓ M-UE-1)

Clinical notes

- This is a serious and dangerous pattern and should be managed in a hospital.

SUMMARY OF GUIDING FORMULAE FOR SUDDEN TURMOIL

Cold, Cold Damp - *Huo Xiang Zheng Qi San* 藿香正气散
- severe Cold - *Li Zhong Wan* 理中丸
- with oedema and scanty urine - *Wei Ling Tang* 胃苓汤
- *yang* collapse - *Si Ni Jia Ren Shen Tang* (*Frigid Extremities Decoction plus Ginseng* 四逆加人参汤

Heat - *Ran Zhao Tang* 燃照汤
- Damp Heat - *Lian Po Yin* 连朴饮
- Heat greater than Damp - *Gui Ling Gan Lu Yin* 桂苓甘露饮
- persistent - *Zhu Ye Shi Gao Tang* 竹叶石膏汤
- with muscle spasms - *Can Shi Tang* 蚕矢汤

Dry - *Xing Jun San* 行军散

25. Tooth Abscess

Toxic Heat
Stomach Fire
Chronic abscess

25 TOOTH ABSCESS

ya yong 牙痈

A tooth abscess is a focal pyogenic lesion in the gum or the base of a tooth. Abscesses can be acute, or chronic and recurrent. When acute, they are associated with a localised accumulation of Toxic Heat, with or without systemic Heat. When chronic, the abscess is due to the establishment of a state of equilibrium between weakened *zheng qi* and a residual pathogen. Chronic tooth abscesses can be quite persistent, and are often complicated by Phlegm and/or Blood stagnation and/or *yin* deficiency.

AETIOLOGY

Poor oral hygiene

The most common cause of both acute and chronic tooth abscesses is poor oral hygiene. The systemic elements can make the gums and teeth vulnerable to infection, but in most cases lack of oral hygiene and inadequate dental attention are the main triggers.

Diet

Aspects of the diet can predispose patients to tooth abscess. Eating large quantities of foods that heat the Stomach, specifically items such as chillies and spices, alcohol, coffee and chocolate, cause Heat to accumulate. Once Heat is resident in the Stomach, its natural tendency to rise will affect the structures of the upper body, in particular those associated with the Stomach and Spleen organ systems. This resident Heat sets the scene for a local trauma in the form of tooth decay or rotting food, to ignite in the gum and form an abscess.

Any foods or substances that weaken the Spleen or create Dampness or Phlegm, may promote the generation of a chronic abscess, especially cold raw foods and dairy products, or multiple courses of antibiotics, (given, perhaps for an acute abscess).

Emotion

The most common emotional pattern contributing to tooth abscess is that which affects the Liver, and then the Stomach. Liver *qi* stagnation is caused by repressed emotion, frustration, anger and resentment. These emotions, especially when chronically unexpressed, can gradually lead to the development of stagnant Heat as the pressure builds up behind the area of congestion. Once Heat has been generated, either primarily in the Liver and then transmitted to the Stomach, or directly in the Stomach as a result of the repeated insult, it will rise to affect the upper structures of the Stomach organ system.

Liver *qi* stagnation can also disrupt Spleen function and digestive efficiency. Spleen weakness and inefficient digestion will contribute to the pathological residue, Dampness, which in turn may obstruct *qi* circulation and generate Heat.

TREATMENT

As with most acute pyogenic lesions, patients will usually be prescribed antibiotics as their first treatment option. Antibiotic treatment is usually effective when the lesion is of an excess Heat type. The downside of antibiotic therapy is that it effectively cools Heat, but does not disperse the TCM defined pathogen. The pathogen may get locked away and become latent. Lesions may become chronic or recurrent. TCM treatment for acute excess Heat type lesions is also effective, with the added elements of supporting the body and *zheng qi*, and aiding dispersal of the pathogen.

TCM treatment is of particular benefit in the chronic or recurrent lesions that are not dealt with adequately by conventional means.

There will always be some patients who do not respond to TCM treatment, and will require surgical drainage of the abscess. These patients can still derive significant benefit from treatment to support their *zheng qi*, aid recovery, promote complete expulsion of any residual Toxin and prevent recurrence.

Fig. 25.1 *Tooth abscess*

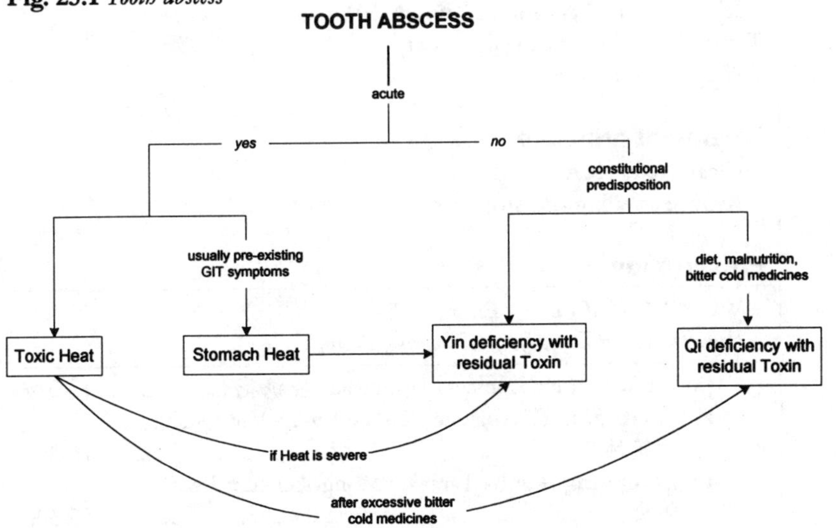

毒热牙痈

25.1 ACUTE ABSCESS

25.1.1 Toxic Heat

Pathophysiology

- Accumulation of Toxic Heat is frequently the basic cause of localised pyogenic lesions. There are various grades of severity associated with Toxic Heat. In the early stages, the Toxic Heat is confined to the affected area and, other than having an abscess in the mouth, the patient feels generally well, that is, there are no systemic signs and symptoms of fever, loss of appetite, etc. When severe, there may be systemic manifestations, but this is less common.
- The mechanism of abscess formation is one of focal pathogenic extravagance. When Heat accumulates at a locus, it will, at a certain point of pressure and intensity, begin to destroy the affected tissues, creating a pocket of pus.

Clinical features

- Focal area in the gum that is throbbing, painful, red, swollen and firm to the touch; the pain is worse for pressure and chewing, and may be relieved with ice. The pain may radiate into the jaw or ear. The swelling usually develops over a period of 3-7 days and is relieved when the abscess ruptures or leaks.
- there may or may not be fever, fever and chills or alternating fever and chills, malaise, nausea, loss of appetite and lethargy
- swollen tender submandibular or cervical nodules
- dry mouth, bad taste in the mouth, halitosis

T red or red tip with a yellow coat
P slippery and rapid

Treatment principle

Clear Toxic Heat
Reduce swelling and stop pain

Prescription

WU WEI XIAO DU YIN 五味消毒饮
(*Five Ingredient Decoction to Eliminate Toxin*)

jin yin hua (Flos Lonicera Japonicae) 金银花 15-30g
zi hua di ding (Herba cum Radice Violae Yedoensitis) 紫花地丁 15-30g
pu gong ying (Herba Taraxaci Mongolici cum Radice) 蒲公英 15-30g

ye ju hua (Flos Chrysanthemi Indici) 野菊花 9-12g
zi bei tian kui (Herba Begoniae Fimbristipulatae)
紫北天葵 9-12g

Method: Decoction. **Jin yin hua** clears Toxic Heat from the *qi* and Blood levels and disperses swelling; **pu gong ying** clears Toxic Heat and cools the Liver; **zi hua di ding** clears Toxic Heat and alleviates deeply rooted sores; **ye ju hua** and **zi bei tian kui** support the other herbs in clearing Toxic Heat. (Source: *Zhong Yi Er Bi Hou Ke Xue*)

Modifications

- It is common practice to take this formula with a small amount of alcohol (10-15mls of vodka or sherry usually suffices). This opens up the local circulation and assists the herbs in penetrating the lesion.
- Enclosed painful lesions generally have a component of Blood stagnation, and the addition of one or two Blood moving herbs is good practice. Select one or two of the following herbs: **dan shen** (Radix Salviae Miltiorrhizae) 丹参 12-18g, **chuan xiong** (Radix Ligustici Chuanxiong) 川芎 6-9g, **mu dan pi** (Cortex Moutan Radicis) 牡丹皮 9-12g or **chi shao** (Radix Paeoniae Rubrae) 赤芍 9-12g.
- If the lesion is difficult to bring to a head, add **bai zhi** (Radix Angelicae Dahuricae) 白芷 9-12g, **wang bu liu xing** (Semen Vaccariae Segetalis) 王不留行 9-12g and **zao jiao ci** (Spina Gleditsiae Sinensis) 皂角刺 9-12g.
- With severe Heat, fever or malaise, add one or two of the following herbs: **da qing ye** (Folium Daqingye) 大青叶 15g, **lian qiao** (Fructus Forsythia Suspensae) 连翘 9-12g, **huang qin** (Radix Scutellariae Baicalensis) 黄芩 9-12g, **ban zhi lian** (Herba Scutellariae Barbatae) 半枝连 15g or **ban bian lian** (Herba Lobeliae Chinensis) 半边莲 15g.
- With Wind Heat, add **lian qiao** (Fructus Forsythia Suspensae) 连翘 9-12g and **fang feng** (Radix Ledebouriellae Divaricatae) 防风 9-12g.
- With severe swelling, add **chan tui** (Periostracum Cicadae) 蝉蜕 9-12g, **fang feng** (Radix Ledebouriellae Divaricatae) 防风 9-12g and **zao jiao ci** (Spina Gleditsiae Sinensis) 皂角刺 9-12g.
- With Heat in the Blood, add **chi shao** (Radix Paeoniae Rubrae) 赤芍 9-12g, **mu dan pi** (Cortex Moutan Radicis) 牡丹皮 9-12g and **sheng di** (Radix Rehmanniae Glutinosae) 生地 12-18g.
- With alternating fever and chills, add **chai hu** (Radix Bupleuri) 柴胡 9-12g and **huang qin** (Radix Scutellariae Baicalensis) 黄芩 9-12g.

Topical treatment

- Boil 15 grams of **huang qin** (Radix Scutellariae Baicalensis) 黄芩 in 1-2 cups of water for 20 minutes and hold the liquid in the mouth for as long as possible.

- With dental caries and relatively severe pain, rinse the mouth with a decoction of **lu feng fang** (Nidus Vespae) 露蜂房 12g and **hai tong pi** (Coretx Erythrinae) 海桐皮 12g.
- *Shuang Liao Hou Feng San* 双料喉风散 (Superior Sore Throat Powder), a powdered patent medicine, can be massaged into the affected area to relieve pain and swelling

Patent medicines

Wu Wei Xiao Du Wan 五味消毒丸 (Wu Wei Xiao Du Wan)
- Toxic Heat

Huang Lian Jie Du Wan 黄连解毒丸 (Huang Lian Jie Du Wan)
- Damp and Toxic Heat; often combined with the above patent medicine for severe abscesses

Chuan Xin Lian Kang Yan Pian 穿心莲抗炎片 (Chuan Xin Lian Antiphlogistic Tablets)
- can be added to any formula to enhance the Toxic Heat clearing action

Ban Lan Gen Chong Ji 板蓝根冲剂 (Ban Lan Gen Chong Ji)

Bei Jing Niu Huang Jie Du Pian 牛黄解毒片 (Peking Niu Huang Chieh Tu Pien) - Toxic Heat in the upper body

Shuang Liao Hou Feng San 双料喉风散 (Superior Sore Throat Powder)
- can be massaged into the affected area to relieve pain and swelling

Acupuncture (select from)

St.44 (*nei ting* -) .... together these points clear Heat from *yang*
LI.4 (*he gu* -) *ming*; they also have a special effect on oral diseases, and are best for abscesses in the lower jaw

Du.10 (*ling tai* -) .... these points have a special effect on pyogenic
Du.12 (*shen zhu* -) lesions

St.42 (*chong yang* -) .... *yuan* point of the Stomach, used for painful abscesses in the upper jaw
LI.11 (*qu chi* -) .... *he* sea point of the Large Intestine, clears Heat and Dampness from the *yang ming* channels
St.6 (*jia che* -) .... local point best for the lower jaw
St.7 (*xia guan* -) .... local point best for the upper jaw

- with high fever, add PC.3 (*qu ze* ↓) and Bl.40 (*wei zhong* ↓)
- with severe pain, add LI.2 (*er jian* -) and SI.5 (*yang gu* -)
- with constipation, add SJ.6 (*zhi gou* -) and St.25 (*tian shu* -)

- *Ear points*: tragus apex, mouth, upper jaw, lower jaw, *shen men*

Clinical notes

- While painful and inconvenient, these types of tooth abscesses usually resolve spontaneously within 10 days, but depending on the state of the gums, mouth, and vitality of the patient, the they can be recurrent.

胃热牙痈

25.1.2 Stomach Heat/Fire

Pathophysiology

- Stomach Heat tooth abscesses are usually associated with the diet. An excess of foods and drink that heat the Stomach, or overconsumption of hot supplementing herbs, can create a rich and ready environment for focal accumulation of Heat in the gums. The lesion itself is an expression of Toxic Heat (a intense focal accumulation of a pathogen that destroys tissue), but the predisposing features and trigger, require a different solution.
- This pattern is characterised by pronounced systemic symptoms in addition to the abscess.

Clinical features

- painful locus of infection in the gum, worse for chewing and pressure; the pain may radiate to the cheek and jaw
- redness, swelling of the gums, possibly ulceration or bleeding
- halitosis, dry mouth, thirst, bad taste in the mouth
- fever, high or afternoon fever
- red flushed face, red lips
- tendency to constipation; rarely, diarrhoea
- copious sweating
- frontal headache
- swollen tender submandibular or cervical nodules

T red and dry with a yellow coat, thicker in the centre of the tongue
P slippery, big and rapid

Treatment principle

Clear Heat and Fire from the Stomach
Clear Toxic Heat, reduce swelling

Prescription

QING WEI TANG 清胃汤
(*Clear the Stomach Decoction*) modified

This formula is suitable when there are clear signs of Stomach Heat without constipation.

shi gao (Gypsum) 石膏 18-30g
huang qin (Radix Scutellariae Baicalensis) 黄芩 9-12g
sheng di (Radix Rehmanniae Glutinosae) 生地 12-15g
mu dan pi (Cortex Moutan Radicis) 牡丹皮 9-12g
huang lian (Rhizoma Coptidis) 黄连 6-9g
sheng ma (Rhizoma Cimicifugae) 升麻 6-9g
jin yin hua (Flos Lonicera Japonicae) 金银花 18-30g

lian qiao (Fructus Forsythia Suspensae) 连翘 12-15g
xuan shen (Radix Scrophulariae Ningpoensis) 玄参 15g

Method: Decoction. **Shi gao** is decocted for 30 minutes prior to the other herbs (*xian jian* 先煎). **Shi gao** clears Heat from the Spleen and Stomach; **huang qin** and **huang lian** clear Heat from the Lungs, Heart and Stomach; **sheng di** cools the Blood and nourishes Stomach *yin*; **mu dan pi** cools the Blood; **sheng ma** rises and disperses Heat, and enables the other cooling herbs to more thoroughly access and clear the Heat; the rising nature of **sheng ma** is nicely balanced by the descending nature of the cooling herbs, thus enabling Heat to be cleared and dispersed without causing damage to *qi* or *yin*; **jin yin hua** and **lian qiao** clear local accumulation of Toxic Heat; **xuan shen** cools the Blood and softens hardness. (Source: *Zhong Yi Er Bi Hou Ke Xue*)

Modifications

- With severe pain, or Blood stagnation, add **dan shen** (Radix Salviae Miltiorrhizae) 丹参 12-18g, **chuan xiong** (Radix Ligustici Chuanxiong) 川芎 6-9g, **mu dan pi** (Cortex Moutan Radicis) 牡丹皮 9-12g and **chi shao** (Radix Paeoniae Rubrae) 赤芍 9-12g.
- With severe redness and swelling of the gums, add two or three of the following herbs: **ma bian cao** (Herba Verbenae Officinalis) 马鞭草 9-12g, **pu gong ying** (Herba Taraxaci Mongolici) 蒲公英 15-30g, **shui niu jiao** (Cornu Bubali) 水牛角 15-30g, **niu bang zi** (Fructus Arctii Lappae) 牛蒡子 9-12g, **niu xi** (Radix Achyranthis Bidentatae) 牛膝 9-12g, **shan zhi zi** (Fructus Gardeniae Jasminoidis) 山栀子 9-12g or **qian cao gen** (Radix Rubiae Cordifoliae) 茜草根 9-12g.
- To encourage the abscess to form a head and rupture, add **bai zhi** (Radix Angelicae Dahuricae) 白芷 9-12g, **wang bu liu xing** (Semen Vaccariae Segetalis) 王不留行 9-12g and **zao jiao ci** (Spina Gleditsiae Sinensis) 皂角刺 9-12g.

Variations and additional prescriptions

Stomach Fire

- In relatively severe cases with pronounced Heat (by convention Fire), the systemic manifestations are quite prominent and the patient is constipated. The features are painful abscessed gum, ulcerations and inflammation of the oral cavity, feelings of heat in the chest, bad breath, irritability, red flushed complexion and lips, red tongue, constipation and concentrated urine. There may be skin rashes. The correct treatment is to purge Stomach Fire down through the bowels with **LIANG GE SAN** (*Cool the Diaphragm Powder* 凉膈散) modified.

  lian qiao (Fructus Forsythia Suspensae) 连翘 15-20g
  da huang (Radix et Rhizoma Rhei) 大黄 6-9g
  mang xiao (Mirabilitum) 芒硝 6-9g
  huang qin (Radix Scutellariae Baicalensis) 黄芩 9-12g

shan zhi zi (Fructus Gardeniae Jasminoidis) 山栀子 9-12g
gan cao (Radix Glycyrrhizae Uralensis) 甘草 6-9g
dan zhu ye (Herba Lophatheri Gracilis) 淡竹叶 9-12g
bo he (Herba Mentha Haplocalycis) 薄荷 6-9g
ban lan gen (Radix Isatidis seu Baphicacanthi) 板蓝根 15-30g
zi hua di ding (Herba cum Radice Violae Yedoensitis)
紫花地丁 9-15g
ku shen (Radix Sophorae Flavescentis) 苦参 9-15g

Method: Decoction. **Bo he** is added near the end of cooking (*hou xia* 后下). **Lian qiao, ban lan gen** and **zi hua di ding** clear Toxic Heat; **shan zhi zi, huang qin** and **ku shen** clear Damp Heat and cool the Stomach; **da huang** and **mang xiao** open the bowels and purge Heat from the Stomach and Intestines; **bo he** promotes Lung function and cools the Lungs and Stomach; **gan cao** clears Heat, moderates the bitter coldness of the other herbs and stops pain; **dan zhu yu** clears Heat from the Heart. (Source: *Zhong Yi Re Bi Hou Ke Xue*)

Topical treatment

See p.847.

Patent medicines

Huang Lian Jie Du Wan 黄连解毒丸 (Huang Lian Jie Du Wan)
- Damp and Toxic Heat

Chuan Xin Lian Kang Yan Pian 穿心莲抗炎片 (Chuan Xin Lian Antiphlogistic Tablets)
- can be added to the above patent medicine to enhance the Toxic Heat clearing action

Niu Huang Qing Huo Wan 牛黄清火丸 (Niu Huang Qing Huo Wan)
- with constipation

Shuang Liao Hou Feng San 双料喉风散 (Superior Sore Throat Powder)
- can be massaged into the affected area to relieve pain and swelling

Acupuncture (select from)

St.44 (*nei ting* -) .... together these points clear Heat from *yang ming*; they also have a special effect on oral diseases, best for abscesses in the lower jaw
LI.4 (*he gu* -)

Du.10 (*ling tai* -) .... these points have a special effect on pyogenic lesions
Du.12 (*shen zhu* -)

St.42 (*chong yang* -) .... *yuan* point of the Stomach, used for painful abscesses in the upper jaw
LI.11 (*qu chi* -) .... *he* sea point of the Large Intestine, clears Heat and Dampness from the *yang ming* channels

Ren.12 (*zhong wan* -) .... *mu* point of the Stomach, clears Heat from the Stomach
PC.8 (*lao gong* -) .... *rong* spring and Fire point of the Pericardium, drains Heat from the Stomach channel, cools the Blood and Heart Fire
St.6 (*jia che* -) .... local point best for the lower jaw
St.7 (*xia guan* -) .... local point best for the upper jaw

- with high fever, add PC.3 (*qu ze* ↓) and Bl.40 (*wei zhong* ↓)
- with severe pain, add LI.2 (*er jian* -) and SI.5 (*yang gu* -)
- with constipation, add SJ.6 (*zhi gou* -) and St.25 (*tian shu* -)
- *Ear points*: tragus apex, mouth, upper jaw, lower jaw, *shen men*

Clinical notes

- Abscesses of this type are usually self limiting and resolve within 7-10 days. The systemic aspect that encourages the abscess, Stomach Heat, will take longer to correct and requires dietary modification.
- For dietary recommendations, see p.882.

正虚邪实

25.2 CHRONIC, RECURRENT TOOTH ABSCESS

25.2.1 Qi deficiency with residual Toxin

Pathophysiology

- Chronic abscesses, or non healing lesions, occur in weak patients, diabetics, the elderly and in those with a pre-existing deficiency of *qi* and Blood. These lesions may also result after multiple courses of antibiotic or bitter cold medications for excess Heat type acute abscesses.
- Essentially the patient's *zheng qi* and the pathogen reach a state of equilibrium, with *zheng qi* unable to overcome the residual pathogen and fully expel it. This 'containment' costs *qi* and the patient's *qi* reserves gradually decline.
- This pattern may be complicated by localised Phlegm accumulation.

Clinical features

- chronic or recurrent focal swelling, ache or pain in the jaw; the lesion is not especially red and may feel soft or rubbery
- pale complexion
- easy sweating, frequent coughs and colds
- loss of appetite, abdominal distension, early satiety
- fatigue, weakness
- low voice, reluctance to speak
- possibly mild feverishness in the morning
- rubbery, non-tender submandibular or cervical nodules

T pale, swollen, thin white coat
P thready, weak

Treatment principle

Support *qi* and Blood
Aid discharge of pus, promote healing
Transform Phlegm

Prescription

TUO LI XIAO DU SAN 托里消毒散
(*Powder to Support the Interior and Eliminate Toxin*)

jin yin hua (Flos Lonicera Japonicae) 金银花 12-15g
huang qi (Radix Astragali Membranacei) 黄芪 12-30g
dang shen (Radix Codonopsis Pilosulae) 党参 12-15g
fu ling (Sclerotium Poriae Cocos) 茯苓 12-15g
bai zhu (Rhizoma Atractylodes Macrocephalae) 白术 9-15g
dang gui (Radix Angelicae Sinensis) 当归 9-12g
bai shao (Radix Paeoniae Lactiflorae) 白芍 12-15g

zao jiao ci (Spina Gleditsiae Sinensis) 皂角刺 9-12g
jie geng (Radix Platycodi Grandiflori) 桔梗 6-9g
gan cao (Radix Glycyrrhizae Uralensis) 甘草 6-9g

Method: Decoction. **Jin yin hua** clears residual Toxic Heat and does not damage the Spleen; **huang qi, dang shen, fu ling, bai zhu** and **gan cao** strengthen the Spleen and supplement *qi*; **dang gui** and **bai shao** nourish and regulate Blood; **zao jiao ci** and **jie geng** aid in discharging residual pus. (Source: *Zhong Yi Er Bi Hou Ke Xue*)

Modifications

- With thin watery exudate, double the dose of **huang qi**.
- With continued pus production, double the dose of **jin yin hua** and add **pu gong ying** (Herba Taraxaci Mongolici cum Radice) 蒲公英 15g.
- With Blood stagnation, add **tao ren** (Semen Persicae) 桃仁 9-12g and **hong hua** (Flos Carthami Tinctorii) 红花 9-12g.
- With obvious Blood deficiency, add **shu di** (Radix Rehmanniae Glutinosae Conquitae) 熟地 12-18g and **rou gui** (Cortex Cinnamomi Cassiae) 肉桂 3-6g.
- When Phlegm complicates the primary pathology, it should be moistened and softened with salty herbs so as to facilitate its dispersal. Add **xuan shen** (Radix Scrophulariae) 玄参 15-18g, **zhe bei mu** (Bulbus Fritillariae Thunbergii) 浙贝母 9-12g and **mu li** (Concha Ostreae) 牡蛎 15-20g.

Variations and additional prescriptions

With yang deficiency

- In elderly or *yang* deficient patients, the abscess may become cold and sealed off from the healing *yang* of the body. The resistance of the lesion to resolve may be associated with the congealing of Phlegm at the site. This pattern may occur as a result of deterioration of *qi* deficiency, or more likely may occur in patients with a pre-existing *yang* weakness. The main feature is a chronic, localised, aching or painful swelling in the gums. The gums are not ulcerated, red or inflamed. In addition, the patient is cold intolerant, has a pale, swollen tongue and a deep weak pulse. The treatment aims to warm *yang*, supplement the Blood and disperse Cold and Phlegm with **YANG HE TANG** (*Yang Heartening Decoction* 阳和汤).

shu di (Radix Rehmanniae Glutinosae Conquitae) 熟地 15-30g
lu jiao jiao (Gelatinum Cornu Cervi) 鹿角胶 6-9g
rou gui (Cortex Cinnamomi Cassiae) 肉桂 1-3g
pao jiang (quick fried Rhizoma Zingiberis Officinalis) 1-2g
ma huang (Herba Ephedra) 麻黄 1-2g
bai jie zi (Semen Sinapsis Albae) 白芥子 3-6g
gan cao (Radix Glycyrrhizae Uralensis) 甘草 1-3g

Method: Decoction. **Lu jiao jiao** is melted before being added to the strained decoction (*yang hua* 烊化). The large dose of **shu di** supplements the Blood and Kidneys; **lu jiao jiao** warms *yang* and assists the **shu di** in supplementing Blood; **rou gui** and **pao jiang** warm *yang* and invigorate the transformation of fluids to assist in transforming Phlegm and clearing areas of stagnation; **bai jie zi** transforms Phlegm; **ma huang** promotes movement of *qi*, assists the dispersing function of the Lungs and dispels Cold; **gan cao** protects the Stomach and harmonises the prescription. With severe Cold, add **zhi fu zi** (Radix Aconiti Carmichaeli Praeparata) 制附子 6g.

Patent medicines

Bu Zhong Yi Qi Wan 补中益气丸 (Bu Zhong Yi Qi Wan, Central Qi Pills) - *qi* deficiency

Xiang Sha Liu Jun Zi Wan 香砂六君子丸 (Xiang Sha Liu Jun Wan, Aplotaxis-Ammomum Pills, Six Gentlemen Tea Pills)
- Spleen *qi* deficiency with Phlegm Damp

Shi Quan Da Bu Wan 十全大补丸 (Shi Quan Da Bu Wan, Ten Flavour Tea) - *qi* and Blood deficiency

Wu Ji Bai Feng Wan 乌鸡白凤丸 (Wu Chi Pai Feng Wan)
- Blood and *yang* deficiency

Li Zhong Wan 理中丸 (Li Zhong Wan)
- Spleen *yang* deficiency

Hai Zao Wan 海藻丸 (Hai Zao Wan)
- add with Phlegm

Acupuncture (select from)

Ren.12 (*zhong wan* +▲) .. *mu* point of the Stomach, strengthens the Stomach and Spleen

Ren.4 (*guan yuan* +▲) ..... warms the Kidneys and supplements *yuan qi*

LI.4 (*he gu*) .... *yuan* point of the Large Intestine, a special point for all oral disorders; assists in clearing any residual pathogen

LI.11 (*qu chi* +▲) .... *he* sea point of the Large Intestine, warms *yang ming* and stimulates *yang qi* in general when moxaed

St.36 (*zu san li* +▲) .... *he* sea point of the Stomach, powerfully warms and strengthens the Spleen and Stomach and supplements *qi* and Blood

Sp.6 (*san yin jiao* +▲)...... strengthens the Spleen and Kidney, invigorates and supplements *qi* and Blood

Bl.20 (*pi shu* +▲) .... *shu* points of the Spleen and Stomach, warm,
Bl.21 (*wei shu* +▲) supplement and regulate middle *jiao qi*

St.6 (*jia che*) .... local points to reinforce circulation of *qi* and
St.7 (*xia guan*) Blood
St.4 (*di cang*)
Du.26 (*ren zhong*)

- with Kidney deficiency, add Bl.23 (*shen shu* +▲), Du.4 (*ming men* +▲) and Kid.3 (*tai xi* +)
- *Ear points*: mouth, upper jaw, lower jaw, spleen, stomach, *shen men*

Clinical notes

- These chronic abscesses will often take weeks to months to completely clear, in association with good nutrition and appropriate dental hygiene.
- Patients will often need to increase protein intake, particularly if there is *yang* and Blood deficiency. For dietary recommendations, see p.870-873.

25.2.2 Yin deficiency with residual Toxin

陰虛留邪

Pathophysiology

- An abscess may develop in a patient with a pre-existing *yin* deficiency pattern or constitution It may also be the result of *yin* damage associated with the Heat generated during the acute phase of the abscess. The complication of *yin* deficiency means that care must be taken in the use of bitter cold herbs, as they can aggravate the already damaged *yin*.

Clinical features

- chronic or recurrent tooth and gum abscess; the lesion may be slightly red with only mild swelling and a dull aching that increases towards the end of the day
- loose teeth, atrophy of the gums, difficulty or weakness in chewing
- dizziness, tinnitus
- blurred vision, poor memory
- insomnia, restlessness at night
- malar or facial flushing, nightsweats
- sensation of heat in the palms and soles ('five hearts hot')
- lower back ache or weakness
- rubbery, non-tender submandibular or cervical nodules

T red and dry with little or no coat
P thready and rapid

Treatment principle

Nourish and supplement Stomach and Kidney *yin*
Aid discharge of pus, promote healing

Prescription

ZHI BAI BA WEI WAN 知柏八味丸
(*Anemarrhena, Phellodendron and Rehmannia Formula*) modified

shu di (Radix Rehmanniae Glutinosae Conquitae) 熟地...... 24-30g
shan yao (Radix Dioscoreae Oppositae) 山药 12-18g
shan zhu yu (Fructus Corni Officinalis) 山茱萸 12-15g
fu ling (Sclerotium Poria Cocos) 茯苓 9-12g
mu dan pi (Cortex Moutan Radicis) 牡丹皮 9-12g
ze xie (Rhizoma Alismatis Orientalis) 泽泻 9-12g
zhi mu (Rhizoma Anemarrhenae Asphodeloidis) 知母 9-12g
huang bai (Cortex Phellodendri) 盐黄柏 9-12g
jie geng (Radix Platycodi Grandiflori) 桔梗 6-9g
yu xing cao (Herba cum Radice Houttuyniae Cordatae)
鱼腥草 15-24g
xuan shen (Radix Scrophulariae Ningpoensis) 玄参 15-18g

Method: Grind the herbs to powder and form into 9-gram pills with honey. The dose is 2-3 pills daily. May also be decocted with quantities as shown. **Shu di** supplements Blood, and Liver and Kidney *yin*; **shan yao** strengthens the Spleen; **shan zhu yu** supplements Liver *yin*; **fu ling**, **ze xie** and **mu dan pi** prevent the supplementing herbs from clogging up the digestive system; **mu dan pi** invigorates Blood and eliminates stagnant Blood; **zhi mu** and **huang bai** clear deficient Heat; **huang bai** and **yu xing cao** clear Damp and Toxic Heat; **jie geng** aids discharge of pus; **xuan shen** nourishes *yin* and softens hardness. (Source: *Zhong Yi Re Bi Hou Ke Xue*)

Modifications

- With pain, add **gu sui bu** (Rhizoma Drynariae) 骨碎补 15g and **di gu pi** (Cortex Lycii Radicis) 地骨皮 15g.
- With loose teeth, add **gu sui bu** (Rhizoma Drynariae) 骨碎补 15g and **gou ji** (Rhizoma Cibotii Barometz) 狗脊 15g.
- With Blood deficiency, add **dang gui** (Radix Angelicae Sinensis) 当归 9-12g and **bai shao** (Radix Paeoniae Lactiflorae) 白芍 12-18g.
- With Phlegm, add **zhe bei mu** (Bulbus Fritillariae Thunbergii) 浙贝母 12g and **mu li** (Concha Ostreae) 牡蛎 15-20g.

Patent medicines

Zhi Bai Ba Wei Wan 知柏八味丸 (Zhi Bai Ba Wei Wan, Chih Pai Pa Wei Wan) - with deficient Heat

Tian Wang Bu Xin Dan 天王补心丹 (Emperors Tea, Tien Wang Pu Hsin Tan) - with Phlegm complication

Nei Xiao Luo Li Wan 内消瘰疬丸 (Nei Xiao Luo Li Wan)
- add to one of the above formulae when Phlegm is clearly established

Acupuncture (select from)

Ren.12 (*zhong wan*) .... *mu* point of the Stomach, nourishes Stomach *yin*, regulates the Stomach and clears Heat
Ren.4 (*guan yuan* +) .... meeting point of the *yin* channels, nourishes *yin* of whole body, with Sp.6
St.36 (*zu san li* +) .... *he* sea point of the Stomach channel, powerfully strengthens the Spleen and Stomach and supplements *qi* and *yin*
Sp.6 (*san yin jiao* +) .... with Ren.4, nourishes *yin* of the whole body

Kid.6 (*zhao hai* +) .... together these points open *yin qiao mai* and *ren*
Lu.7 (*lie que* +) *mai*, nourish *yin* and benefit the mouth

LI.4 (*he gu*) .... *yuan* point of the Large Intestine, a special point for all oral disorders
Kid.3 (*tai xi* +) .... *yuan* point to nourish Kidney *yin*

Bl.21 (*wei shu* +) .... these points nourish Stomach and Spleen *yin*
Bl.20 (*pi shu* +)

St.6 (*jia che*) .... local points to reinforce circulation of *qi* and
St.7 (*xia guan*) Blood
St.4 (*di cang*)
Du.26 (*ren zhong*)

- *Ear points*: mouth, upper jaw, lower jaw, kidney, stomach, *shen men*

Clinical notes

- *Yin* deficiency chronic abscess respond variably, depending on the longevity of the condition. For those that respond, the treatment will usually need to be lengthy. Six to nine months may be required to clear any residual pathogen and rebuild the *yin* sufficiently to prevent recurrence.
- For dietary recommendations, see p.876.

SUMMARY OF GUIDING FORMULAE FOR TOOTH ABSCESS

Acute patterns

Toxic Heat - *Wu Wei Xiao Du Yin* 五味消毒饮

Stomach Heat/Fire - *Qing Wei Tang* 清胃汤
- with constipation - *Liang Ge San* 凉膈散

Chronic or recurrent patterns

Qi deficiency with residual Toxin - *Tuo Li Xiao Du San* 托里消毒散
- *Yang* deficiency - *Yang He Tang* 阳和汤

Yin deficiency - *Zhi Bai Ba Wei Wan* 知柏八味丸

26. The Diet

26 THE DIET

There is nothing more fundamental to gastro-intestinal and indeed general health, than an appropriately balanced diet. Unfortunately for many people in the developed world, what is thought to be a good diet is often influenced by a confusing and conflicting jumble of fads, fallacies and misinformation.

TCM recognises that patients with different constitutions and problems require unique dietary solutions. The structure and content of the diet can be manipulated to help correct pathological imbalances in most instances. In all patients, the aim of diet therapy is to gradually move from whatever dietary approach is suitable to correct a particular imbalance, towards a Spleen and Stomach *qi* strengthening diet. A healthy Spleen and Stomach function is necessary for all aspects of life and health, including tissue growth and repair, metabolism, defence and reproduction. Maintenance of healthy Spleen and Stomach function is central to the treatment and management of all internal disorders.

A detailed description of the mechanics of diet from a TCM point of view is beyond the scope of this text, but see Pitchfords' *Healing with Whole Foods: Oriental Traditions and Modern Nutrition*, and Leggetts' *Helping Ourselves: A Guide to Traditional Chinese Food Energetics* and *Recipes for Self Healing*, all excellent sources of information on this topic.

There are two main aspects of diet to be considered, the type of food ingested and the way it is consumed.

1. THE TYPE OF FOOD CONSUMED

There is no single diet that is appropriate for everyone. Different constitutional types and pathological patterns require different types of food.

Food groups and achieving the right balance

There are three general groups of foods that we are concerned with in TCM, carbohydrates, proteins and fruits and vegetables. Each group is composed of diverse items with their own unique functions and flavours, but each group as a whole has a specific nutritional and energetic activity. In general the carbohydrates are sweet and warm, strengthen the Spleen and build *qi*. The protein group nourish *qi*, Blood, *yin* and *jing* and tend to be warmer than the carbohydrates. Fruits and vegetables tend to be cooling, clearing and mobilising in nature, providing a dietary counterpoint to the supplementing, building elements of the other two groups. As TCM practitioners, our aim is to construct the appropriate mix of these components to suit our patients' specific needs. By varying the proportions we can achieve quite different outcomes. Patients with deficiency patterns will benefit from a diet based on the supplementing elements, the carbohydrates and proteins. The balance of carbohydrate and protein can be varied depending on the type of

Figure 26.1 *Characteristics of food groups*

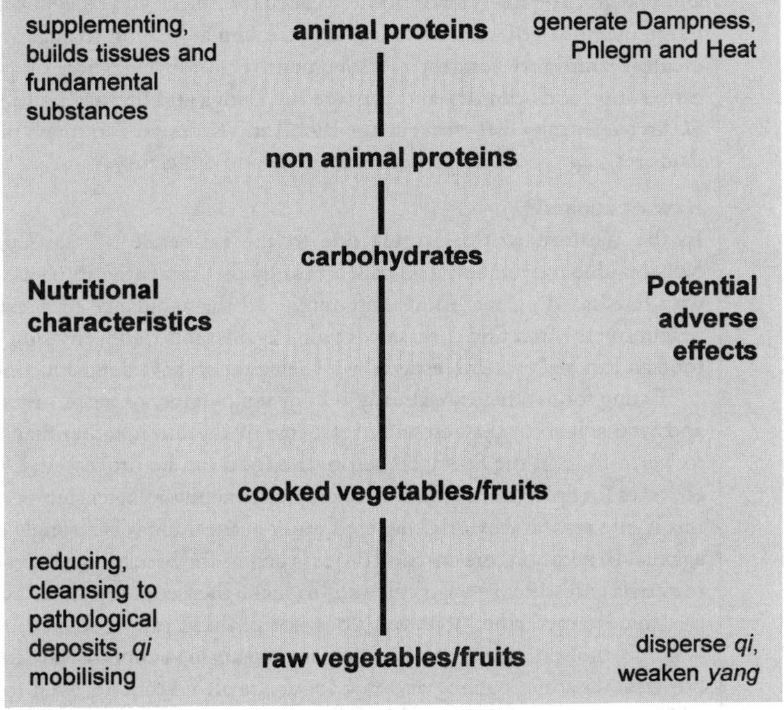

deficiency. *Qi* deficiency, as an example, needs more carbohydrate, whereas Blood deficiency benefits from a higher proportion of animal protein. Those tending to excess patterns will benefit from a higher proportion of fruits and vegetables. Vegetables and fruit can be modified or enhanced in their reducing action depending on how they are prepared.

In general, the average diet of the developed world is animal protein rich and thus overly supplementing, especially to Blood and *yin*. The negative effect of excessive supplementation is the development of Dampness and Phlegm, often with Heat. Phlegm Damp can be deposited in various locations, including the cardiovascular system, where it may contribute to the most significant causes of mortality in the developed world, heart disease and stroke.

The correct proportions are important in structuring an appropriate diet. People should aim for a good overall balance of the correct groups, without undue emphasis on individual items in any group. Too much of any group or one item will cause imbalance. As in all endeavours in Chinese medicine, striking the balance is the goal. A meat and protein rich diet will be too supplementing for some people and will generate and aggravate Dampness and Phlegm. Too many sweet foods weaken the Spleen and create Dampness. Large quantities of carbohydrates act in a similar fashion to sugar and can create Damp and congest *qi* movement. Excessive heating or pungent dispersing foods can dry and damage the Lungs and Stomach and weaken *qi*. An overly salty diet weakens the Blood and Kidneys. Too much raw food damages *yang*. Too little protein leads to Blood deficiency.

Raw or cooked?

In the Western world, largely due to the influence of the European naturopathic movement, a so called healthy diet has come to be associated with one based on raw foods and juices and the avoidance of meat. TCM practitioners often find themselves going against this trend, advising cooked food and animal proteins, especially if their patients have deficient conditions.

Eating foods which are already at body temperature or more, saves Spleen and Stomach *qi* for the demanding process of digestion, rather than using it to warm food in the Stomach before the food can be processed. Digestive enzymes (or Spleen and Stomach *qi*) only work at physiological temperatures–this is one reason why drinking iced water at meal times is strongly advised against. In addition, the cooking process begins the breakdown of vegetable materials and softens tough cell walls to make their contents more available.

Chinese medicine, however, does not prohibit raw food. Robust, hot, *yang* constitutions require the cooling and cleansing action of raw foods. In hot weather some cooling and raw foods are also desirable, even for those with some Spleen *qi* deficiency, but never for those with Spleen *yang* deficiency.

Quality of ingredients

It goes without saying that what we put into our bodies determines the quality of *qi*, Blood and tissues. All produce should be the best quality available. Where health and vitality are concerned, it never pays to cut corners and quality ingredients do not always cost more than processed foods. All meat should be as chemical, hormone and antibiotic free as possible. Food should appeal to the senses, being vibrant in colour and aroma, bursting with vitality and *qi*. It is important to buy fresh produce frequently, rather than letting large amounts wilt in the refrigerator. Locally grown and seasonal produce is better than that grown artificially in hothouses in a distant locations or country.

Vegetarian or meat diet?

A vegetarian diet is, by nature, quite *yin*, and therefore suitable for those with *yang* conditions. The TCM practitioner may recommend a vegetarian diet to those with a Hot or Damp Heat constitution or condition. It is unsuitable for those with Blood and/or *yin* deficiency. Being strictly vegetarian and meeting all nutritional needs presents certain challenges in the modern world. The major consideration is getting sufficient protein and an adequate supply of vitamin B_{12}.

Thermal nature and flavours of foods

The thermal nature and the flavours of food are a way of describing the properties of foods and their effects upon the body. The actual oral sensation and tastes of some foods do not necessarily correspond to their designated thermal nature or flavour. For example, beef and chicken are classified as sweet, lettuce and broccoli as bitter.

Foods that warm the body

Warm and hot natured foods warm the body, encourage the ascent of *qi*, promote circulation, stimulate *yang* and increase metabolism. Cooking increases the warmth of foods, especially prolonged stewing, roasting and deep frying. Warm foods are suitable for deficiency and Cold conditions, while too much can aggravate Heat or excess patterns

Foods that cool the body

Cool and cold thermal natured foods cool the body and clear Heat. They tend to direct *qi* inwards and downwards, and in general slow down metabolic processes. Raw foods are the coolest, but some cooking methods, such as quick stir frying, steaming and blanching, preserve most of the cool nature of foods while making them Spleen friendly and easy to digest. Cooling foods are indicated in Heat patterns, but too much can weaken *yang* and create stagnation.

Sweet

Sweet flavours are *yang* and have an affinity for the Spleen. In proper amounts sweet flavours are stimulating and beneficial to the digestive process and relax spasm in smooth muscles. Sweet, warm flavours are on the whole strengthening, and tend to supplement *qi* and *yang* and build *yin* and Blood. Sweet cool flavours tend to be moistening and cleansing.

An overly sweet diet causes accumulation of Dampness and Phlegm and may aggravate tissue proliferation, as occurs in obesity and various growths, plaques and tumours. Many root vegetables, grains and meats are sweet and warm or sweet and neutral; fruit tends to be sweet and cool. Sweet flavours are emphasised in deficiency patterns.

Sour

Sour flavours are *yin*, contracting and astringing, and tend to be cooling. Sour flavours benefit the Liver and assist in toning and tightening tissues, and stopping fluid leakage, as in sweating and frequent urination.

An excessively sour diet can retard the metabolism and expulsion of pathogens, so sour food should be used sparingly when Dampness or lingering pathogens are present. Too much sour flavour may cause dryness and injure the Tendons. Many fruits are sour, as are tomato, lemon, leek, yogurt, sourdough bread, vinegar, pickles and wine.

Salty

Salty flavours are *yin*, cooling and moistening and tend to focus their effects inward and downward. Salty flavours have a descending and contracting tendency with a special effect on the Kidney system. They also soften areas of hardness, such as masses and nodules.

An overly salty diet can aggravate Dampness, damage the bones and Blood and disrupt fluid metabolism. Foods with a salty flavour include many seafoods, kelp and other seaweeds, fermented soy products, millet, parsley and of course, salt.

Pungent

Pungent flavours are *yang*, dispersing, and direct *qi* upwards and out towards the surface. They are particularly beneficial to the Lungs and assist the Spleen in the digestion and processing of rich, supplementing foods. Pungent flavours promote sweating, help break up Phlegm, invigorate the circulation of *qi* and Blood, and assist in dispersing stagnation of *qi* and Blood.

An excessively pungent diet will tend to dissipate *qi* and *yin*, and cause dryness, especially of the Lungs and Stomach. Large quantities are not suitable for deficiency states. Pungent food can be warm or cool. Pungent warm foods are the onion family, chilli, ginger, pepper, cinnamon and many kitchen spices. Examples of pungent cooling foods are radish, watercress, cabbage, celery and peppermint. Pungency is diminished by cooking. When this aspect is desired light cooking or no cooking is appropriate.

Bitter

Bitter flavours are *yin*, drying, descending, often cooling and specifically aligned with the Heart. Bitter flavours dry Dampness and in small amounts assist the Spleen and encourage Stomach *qi* to descend. As a component of a diet, bitter flavours help maintain the *qi* mechanism. Bitter cool foods are good for clearing Heat and Damp Heat, while bitter warm flavours dry Damp.

An overly bitter diet, while rather uncommon, can weaken the Spleen, damage *yin* and Blood and cause dryness. Bitter flavours include coffee, tea, oats and rye, lettuce, bamboo shoot, broccoli and bitter melon.

2. THE WAY FOOD IS CONSUMED

Chinese medicine recognises the fact that the way food is consumed is as important as the food itself. Eating a nutritious and well balanced diet will not guarantee healthy *qi* if the Spleen and Stomach are compromised by other factors that affect their performance. There are several factors which influence the efficiency of the Spleen and Stomach.

Timing of eating

The Spleen and Stomach function best with a regular routine. According to their own internal cycle, they prepare themselves, in association with the Liver, to receive and process food at specific times. If meals are missed frequently, or the timing of eating is erratic, as commonly occurs in shift workers, the function of the Spleen and Stomach can be severely compromised. The optimum times of eating will vary from person to person. However, larger, and more carbohydrate rich meals should be consumed earlier in the day, to provide a steady supply of *yang qi* for the day's activities. The best time for the main carbohydrate meals is between 7am and 11am, the Spleen and Stomach time. Smaller meals are recommended towards the end of the day, as the transition from the *yang* active phase of the day proceeds into the *yin* quiet phase, and the body prepares for rest. Patients with deficient *qi* may find that they need to eat small amounts more frequently, every 2-3 hours. Eating large meals late at night can be particularly taxing to the Spleen and may disrupt sleep.

Eating in a relaxed state

Digestion is an energy demanding process. If *qi* is diverted from the Spleen and Stomach into some other activity when it should be concentrated in the middle *jiao*, there is less *qi* available for the transformation of raw materials into *qi* and Blood. Even seemingly benign activities, such as reading or watching TV while eating, can have an impact on the digestive function by diverting *qi* from the Spleen and Stomach to the Liver and eyes. Energy intensive activities, such as working breakfasts, working through lunch, and eating on the run, can have significant negative impact on the function of the Spleen.

Enjoyment

An essential feature of good digestion is the enjoyment of food. Flavours and textures of food should be pleasing to the palate, while colour, variety and presentation of food should be pleasing to the eye. Even the most nutritious and well balanced diet will fail if eating it is a chore or merely tolerated. A healthy diet should not be a chore. It is particularly important for patients with Spleen deficiency patterns to note, as they can tend to become obsessive about diets. Very rigid or restrictive diets will feed the Spleen imbalance, and can create a destructive cycle of food obsession and further weakness. Pleasure in eating a fine healthy meal settles the Liver, eases the Stomach and facilitates the whole digestive process.

Over eating

In the developed world we tend to eat too much for our predominantly sedentary lives. It is estimated that on average, 30% excess calories per day are consumed in Australia and the USA, hence the epidemic of obesity. It was traditional wisdom to leave the table feeling we could eat a little more, but that rarely occurs now. For many people, especially those with excess patterns (Heat, Damp Heat, Phlegm, *qi* or food stagnation) reducing the amount of food eaten is helpful. This can be achieved by having smaller meals, having two meals per day rather than the usual three or by an occasional fast. On the other hand, people with *qi* deficiency patterns generally need to have small but regular and frequent meals.

Undereating, dieting

Skipping meals or severely restricting calorie intake in an attempt to lose weight can easily damage Spleen *qi* and *yang*. The quick rebound gain of more weight than was lost when normal calorie intake is resumed is evidence of this. Chinese medicine advocates eating sufficient of the right foods at the right time, in combination with appropriate activity, to maintain the ideal weight. When Spleen *qi* is strong, good metabolism will help guard against weight gain.

Fasting

Fasting is not a common practice among the Chinese, but has a valuable therapeutic role in some situations. Fasting is beneficial for patients with excess conditions, especially Dampness, Phlegm and Damp Heat. Fasting here is usually defined as no solid foods, however vegetable juices and light broths are acceptable. This type of fast is quite different in intent and execution to the fast carried out by those pursuing spiritual goals.

In general, we don't recommend multiple days of fasting, but a day's fast every now and then can accelerate the elimination of pathogens. In most cases of excess, a day's fast every seven days or so (Sunday is convenient) for a period of a few weeks is sufficient. In severe cases a slightly longer period of fasting (2-3 days) may be beneficial at greater intervals, say every 3-4 weeks.

Fasting is not recommended at all for patient's with deficiency patterns, and in fact can contribute significantly to an aggravation of the problem. Many TCM practitioners have had the experience of trying to mend the damage done to Spleen *qi* and *yang* deficient patients who return from a week of juice fasting at the health farm. Rather than the hoped for weight loss, there is often an increase in fluid retention, fatigue and digestive weakness. Patients with mixed deficiency and excess patterns may tolerate a mild fast now and then. Fasting is not recommended during cold weather, for children, during pregnancy or when lactating.

Modifying a diet

Food plays many social roles in addition to its main nutritional roles. It is a social lubricant, used in ritual and celebration and for emotional comfort. Thus major changes in a diet cannot, and should not, happen too suddenly.

Modifications, additions and subtractions to the diet should be made gradually to allow time for both physical and mental adaptation. Keep in mind that fundamental changes to the diet often contribute to digestive symptoms while the system adjusts. Constipation is quite a common manifestation.

QI DEFICIENCY

General principles

A diet which strengthens Spleen *qi* focuses on well cooked, simple food, with relatively few components in each meal. The basis of the diet is complex carbohydrates with the addition of small amounts of high quality protein and lightly cooked vegetables. To get the best quality *qi* from food, the food itself should be fresh and vibrant, and should appeal to the eye as well as the palate. Locally grown, seasonal produce has the best *qi*.

Even though all food should be cooked, overcooking to the point of sogginess is not recommended. Depending on the food, light cooking, leaving a residual crunch is sufficient. Green leafy and delicate vegetables, like broccoli and beans require light cooking only, while root vegetables and grains will retain their shape, texture and *qi* with long slow cooking.

The digestive process begins in the mouth and food should be well chewed and savoured slowly. The food must be enjoyed. Rigid or boring diets are detrimental to the Spleen.

The preparation of food can be a significant factor in it's overall *qi* quality and benefit. It goes without saying that meals prepared with pleasure and love, taste better than those that are store bought, or made in haste or resentment. This can be difficult as not everyone likes to cook or has the time. However, making the time and effort to nurture can be an important part of the therapeutic process. Setting aside time on weekends to prepare hearty soups, stocks and stews for the coming week is a way of actively participating in the Spleen strengthening process, and has mental benefits that also assist the Spleen.

Figure 26.2 *Recommended proportions for building qi and yang*

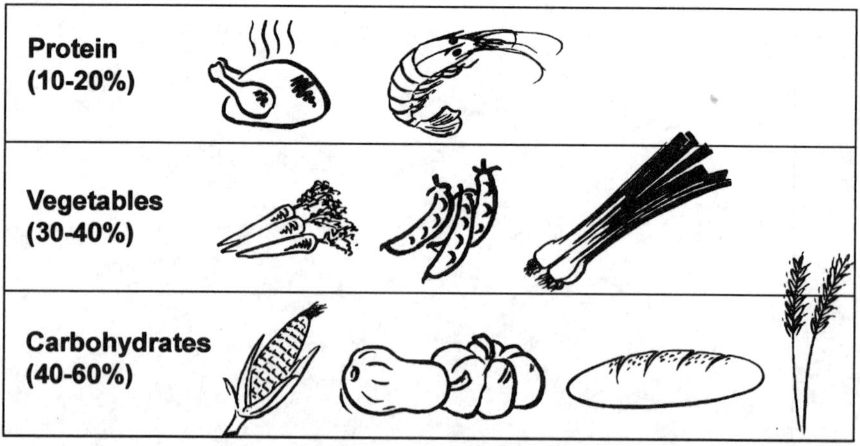

Qi deficiency

General principles	**Yes:** All food cooked and warm, long slow cooking; soups, broths and stews; thorough chewing; simple combinations of a few ingredients; smaller meals more often; regular meal times; high complex carbohydrate and vegetable, low meat **No:** excessive fluids with meals; overeating; missing meals; eating while working
Beneficial	**Neutral or sweet, warm flavours:** light grains especially white rice and rice porridge [congee], oats, roasted barley, sweet rice, spelt, pumpkin, sweet potato, celeriac, squash, carrot, corn, parsnip, chick peas, black beans, kumera, yams, peas, walnuts, stewed fruit, chicken, beef, lamb, liver, kidney, mackerel, tuna, anchovy **Pungent flavours (small amounts):** onion, leek, garlic, turnip, pepper, fresh ginger, cinnamon, nutmeg, fennel, kitchen spices **Complex sweet flavours (small amounts):** molasses, dates, rice syrup, barley malt, palm sugar
Restrict or avoid	**Cold natured, uncooked and raw food:** salads, raw fruits (whole and juiced, especially citrus), wheat, sprouts and cereal grasses, raw vegetables, tomato, spinach, swiss chard, tofu, millet, seaweeds, salt, too many sweet foods and concentrated sweeteners, brown rice, antibiotics, vitamin C (over 1-2 grams per day), beer **Congesting, Damp generating:** ice cream and dairy foods (except a little butter and yogurt), sugar, chocolate, nuts and seeds (except walnuts) and nut butters

The Lungs are an important partner of the Spleen in the *qi* production process. Strengthening the Spleen will benefit the Lungs through the generating (*sheng* 生) cycle. Moderate exercise and deep breathing help to strengthen the Lungs. In terms of foods, the Lungs specifically benefit from the addition of a small amount of pungent foods which assists their natural function of dispersing and descending. Care must be exercised with these items in cases with significant deficiency, especially in the early stages of dietary modification, as they may be too dispersing and further weaken *qi*.

Proportions

Easily digested carbohydrates, such as white rice, oats and starchy root vegetables, should make up the bulk of the material ingested, around 40-60%. The remainder is composed of cooked green, red and yellow vegetables (30-40%) and a small proportion (~10-20%) of high quality protein. This is especially important in the early stages of a treatment. As the Spleen strengthens, of course, other elements can be introduced. Care with the volume of carbohydrates is necessary, however, when there is significant Dampness. Small amounts of salad vegetables (on sandwiches etc.), may be added as the Spleen strengthens or in hot climates.

YANG DEFICIENCY

General principles

The overall principles for treating *yang* deficiency with diet are the same as for *qi* deficiency. Maintenance of vigorous Spleen function is the primary goal. The major difference is the addition of some specific warming foods for the Spleen and Kidney, and the absolute avoidance of all raw food, including salad vegetables. The proportions of the various food groups are the same as for Spleen *qi* deficiency.

Spleen yang deficiency

Spleen *yang* deficiency is a degree more severe than Spleen *qi* deficiency, with the overall result that digestive power is significantly reduced. The basic diet structure is the same with the addition of more warming foods and spices (*see* chart below).

Kidney yang deficiency

Kidney *yang* must be warmed and strengthened through the Spleen, using a diet which strengthens Spleen *yang*. In addition, adding some specific foods that warm the Kidneys is beneficial. If oedema is a feature, some diuretic foods such as cooked celery and lettuce can be added.

Yang deficiency	
General comments	The general principles are as for *qi* deficiency
Spleen	In addition to the foods suitable for *qi* deficiency, an emphasis on the more warming items such as rice, (especially as porridge), oats, parsnip, sweet potato, onion, leek, stocks and broths, lamb, beef, chicken, prawn, mantis shrimp, stewed fruit, chestnut. In addition, add a greater proportion of warming spices such as dry ginger, clove, cayenne, cardamon, cinnamon, rosemary, turmeric, star anise and nutmeg.
Kidney	clove, fenugreek, fennel seed, black pepper, cinnamon bark, dry ginger, rosemary, star anise, walnut, chestnut, pistachio, lamb, salmon, black beans, onion, leek, chives, mussel, lamb and beef kidney
Avoid (for all types)	raw fruits and vegetables, sprouts and salads, spinach, tomato, soybean, tofu, glutinous rice, millet, kelp, excessive salt and sweet food, dairy products, vinegar, nuts and seeds, soymilk, refrigerated or iced drinks

BLOOD DEFICIENCY

General principles

Building Blood requires specific nutrients that generate Blood, and adequate absorption of those nutrients. Absorption of nutrients is maximised by encouraging healthy Spleen *qi*. The principles associated with maintaining good Spleen function apply to building Blood.

In addition, Blood building requires a greater protein intake. The best sources of protein for Blood building are animal proteins, in particular chicken. It is possible to build Blood on a vegetarian diet, but the results are much slower. The old adage that it takes '40 parts of *qi* to make 1 part of Blood' applies, and the best Blood foods are those that have concentrated *jing*, the animal proteins. Stocks and soups can be made with organic chicken or beef bones which release pure *jing* from their bone marrow. When animal protein is not appropriate, some form of supplementation, in the form of tablets or liquid, may be useful, at least in the short term.

Green leafy vegetables, that is, those that are chlorophyll rich are especially beneficial, as they not only contain iron, but have other components that assist in the absorption and utilisation of iron, and manufacture of Blood.

Blood quality is also directly affected by the level of additives in food, especially hormones and excessive sugar and salt. Meat should be organic, or at least chemical free. Where this is not possible, it is better to have some lesser quality meat than none at all. When liver is used it must be organic, as the liver concentrates additives in animal feed.

Figure 26.3 *Recommended proportions for building Blood*

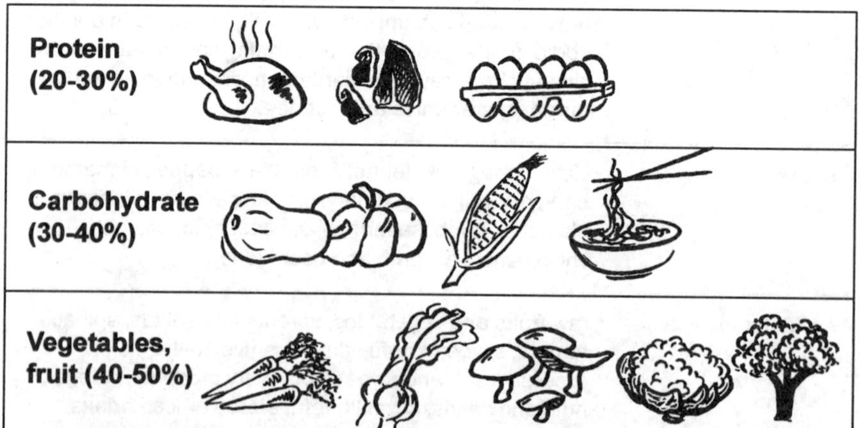

Blood deficiency	
General comments	Same basic approach as for Spleen *qi* deficiency (as the Spleen produces Blood), iron and protein rich food; folic acid and vitamin B_{12}. In strict vegetarian diets, B_{12} may need to be supplemented in tablet form.
Beneficial	high quality protein, meat (especially chicken meat and soup, beef and pork liver and pork trotter), pigeon, oyster, mussel, shark, eel, stocks and broths, bone marrow, eggs, legumes, black bean, green leafy vegetables, wheatgrass, spinach, carrots, beetroot, parsley, molasses, fermented bean products, miso, tempeh, seaweed, spirulina, black sesame seed, lychee, coconut, rice, stout, Guiness, vegemite, marmite
Liver Blood def.	as for general Blood deficiency, plus lycium fruit (gou qi zi, excellent cooked with chicken or in rice porridge)
Restrict or avoid	As for Spleen *qi* deficiency; plus bitter, sour, salty and pungent/hot foods, refined sugars, chemical additives, hormones

Proportions

The emphasis of a Blood building diet should be towards green leafy vegetable matter (~30-40%) and high quality, preferably organic, animal, protein (~20-30%), with around 30-40% as complex carbohydrates (rice, wheat, oat, starchy root vegetables, etc.). As the Blood is replenished the overall proportions of the diet can be altered to reflect the general Spleen strengthening proportions.

YIN DEFICIENCY

General principles

In treating *yin* deficiency, we recommend foods which supply concentrated nutrition to maintain or improve tissue integrity, and encourage increased fluid and moisture levels. In general principles the *yin* nourishing diet is similar to that used to nourish Blood–a higher proportion of protein, a wide range of green leafy and root vegetables and the more nourishing grains such as wheat. In addition, moistening and lubricating elements are useful. The concentrated nutrition and oils in seeds and beans both build and lubricate. Animal proteins are ideal, although excessive amounts or highly concentrated forms such as eggs, cheese and bone marrow, can cause overheating and Phlegm accumulation. It is wise to use a mixture of soy and leguminous proteins, and animal proteins.

As with the manufacture of *qi* and Blood, *yin* must be extracted from food by the Spleen and Stomach. The diet therefore follows the previously mentioned principles for maintaining a healthy Spleen, with the addition of some specific foods.

The foods listed in the beneficial section are suitable for all types of *yin* deficiency. Those listed under the various subheadings are thought to be especially good for the relevant organ system, however there is a degree of overlap and the distinctions should not be relied upon too much.

Proportions

Complex carbohydrates from a grain or vegetable source, and green leafy vegetables, watery vegetables and fruits should be in about equal proportions.

Figure 26.4 *Recommended proportions for nourishing yin*

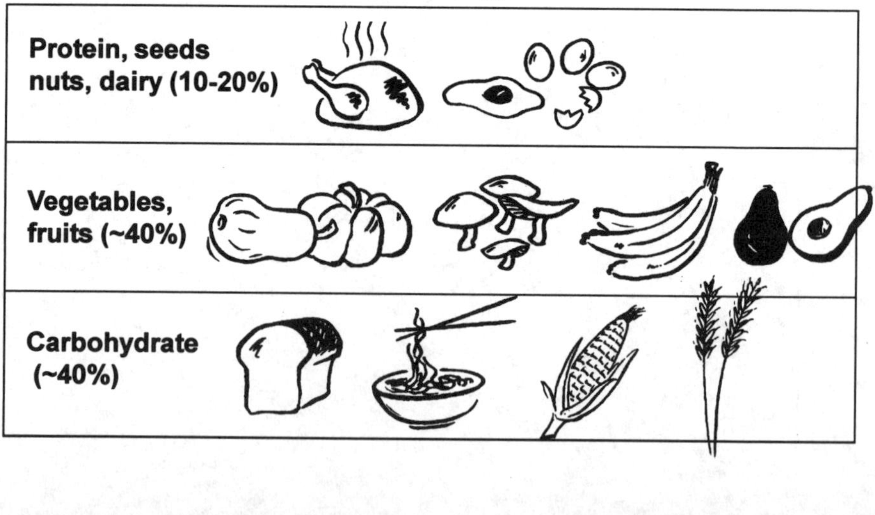

Yin deficiency	
General comments	The focus of a *yin* nourishing diet is towards concentrated nourishment: seeds and beans, a higher proportion of high quality protein. Use plenty of water in cooking, lots of soups and stews.
Beneficial	wheat, oats, rice, millet, barley, pork, chicken, duck, pigeon, bone marrow, eggs, butter, milk and cheese in small amounts, yogurt, tofu, tempeh, nuts and seeds, spanish mackerel, sardine, oyster, mussel, clam, cuttlefish, squid, kelp, spirulina, zucchini, marrow, squash, potato, sweet potato, melon, string bean, beetroot, mushroom, white and black fungus (wood ears), aduki beans, black beans, apple, banana, mulberry, mango, coconut, mung bean, peanut, olive oil, flaxseed oil, almond oil
Stomach *yin*	slippery elm powder, white wood ears, barley, millet, tofu, mung beans, asparagus, sweet potato, butter, milk, orange, mandarin, lychee, apple, banana, pineapple, plum, pomegranate
Lung *yin*	pears, peach, apple, banana, fig, pawpaw, strawberry, tomato, string bean, seaweed, kelp, white and black fungus (wood ears), spirulina, soy milk, tofu, tempeh, pork, oyster, butter, milk, cheese, pine nuts
Kidney *yin*	pork, pork kidney, duck, millet, barley, tofu, string bean, black bean, black soybean, kidney bean, black sesame seed, blueberry, blackberry, seaweed, black fungus (wood ears)
Restrict or avoid	warming, drying, bitter, pungent items: chillies, curry and spices, cinnamon, garlic, ginger, onion, shallots (scallion), leeks, basil, clove, wasabi, coffee, lamb, prawns (shrimp), veal, pigeon, game birds, vinegar, citrus, pickles, coffee, tea, cigarettes, alcohol, vitamin B, corticosteroids, recreational stimulants (amphetamines, cocaine, ecstasy), non steroidal anti-inflammatories (Stomach *yin*)

The remainder is made up of high quality proteins (legume and animal protein), and nuts and seeds. Small amounts of good quality dairy products such as organic cheese, cow or goat milk, yogurt and butter are beneficial, especially when there is dryness.

LIVER QI STAGNATION

General principles

Qi stagnation is mostly associated with dysfunction of the Liver. From a biomedical point of view, the liver is the detoxification factory of the body and all substances that enter the gastro-intestinal system initially pass through the liver. The liver processes and metabolises natural and synthetic compounds. With the ever increasing load of synthetic substances (preservatives, colouring agents, pharmaceuticals and so on) in the modern diet, the liver is often overloaded. This can contribute to some of the symptoms we recognise in TCM as Liver *qi* stagnation.

The Liver can be affected by the ingestion of too much food or by eating too frequently, before the previous meal has been processed. Even though the primary organ of digestion is the Spleen, it is the Liver that regulates the timing and distribution of resources to the Spleen, so that it can function efficiently. Overloading the Spleen will have a knock on effect on the movement of Liver *qi*.

Astringing and congesting foods should be avoided if there is Liver *qi* stagnation. Foods which have a mild pungent, dispersing nature should be favoured. Patients should eat less (leave the table feeling as though they could continue eating) and take the last meal in the late afternoon or early evening. Turbulent or volatile emotions at meal times are especially detrimental, and meals should be eaten in a calm and relaxed environment.

Proportions

The emphasis of the diet should be towards vegetable matter, with plenty of

Figure 26.5 *Recommended proportions for alleviating Liver qi stagnation*

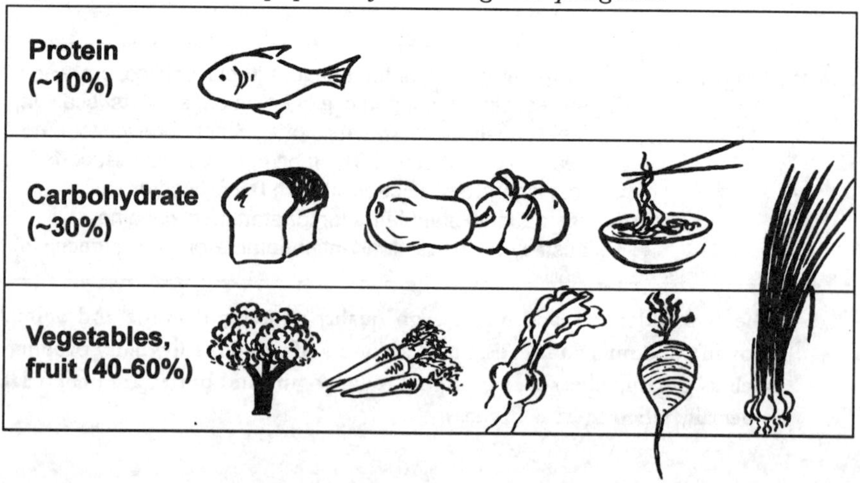

Qi stagnation	
General comments	**Yes:** eat less; main meals earlier in the day; concentrate on light and mildly spicy foods; stir fry, poaching and steaming; high vegetable, low carbohydrate, low meat **No:** processed, junk or adulterated food; unnecessary drugs or intoxicants; eating when upset or under pressure, skipping meals, eating quickly, overeating
Beneficial	**Mild dispersing, pungent flavours:** spices, onions, garlic, mustard greens, watercress, turmeric, basil, mint, peppermint, horseradish, pepper, cardamon, cumin, fennel, dill, ginger, small quantities of grape or rice wine (red is best), coffee (1 per day); care with the warming foods when there is stagnant Heat. **Sour flavours (small amounts):** citrus, vinegar, pickles, sour cherry, plums **Other:** plenty of fresh vegetables, some fruits; sprouted grains, asparagus, taro, cabbage, turnip, cauliflower, broccoli, brussel sprouts, beetroot, jerusalem artichoke, sourdough rye bread, extra virgin olive oil, molasses, small amounts of high quality meat protein and fish
Restrict or avoid	**Food high in saturated fats and oils:** cheese, eggs, cream, ice cream, red meats, lard, shortening, margarine, nuts, pizza, hot chips **Excessively hot and pungent flavours:** hot chillies and peppers, spirits **Excessive cold or refrigerated food:** ice cream, beer, salads and raw vegetable juices, white wine **Artificial, synthetic substances:** preservatives, colourings, pharmaceuticals (as appropriate)

greens, yellows and reds, complemented by the pungent, dispersing items noted above. Lightly spiced foods, such as curries and Asian style dishes help circulate the *qi*. Carbohydrates and proteins should be secondary, together constituting less than half the diet.

DAMPNESS AND PHLEGM

General principles

To treat Dampness and Phlegm, with diet two aspects must be considered. Firstly, foods which create Dampness and Phlegm, such as dairy, processed carbohydrates, sweets and rich or overly supplementing foods, should be avoided. Secondly, a diet which supports peak Spleen and Stomach function must be adhered to.

Where complete removal of offending foods is too restrictive, certain modifications and combinations can be made. Specifically, bitter, pungent or drying foods can be added to rich or cloying foods to prevent Dampness from forming. Common examples of this approach include combining meats with mustard, horseradish or bitter and pungent vegetables such as turnips and pumpkin, using pungent toppings on pasta (made with plenty of onions and garlic, or pesto), combining cheese and chutney, sipping wine with meat meals, green tea with fried food, and selecting bitter ales. With a little thought, it is actually quite easy to modify a typical western diet so that it is less deleterious and Damp generating.

Proportions

Carbohydrates should be used moderately as they tend to be sweet, and an excessive amount can create or aggravate Dampness. In general, between 30-40% of the dietary bulk can be composed of carbohydrates. The best sources are the more drying varieties–rice, rye, barley, millet and oats.

Vegetables, with a mixture of sweet, bitter and pungent varieties, can make up 40-50% of the diet. The remainder can be a small amount of high

Figure 26.6 *Recommended proportions for drying and transforming Dampness and Phlegm*

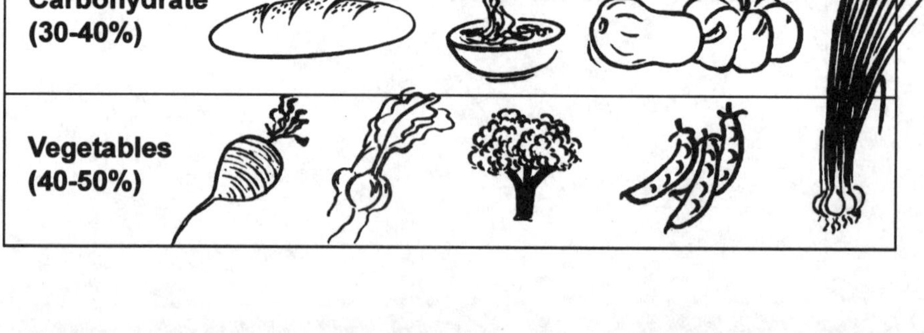

Dampness and Phlegm

General comments	The general principles and foods that apply to maintaining healthy Spleen *qi* are also applicable. **Yes:** Emphasise bitter and pungent flavours; all food cooked and warm; low intake of fats and oils, dairy and sugar; eat less at each sitting **No:** late night meals, deep fried and junk food.
Beneficial	buckwheat, barley, corn, rye, sourdough bread, caraway rye, pumpernickel, dry roasted oats, lettuce, celery, pumpkin, onion, shallot (scallion), garlic, turnip, watercress, aduki bean, broad bean, radish, extra virgin olive oil, mustard, horseradish, quail, clam, lean meat, white and black pepper, clove, cardamon, nutmeg, dill seed, coriander (cilantro) leaf, oregano, thyme, basil, fresh ginger **Sparingly:** sweet potato, yams, kumera, potato, red and green tea
Lungs, sinuses	radish, daikon, turnip, onion, shallot (scallion), garlic, mustard greens, horseradish, ginger, fenugreek, fennel seed, cayenne, watercress
Urinary Bladder	aduki bean, fennel seed, ginger, fenugreek, peas
Restrict or avoid	wheat, ice cream and dairy products (except raw goat's milk and yogurt), sugar and concentrated sweeteners, fatty meat (especially pork and duck), eggs, tofu, tempeh, soy milk, lard, butter, margarine, chocolate, nuts and seeds (especially peanuts), avocado, raw and dried fruit (especially banana and tropical fruits), salt, vinegar, beer

quality animal protein, around 10% is right. Soy proteins, especially tofu, can be too cooling and moistening when used in excessive amounts. Nuts and seeds should be avoided.

HEAT, FIRE

General principles

Bitter, cool, pungent foods are beneficial. In general, a higher proportion of raw foods–vegetables and fruits–is appropriate. This approach to diet is also beneficial for people who are constitutionally hot or *yang* excess, even in the absence of specific symptoms.

Acute Heat patterns

During acute Heat patterns, such as those characterised by acute fever, sweating and thirst, keeping up fluids is essential. The best strategy is to use plenty of liquids like fruit and vegetable juices, herbal teas and broths or light soups. Warm or room temperature liquids are preferred. Iced or cold liquids should be avoided as they can impact negatively on the Spleen.

During an attack of Wind Heat, the Heat is trapped in the superficial layers of the body (*wei* level) and requires opening of the pores (diaphoresis) to release the pathogen. Wind Heat patterns are acute and self limiting, so dietary approaches are generally only used for a few days. Pungent, cool, dispersing foods are useful as teas or in soups, particularly peppermint, pear, radish, watercress and cabbage. Warming and supplementing foods, such as lamb, beef, chicken, shellfish and warming spices should be avoided.

Chronic Heat patterns

Cooking methods that increase the warming thermal nature of foods, such as roasting, frying and deep frying are not appropriate. Light cooking, such as steaming and stir frying is recommended. Some whole raw foods are useful (except in Stomach Heat, *see* below), relative to any accompanying degree of deficiency. Combine raw foods with cooked foods, or use light

Figure 26.7 *Recommended proportions for cooling Heat*

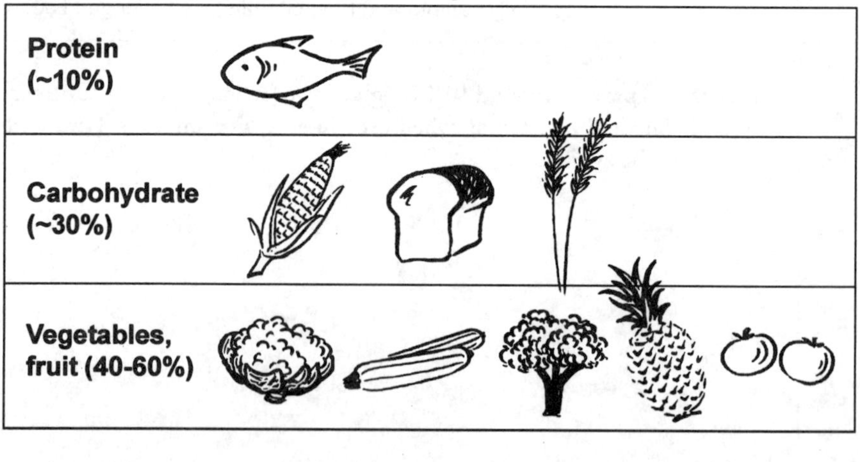

Heat, Fire	
General comments	Yes: short cooking times, cooking in plenty of water, steaming, stir frying; water soups with plenty of vegetables, some raw foods (especially salad items, sprouts, juices); more liquids in general No: deep frying, BBQ or roasting; overeating
Beneficial	celery, spinach, swiss chard, cucumber, lettuce, radish, asparagus, eggplant (aubergine), savoy and chinese cabbage, tomato, broccoli, cauliflower, zucchini, apple, pear, watermelon, millet, wheat, barley, tofu, tempeh, soy milk, yogurt, mung bean and alfalfa sprouts, kelp, spirulina, crab
Stomach Heat	Mucilaginous foods to cool, moisten and line the Stomach: rice, barley, millet or oat porridge, banana, avocado, cucumber, spinach, lettuce, rocket (arugula), watercress, cabbage (juiced as well as cooked), tofu, soy milk, yogurt
Liver Heat	peppermint, mung beans and sprouts, celery, radish, daikon, kelp, lettuce, dandelion, cucumber, watercress, millet, tofu
Heat in the Lungs	watercress, apple, pear, peach, strawberry, lemon, radish, carrot, pumpkin, cabbage, cauliflower, spinach, swiss chard, white fungus (wood ear)
Heat in the Blood	Cooling and haemostatic foods for bleeding: eggplant (aubergine), spinach, swiss chard, persimmon, lemon, celery, lettuce, olive
Restrict or avoid	chillies, cinnamon, ginger, black pepper, garlic, mustard, horseradish, coffee, chocolate, heated (usually cheap) vegetable oils, red meat (especially lamb), chicken, alcohol, vinegar, prawns, mantis shrimp, cheese, eggs, excessive salt, peanuts

blanching to slightly warm food while retaining freshness.

Avoid heating and stimulating substances, in particular alcohol, coffee, red meats, rich, creamy food and deep fried food. Diuretic foods such as celery, cucumber and beetroot, are useful to stimulate urination and provide an escape route for the Heat.

Stomach Heat

In Stomach and Intestinal Heat patterns, whole raw foods may be too physically abrasive and irritating to already inflamed tissues. Juices are generally well tolerated. Other foods may need to be well cooked and soft, or even mashed in severe cases, until the Heat and inflammation clears and the Stomach strengthens.

Damp Heat

The principles are similar to those applicable to the Heat clearing and Damp drying diet, depending on the mixture of Dampness and Heat. Proportions are similar to those for Heat in general, with a little less carbohydrate (20-30%) and more pulses and soy proteins in place of animal proteins. Raw foods may or may not be appropriate depending on the degree of Dampness present. Individuals will vary in their responses, and experimentation with varying mixtures of raw, cooked and carbohydrate rich food is necessary.

Damp Heat

General comments	Eat less; light simple foods, some raw foods and juices; plenty of lightly cooked leafy greens
Beneficial	millet, wheat, barley, aduki beans, celery, carrot, spinach, swiss chard, eggplant (aubergine), chinese cabbage, tomato, broccoli, peas, cauliflower, asparagus, lemon, cranberry, watercress, rocket (arugula), lettuce, radish, daikon, legumes, mung bean and alfalfa sprouts, tofu, tempeh, green and red tea, water Sparingly: olive oil, root vegetables
Liver/Gallbladder	mung bean, mung bean and alfalfa sprouts, celery, kelp, lettuce, tofu, leafy greens, shiitake mushroom, peppermint tea, chrysanthemum tea, dandelion tea
Urinary Bladder	aduki bean, mung bean, barley water, celery, asparagus, diluted lemon juice, cranberry juice, blueberries, watermelon, dandelion tea, green tea
Restrict or avoid	alcohol, greasy or oily food, deep fried food, fatty meat, eggs, cheese, sugar, concentrated sweeteners, chocolate, 'junk food', nuts and seeds (especially peanuts), chillies, cinnamon, ginger, black pepper, garlic, mustard, horseradish, coffee, vinegar, prawns, mantis shrimp, excessive salt

A major feature of a Damp Heat diet is avoidance of the specific foods that aggravate Damp Heat, notably alcohol, cheese, deep fried food and fatty meats.

Phlegm Heat

The general structure of a Phlegm Heat clearing diet is similar to that applicable for Damp Heat. Foods that are specific for Phlegm Heat can be added as appropriate. Phlegm Heat tends to congeal in the Lungs, therefore specific foods with an affinity for the Lungs, such as pears, are helpful.

Phlegm Heat	
General comments	Eat less; light simple foods, some raw foods and juices; plenty of lightly cooked leafy greens
Beneficial	bamboo shoots, watercress, radish, kelp and seaweed, turnip, persimmon, shiitake mushroom, rice milk
Restrict or avoid	all dairy products, ice cream, sugar, fatty, meat, eggs, tofu, tempeh, soy milk, soy sauce, nuts and seeds (especially peanuts), bananas, avocado, pineapple, salt, coffee, alcohol, chocolate

BLOOD STAGNATION

General principles

The main principles of nutrition for Blood stagnation patterns are similar to those of *qi* stagnation. Foods and practices that congest the Liver, impair the circulation of *qi* and Blood, or cool and constrict the vessels should be avoided.

Foods that disperse stagnant Blood are, in general, pungent and/or warming. The warmer elements like cayenne, ginger and garlic should be used with caution when there is complicating Heat or *yin* deficiency. Care must also be taken with an overly dispersing diet when Blood stagnation is complicated or caused by *qi* or *yang* deficiency. In general, Blood stagnation will be a complication of, or be complicated by, other pathologies. In such cases, rather than emphasising Blood moving foods as a primary theme of the diet, a few appropriate foods from the list below can be added to whatever diet is suitable. Of course, if Blood stagnation is the primary pathology, a stronger emphasis may be placed on dispersing foods initially, until the stagnation begins to shift. As the patient improves, the diet can then be adjusted accordingly.

Certain foods are though to be especially beneficial for various types of cancer. This may be because they are salty, and therefore soften hardness and aid in the dispersal of masses, or because they have immune stimulating properties. Others are known to have high levels of natural antioxidants. The addition of one or more of these items to an appropriate diet may be useful.

Blood stagnation	
General comments	The same principles, proportions and foods as for *qi* stagnation. In addition, avoid cold raw foods that freeze and constrict the circulation.
Beneficial	turmeric, shallot (scallion), leek, chives, garlic, ginger, taro, eggplant, basil, cayenne, nutmeg, oregano, rosemary, white pepper, aduki bean, chestnut, crab, red wine
Uterus	eggplant (aubergine), kelp, seaweeds, black fungus (wood ears)

Anticancer	
Generally beneficial	green tea, oolong tea, radish, ginger, pepper, vinegar, light salting, a little wine, watermelon, tomatoes, pears, waterchestnuts, fungus of all kinds (mushrooms, wood ears, etc.), aduki beans, lotus seeds, chinese barley (job's tears)
Salty, to soften masses	crab, jellyfish, kelp, laver, mussel, clam, sea cucumber (beche de mer, trepang), abalone, hawthorn

DRYNESS

General principles

Dryness primarily affects the Lungs and Stomach and their associated structures. Dryness may, or may not, be associated with a deficiency of *yin*. Patients can experience dryness without *yin* deficiency, but rarely *yin* deficiency without some dryness. Normal body fluids are the most superficial of the body's *yin*, and the most easily damaged and replenished. Foods to moisten dryness tend to be lubricating and mucilaginous, and thus are different from those that build *yin*, which tend to be deeply nourishing and protein rich. Some foods that benefit *yin* however will also moisten dryness.

Dryness	
Lungs	small quantities of milk and dairy products such as butter and yogurt, pear, apple, banana, tofu, tempeh and soymilk, barley, millet, black and white fungus (wood ears), almond, pinenut, peanut, sesame seed, eggs, pork, herring
Stomach	white fungus (wood ear), tofu, asparagus, slippery elm powder, barley, millet, rice, sweet rice, oats, roasted barley, mung beans, sweet potato, pear, spirulina, spanish mackerel, sardine
Restrict or avoid	hot, pungent, bitter and dispersing substances; tobacco, chillies, coffee, bitter melon, lemon

CHARACTERISTICS OF COMMON FOODS

Grains

Barley	Sweet, cool; strengthens the Spleen and Stomach, supplements *qi*, dries Dampness, promotes urination. ✔ Weak digestion, poor appetite, convalescence, diarrhoea, difficult or painful urination, oedema, fever with thirst, Summerheat, Spleen deficiency with Damp Heat. ✗ Constipation.
Buckwheat	Sweet, cool; strengthens the Spleen and Stomach, dries Dampness, clears Heat. ✔ Food stagnation with abdominal distension and pain, Spleen deficiency with Damp Heat, chronic diarrhoea, dysenteric disorder, anorectic dysenteric disorder, leucorrhoea.
Corn, maize	Sweet, neutral; strengthens the Spleen and Stomach, promotes urination. ✔ Spleen and Stomach weakness, reduced appetite, difficult urination, oedema.
Millet	Sweet, salty, cool; Benefits the Spleen and Kidneys, clears Heat, promotes urination. ✔ Spleen and Stomach weakness, reduced appetite, diarrhoea, vomiting, indigestion, diabetes, spontaneous sweating, weakness, convalescence. Good for young children.
Oats	Sweet, bitter, warm; strengthens the Spleen and Stomach, supplements *qi*, benefits the Heart. ✔ Spleen and Stomach weakness, generalised deficiency, reduced appetite, nervous debility, dysentery, diabetes, indigestion, abdominal distension. ✗ Can aggravate a tendency to Dampness in some people; avoid combining with sugar and milk, dry roast before cooking.
Rice, white	Sweet, neutral; strengthens the Spleen and Stomach, supplements *qi*. ✔ Spleen and Stomach weakness, generalised weakness, reduced appetite, nausea and vomiting, post febrile *yin* damage, thirst and oral dryness. NB: Rice porridge (congee or jook), is ideal for convalescence and is easily digested. Other properties can be added by including one or more appropriate ingredients. Generally considered to be the most well balanced grain.
Rice, basmati	Similar to white rice, but more fragrant and slightly dispersing, and thus better for Damp accumulation.

Rice, brown	Similar in property to white rice but considerably more difficult to digest. Not suitable for Spleen and Stomach deficiency patterns, Cold accumulation, food stagnation, or digestive weakness of any kind, although prolonged cooking (2 hours+) renders it more easily digested.
Rice, glutinous	Sweet, warm, mildly astringent; strengthens the Spleen and Stomach, supplements *qi*. ✔ Spleen and Stomach weakness, generalised weakness, convalescence, diarrhoea, spontaneous sweating, frequent and excessive urination. ✗ Phlegm Heat patterns.
Rye	Bitter, neutral; dries Dampness, moves Liver *qi*. ✔ Damp conditions, balances Damp foods like cheese, *qi* stagnation conditions (sourdough rye bread).
Wheat	Sweet, cool, mildly astringent; nourishes the Heart, calms the shen. ✔ Heart *qi* deficiency, shen disturbance, spontaneous sweating, night sweats, diabetes, difficult urination with Heat. ✗ Spleen *qi* and *yang* deficiency. NB: Wheat, being cool, may be hard for patients with Spleen deficiency to digest and is best avoided or minimised when there are symptoms of digestive weakness.

Vegetables, vegetable fruits

Alfalfa, sprouts	Bitter, neutral; dries Dampness, promotes urination, benefits the Kidney. ✔ Oedema, osteo-arthritis, urinary tract stones, chronic sore throat, flatulence, gastric ulcers, insufficient lactation. ✗ Spleen *qi* and *yang* deficiency (uncooked), auto-immune disorders.
Artichoke, globe	Bitter, neutral; dries Dampness, benefits the Liver and Gallbladder, stimulate bile secretion, benefits Blood. ✔ Damp conditions, chronic Damp Heat in the Liver, Liver *qi* stagnation, hangover, intolerance to fats and oils, ✗ Not recommended while breast-feeding as the bitterness can pass into the milk.
Artichoke, jerusalem	Sweet; benefits the Spleen, Lungs and Intestines. ✔ Constipation, diabetes, asthma. Reputed to be good for repairing the intestinal lining following damage by antibiotics or nonsteroidal anti-inflammatory drugs (NSAIDS).

Asparagus	Bitter, pungent, cool; promotes urination, increases *yin* fluids, benefits the Kidneys. ✔ Stomach and Kidney *yin* deficiency patterns, Kidney *qi* deficiency, Damp accumulation, oedema, painful urination, urinary dysfunction, constipation. ✗ Too much asparagus may irritate the Kidneys.
Avocado	Sweet, cool; nourishes *yin* and Blood, moistens the Lungs and Intestines. ✔ Dryness of the Lungs, Intestines and skin. ✗ Phlegm Damp.
Bamboo shoot	Sweet, bitter, cold; clears Heat, transforms Phlegm, laxative. ✔ Phlegm Heat cough, Stomach Heat disorders, constipation (uncooked). ✗ Spleen *qi* deficiency, diarrhoea.
Beans (string)	Sweet, neutral; strengthens the Spleen and Kidneys, increases *yin* fluids. ✔ Spleen and Kidney *qi* and *yin* deficiency patterns, dry cough, diabetes, frequent urination, thirst and oral dryness, diarrhoea, leucorrhoea. ✗ Can aggravate a tendency to constipation.
Beetroot	Sweet, neutral; benefits the Liver and Blood, moistens the Intestines, strengthens the Heart. ✔ Liver disorders, *qi* stagnation, Blood deficiency, menopausal symptoms, insomnia, anxiety and nervousness, dry constipation.
Bitter melon	Bitter, cold; clears Heat and Summerheat, improves vision. ✔ Hot diseases, Summerheat, Liver Heat eye disorders ✗ Spleen *qi* and *yang* deficiency
Broccoli	Sweet, bitter, neutral; clears Summerheat, benefits the Liver, alleviates stagnant *qi*, improves vision. ✔ abdominal pain, gastric ulcers, eye inflammation, visual weakness, thirst and fever during a Summerheat disorder.
Brussel sprouts	Similar to savoy cabbage.
Cabbage, savoy	Sweet, pungent, warm; moistens the Intestines, benefits the Stomach and digestion ✔ Constipation, common cold, whooping cough (soup); intestinal parasites, gastric ulcers (fresh juice); mastitis and skin eruptions (topical).

Cabbage, Chinese	Sweet, cool; clears Heat, promotes urination. ✔ Lung and Stomach Heat, thirst, cough, constipation, painful or difficult urination (juice or in soup). ✗ Spleen *qi* deficiency (uncooked).
Capsicum	Sweet, cool; benefits digestion, supplements *qi*. ✔ Digestive weakness, reduced appetite, indigestion, poor circulation. ✗ Spleen *qi* and *yang* deficiency (uncooked).
Carrot	Sweet, neutral; Strengthens the Spleen and aids digestion, benefits the Liver, improves vision, directs *qi* downwards, stops cough. ✔ Indigestion, weak digestion, abdominal distension, constipation, diarrhoea (well cooked), visual weakness, night blindness; Lung Heat cough and whooping cough (fresh juice), assists in the rash disorders of childhood (measles and chicken pox), dysentery (grated uncooked). ✗ Spleen *yang* deficiency (uncooked and juiced). The juice is quite sweet and excessive consumption may aggravate Dampness.
Cauliflower	Similar to broccoli (and other members of the Brassica family).
Celery	Sweet, pungent, cool; cools the Liver, clears Heat, promotes urination and dries Dampness, directs Stomach *qi* downwards. ✔ Heat patterns and excess *yang* affecting the Liver and Stomach causing high blood pressure, red, sore eyes, gum disease, headaches, vomiting, childhood fever, painful and turbid urination, blood in the urine, mouth ulcers, hangover. Used uncooked, juiced and lightly cooked in stir fries.
Chilli	Pungent, hot; warms the Spleen and Stomach, dispels Cold, dries Dampness, diaphoretic, benefits the Lungs. ✔ Spleen and Stomach *yang* deficiency, abdominal pain, watery diarrhoea, Cold Damp or Phlegm congestion in the Lungs and digestive system, Cold Damp *bi* syndrome, Wind Cold exterior pattern. ✗ Yin deficiency, internal Heat, bleeding, haemorrhoids, gastric ulcers, dry cough, tendency to boils, eczema and psoriasis.
Chive	Pungent, sweet, warm; warms and strengthens Kidney *yang*, warms the Stomach (lightly cooked), eliminates stagnant Blood (uncooked). ✔ Impotence, frequent urination, nocturia, lower back ache, dysphagia, regurgitation, reduced appetite, chest pain. ✗ Yin deficiency, internal Heat, boils and skin disorders, eye disorders.

Coriander	Also known as cilantro. Pungent, warm; Regulates *qi*, benefits the Stomach, diaphoretic. ✔ reduced appetite, nausea, Wind Cold exterior pattern, early stage of measles, incomplete expression of measles ✗ Eye disease.
Cucumber	Sweet, cool; clears Heat, stops thirst, promotes urination. ✔ Summerheat invasion, oedema, difficult urination, Stomach Heat. ✗ Spleen *yang* deficiency, diarrhoea, Phlegm Damp.
Eggplant	Also known as aubergine. Sweet, cool; clears Heat, cools the Blood and stops bleeding, eliminates stagnant Blood, laxative. ✔ Bleeding haemorrhoids, rectal bleeding, Intestinal Wind, blood in the urine, stagnant Blood in the uterus, dysmenorrhoea, fibroids, tendency to constipation. ✗ Pregnancy (thought to contribute to miscarriage).
Garlic	Pungent, sweet, warm; warms the Spleen and Stomach, improves digestion, kills parasites. ✔ Intestinal worms, amoebic and bacterial dysentery, Wind Cold exterior pattern, sore throat (uncooked); whooping cough, TB (in porridge); indigestion (pickled). ✗ Yin deficiency, internal Heat, boils and skin disorders, eye disorders.
Ginger	Pungent, warm; warms the Spleen, Stomach and Lungs, stops vomiting, diaphoretic. ✔ Nausea, weak digestion, reduced appetite, Spleen *qi* and *yang* deficiency, Lung congestion, productive cough, Phlegm Damp accumulation, Wind Cold exterior pattern ✗ Eye disease, *yin* deficiency, internal Heat, haemorrhoids.
Kelp, kombu	Salty, cold; moistens dryness, increases *yin* fluids, softens hardness, transforms Phlegm and clears Phlegm Heat, promotes urination. ✔ Phlegm type nodules and swellings, goitre, prostate swelling, lymphatic swelling, hypertension, oedema, dysphagia, testicular swelling and pain, shan *qi* disorders. ✗ Pregnancy, Spleen *qi* and *yang* deficiency, emaciated patients.
Leek	Pungent, sour, warm; regulates *qi* and Blood, warms the Spleen and Stomach, stops bleeding, benefits the Liver. ✔ Dysphagia, chronic diarrhoea and dysentery, rectal bleeding, bleeding haemorrhoids.

Lettuce	Bitter, sweet, cool; promotes urination, dries Dampness. ✔ Oedema, haemorrhoids, blood in the urine, difficult urination, insufficient lactation. ✗ Spleen *qi* and *yang* deficiency, eye disease.
Mustard greens	Pungent, warm; transforms Phlegm, regulates *qi*, warms the Spleen and Stomach, dispels Cold, diaphoretic. ✔ Cold Phlegm congestion in the Lungs, productive cough, reduced appetite, nausea and vomiting, Wind Cold exterior pattern. ✗ Eye disease, boils, haemorrhoids, internal Heat.
Onion	Pungent, warm; transforms Phlegm, stimulates the Lungs, benefits digestion, regulates *qi* and Blood. ✔ Phlegm congestion in the Lungs and sinuses, Damp accumulation, Wind Cold exterior pattern, high blood pressure.
Parsley	Pungent, warm, bitter, salty; improves digestion, promotes urination, strengthens the teeth. ✔ Kidney and urinary problems, weak digestion, indigestion, dental problems, incomplete expression of measles. ✗ Not recommended during lactation as it can dry up milk.
Peas	Sweet, neutral; strengthens the Spleen, harmonises the Liver and Spleen, directs Stomach *qi* downwards. ✔ hiccoughs, vomiting, belching, constipation.
Potato	Sweet, neutral; strengthens the Spleen and Stomach, benefits *qi*, stops pain. ✔ Weak Spleen and Stomach, *qi* deficiency, indigestion; epigastric and abdominal pain, gastric ulcers (fresh juice). ✗ Avoid green and sprouted potatoes, which contain the toxic alkaloid solanine.
Pumpkin	Sweet, bitter, neutral; strengthens the Spleen and Stomach, benefits *qi*, dries Dampness, transforms Phlegm, aids in discharge of pus, expels worms (pumpkin seeds). ✔ Weak Spleen and Stomach, *qi* deficiency, Phlegm congestion, chronic asthma, chronic Heat and Phlegm Heat in the Lungs, roundworms (seeds), diabetes, helps to stabilise foetus in the womb.
Radish, red & daikon	Pungent, sweet, cool; clears Heat, transforms Phlegm, cools the Blood, promotes urination, directs *qi* downwards, improves digestion. ✔ Phlegm Heat cough, Heat in the Lungs, febrile illness, diabetes, painful urination, urinary tract stones, difficult urination (juice); indigestion, abdominal distension, mucus congestion (cooked).

	✗ Spleen deficiency (uncooked); concurrent use with supplementing herbs, especially ginseng.
Shallot (scallion)	Pungent, warm; diaphoretic, promotes circulation of *yang qi* in the chest, dispels Cold. ✔ Wind Cold exterior pattern, Cold type abdominal pain, abdominal pain from worm infestation, mastitis and boils (crushed and applied topically as well). Use uncooked or added at the very end of cooking. ✗ Weak patients with spontaneous sweating.
Spinach	Sweet, cool; moistens and lubricates the Intestines, clears Heat, increases *yin* fluids and stops thirst, nourishes the Liver and improves vision. ✔ Constipation from dryness, deficiency and in the elderly, diabetes, Stomach Heat and *yin* deficiency, Liver Heat or *yin* deficiency visual disorders. ✗ Because spinach is rich in oxalic acid, it should avoided by those prone to kidney stones. Should not be cooked with calcium rich items, such as tofu, to avoid excessive calcium oxalate formation.
Squash, Summer	Sweet, cool; increase *yin* fluids, promote urination. ✔ Summerheat disorders, oedema, difficult urination. ✗ Spleen *qi* and *yang* deficiency.
Squash, Winter	Sweet, warm, strengthens the Spleen and Stomach, benefits *qi*. ✔ Weak Spleen and Stomach, *qi* deficiency.
Sweet potato	Also known as yam or kumera. Sweet, neutral or cool (uncooked); strengthens the Spleen and Stomach, laxative, (cooked), increases *yin* fluids. ✔ Weak Spleen and Stomach, *qi* deficiency, insufficient lactation, visual weakness, constipation; fever and thirst (uncooked). ✗ Spleen *qi* and *yang* deficiency (uncooked). As sweet potatoes are very sweet, overuse (both uncooked and cooked) can aggravate Dampness and cause indigestion and abdominal distension.
Taro	Sweet, pungent, neutral, slightly toxic; strengthens the Spleen and Stomach, invigorates *qi* and Blood, dissipates nodules. ✔ Reduced appetite, weak digestion, nodules in the neck. ✗ Always used cooked as uncooked taro is slightly toxic and irritates mucus membranes. Overuse can cause *qi* stagnation and weaken the Spleen.
Tomato	Sweet, sour, cool; clears Heat, increases *yin* fluids, cools the Blood, benefits the Liver. ✔ Post febrile Stomach *yin* deficiency, thirst and oral dryness;

	Liver *yin* deficiency visual disorders, dry eyes and night blindness; epistaxis, bleeding gums; May be used in sauces, uncooked or juiced. Cooked tomatoes are thought to be good for some types of cancer (especially prostate) due to high antioxidant content.
Turnip	Pungent, sweet, bitter, neutral; invigorates *qi* and Blood, diaphoretic, transforms Phlegm, dries Dampness, benefits digestion. ✔ Indigestion, Phlegm congestion in the Lungs and sinuses, wheezing, diabetes, Spleen Damp. Light cooking retains the therapeutic benefit.
Watercress	Pungent, bitter, cool; clears Heat and Dampness, promotes urination, regulates *qi*. ✔ Jaundice, painful urination, Phlegm Heat cough, sore throat, halitosis, flatulence, *qi* and Damp Heat accumulation in the Spleen and Stomach. Used uncooked in salads, juices or lightly cooked in soup. ✗ Frequent urination, nocturia, incontinence.
Zucchini	*See* Summer squash.

Fruit

(used uncooked unless otherwise specified; cooking increases warmth)

Apple	Sweet, sour, cool; increases *yin* fluids and stops thirst; clears Heat, benefits the Spleen and Stomach, stops diarrhoea. ✔ Indigestion, reduced appetite, diarrhoea, indeterminate gnawing hunger; fever and thirst, hangover, Lung Heat from cigarettes.
Apricot	Sweet, sour, neutral; moistens the Lungs, increases *yin* fluids. ✔ Dryness of the Lungs and throat, thirst, dry cough, chronic wheezing, constipation. ✗ Diarrhoea, Phlegm Damp congestion. Overconsumption can damage the teeth and aggravate skin problems, boils and eczema.
Banana	Sweet, cool, astringent (unripe); benefits Stomach and Intestinal *yin*, increases *yin* fluids, moistens dryness. ✔ Stomach *yin* deficiency, thirst, oral dryness, indeterminate gnawing hunger, febrile illness, high blood pressure, constipation, bleeding haemorrhoids, dryness of the Lungs, dry cough (fresh, ripe); diarrhoea (steamed unripe). ✗ Diarrhoea (ripe), Phlegm Damp congestion.
Cherry	Sweet, warm; strengthens the Spleen, benefits *qi* and Blood,

	expels Wind Cold Damp. ✔ Joint pain, arthritis, gout, Cold bi syndrome, Blood deficiency.
Date	Sweet, neutral; strengthens and supplements Spleen *qi*, nourishes Blood, moistens the Lungs and Intestines. ✔ Digestive weakness, *qi* deficiency, reduced appetite, fatigue, dizziness, dry cough, dry type constipation. ✗ Dates are very sweet and should be used sparingly as they can aggravate Phlegm Damp conditions and cause abdominal distension.
Fig	Sweet, neutral; strengthens the Spleen and Stomach, moistens the Lungs and Intestines. ✔ Indigestion, digestive weakness, dry cough, sore throat, postpartum weakness and insufficient lactation, dry type constipation, bleeding haemorrhoids. ✗ Phlegm Damp conditions.
Grape	Sweet, sour, neutral; supplements the Liver and Kidney, benefits *qi* and Blood, increases *yin* fluids, promotes urination. ✔ Lower back ache and weakness, palpitations, nightsweats, thirst, oral dryness, hepatitis, oedema, concentrated urine, difficult and painful urination, blood in the urine, joint pain, arthritis. ✗ Excessive use may weaken the eyes.
Grapefruit	Sweet, sour, cool; stimulates digestion, directs *qi* downwards. ✔ Indigestion, flatulence, belching, hangover, reduced appetite during pregnancy. ✗ An excessive amount of grapefruit can damage *yin* and Blood.
Lemon, lime	Very sour, astringent, cool; clears Heat and Summerheat, increases *yin* fluids, benefits the Stomach and Liver. ✔ Summerheat disorder, Stomach Heat with thirst, nausea, vomiting, morning sickness, Phlegm Heat cough, indigestion, flatulence. ✗ An excessive amount of lemon or lime can damage *yin* and Blood, and aggravate dryness. May aggravate gastric ulcers.
Lychee	Sweet, sour, warm; increases *yin* fluids and stops thirst, supplements Spleen *qi*, benefits Blood. ✔ Stomach *yin* deficiency thirst and oral dryness, indeterminate gnawing hunger (fresh); weak digestion, reduced appetite, nausea, vomiting, diarrhoea (dried); Blood deficiency, insomnia, palpitations, dizziness (with rice porridge). ✗ Yin deficiency with lots of Heat, excess Heat patterns.
Mandarin	Sweet, sour, cool; increases *yin* fluids, promotes urination. ✔ Stomach Heat, thirst, oral dryness, hangover, difficult urination.

	✗ Spleen and Stomach deficiency, Cold type cough.
Mango	Sweet, sour, cool; clears Heat and sedates *yang*, increases *yin* fluids and stops thirst, promotes urination ✔ Hot type oedema and difficult urination; Stomach *yin* deficiency, thirst, nausea and vomiting, Summerheat disorders. Used in large quantities in India to eliminate intestinal parasities ✗ Thought to be slightly toxic. Common cold, indigestion; overconsuption may cause itching and skin rash
Mulberry	Sweet, sour, cold; directs *qi* downward, supplements *qi* and Blood, clears Heat, nourishes the Liver and Kidneys, extinguishes Wind, laxative ✔ *Yin* and Blood deficiency visual problems, dizziness, insomnia, diabetes, constipation, anaemia, high blood pressure. ✗ Spleen deficiency, diarrhoea.
Orange	Sweet, sour, cool; benefits digestion, increases *yin* fluid, directs *qi* downwards. ✔ Stomach *qi* and *yin* deficiency, thirst and oral dryness, indeterminate gnawing hunger, hangover, reduced appetite, nausea, vomiting, arthritis. ✗ Wind Cold exterior pattern, Phlegm Damp cough. Oranges can cause irritability, restlessness and allergic symptoms in children and should be limited.
Pawpaw	Also known as papaya. Sweet, bitter, neutral; benefits the Stomach and digestion, moistens the Lungs, transforms Phlegm, kills worms. ✔ Indigestion, dysentery, Phlegm congestion, joint pain; Intestinal parasites (unripe fruit and seeds).
Peach	Sweet, sour, neutral; benefits the Stomach, moistens the Lungs and Intestines, increases *yin* fluids. ✔ Stomach *yin* deficiency, indeterminate gnawing hunger, constipation, dry cough. Used both fresh and stewed.
Pear	Sweet, sour, cool; clears Heat, increases *yin* fluids, moistens dryness and benefits the Lungs. ✔ Thirst and dehydration during fever, diabetes, Lung Heat or dryness cough and sore dry throat, hoarse voice, dysphagia, constipation, hangover. ✗ Spleen *qi* and *yang* deficiency, diarrhoea, cough without Heat or dryness.
Persimmon	Sweet, astringent (unripe), cool; moistens and cools the Lungs and transforms Phlegm, astringes the Intestines, increases *yin* fluids and stops thirst.

	✔ Lung Heat or dryness cough, Stomach *yin* deficiency and dryness, mouth ulcers, indeterminate gnawing hunger (ripe fruit); chronic diarrhoea and dysentery, bleeding from the bowel, bleeding haemorrhoids, haemoptysis, haematemesis, haematuria (diarrhoea & bleeding, use the unripe fruit). ✗ Spleen *qi* and *yang* deficiency (ripe), Phlegm Damp cough.
Pineapple	Sweet, sour, cold; increases *yin* fluids and stops thirst, promotes urination. ✔ Hot type oedema and difficult urination; Stomach *yin* deficiency, thirst, reduced appetite, nausea and vomiting, Summerheat disorders. ✗ Gastric ulcers. Excess can cause mouth ulcers and damage the teeth.
Plum	Sweet, sour, cool; cools the Liver, increases *yin* fluids. ✔ Liver Heat and *yin* deficiency patterns, bone steaming, constipation, thirst, oral dryness, hypochondriac pain. ✗ Gastric ulcers, Spleen deficiency, weak digestion.
Pomegranate	Sweet, sour, astringent, neutral; increases *yin* fluids, stops thirst, astringes the Intestines and stops diarrhoea. ✔ Stomach *yin* deficiency and dryness, thirst, indeterminate gnawing hunger, gingivitis, mouth ulcers; chronic diarrhoea and dysentery, leucorrhoea, rectal prolapse (pomegranate skin).
Strawberry	Sweet, sour, cool; moistens the Lungs, increases *yin* fluids. ✔ Sore dry throat, hoarse voice, thirst, reduced appetite, difficult urination. ✗ Wind Damp Heat *bi* syndrome, gout
Watermelon	Sweet, cold; clears Heat and Summerheat, increases *yin* fluids, stops thirst, promotes urination. ✔ Summerheat disorders, fever with thirst and dryness, Heart Fire, mouth and tongue ulcers, painful, scanty and difficult urination. ✗ Spleen *qi* and *yang* deficiency, frequent urination.

Fungi

Black fungus	Also known as black wood ears. Sweet, neutral; moisten the Lungs and increase *yin* fluids, stop bleeding. ✔ Lung *yin* deficiency dry cough and wheezing, mild haemoptysis, rectal bleeding, bleeding haemorrhoids, uterine bleeding, vomiting blood; Stomach *yin* deficiency, thirst, oral dryness, constipation. ✗ Loose stools or diarrhoea. Less cloying then white fungus.

Button mushroom	Sweet, cool; supplements Spleen *qi*, moistens dryness, nourishes Lung *yin*, transforms Phlegm. ✔ Spleen and Stomach deficiency, reduced appetite, weakness, insufficient lactation, Lung *yin* deficiency dry cough, weak immunity, chronic hepatitis.
Shiitake mushroom	Sweet, neutral; Strengthens the Spleen and Stomach, benefits *qi*. ✔ Spleen and Stomach deficiency, reduced appetite, weakness and fatigue, frequent urination, diabetes, hypertension, chronic hepatitis, leucopenia, high cholesterol, stomach and cervical cancer, weak immunity.
White fungus	Also known as white wood ears. Sweet, neutral; nourishes *yin*, moistens the Lungs, increases *yin* fluids, stops bleeding. ✔ Lung *yin* deficiency and dry cough and wheezing, mild haemoptysis, rectal bleeding, bleeding haemorrhoids, uterine bleeding, vomiting blood; Stomach *yin* deficiency, thirst, oral dryness, constipation. ✗ Phlegm Damp cough, loose stools or diarrhoea.

Legumes, nuts and seeds

Aduki bean	Sweet, neutral; Strengthens the Spleen, promotes urination, eliminates stagnant Blood. ✔ Spleen deficiency oedema, Heat and Damp Heat type painful urination, diarrhoea, leucorrhoea, Intestinal abscess, haemorrhoids, bleeding from the bowel. ✗ *Yin* deficiency and dryness
Almond	Sweet, warm; regulates Lung *qi*, transforms Phlegm, stops cough, moistens the Intestines. ✔ Cough, wheezing, dry type constipation. ✗ Phlegm Damp, loose stools, diarrhoea.
Black bean	Sweet, warm; benefits the Kidneys, promotes urination, nourishes *yin* and Blood. ✔ Low back and leg aching, infertility, kidney stones, difficult urination, menopausal flushing.
Black sesame	Sweet, neutral; nourishes *yin*, Blood, Liver and Kidneys, moistens the Intestines. ✔ Visual weakness, tinnitus, dizziness, hair loss, grey hair, dry type constipation, insufficient lactation, numbness. ✗ Spleen deficiency, diarrhoea.
Chestnut	Sweet, warm; strengthens the Spleen, Stomach and Kidneys, stops bleeding.

	✔ Spleen deficiency, digestive weakness, diarrhoea, regurgitation, low back ache, weak legs (roasted); haematemesis, bleeding from the bowel, epistaxis (uncooked).
Chick peas	Also known as garbanzo beans. Sweet; benefits the Spleen and *qi*, dries Dampness. ✔ Digestive and *qi* weakness, Damp accumulation.
Coconut	Sweet, warm; nourishes *yin* and Blood. ✔ Weakness, emaciation, malnutrition, dry skin and hair. ✗ Coconut (especially the milk) can generate Phlegm Damp.
Kidney bean	Sweet, neutral; benefits the Kidneys, promotes urination. ✔ Weakness, urinary dysfunction, oedema, diabetes.
Mung bean	Sweet, cool; clears Heat and expels Summerheat, promotes urination, alleviates Toxin. ✔ Acute Summerheat disorder, Heat and Damp Heat painful and difficult urination, Stomach Heat, oedema, dysentery, food poisoning, aconite or croton seed poisoning, lead poisoning, conjunctivitis, high blood pressure. Usually used as a tea.
Mung bean sprouts	Sweet, cold; increase *yin* fluids, clear Heat. ✔ Similar to mung bean, but colder. ✗ Spleen *qi* and *yang* deficiency (uncooked).
Peanut	Sweet, neutral (raw), warm (roasted); supplements Spleen *qi*, moistens the Lungs, benefits *yin*. The whole peanut, including the brown skin, is used. ✔ Postpartum *qi* and Blood deficiency, insufficient lactation (in soup); chronic dry cough, haematuria (uncooked), ✗ Loose stools and diarrhoea, Phlegm Damp, atopic patients
Pinenut	Sweet, warm; moistens the Lungs and Intestines. ✔ Dry cough, constipation.
Pumpkin seed	Sweet, bitter, neutral; kills worms. ✔ Round worm and tapeworm infestation, motion sickness, prostatic swelling, difficult urination.
Soy bean	Sweet, cool; strengthens the Spleen, promotes urination, alleviates toxin. ✔ Qi and Blood deficiency, emaciation, malnutrition, oedema. **NB:** Soy beans are quite difficult to digest which is why they are generally consumed in the more digestible processed and fermented forms (tofu, miso, soy sauce, tempeh). Very young soy beans (in the pod) are digestible and popular steamed in Japan and China as a bar snack.

Soy bean, black	Sweet, neutral; benefits the Spleen and Kidneys, invigorates Blood, promotes urination, expels Wind. ✔ Abdominal distension, oedema, jaundice, diabetes, Wind Damp bi syndrome, postpartum convulsions, boils. ✗ Not suitable for children or severely debilitated patients.
Soymilk	Sweet, cool; benefits the Spleen and Stomach, supplements *qi*. Similar nutritionally to whole soybean, but more digestible. Also used for patterns of dryness, Heat and *yin* deficiency. Excessive use will weaken Spleen *yang* and can generate Dampness.
Sunflower seed	Sweet, neutral; benefits the Spleen, moistens the Intestines. ✔ Constipation, incomplete eruption of measles (as tea).
Tempeh	Sweet, warm; supplements *qi* and Blood. ✔ An excellent source of protein and a good alternative to meat .
Tofu	Sweet, cool; benefits *qi* and *yin*, increases *yin* fluids, moistens dryness, clears Heat. ✔ Chronic or recurrent dysentery, diabetes, damage associated with excessive alcohol consumption, Stomach and Liver Heat, *qi* deficiency; Stomach and Kidney *yin* deficiency, thirst and oral dryness, indeterminate gnawing hunger. ✗ Best in moderate amounts only. Tofu is quite cooling (even when cooked) and can deplete Spleen and Kidney *yang* if overused.
Walnut	Sweet, warm; warms and supplements Kidney *yang*, moistens the Intestines. ✔ Low back and leg aching, frequent urination, impotence, low libido, frequent urination, chronic asthma and cough, urinary tract stones, dry type constipation. ✗ Diarrhoea, Phlegm and Phlegm Heat asthma, *yin* deficiency. Overconsumption can aggravate Heart Fire and cause mouth ulcers.

Animal products

Beef	Sweet, warm; strengthens the Spleen and Stomach, supplements *qi* and Blood. ✔ Spleen and Stomach *qi* and *yang* deficiency, Blood deficiency, anaemia, emaciation, reduced appetite, diarrhoea, general weakness, convalescence, lack of vitality. ✗ Damp Heat conditions, internal Heat, psoriasis, hot skin diseases.
Beef liver	Sweet, neutral; supplements the Liver, nourishes Blood and improves vision. ✔ General Blood deficiency, anaemia, visual problems.

Beef kidney	Sweet, neutral; strengthens the Kidneys. ✔ Impotence, low libido, low back and leg aching.
Beef tripe	Sweet, neutral; strengthens the Spleen and Stomach. ✔ General *qi* deficiency, weak digestion, reduced appetite, convalescence after illness, weakness, loose stools.
Chicken	Sweet, warm; strengthens the Spleen and Stomach, supplements *qi* and Blood, supplements the Kidneys, benefits *jing*. ✔ Postpartum Blood deficiency, insufficient lactation, convalescence, general *qi* and Blood deficiency states, jing deficiency ✗ Excess conditions, residual pathogens. **NB**: The black boned chicken is considered by the Chinese to be nutritionally superior to the ordinary domestic chicken. It has the additional action of clearing deficient Heat to treat night sweats and bone steaming from *yin* and Blood deficiency. It forms the basis of the popular White Phoenix Pills.
Chicken liver	Sweet, warm; supplements the Liver and Kidneys and improves vision. ✔ Liver and Kidney deficiency visual problems, night blindness, childhood gan syndrome.
Chicken egg	Sweet, neutral; nourishes *yin* and Blood. ✔ Convalescence after illness and pregnancy, insufficient lactation, Blood deficiency during pregnancy, diarrhoea, tendency to miscarriage, emaciation. ✗ Phlegm Damp.
Cows milk	Sweet, neutral; moistens dryness, benefits the Lungs and Stomach. ✔ General debility, convalescence, emaciation, *yin* deficient and dry conditions especially of the Lungs, Stomach and Intestines, dry cough, dysphagia, regurgitation, gastric ulcers, constipation, diabetes. ✗ Spleen *yang* deficiency, Phlegm Damp, diarrhoea. Milk is subject to considerable contamination from antibiotics, hormones and other food additives. The benefit of milk is retained in organic and unprocessed varieties.
Duck	Sweet, salty, neutral; nourishes *yin*, benefits the Stomach, promotes urination, alleviates oedema. ✔ Yin deficient fever, cough and dry throat, oedema, difficult urination. ✗ Early stage of an exterior syndrome, loose stools or diarrhoea.
Goat	See Sheep

Goats milk	Sweet, warm; supplements deficiency, moistens dryness. ✔ General debility, convalescence, emaciation, gastric ulcers, dryness of the Stomach and Intestines, thirst, oral dryness, constipation, diabetes, regurgitation.
Pigeon	Salty, neutral; supplements the Liver and Kidneys, nourishes *yin* and Blood. ✔ Liver and Kidney *yin* deficiency, diabetes, weakness, lack of vitality, amenorrhoea, scanty periods, *qi* deficiency, reduced appetite.
Pork	Sweet, salty, neutral; nourishes *yin* and Blood, moistens dryness. ✔ Lung *yin* deficiency or dryness cough, dryness of the mouth and throat, general *qi* and Blood deficiency states, convalescence following illness and pregnancy, constipation. ✗ Damp Heat and Phlegm conditions.
Pork kidney	Salty, neutral; supplements the Kidney. ✔ Kidney deficiency backache, chronic diarrhoea.
Pork liver	Sweet, bitter, warm; supplements Liver Blood and improves vision. ✔ Liver Blood deficiency visual problems, general Blood deficiency.
Pork tripe	Sweet, warm; strengthens the Spleen and Stomach. ✔ General *qi* deficiency, weak digestion, reduced appetite, convalescence after illness, childhood malnutrition, weakness, loose stools.
Pork trotter	Sweet, salty, neutral; Nourishes Blood, promotes lactation. ✔ Qi and Blood deficiency insufficient lactation.
Quail	Sweet, neutral; supplements the Spleen and *qi*, promotes urination, dries Dampness. ✔ Digestive weakness, general debility, oedema, diarrhoea, lower back and leg weakness and aching, Damp bi syndrome.
Quail egg	Sweet, neutral; supplements *qi* and Blood, strengthens tendons and bones. ✔ Debility following chronic illness or in the elderly, insomnia, poor memory, reduced appetite, fatigue, *bi* syndrome.
Rabbit	Sweet, cool; strengthens the Spleen, supplements *qi*. ✔ Spleen and Stomach *qi* deficiency patterns, diabetes. ✗ Spleen *yang* deficiency.
Sheep, goat	Sweet, warm to very warm; warms the Spleen and Kidneys, supports *yang*, supplements *qi* and Blood. The younger the animal the warmer the meat.

✔ Kidney *yang* deficiency backache, sexual dysfunction, impotence, low libido, cold intolerance, nocturia and urinary disorder, postpartum abdominal pain, dysmenorrhoea, Spleen deficiency diarrhoea.
✗ Exterior syndromes, fever, hot disorders, hot constitutions.

Seafood

Anchovy	Salty, warm; benefits *qi* ✔ Spleen *qi* deficiency, general weakness, indigestion, reduced appetite. ✗ Excessive amounts of preserved or salted anchovies can weaken the Kidneys and damage the bones.
Carp	Sweet, neutral; promotes urination and lactation. ✔ Oedema, difficult urination, jaundice, insufficient lactation, chronic cough and wheezing.
Clam	Salty, cool; moistens dryness, benefits *yin*, transforms Phlegm and Damp. ✔ Phlegm Damp accumulation, productive cough, sinus congestion, oedema, leucorrhoea, goitre, haemorrhoids.
Crab	Salty, cold (depending on the type of crab, they can be cold or warming; most types however are cold); invigorates Blood and eliminates stagnant Blood, promotes healing, dries Dampness. ✔ Traumatic injury, broken bones, Damp Heat jaundice. ✗ Exterior syndromes, early stage of colds and flu.
Cuttlefish	Sweet, neutral; supplements the Liver and Kidneys, nourishes *yin* and Blood. ✔ Liver and Kidney deficiency, Blood deficiency, amenorrhoea, insufficient lactation.
Eel	Sweet, neutral or warm; supplements *qi* and Blood, strengthens Tendons and bones, expels Wind Damp. ✔ General *qi* and Blood deficiency patterns, chronic dysentery, haemafecia, bleeding haemorrhoids, chronic Wind Damp bi syndrome, joint pain, postpartum painful urination.
Garfish	Sweet, neutral; nourishes *yin*, supplements *qi*. ✔ Yin deficiency fever, night sweats, flushing, chronic non-healing ulcers and sores.
Mantis shrimp	Also known as Dublin Bay prawns. Sweet, salty, astringent, warm; supplements Kidney and Spleen *yang*. ✔ Frequent urination, nocturia, impotence, lower back and leg ache, spontaneous sweating, chronic diarrhoea, insufficient lactation.

	✗ Skin diseases, early stage of external disorders, latent pathogens.
Mussel	Salty, warm; supplements the Liver and Kidneys, nourishes *yin* and Blood, benefits jing, softens hardness, stops diarrhoea. ✔ Impotence, wasting disease, convalescence, lower back ache, anaemia, chronic diarrhoea and dysentery, goitre, swelling and nodules in the neck, menorrhagia, uterine bleeding, night sweats, high blood pressure, frequent urination.
Oyster	Sweet, salty, neutral; nourishes *yin* and Blood. ✔ Anaemia, nervous conditions, dry skin, hair and eyes, insomnia, feverishness following excessive alcohol consumption. ✗ Skin diseases.
Prawn	Also known as shrimp. Sweet, warm; Strengthens Kidney *yang*, promotes lactation, encourages full expression of rashes. ✔ Impotence, insufficient lactation, nervous conditions, joint pain, failure of rash to express sufficiently in weak patients. ✗ Skin diseases, early stage of external disorders, latent pathogens.
Sardine	Sweet, salty, neutral; benefits *qi* and *yin*, strengthens Tendons and bones. ✔ Spleen and Stomach *qi* and *yin* deficiency, convalescence, recovery after fever, arthritis, joint pain. ✗ Excessive amounts can aggravate Phlegm Damp congestion and internal Heat.
Shark	Sweet, salty, neutral; supplements *qi* and Blood; ✔ General *qi* and Blood deficiency patterns, chronic non-healing ulcers and sores.
Spanish mackerel	Sweet, neutral; nourishes *yin*, moistens dryness, benefits the Spleen and Stomach. ✔ Lung *yin* deficiency, dry cough, dry mouth and throat, tidal fever, night sweats, flushing, dysphagia, regurgitation, nausea, dry retching, indeterminate gnawing hunger. ✗ Spleen and Lung *yang* deficiency, Phlegm Damp.
Tuna	Sweet, neutral (raw), warm (cooked); supplements *qi* and Blood. ✔ Spleen and Stomach *qi* deficiency, Blood deficiency, anaemia, emaciation, reduced appetite, diarrhoea, general weakness, convalescence, lack of vitality.

Condiments, spices and miscellaneous items

Beer	In general, beer is bitter and cool, and tends to generate Dampness. This tendency is dose related. In small amounts its

	bitterness counteracts its Dampness producing qualities. In large quantities, the warmth of the alcohol combines with the Damp tendency to produce Damp Heat. The darker beers (stout, Guinness) are more therapeutic and can nourish Blood. Best avoided by those with Damp conditions.
Black pepper	Pungent, hot; warms the Spleen and Stomach, dispels Cold, stimulates the appetite. ✔ Reduced appetite, abdominal pain, nausea, vomiting, diarrhoea, early stage of colds and flu, congestion in the Lungs. ✗ Yin deficiency, eye disease, Heat patterns, haemorrhoids.
Coffee	Bitter, very warm; regulates *qi*, promotes urination, dries Dampness, stimulates digestion. ✔ In small quantities (1-2 cups daily) coffee stimulates *yang*, activates the brain and assists digestion. It is beneficial for congestion in the Lungs and for *qi* and Damp accumulation. Treats productive cough and asthma. Balances a rich meal. ✗ Yin and Blood deficiency, Heat and dryness patterns. Irritates the digestive tract and can cause nausea. Easily overheats the Heart and shen causing insomnia and mouth ulcers.
Mustard	Pungent, hot; strengthens the Spleen, disperses stagnant *qi*, dries Dampness, transforms Phlegm. ✔ Weak digestion, Spleen Damp, indigestion, diarrhoea, congestion in the Lungs, productive cough, sinus congestion, chronic non-healing sores. ✗ Yin and Blood deficiency, Heat and dryness patterns.
Salt	Salty, neutral; benefits the Kidneys, moistens dryness, softens hardness. ✔ Salt is an essential part of any diet, and quality unprocessed sea salt is recommended. A small amount assists the Kidneys, benefits digestion, promotes bowel movements. ✗ Oedema, diabetes, high blood pressure. Excessive salt damages the Blood and weakens the bones.
Spices	The kitchen spices include flavouring items and those that are classed as medicinal herbs, such as cloves, cinnamon, fennel seed, caraway, nutmeg, dill seed, cardamon, coriander leaf and seed, cumin seed, ginger, bay, rosemary, oregano and basil. In the kitchen, they are used in a different fashion than when used with a specific therapeutic purpose. Usually only small amounts are used, and always in combination with an appropriate dish. As a group they tend to be warm, drying and dispersing and act to improve the flavour, digestibility and metabolism of Damp creating foods. They are especially beneficial for Cold or Damp individuals.

Spirits	Similar in action to wine, but more concentrated. In small quantities, spirits are beneficial to the joints and improve circulation. Spirits are often used as a medium for Wind Damp expelling herbs.
Tea, green, red & black	Sweet, bitter, cool; improves digestion, promotes urination, benefits the eyes. Green tea is cooler than red and black tea. ✔ Wind Heat headache and visual disturbances, Summerheat disorder, thirst, indigestion from rich food, painful urination, scanty urination, dysentery, diarrhoea; mouth ulcers, herpes (topical). ✗ Excessive tea can generate Phlegm Damp and weaken the Kidneys. Not recommended for those suffering from insomnia or gastric ulcers.
Vinegar, brewed	Sour, bitter, warm; improves digestion, disperses stagnant Blood, stops bleeding. ✔ Food stagnation, balances rich and oily foods, abdominal and hypochondriac masses and accumulations, haematemesis, haemafecia, epistaxis, postpartum dizziness and fainting, food poisoning. ✗ Weak digestion, Damp accumulation, Damp bi syndrome, wei syndrome, early stage of an exterior pattern.
White sugar	Sweet, neutral; moistens the Lungs, increases *yin* fluids, benefits the Spleen. ✔ Dry cough, thirst, dry throat, dull abdominal pain. The effects of white sugar are dose related. Quite small amounts are therapeutic and can balance other flavours, however it quickly becomes problematic at higher doses. ✗ Phlegm Damp, Damp Heat, diabetes.
Wine (grape)	In general wine is sweet, sour and warm, red wine being warmer than white. In small quantities, wine is very beneficial, improving digestion and invigorating the circulation of *qi* and Blood. The deleterious effects, generation of Damp Heat and damage to *yin*, are dose related. In general, 1-2 small glasses daily is beneficial, depending on the size and constitution of the individual. Therapeutically, wine helps with *bi* syndrome and poor circulation (red wine in particular).

Supplements

Spirulina	Salty, cool; increases *yin* fluids, nourishes Blood, benefits the Liver. ✔ Anaemia, diabetes, hypoglycaemia, chronic dry skin, dry skin diseases, hepatitis, recovery from alcohol and drug abuse,

depression, chronic Damp Heat patterns, Stomach *yin* deficiency.
✗ Spleen *qi* and *yang* deficiency, Phlegm Damp.

Vitamin A	Benefits the Liver and improves vision; overdose weakens Blood.
Vitamin C	Clears Heat, strengthens *wei qi*; large doses can be quite hard on the Spleen and overuse will damage Spleen *yang* and cause diarrhoea.
Vitamin B	The B group of vitamins are generally warm and dispersing, can regulate and move Liver *qi* and nourish Blood. They can be too warming however, and cause some people (especially those with pre-existing Heat) to overheat. In excess they may damage *yin*.
Vitamin D	Strengthens the Kidneys, benefits the bones.
Vitamin E	Nourishes Liver Blood.

Pharmaceuticals

Amphetamines	Warm and dispersing; seriously plunder *yin* and *jing*.
Antibiotics	Bitter and cold, clear Heat; excellent for acute excess Heat patterns, but will weaken Spleen *yang* and create Dampness when used inappropriately or repeatedly.
Cocaine	Warm and dispersing; seriously plunders *yin* and *jing*.
Corticosteroids	Warm and dispersing, promote circulation of *yang*, disperse accumulation of *qi*; deplete *yin* and *yang* in the long term. Steroids (especially oral) seem to block the effects of acupuncture.
NSAIDS	Cool and dispersing, clear Heat, disperse stagnation of *qi* and Blood; easily damage Stomach *qi* and *yin*.
Salbutamol	Warm and dispersing, disperses Lung *qi* accumulation; weakens Lung *qi* over time.

APPENDIX 1. Extra Prescriptions

GUI ZHI FU LING WAN 桂枝茯苓丸 (*Cinnamon and Hoelen Formula*)

gui zhi (Ramulus Cinnamomi Cassiae) 桂枝 9-12g
fu ling (Sclerotium Poriae Cocos) 茯苓 12-15g
chi shao (Radix Paeoniae Rubrae) 赤芍 9-12g
tao ren (Semen Persicae) 桃仁 9-12g
mu dan pi (Cortex Moutan Radicis) 牡丹皮 9-12g

Method: Grind the herbs to powder and form into 9-gram pills with water. The dose is one pill 2-3 times daily.

JIN SUO GU JING WAN 金锁固精丸
(*Metal Lock Pill to Stabilize the Essence*)

sha yuan ji li (Semen Astragali Complanati) 沙苑蒺藜 90g
qian shi (Semen Euryales Ferocis) 芡实 90g
lian xu (Stamen Nelumbinis Nucifera) 莲须 90g
duan long gu (calcined Os Draconis) 煅龙骨 30g
duan mu li (calcined Concha Ostreae) 煅牡蛎 30g

Method: Grind the herbs to a fine powder and form into 9-gram pills with honey. The dose is three pills daily. May also be decocted with an 80% reduction in quantities.

JING FANG BAI DU SAN 荆防败毒散
(*Schizonepeta and Ledebouriella Powder to Overcome Pathogenic Influences*)

jing jie (Herba seu Flos Schizonepetae Tenuifolia) 荆芥 9-12g
fang feng (Radix Ledebouriellae Divaricatae) 防风 9-12g
jie geng (Radix Platycodi Grandiflori) 桔梗 9-12g
qian hu (Radix Peucedani) 前胡 9-12g
qiang huo (Rhizoma et Radix Notopterygii) 羌活 9-12g
zhi ke (Fructus Citri Aurantii) 枳壳 9-12g
du huo (Radix Angelicae Pubescentis) 独活 6-9g
chuan xiong (Radix Ligustici Chuanxiong) 川芎 6-9g
chao xing ren (dry fried Semen Pruni Armeniacae) 炒杏仁 6-9g
sheng jiang (Rhizoma Zingiberis Officinalis Recens) 生姜 6-9g

Method: Decoction. The herbs should be gently simmered for no longer than 20 minutes. Take hot or follow with hot porridge to induce sweating.

QI JU DI HUANG WAN 杞菊地黄丸
(*Lycium, Chrysanthemum and Rehmannia Formula*)

shu di (Radix Rehmanniae Glutinosae Conquitae) 熟地 240g
shan yao (Radix Dioscoreae Oppositae) 山药 120g
shan zhu yu (Fructus Corni Officinalis) 山茱萸 120g
fu ling (Sclerotium Poria Cocos) 茯苓 90g
ze xie (Rhizoma Alismatis Orientalis) 泽泻 90g

mu dan pi (Cortex Moutan Radicis) 牡丹皮 90g
gou qi zi (Fructus Lycii) 枸杞子 90g
ju hua (Flos Chrysanthemi Morifolii) 菊花 90g
Method: Grind the herbs to powder and form into 9-gram pills with honey. The dose is 2-3 pills daily. May also be decocted with a 90% reduction in dosage.

SHA SHEN MAI MEN DONG TANG 沙参麦门冬汤
(*Adenophora and Ophiopogon Combination*)

sha shen (Radix Adenophorae seu Glehniae) 沙参 9-12g
mai dong (Tuber Ophiopogonis Japonici) 麦冬 9-12g
yu zhu (Rhizoma Polygonati Odorati) 玉竹 9-12g
sang ye (Folium Mori Albae) 桑叶 6-9g
tian hua fen (Radix Trichosanthes Kirilowii) 天花粉 6-9g
bai bian dou (Semen Dolichoris Lablab) 白扁豆 9-12g
gan cao (Radix Glycyrrhizae Uralensis) 甘草 3-6g
Method: Decoction.

SHENG MAI SAN 生脉散 (*Generate the Pulse Powder*)

ren shen (Radix Ginseng) 人参 9-15g
mai dong (Tuber Ophiopogonis Japonici) 麦冬 15-24g
wu wei zi (Fructus Schizandrae Chinensis) 五味子 6-9g
Method: Grind the herbs to powder and form into 9-gram pills with honey. The dose is 2-3 pills daily. May also be decocted.

TAO HONG SI WU TANG 桃红四物汤
(*Dang Gui Four Combination with Persica and Carthamus*)

shu di (Radix Rehmanniae Glutinosae Conquitae) 熟地 12-24g
bai shao (Radix Paeoniae Lactiflora) 白芍 12-18g
dang gui (Radix Angelicae Sinensis) 当归 9-12g
chuan xiong (Radix Ligustici Chuanxiong) 川芎 6-9g
tao ren (Semen Persicae) 桃仁 9-12g
hong hua (Flos Carthami Tinctorii) 红花 9-12g
Method: Decoction.

WU LING SAN 五苓散 (*Hoelen Five Formula*)

ze xie (Rhizoma Alismatis Orientalis) 泽泻 12-15g
fu ling (Sclerotium Poriae Cocos) 茯苓 12-15g
zhu ling (Sclerotium Polypori Umbellati) 猪苓 12-15g
bai zhu (Rhizoma Atractylodes Macrocephalae) 白术 12-15g
gui zhi (Ramulus Cinnamomi Cassiae) 桂枝 6-9g
Method: Decoction.

XIAO LUO WAN 消瘰丸 (*Reduce Scrophula Pill*)

xuan shen (Radix Scrophulariae) 玄参 100g
zhe bei mu (Bulbus Fritillariae Thunbergii) 浙贝母 100g

mu li (Concha Ostreae) 牡蛎 100g

Method: Grind the herbs to powder and form into 9-gram pills with honey. The dose is 2-3 pills daily. May also be decocted with a 80%-90% reduction in quantities.

ZHEN WU TANG 真武汤 (*True Warrior Decoction*)

zhi fu zi (Radix Aconiti Carmichaeli Praeparata) 制附子 9-12g
bai zhu (Rhizoma Atractylodes Macrocephalae) 白术 9-12g
fu ling (Sclerotium Poriae Cocos) 茯苓 12-15g
sheng jiang (Rhizoma Zingiberis Officinalis Recens) 生姜 9-12g
bai shao (Radix Paeoniae Lactiflora) 白芍 9-12g

Method: Decoction. **Zhi fu zi** is cooked for 30 minutes before adding the other herbs (*xian jian* 先煎).

ZHI GAN CAO TANG 炙甘草汤 (*Baked Licorice Combination*)

sheng di (Radix Rehmanniae Glutinosae) 生地 24g
zhi gan cao (honey fried Radix Glycyrrhizae Uralensis) 炙甘草 12g
ren shen (Radix Ginseng) 人参 6g
gui zhi (Ramulus Cinnamomi Cassiae) 桂枝 9g
mai dong (Tuber Ophiopogonis Japonici) 麦冬 9g
e jiao^ (Gelatinum Corii Asini) 阿胶 6g
huo ma ren (Semen Cannabis Sativae) 火麻仁 9g
sheng jiang (Rhizoma Zingiberis Officinalis) 生姜 9g
da zao (Fructus Zizyphi Jujubae) 大枣 5pce

Method: Decoction. **E jiao** is melted in the hot strained decoction (*yang hua* 烊化).

APPENDIX 2. The Primary Pathological Triad (PPT)

The Primary Pathological Triad represents three patterns of pathology which are commonly found to occur simultaneously in gastro-intestinal disorders. These pathologies are mutually engendering. The PPT comprises Spleen deficiency, Liver *qi* stagnation and Heat, usually Damp Heat or stagnant Heat.

In chronic cases there may be further complication by Blood and *yin* deficiency, Blood stagnation, disruption to communication between the Heart and Kidney, and Phlegm.

The three main patterns of the PPT reinforce each other in the following way. Liver *qi* stagnation impacts on the Spleen and Stomach, weakening their function and encouraging the generation of Dampness. Dampness is heavy in nature and tends to sink downwards into the depths of the gastro-intestinal system. *Qi* stagnation, and the increase in *qi* pressure behind an obstruction,

Figure 1. *The Primary Pathological Triad*

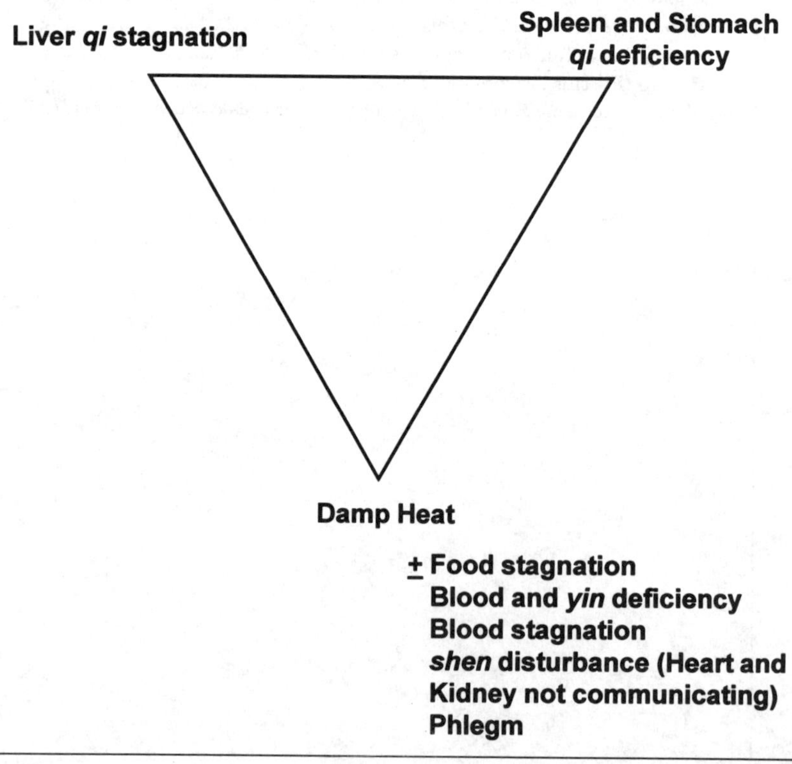

tend to generate Heat, as temperature and pressure are directly related. Stagnant Heat, once present and applied to pre-existing Dampness creates Damp Heat. Damp on its own, as a consummate stagnator, can also generate Heat and become Damp Heat. This combined pathology has been described in the classical literature as *yin* Fire, originally by Li Dong-yuan in the *Pi Wei Lun* (Treatise on the Spleen and Stomach).

The Western lifestyle seems to be particularly attuned to producing the PPT. A combination of stress, inappropriate diet and eating habits, sedentary occupations, and overuse of pharmaceuticals (in particular antibiotics and analgesics) all contribute.

It is because this combination of pathologies is so prevalent that the 'harmonising' category of prescriptions is the most widely used group of formulations worldwide. Harmonising prescriptions combine herbs with several different, often opposing, actions. They are typically complex, utilising pungent hot, bitter cold and sweet warm substances.

Treatment

To successfully treat this triad of pathological patterns, each pattern must be addressed at the same time or the condition will either not improve or will quickly relapse. For example, if only the Spleen is treated, the repeated insult of the Liver will continue to weaken it and the Spleen will be damaged again. If only Damp Heat is treated, the weakened Spleen will continue to produce Dampness and will likely be damaged by the bitter cold medicines used to clear the Damp Heat.

The major prescriptions for the various elements of the PPT can be mapped according to the hierarchy of therapeutic features they display. Figure 2 charts twelve prescriptions used to treat many different disorders, but primarily those of the gastro-intestinal system. From their position inside the triangle which represents the relationship between Spleen *qi* deficiency, Liver *qi* stagnation and Damp Heat, one can see at a glance the relative balance of the action of the prescription.

For example, **XIAO CHAI HU TANG** (*Minor Bupleurum Combination* 小柴胡汤) can be mapped in the centre of the triangle (Fig.2) as it is equally balanced between the three major principles of treatment. It strengthens the Spleen and supplements *qi*, regulates Liver *qi* and clears Damp Heat, in about equal proportions. This accounts for the popularity of this prescription as a 'clearing' prescription. **XIAO CHAI HU TANG** can be prescribed for complex syndromes with many and various contradictory signs and symptoms in an attempt to 'clear' the picture. As its therapeutic action takes effect, contradicting signs and symptoms are reduced and a primary pathology emerges.

Selection of the appropriate guiding prescription is based on a clinical

Figure 2. *Approximate location of prescriptions on the PPT diagram*

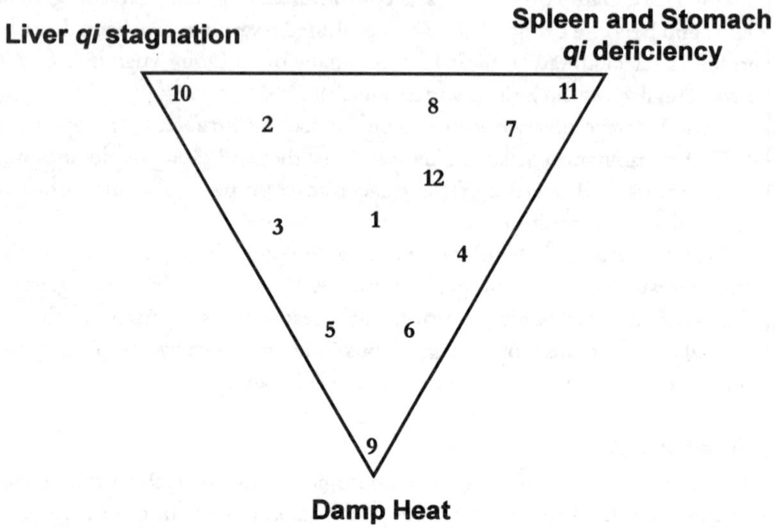

1. **XIAO CHAI HU TANG** (*Minor Bupleurum Combination*)
2. **XIAO YAO SAN** (*Bupleurum and Dang Gui Formula*)
3. **DAN ZHI XIAO YAO SAN** (*Bupleurum and Paeonia Formula*)
4. **BAN XIA XIE XIN TANG** (*Pinellia Combination*)
5. **SHAO YAO TANG** (*Peony Combination*)
6. **ZHONG MAN FEN XIAO WAN** (*Separate and Reduce Fullness in the Middle Pill*)
7. **BU ZHONG YI QI TANG** (*Ginseng and Astragalus Combination*)
8. **XIANG SHA LIU JUN ZI TANG** (*Saussurea and Cardamon Combination*)
9. **HUANG LIAN JIE DU TANG** (*Coptis and Scute Combination*)
10. **SI NI SAN** (*Bupleurum and Zhi Shi Combination*)
11. **SI JUN ZI TANG** (*Six Major Herbs Combination*)
12. **WU MEI WAN** (*Mume Pill*)

assessment of the relative importance and dominance of any pathology.

The three primary principles of treatment are
- to strengthen the Spleen to bolster *qi* with sweet and warms herbs
- to regulate the Liver, invigorate *qi* and stimulate the correct functioning of the *qi* mechanism with pungent dispersing herbs)
- to clear Heat or Damp Heat with bitter cold herbs

The above principles are prioritised according to the symptom picture and the diagnosis.

Take, for example, a patient with chronic bloody diarrhoea (associated with ulcerative colitis). At the time of presentation, the Damp Heat elements (bloody diarrhoea, night sweats, etc.) are dominant, with the Spleen deficiency and Liver *qi* stagnation components secondary. The guiding prescription is selected from the Damp Heat end of the map. In this example, **SHAO YAO TANG** (*Peony Combination* 芍药汤) would be selected if pain is a dominant feature, while **ZHONG MAN FEN XIAO WAN** (*Separate and Reduce Fullness in the Middle Pill* 中满分消丸) might be chosen if abdominal bloating is a main feature. As the Damp Heat elements resolve, the balance of the pathology will shift and another appropriate prescription selected. To follow the case above, as the Damp Heat clears, the Liver *qi* stagnation component emerges as the dominant pathology and a prescription that reflects this is selected, say **DAN ZHI XIAO YAO SAN** (*Bupleurum and Paeonia Formula* 丹栀逍遥散). If Spleen deficiency had emerged as the major feature, **XIANG SHA LIU JUN ZI TANG** (*Saussurea and Cardamon Combination* 香砂六君子汤) may have been selected.

Whatever prescription is selected, it will be suitably modified depending on any other complicating features. Modifications are generally few in number and tightly focused, so as not to dilute the main thrust of the guiding prescription.

APPENDIX 3. Herb Delivery, dosage and processing

Method of decoction

The prescriptions in this volume describe raw herbs and the quantities given are generally sufficient for two days doses. One packet of herbs is usually decocted twice, although supplementing herbs may be decocted three times. The amount of water required will vary depending on the type of herbs used and the purpose of the formula, but in general, enough water to cover the herbs by about one centimetre is correct (usually about 3-4 cups) with the aim of providing two cups of decoction per day. Keep in mind that some dry ingredients are absorbent and will soak up a considerable amount of the water, while others, like minerals and shells, will absorb none. During the first boil the decoction is reduced to about two cups. The decoction is strained and usually taken on an empty stomach. For the second boil, 2½ - 3 cups of water are added to the same herbs and reduced to two cups. The results of the two boilings can be combined to maintain consistency of strength. The dose is two cups daily. In severe or emergency situations, the dose can be doubled and a cup can be taken every two hours. For patients unable to ingest the medicine, the herbs may be give via a nasogastric tube or retention enema. Diaphoretic and purgative formulae are generally discontinued once sweating or purgation occurs.

The pot used should preferably be ceramic, although stainless steel is also acceptable. Aluminium, iron and copper pots should not be used. A tight fitting lid is necessary to prevent the escape of volatile oils. Plant materials should be soaked in cold water for at least 20–30 minutes before cooking. This allows the plant cells to expand and to release their contents when boiled. If the herbs are boiled before they are soaked, the boiling water can seal in the active components by toughening the cell walls.

For busy people, the traditional decoction method can be time consuming and inconvenient. To increase patient compliance, variations to the traditional decoction regime can be made. Several packets of herbs can be decocted at one time and the second boiling avoided by beginning with more water and boiling for longer (other than for those exceptions listed below). For example, two packets of herbs can be cooked with 9-10 cups of water and reduced to around 8 cups, yielding four days doses (at two cups daily). The strained decoction can be stored in a covered plastic container in the refrigerator and warmed by the addition of boiling water before ingestion. Stored in this way, the herbs will keep for up to a week.

Cooking time

Most general prescriptions can be cooked for 30-40 minutes. Prescriptions for dispersing external Wind, clearing Heat or those containing ingredients with volatile oils should be simmered in a lidded pot for a relatively short time, 10-15 minutes. Supplementing herbs, minerals and shells can stand long slow simmering (more than one hour) to extract all their goodness. Certain herbs in a prescription, such as hard or delicate herbs, may require different treatment than the bulk of the ingredients and can be packaged separately for convenience. Where individual herbs require different treatment, it is noted in the method section beneath the prescription.

The issue of dosage

Correct dosage and balance of different herbs in a prescription can be complex and may depend on several factors. These factors include an intimate knowledge of the action and capabilities of a particular herb at a particular dose and how it may interact with other herbs in a prescription. Recommending a particular dose is not a straightforward matter and we have therefore chosen to give a standard dosage range for most of the herbs listed. Sometimes however, a specifically high or low dose is given because we wish to elicit a particular action of that herb. For example small doses (1-2 grams) of **da huang**, usually prescribed as a purgative, can actually astringe and stop diarrhoea. Another example is **huang qi**, which is usually used in the range of 18-30 grams in decoction, but 60 grams or more are often required for problems such as the sequelae of Wind Stroke or rectal prolapse. The normal dosage range is relatively ineffective for conditions such as these. The various elements in a principle of treatment must be carefully considered so that one component can be emphasised and others de-emphasised as appropriate, by varying the doses of individual components. This level of finesse can never be fully conveyed in a book and must be learnt through clinical instruction and experience. Doses will vary depending on the physical mass, age and sensitivity of a patient. Large people in general require higher doses than smaller individuals. Some people are by nature more receptive to herbs and acupuncture (the good responders) and require less to get satisfactory results. Certain patterns do better with small doses over a prolonged period of time. These are the deep *yin* and *jing* deficiency states, and to a lesser extent, Blood deficiency. The aim of treatment in these cases is to gradually rebuild or repair damaged tissues and organs, and this process cannot be forced by big doses.

Concentrated herbal extracts

Concentrated herbal extracts are a relatively recent and popular method of herb preparation. Concentrated, desiccated extracts now constitute the primary method of prescribing herbs in Japan, Taiwan and the West. Concentrated granules are produced by making large batches of single or mixed herbs as decoctions, then draining the liquid from the dregs. The liquid is then evaporated and concentrated by gentle heating or vacuum extraction. The concentrate is added to an excipient filler, such as corn starch or the dregs of the decoction, to form a paste. The paste is then spray dried and the remaining water evaporated, leaving a dry powder.

The concentration factor varies from one herb to another and from one formula to another, but on average is around a 6:1 concentration of the ingredients of the crude herbs. What this means is that about 600 grams of raw herbs go into 100 grams of concentrated powder. The typical dose for these granules is from 6-12 grams per day, which is equivalent to about 40-80 grams of raw herb.

Because the herbs are concentrated, the quantity taken each day is relatively small. The production process for the major manufacturers (located in China, Japan, Taiwan and the United States) is regulated by Good Manufacturing Practice (GMP), which ensures quality control and consistency of active ingredients across batches. In the raw herb market place in China many substitutions are made–sometimes inferior or wrong herbs may be purchased inadvertently by the unwary doctor. For Western practitioners who perhaps don't have the training or experience to correctly identify a herb in its natural form, the security of using a product which has been identified and analysed by experts before and after processing gives not only better therapeutic effect but also a greater margin of safety.

Concentrated powders are taken as a tea after being reconstituted in hot water or as a draft washed down with water. Powders can also be packed into gelatin capsules. Patient compliance is high, and as the powders are often more bland than fresh decoctions, they are excellent for children. The extraction technology is improving all the time and the quality of these products is usually high.

We have found that the newest generation of concentrated herb granules, which contain no extraneous additives or fillers, have a potency very close to that of the decocted raw herbs. When increasing frequency of administration and compliance is taken into account their clinical effectiveness is sometimes greater. Having said that, for acute conditions which require quick alteration of prescription, nothing works quite so well and rapidly as that strong smelling freshly cooked brew!

Processing methods

Many herbs are processed before use in order to modify their nature and therapeutic effect. These processing methods are usually done by the wholesaler or retail outlet, and are specified by the prescribing physician when writing the prescription. Processing can have a dramatic effect on the action of some herbs, so it is important to specify the correct state of the herb.

Zhi 炙 (frying with liquids)

Mixing the herb with a liquid and stir frying.

- Frying with honey (*mi zhi* 蜜炙) increases the tonifying, Lung moistening and cough stopping effects. Usually, if no particular medium is specified, writing *zhi* alone will result in honey frying.
- Frying with vinegar (*cu zhi* 醋炙) increases the effects on the Liver, and enhances the analgesic, astringent and Blood invigorating qualities; it also modifies unpleasant odours and tastes.
- Frying with wine (*jiu zhi* 酒炙) increases Blood invigorating, channel clearing action, and leads the herb to the upper body.
- Frying with salt water (*yan zhi* 盐炙) leads the herb to the Kidney, and can improve the Kidney Fire clearing nature.
- Frying with ginger juice (*jiang zhi* 姜炙) reduces the tendency of bitter and cold herbs to injure Stomach *qi*, can enhance the action of stopping nausea and vomiting and can modify the toxic nature of herbs such as **ban xia** (Rhizoma Pinelliae Ternatae) 半夏, and **tian nan xing** (Rhizoma Arisaema) 天南星.

Chao 炒 (dry frying)

Browning and drying the herb in a wok. There are several degrees of dry frying:

- Mild dry frying, the most common method, is denoted by the character **chao** before the herb. The herb is dry fried until a light yellow brown. This method increases the warmth and digestibility of a herb, and improves the Stomach strengthening effect. Commonly used with Spleen tonics.
- Frying over high heat until dark brown or black on the outside. This method is usually used with food stagnation herbs, as it strongly improves digestion. Denoted by the character **jiao** (焦) before the herb.
- Frying over high heat until blackened and charred on the outside. This increases the astringent nature, and is used to improve the haemostatic effect of various herbs. Denoted by the character **tan** (炭) after the herb.

Duan 煅 (calcining)

- Calcining involves placing the substance, usually a mineral or shell in a fire until it is heated red hot. It becomes brittle and is easily broken up. The substance's active ingredients are then made more available when decocted.

Wei 煨 (roasting in ashes)

- The herb is wrapped in a coating of wet paper, mud or flour paste and roasted in hot coals until the coating is blackened and cracked; the substance inside has been cooked at a high temperature without burning. Usually used to modify the irritant or toxic natures of certain herbs.

Modifications to prescription

Different terms need to be added to a prescription depending on the specialised treatment some herbs require. The characters denoting these requirements are usually placed in brackets below the herb characters when written from top to bottom in the traditional script format. Common examples are listed in Table A3.1.

Hou xia 后下 (added towards the end)

- This instruction is used for herbs and substances that are added at the end of cooking or a few minutes before the end of cooking. These herbs usually contain volatile oils and the short cooking prevents the oils from evaporating off. The herbs are wrapped separately by the dispenser. This group includes light and aromatic herbs and herbs that change in action with different cooking times, like **da huang** (Radix et Rhizoma Rhei) 大黄, which purges more the less it is cooked.

Xian jian 先煎 (cooked first)

- This instruction applies to herbs and substances that require pre-cooking. This group includes toxic herbs like **fu zi** (Radix Aconiti Carmichaeli) 附子 that are rendered safer by long cooking (usually at least one hour), and minerals and shells like **mu li** (Concha Ostrea) 牡蛎, **long gu** (Os Draconis) 龙骨 and **ci shi** (Magnetitum) 磁石. The herbs are wrapped separately by the dispenser and usually cooked for about 30 minutes before the rest of the prescription is added.

Chong fu 冲服 (added to, or followed by, the strained decoction)

- This instruction applies to herbs and substances that are not cooked at all. They are wrapped separately by the dispensing herbalist, and dissolved in the hot liquid after straining or taken powdered and chased by the decoction. It is used for substances like **mang xiao** (Mirabilitum) 芒硝 and **san qi** (Radix Notoginseng) 三七.

Bao jian 包煎 (cooked in a cloth bag)

- Due to the presence of hairs or other irritants and the small size of certain seeds, some herbs should be cooked in a cloth or muslin bag. Often the whole formula will be placed in the bag by the dispenser.

Yang hua 烊化 (melted before adding to the strained decoction)

- Very sticky or viscous substances that may stick to the pot or the other herbs in the decoction are melted separately and added to the strained decoction. These substances can be gently boiled to aid their melting. Herbs that require this treatment include **e jiao** (Gelatinum Corii Asini) 阿胶 and **yi tang** (Saccharum Granorum) 饴糖.

Table A3.1 *Herbs requiring individual treatment when decocted*

Treatment variation	Herb
added at the end of cooking hou xia 后下 *cooked no more than 5 minutes °cooked no more than 10 minutes	bai dou kou* (Fructus Amomi Kravanh) bo he* (Herba Mentha Haplocalycis) chuan xiong° (Radix Ligustici Chuanxiong) da huang (Radix et Rhizoma Rhei) gou teng° (Ramulus Uncariae cum Uncis) huo xiang° (Herba Agastaches seu Pogostei) qing hao° (Herba Artemisiae Annuae) sha ren* (Fructus seu Semen Amomi)
cooked for 30 minutes before the other herbs xian jian 先煎	ci shi (Magnetitum) dai zhe shi (Haematitum) fu zi (Radix Aconiti Carmichaeli) long gu (Os Draconis) mu li (Concha Ostreae) shi gao (Gypsum) shi jue ming (concha Haliotidis) zhen zhu mu (Concha Margaritaferae)
cooked in a muslin bag bao jian 包煎	che qian zi (Semen Plantaginis) hua shi (Talc) pi pa ye (Folium Eryobotryae Japonicae) xuan fu hua (Flos Inulae)
best taken seperately in pill or powder form	bing pian (Borneol) di long (Lumbricus) ge jie (Gecko) hu po (Succinum) ji nei jin (Endothelium Corneum Gigeraiae Galli) lu rong (Cornu Cervi Parvum) niu huang (Calculus Bovis) quan xie (Buthus Martensi) san qi (Radix Pseudoginseng su he xiang (Styrax Liquidis) wu bei zi (Galla Rhois Chinensis) wu gong (Scolopendra Subspinipes) zhu li (Succus Bambusae) zhu sha (Cinnabaris) zi he che (Placenta Hominis)
dissolved in the strained decoction chong fu 冲服	e jiao (Gelatinum Corii Asini) mang xiao (Mirabilitum) yi tang (Maltose)

PIN YIN	BENSKY AND GAMBLE	MACLEAN AND LYTTLETON
Ai Fu Nuan Gong Wan 艾附暖宫丸	Mugwort and Prepared Aconite Pill for Warming the Womb	Mugwort and Prepared Aconite Pill for Warming the Womb
Ba Xian Chang Shou Wan 八仙长寿丸	Eight Immortal Pill for Longevity	Rehmannia, Schizandra and Ophiopogon Combination
Ba Zhen Tang 八珍汤	Eight Treasure Decoction	Ginseng and Dang Gui Eight Combination
Ba Zheng San 八正散	Eight Herb Powder for Rectification	Dianthus Formula
Bai He Gu Jin Tang 百合固金汤	Lily Bulb Decoction to Preserve the Metal	Lily Combination
Bai Hu Tang 白虎汤	White Tiger Decoction	Anemarrhena and Gypsum Combination
Bai Tou Weng Tang 白头翁汤	Pulsatilla Decoction	Pulsatilla Decoction
Ban Liu Wan 半硫丸		Pinellia and Sulphur Pill
Ban Xia Bai Zhu Tian Ma Tang 半夏白术天麻汤	Pinellia, Atractylodes Macrocephala and Gastrodia Decoction	Pinellia and Gastrodia Combination
Ban Xia Hou Po Tang 半夏厚朴汤	Pinellia and Magnolia Bark Decoction	Pinellia and Magnolia Combination
Ban Xia Xie Xin Tang 半夏泻心汤	Pinellia Decoction to Drain the Epigastrium	Pinellia Combination
Bao He Wan 保和丸	Preserve Harmony Pill	Citrus and Crategus Formula
Bao Yuan Tang 保元汤	Preserve the Basal Decoction	Preserve the Basal Decoction
Bao Zhen Tang 保真汤		Preserve the True Decoction
Bei Xie Fen Qing Yin 萆解分清饮	Dioscorea Hypoglauca Decoction to Separate the Clear	Tokoro Combination
Bei Xie Shen Shi Tang 萆解渗湿汤		Dioscorea Hypoglauca Decoction to Leach Out Dampness
Bi Yun San 碧云散	Jasper Powder	Blue Cloud Powder
Bing Lian San 冰连散		Borneol and Coptis Powder
Bing Peng San 冰硼散		Borneol and Borax Powder
Bu Fei E Jiao Tang 补肺阿胶汤	Tonify the Lungs Decoction with Ass-Hide Gelatin	Tonify the Lungs Decoction with Ass-Hide Gelatin
Bu Fei Tang 补肺汤	Tonify the Lungs Decoction	Tonify the Lungs Decoction
Bu Gu Zhi Wan 补骨脂丸		Psoraleae Pills
Bu Nao Wan 补脑丸		Brain Tonic Pills

Bu Qi Yun Pi Tang 补气运脾汤		Decoction to Supplement Qi and Invigorate the Spleen
Bu Tian Da Zao Wan 补天大造丸		Tonify Heaven Great Creation Pill
Bu Yang Huan Wu Tang 补阳还五汤	Tonify the Yang to Restore Five [Tenths] Decoction	Tonify the Yang to Restore Five [Tenths] Decoction
Bu Zhong Yi Qi Tang 补中益气汤	Tonify the Middle and Augment Qi Decoction	Ginseng and Astragalus Combination
Can Shi Tang 蚕矢汤		Arrowlike Decoction of Silkworm
Cang Er Zi San 苍耳子散	Xanthium Powder	Xanthium Formula
Cao Guo Yin 草果饮		Tsaoko Decoction
Chai Hu Gui Zhi Tang 柴胡桂枝汤	Bupleurum and Cinnamon Twig Decoction	Bupleurum and Cinnamon Combination
Chai Hu Jia Long Gu Mu Li Tang 柴胡加龙骨牡蛎汤	Bupleurum plus Dragon Bone and Oyster Shell Decoction	Bupleurum and Dragon Bone Combination
Chai Hu Qing Gan Tang 柴胡清肝汤	Bupleurum Decoction to Clear the Liver	Bupleurum Liver Clearing Decoction
Chai Hu Shu Gan San 柴胡舒肝散	Bupleurum Powder to Spread the Liver	Bupleurum and Cyperus Formula
Chai Hu Zhi Jie Tang 柴胡枳桔汤	Bupleurum, Bitter Orange and Platycodon Decoction	Bupleurum, Bitter Orange and Platycodon Decoction
Chai Ling Tang 柴苓汤		Bupleurum and Hoelen Combination
Chen Xiang San 沉香散		Aquillaria Powder
Cheng Shi Bei Xie Fen Qing Yin 程氏萆解分清饮		Tokoro Formula [from the Cheng Clan]
Chong He Gao 冲和膏		Flush and Harmonise Ointment
Chuan Xiong Cha Tiao San 川芎茶调散	Ligusticum Chuanxiong Powder to be Taken with Green Tea	Cnidium and Tea Formula
Cong Bai Qi Wei Yin 葱白七味饮	Scallion Decoction with Seven Ingredients	Shallot and Seven Herb Drink
Cui Gan Wan 摧肝丸		Broken Liver Pills
Da Ban Xia Tang 大半夏汤		Major Pinellia Decoction
Da Bu Yin Wan 大补阴丸	Great Tonify the Yin Pill	Great Tonify the Yin Pill
Da Bu Yuan Jian 大补元煎	Great Tonify the Basal Decoction	Great Tonify the Basal Decoction
Da Chai Hu Tang 大柴胡汤	Major Bupleurum Decoction	Major Bupleurum Combination
Da Cheng Qi Tang 大承气汤	Major Order the Qi Decoction	Major Rhubarb Combination

PIN YIN	BENSKY AND GAMBLE	MACLEAN AND LYTTLETON
Da Ding Feng Zhu 大定风珠	Major Arrest Wind Pearl	Major Arrest Wind Pearl
Da Fen Qing Yin 大分清饮		Major Distinguishing Decoction
Da Huang Fu Zi Tang 大黄附子汤	Rhubarb and Prepared Aconite Decoction	Rhubarb and Prepared Aconite Decoction
Da Huang Huang Qin Xie Xin Tang 大黄黄芩泻心汤		Rhubarb and Scute Decoction to Drain the Epigastrium
Da Huang Mu Da Pi Tang 大黄牡丹皮汤	Rhubarb and Moutan Decoction	Rhubarb and Moutan Decoction
Da Huang Zhe Chong Wan 大黄蛰虫丸	Rhubarb and Eupolyphaga Pill	Rhubarb and Eupolyphaga Pill
Da Jian Zhong Tang 大建中汤	Major Construct the Middle Decoction	Major Zanthoxylum Combination
Da Qin Jiao Tang 大秦艽汤	Major Gentiana Qinjiao Decoction	Major Gentiana Qinjiao Decoction
Da Qing Long Tang 大青龙汤	Major Bluegreen Dragon Decoction	Major Blue Dragon Combination
Dai Di Dang Wan 代抵当丸		Substituted Resistance Pill
Dai Ge San 黛蛤散		Indigo and Conch Powder
Dan Dao Qu Hui Tang 胆道驱蛔汤	Drive Roundworms from the Biliary Tract Decoction	Decoction for Expelling Roundworms from the Bile Duct
Dan Shen Yin 单身饮	Salvia Decoction	Salvia Decoction
Dan Xi Bi Yuan Fang 丹溪鼻渊方		Dan Xi's Nasal Congestion Formula
Dan Zhi Xiao Yao San 丹栀逍遥散	Augmented Rambling Powder	Bupleurum and Paeonia Formula
Dang Gui Bu Xue Tang 当归补血汤	Tangkuei Decoction to Tonify the Blood	Dang Gui Blood Tonic Decoction
Dang Gui Liu Huang Tang (Wan) 当归六黄汤 (丸)	Tangkuei and Six-Yellows Decoction	Dang Gui and Six Yellow Pills
Dang Gui Long Hui Wan 当归龙荟丸	Tangkuei, Gentiana Longdancao and Aloe Pill	Dang Gui, Gentiana Longdancao and Aloe Pill
Dang Gui Shao Yao San 当归芍药散	Tangkuei and Peony Powder	Dang Gui and Peony Formula
Dang Gui Si Ni Tang 当归四逆散	Tangkuei Decoction for Frigid Extremities	Dang Gui Decoction for Frigid Extremities
Dao Chi San 导赤散	Guide Out the Red Powder	Rehmannia and Akebia Formula
Dao Qi Tang 导气汤	Conduct the Qi Decoction	Conduct the Qi Decoction
Dao Tan Tang 导痰汤	Guide Out Phlegm Decoction	Guide Out Phlegm Decoction

Di Huang Yin Zi 地黄饮子	Rehmannia Decoction	Rehmannia Decoction
Di Tan Tang 涤痰汤	Scour Phlegm Decoction	Scour Phlegm Decoction
Di Yu San 地榆散	Sanguisorba Powder	Sanguisorba Powder
Dian Xian San 癫痫散		Epilepsy Powder
Ding Chuan Tang 定喘汤	Arrest Wheezing Decoction	Stop Wheezing Decoction
Ding Kou Li Zhong Wan 丁蔻理中丸		Regulate the Middle Pill with Clove and Cardamon
Ding Xian Wan 定痫丸	Arrest Seizures Pill	Arrest Seizures Pill
Ding Xiang San 丁香散		Clove Powder
Ding Xiang Tou Ge San 丁香透膈散		Clove Powder to Penetrate the Diaphragm
Ding Zhi Wan 定志丸	Settle the Emotions Pill	Settle the Emotions Pill
Du Huo Ji Sheng Tang 独活寄生汤	Angelica Pubescens and Sangjisheng Decoction	Tu-huo and Vaecium Combination
Er Chen Wan 二陈丸	Two-Cured Decoction	Citrus and Pinellia Combination
Er Long Zuo Ci Wan 耳聋左慈丸	Pill for Deafness that is Kind to the Left (Kidney)	Pill for Deafness that is Kind to the Left (Kidney)
Fang Feng Tong Sheng San 防风通圣丸	Ledebouriella Powder that Sagely Unblocks	Siler and Platycodon Formula
Fang Ji Huang Qi Tang 防己黄芪汤	Stephania and Astragalus Decoction	Stephania and Astragalus Combination
Fei Er Wan 肥儿丸	Fat Baby Pill	Fat Baby Pill
Fu Yuan Huo Xue Tang 复元活血汤	Revive Health by Invigorating the Blood Decoction	Revive Health by Invigorating the Blood Decoction
Fu Zi Li Zhong Wan 附子理中丸	Prepared Aconite Pill to Regulate the Middle	Aconite, Ginseng and Ginger Combination
Gan Cao Xie Xin Tang 甘草泻心汤	Licorice Decoction to Drain the Epigastrium	Pinellia and Licorice Combination
Gan Jiang Ling Zhu Tang 干姜苓术汤		Licorice, Ginger, Hoelen and Atractylodes Decoction
Gan Lu Xiao Du Dan 甘露消毒丹	Sweet Dew Special Pill to Eliminate Toxin	Sweet Dew Special Pill to Eliminate Toxin
Gan Lu Yin 甘露饮		Sweet Dew Decoction
Gan Mai Da Zao Tang 甘麦大枣丸	Licorice, Wheat and Jujube Decoction	Licorice and Jujube Combination
Ge Gen Huang Qin Huang Lian Tang 葛根黄芩黄连汤	Kudzu, Coptis and Scutellaria Decoction	Kudzu, Coptis and Scute Combination

PIN YIN	BENSKY AND GAMBLE	MACLEAN AND LYTTLETON
Ge Gen Jia Ban Xia Tang 葛根加半夏汤	Kudzu Decoction plus Pinellia	Kudzu Decoction plus Pinellia
Ge Gen Tang 葛根汤	Kudzu Decoction	Pueraria Combination
Ge Hua Jie Cheng Tang 葛花解醒汤		Pueraria Flower Decoction to Alleviate Hangover
Ge Xia Zhu Yu Tang 膈下逐瘀汤	Drive Out Blood Stasis Below the Diaphragm Decoction	Drive Out Blood Stasis Below the Diaphragm Decoction
Gu Chong Tang 固冲汤	Stabilise Gushing Decoction	Stabilise Gushing Decoction
Gua Di San 瓜蒂散	Melon Pedicle Powder	Melon Pedicle Powder
Gua Lou Xie Bai Ban Xia Tang 瓜楼薤白半夏汤	Trichosanthes Fruit, Chinese Chive and Pinellia Decoction	Trichosanthes, Bakeri and Pinellia Combination
Guan Xin Su He Xiang Wan 冠心苏合香丸		Liquid Styrax Pills for Coronary Heart Disease
Gui Ling Gan Lu Yin 桂苓甘露饮	Cinnamon and Poria Sweet Dew Decoction	Cinnamon and Poria Sweet Dew Decoction
Gui Pi Tang 归脾汤	Restore the Spleen Decoction	Ginseng and Longan Combination
Gui Zhi Fu Ling Wan 桂枝茯苓丸	Cinnamon Twig and Poria Pill	Cinnamon and Hoelen Formula
Gui Zhi Gan Cao Long Gu Mu Li Tang 桂枝甘草龙骨牡蛎汤	Cinnamon, Licorice, Dragon Bone and Oyster Shell Decoction	Cinnamon, Licorice, Dragon Bone and Oyster Shell Decoction
Gui Zhi Jia Hou Po Xing Ren Tang 桂枝加厚朴杏仁汤	Cinnamon Twig Decoction plus Magnolia Bark and Apricot Kernel	Cinnamon, Magnolia and Apricot Seed Combination
Gui Zhi Jia Long Gu Mu Li Tang 桂枝加龙骨牡蛎汤	Cinnamon Twig Decoction plus Dragon Bone and Oyster Shell	Cinnamon and Dragon Bone Combination
Gui Zhi Tang 桂枝汤	Cinnamon Twig Decoction	Cinnamon Combination
Gun Tan Wan 滚痰丸	Vaporize Phlegm Pill	Vaporize Phlegm Pill
Hao Qin Qing Dan Tang 蒿芩清胆汤	Artemesia Annua and Scutellaria Decoction to Clear the Gallbladder	Artemesia Annua and Scutellaria Decoction to Clear the Gallbladder
He Che Da Zao Wan 河车大造丸		Placenta Great Creation Pills
He Jian Shao Yao Huang Lian Tang 河间芍药黄连汤		Peony and Coptis Decoction to Bolster the River
Hei Xi Dan 黑锡丹	Lead Special Pill	Lead Special Pill

Hua Gai San 华盖散	Canopy Powder	Canopy Powder
Hua Gan Jian 化肝煎		Transform the Liver Decoction
Huai Hua San 槐花散	Sophora Japonica Flower Powder	Sophora Japonica Flower Powder
Huai Jiao Wan 槐角丸	Sophora Japonica Fruit Powder	Sophora Japonica Fruit Powder
Huang Lian E Jiao Tang 黄连阿胶汤	Coptis and Ass-Hide Gelatin Decoction	Coptis and Ass-Hide Gelatin Decoction
Huang Lian Jie Du Tang 黄连解毒汤	Coptis Decoction to Relieve Toxicity	Coptis and Scute Combination
Huang Lian Wen Dan Tang 黄连温胆汤	Coptis Decoction to Warm the Gallbladder	Coptis Decoction to Warm the Gallbladder
Huang Lian Xiang Ru Yin 黄连香薷饮		Coptis and Elsholtzia Decoction
Huang Long Tang 黄龙汤	Yellow Dragon Decoction	Yellow Dragon Decoction
Huang Qi Jian Zhong Tang 黄芪建中汤	Astragalus Decoction to Construct the Middle	Astragalus Decoction to Construct the Middle
Huang Qi Tang 黄芪汤		Astragalus Decoction
Huang Tu Tang 黄土汤	Yellow Earth Decoction	Yellow Earth Decoction
Huo Dan Wan 藿胆丸		Agastache and Pig Bile Pills
Huo Luo Xiao Ling Dan 活络校零担	Fantastically Effective Pill to Invigorate the Collaterals	Fantastically Effective Pill to Invigorate the Collaterals
Huo Xiang Zheng Qi San 藿香正气散	Agastache Powder to Rectify the Qi	Agastache Formula
Huo Xue Hua Yu Tang 活血化瘀汤		Decoction to Regulate Blood and Disperse Stagnant Blood
Ji Chuan Jian 济川煎	Benefit the River (Flow) Decoction	Benefit the River Decoction
Ji Jiao Li Huang Wan 已椒苈黄丸	Stephania, Zanthoxylum, Descurainia and Rhubarb Pill	Stephania, Zanthoxylum, Descurainia and Rhubarb Pill
Ji Sheng Shen Qi Wan 济生肾气丸	Kidney Qi Pill from Formulas to Aid the Living	Kidney Qi Pill from Formulas to Aid the Living
Jia Jian Wei Rui Tang 加减葳蕤汤	Modified Polygonatum Odoratum Decoction	Modified Yu Zhu Tang

PIN YIN	BENSKY AND GAMBLE	MACLEAN AND LYTTLETON
Jia Wei Er Miao San 加味二妙散		Augmented Two Marvel Powder
Jian Pi Wan 健脾丸	Strengthen the Spleen Pill	Strengthen the Spleen Pill
Jiao Ai Tang 胶艾汤	Ass-Hide Gelatin and Mugwort Decoction	Ass-Hide Gelatin and Mugwort Decoction
Jiao Gui Tang 椒桂汤		Sichuan Pepper and Cinnamon Decoction
Jie Gan Jian 解肝煎		Loosen the Liver Decoction
Jie Geng Tang 桔梗汤		Platycodon Decoction
Jie Yu Dan 解语丹		Relax the Tongue Special Pill
Jin Fei Cao San 金沸草散		Inula Powder
Jin Kui Shen Qi Wan 金匮肾气丸	Kidney Qi Pill from the Golden Cabinet	Rehmannia Eight Formula
Jin Suo Gu Jing Wan 金锁固精丸	Metal Lock Pill to Stabilize the Essence	Metal Lock Pill to Stabilize the Essence
Jing Fang Bai Du San 荆防败毒散	Schizonepeta and Ledebouriella Powder to Overcome Pathogenic Influences	Schizonepeta and Ledebouriella Powder to Overcome Pathogenic Influences
Ju He Wan 橘核丸	Tangerine Seed Pill	Tangerine Seed Pill
Ju Pi Zhu Ru Tang 橘皮竹茹汤	Tangerine Peel and Bamboo Shavings Decoction	Tangerine Peel and Bamboo Shavings Decoction
Kai Jin San 开噤散		Powder for Treating Anorectic Dysentery
Ke Xue Fang 咳血方	Coughing of Blood Formula	Coughing of Blood Formula
Lan Wei Jie Du Tang 阑尾解毒汤		Detoxify the Appendix Decoction
Lan Wei Qing Hua Tang 阑尾清化汤		Appendix Cooling and Transforming Decoction
Li Zhong Wan 理中丸	Regulate the Middle Pill	Ginseng and Ginger Combination
Lian Po Yin 连朴饮	Coptis and Magnolia Bark Decoction	Coptis and Magnolia Bark Decoction
Liang Fu Wan 良附丸	Galangal and Cyperus Pill	Galangal and Cyperus Pill
Liang Ge Qing Chang San 凉膈清肠散		Cool the Diaphragm, Clear the Intestine Powder
Liang Ge San 凉膈散	Cool the Diaphragm Powder	Cool the Diaphragm Powder
Liang Xue Di Huang Tang 凉血地黄汤		Rehmannia Decoction to Cool the Blood
Ling Gui Zhu Gan Tang 苓桂术甘汤	Poria, Cinnamon Twig, Atractylodes Macrocephala and Licorice Decoction	Atractylodes and Hoelen Combination

Liu Jun Zi Tang 六君子汤	Six-Gentlemen Decoction	Six Major Herb Combination
Liu Mo Tang 六磨汤	Six Milled-Herb Decoction	Six Milled-Herb Decoction
Liu Wei Di Huang Wan 六味地黄丸	Six-Ingredient Pills with Rehmannia	Rehmannia Six Formula
Liu Wei Tang 六味丸		Six Flavour Decoction
Long Dan Xie Gan Tang 龙胆泻肝汤	Gentiana Longdancao Decoction to Drain the Liver	Gentiana Combination
Lu Rong Bu Se Wan 鹿茸补涩丸		Deer Horn Pills to Tonify and Astringe
Ma Huang Lian Qiao Chi Xiao Dou Tang 麻黄连翘赤小豆汤		Ma Huang, Forsythia and Aduki Bean Decoction
Ma Huang Tang 麻黄汤	Ephedra Decoction	Ma Huang Combination
Ma Huang Fu Zi Xi Xin Tang 麻黄附子细辛汤	Ephedra, Asarum and Prepared Aconite Decoction	Ma Huang, Asarum and Prepared Aconite Decoction
Ma Xing Shi Gan Tang 麻杏石甘汤	Ephedra, Apricot Kernel, Gypsum and Licorice Decoction	Ma Huang, Apricot Seed, Gypsum and Licorice Combination
Ma Zi Ren Wan 麻子仁丸	Hemp Seed Pill	Apricot Seed and Linum Formula
Mai Men Dong Tang 麦门冬汤	Ophiopogonis Decoction	Ophiopogon Combination
Man Jing Zi San 蔓荆子散		Vitex Powder
Miao Xiang San 妙香散	Marvellously Fragrant Powder	Marvellously Fragrant Powder
Mu Dan Pi San 牡丹皮散		Paeonia Suffruticosa Powder
Mu Li San 牡蛎散	Oyster Shell Powder	Oyster Shell Formula
Mu Xiang Bing Lang Wan 木香槟榔丸	Aucklandia and Betel Nut Pill	Aucklandia and Betel Nut Pill
Mu Xiang Shun Qi Wan 木香顺气丸		Sausurrea Pill to Order the Qi
Niao Lu Pai Shi Tang #1 尿路排石汤一号		Expel Urinary Stones #1
Nuan Gan Jian 暖肝煎	Warm the Liver Decoction	Warm the Liver Decoction
Ping Chen Tang 平陈汤		Calm the Stomach plus Citrus and Pinellia Decoction
Ping Wei San 平胃散	Calm the Stomach Powder	Magnolia and Ginger Formula

PIN YIN	BENSKY AND GAMBLE	MACLEAN AND LYTTLETON
Pu Ji Xiao Du Yin 普济消毒饮	Universal Benefit Decoction to Eliminate Toxin	Universal Benefit Decoction to Eliminate Toxin
Qi Ge San 启隔散		Open the Diaphragm Powder
Qi Ju Di Huang Wan 杞菊地黄丸	Lycium Fruit, Chrysanthemum and Rehmannia Pill	Lycium, Chrysanthemum and Rehmannia Formula
Qi Yang Yu Xin Dan 启阳娱心丹		Arouse yang, Please the Heart Special Pill
Qian Gen San 茜根散		Rubia Decoction
Qian Zheng San 牵正散	Lead to Symmetry Powder	Lead to Symmetry Powder
Qiang Huo Sheng Shi Tang 羌活胜湿汤	Notopterygium Decoction to Overcome Dampness	Notopterygium Decoction to Overcome Dampness
Qin Jiao Bai Zhu Wan 秦艽白术散		Gentiana Macrophylla and Atractylodes Macrocephala Pill
Qing Chang Yin 清肠饮		Cool the Intestine Decoction
Qing Dan Xie Huo Tang 清胆泻火汤	Clear the Gallbladder and Drain Fire Decoction	Clear the Gallbladder and Drain Fire Decoction
Qing Fei Yin 清肺饮		Clear the Lungs Decoction
Qing Hun San 清魂散		Clear the Hun Powder
Qing Huo Di Tan Tang 清火涤痰汤		Clear Fire, Wash Away Phlegm Decoction
Qing Jin Hua Tan Tang 清金化痰汤		Clear Metal, Transform Phlegm Decoction
Qing Qi Hua Tan Wan 清气化痰丸	Clear the Qi and Transform Phlegm Pill	Clear the Qi and Transform Phlegm Pill
Qing Re Jie Du Hua Yu Tang 清热解毒化瘀汤		Heat Clearing, Toxin Eliminating, Blood Stasis Transforming Decoction
Qing Wei San 清胃散	Clear The Stomach Powder	Clear The Stomach Powder
Qing Wei Tang 清胃汤	Clear the Stomach Decoction	Clear the Stomach Decoction
Qing Wen Bai Du Yin 清瘟败毒饮	Clear Epidemics and Overcome Toxin Decoction	Clear Epidemics and Overcome Toxin Decoction
Qing Xin Lian Zi Yin 清心莲子饮		Lotus Seed Combination
Qing Yan Li Ge Tang 清咽利膈汤		Clear the Throat, Benefit the Diaphragm Decoction
Qing Yan Ning Fei Tang 清咽宁肺汤		Clear the Throat and Calm the Lungs Decoction

Qing Ying Tang 清营汤	Clear the Nutritive Level Decoction	Clear the Ying Decoction
Qing Zao Jiu Fei Tang 清燥救肺汤	Eliminate Dryness and Rescue the Lungs Decoction	Eriobotria and Ophiopogon Combination
Qu Feng Dao Tan Tang 祛风导痰汤		Expel Wind and Guide Out the Phlegm Decoction
Qu Tao Tang 驱绦汤	Expel Tapeworm Decoction	Expel Tapeworm Decoction
Ran Zhao Tang 燃照汤		Illuminating Decoction
Ren Shen Ge Jie San 人参蛤蚧散	Ginseng and Gecko Powder	Ginseng and Gecko Powder
Ren Shen Yang Ying Tang 人参养营汤	Ginseng Decoction to Nourish the Nutritive Qi	Ginseng Nutritive Combination
Run Chang Bu Xue Tang 润肠补血汤		Moisten the Intestines and Supplement Blood Pill
Run Chang Wan 润肠丸	Moisten the Intestines Pill	Moisten the Intestines Pill
Run Hou Tang 润喉汤		Moisten the Throat Pill
San Jia Fu Mai Tang 三甲复脉汤	Three Shells Decoction to Restore the Pulse	Three Shells Decoction to Restore the Pulse
San Jin Tang 三金汤	Three Gold Decoction	Three Golden Herbs Decoction
San Ren Tang 三仁汤	Three Nut Decoction	Three Nut Decoction
San Zi Yang Qin Tang 三子养亲汤	Three Seed Decoction to Nourish One's Parents	Three Seed Decoction to Nourish One's Parents
Sang Dan Xie Bai Tang 桑丹泻白汤	Mulberry Leaf and Moutan Decoction to Drain the White	Mulberry Leaf and Moutan Decoction to Drain the White
Sang Ju Yin 桑菊饮	Mulberry Leaf and Chrysanthemum Decoction	Morus and Chrysanthemum Formula
Sang Piao Xiao San 桑螵硝散	Mantis Egg Case Powder	Mantis Egg Case Powder
Sang Xing Tang 桑杏汤	Mulberry Leaf and Apricot Kernel Decoction	Morus and Apricot Seed Combination
Sha Shen Mai Men Dong Tang 沙参麦门冬汤	Glehnia and Ophiopogonis Decoction	Adenophora and Ophiopogon Combination
Shao Fu Hua Yu Tang 少腹化瘀汤		Decoction to Transform Blood Stagnation in the Lower Abdomen
Shao Fu Zhu Yu Tang 少腹逐瘀汤	Drive Out Blood Stasis in the Lower Abdomen Decoction	Drive Out Blood Stasis in the Lower Abdomen Decoction

PIN YIN	BENSKY AND GAMBLE	MACLEAN AND LYTTLETON
Shao Yao Tang 芍药汤	Peony Decoction	Peony Decoction
Shen Fu Tang 参附汤	Ginseng and Prepared Aconite Decoction	Ginseng and Prepared Aconite Decoction
Shen Fu Zai Zao Wan 参附再造丸		Ginseng and Aconite Pills for a New Lease on Life
Shen Ling Bai Zhu San 参苓白术散	Ginseng, Poria and Atractylodes Macrocephala Powder	Ginseng and Atractylodes Formula
Shen Shi Tang 渗湿汤		Leach out Dampness Decoction
Shen Su Yin 参苏饮	Ginseng and Perilla Leaf Decoction	Ginseng and Perilla Combination
Sheng Hua Tang 生化汤	Generation and Transformation Decoction	Generation and Transformation Decoction
Sheng Hui Tang 生慧汤		Promote Wisdom Decoction
Sheng Jiang Xie Xin Tang 生姜泻心汤	Fresh Ginger Decoction to Drain the Epigastrium	Fresh Ginger Decoction to Drain the Epigastrium
Sheng Mai San 生脉散	Generate the Pulse Powder	Generate the Pulse Powder
Shi Hui San 十灰散	Ten Partially Charred Substance Powder	Ten Partially Charred Substance Powder
Shi Pi Yin 实脾饮	Bolster the Spleen Decoction	Magnolia and Atractylodes Combination
Shi Quan Da Bu Tang 十全大补汤	All Inclusive Great Tonifying Decoction	Ginseng and Dang Gui Ten Combination
Shi Wei San 石苇散		Pyrrosia Powder
Shi Xiao San 失笑散	Sudden Smile Powder	Break Into a Smile Powder
Shi Yi Wei Wen Dan Tang 十一味温胆汤	Eleven Ingredient Decoction to Warm the Gallbladder	Eleven Ingredient Decoction to Warm the Gallbladder
Shi Zao Tang 十枣汤	Ten Jujube Decoction	Ten Jujube Decoction
Shou Xing Wan 寿星丸		God of Longevity Pills
Shu Feng Qing Re Tang 疏风清热汤		Dispel Wind, Clear Heat Decoction
Shu Gan Li Pi Tang 疏肝理脾汤	Spread the Liver and Regulate the Spleen Decoction	Spread the Liver and Regulate the Spleen Decoction
Shuang Jie Tong Sheng San 双解通圣散		Doubly Dispersing Powder to Sagely Unblock
Shui Niu Jiao Di Huang Tang 水牛角地黄汤		Water Buffalo Horn and Rehmannia Decoction
Si Jun Zi Tang 四君子汤	Four Gentlemen Decoction	Four Major Herbs Combination

Si Mo Tang 四磨汤	Four Milled-Herb Decoction	Four Milled-Herb Decoction
Si Ni Jia Ren Shen Tang 四逆加人参汤	Frigid Extremities Decoction plus Ginseng	Frigid Extremities Decoction plus Ginseng
Si Ni San 四逆散	Frigid Extremities Powder	Bupleurum and Zhi Shi Formula
Si Ni Tang 四逆汤	Frigid Extremities Decoction	Frigid Extremities Decoction
Si Shen Wan 四神丸	Four Miracle Pills	Four Miracle Pills
Si Wu Tang 四物汤	Four Substance Decoction	Dang Gui Four Combination
Si Wu Xiao Feng San 四物消风散		Eliminate Wind Powder with the Four Substances
Su He Xiang Wan 苏合香丸	Liquid Styrax Pill	Liquid Styrax Pill
Su Ye Huang Lian Tang 苏叶黄连汤		Perilla Leaf and Coptis Decoction
Su Zi Jiang Qi Tang 苏子降气汤	Perilla Fruit Decoction for Directing Qi Downward	Perilla Fruit Combination
Suan Zao Ren Tang 酸枣仁汤	Sour Jujube Decoction	Zizyphus Combination
Tan Bi Tang 痰秘汤		Phlegm Constipation Decoction
Tao He Cheng Qi Tang 桃核承气汤	Peach Pit Decoction to Order the Qi	Persica and Rhubarb Combination
Tao Hong Si Wu Tang 桃红四物汤	Four Substance Decoction with Safflower and Peach Pit	Dang Gui Four Combination with Persica and Carthamus
Tao Hua Tang 桃花汤	Peach Blossom Decoction	Peach Blossom Decoction
Tian Ma Gou Teng Yin 天麻钩藤饮	Gastrodia and Uncaria Decoction	Gastrodia and Gambir Formula
Tian Tai Wu Yao San 天台乌药散	Top Quality Lindera Powder	Top Quality Lindera Powder
Tian Wang Bu Xin Dan 天王补心丹	Emperor of Heaven's Special Pill to Tonify the Heart	Ginseng and Zizyphus Formula
Tiao Wei Cheng Qi Tang 调胃承气汤	Regulate the Stomach and Order the Qi Decoction	Regulate the Stomach and Order the Qi Decoction
Tie Di Wan 铁笛丸		Iron Whistle Pill
Ting Li Da Zao Xie Fei Tang 葶苈大枣泻肺汤	Descurainia and Jujube Decoction to Drain the Lungs	Descurainia and Jujube Decoction to Drain the Lungs
Tong Qiao Huo Xue Tang 通窍活血汤	Unblock the Orifices and Invigorate Blood Decoction	Unblock the Orifices and Invigorate Blood Decoction
Tong Xie Yao Fang 痛泻要方	Important Formula for Painful Diarrhoea	Important Formula for Painful Diarrhoea
Tong You Tang 通幽汤		Open the Pyloric Sphincter Decoction

PIN YIN	BENSKY AND GAMBLE	MACLEAN AND LYTTLETON
Tou Nong San 透脓散	Discharge Pus Powder	Discharge Pus Powder
Tuo Li Tou Nong San 托里透脓散		Decoction to Support the Interior While Discharging Pus
Tuo Li Xiao Du San 托里消毒散		Powder to Support the Interior and Eliminate Toxin
Wai Ba Fang 外八方		External Formula for All Points of the Compass
Wei Jing Tang 苇茎汤	Reed Decoction	Reed Decoction
Wei Ling Tang 胃苓散	Calm the Stomach and Poria Decoction	Magnolia and Hoelen Combination
Wen Dan Tang 温胆汤	Warm the Gallbladder Decoction	Bamboo and Hoelen Combination
Wen Fei Tang 温肺汤		Warm the Lungs Decoction
Wen Fei Zhi Liu Dan 温肺止流丹		Warm the Lungs, Stop the Flow Special Pill
Wen Jing Tang 温经汤	Warm the Menses Decoction	Dang Gui and Evodia Combination
Wu Bi Shan Yao Wan 无比山药丸		Incomparable Dioscorea Pill
Wu Ji San 五积散	Five Accumulation Powder	Five Accumulation Powder
Wu Lin San 五淋散	Five Ingredient Powder for Painful Urinary Dysfunction	Gardenia and Hoelen Formula
Wu Ling San 五苓散	Five Ingredient Powder with Poria	Hoelen Five Formula
Wu Mei Wan 乌梅丸	Mume Pill	Mume Pill
Wu Mo Yin Zi 五磨饮子	Five Milled Herb Decoction	Five Milled Herb Decoction
Wu Tou Chi Shi Zhi Wan 乌头赤石脂丸		Aconite and Halloysium Pills
Wu Wei Xiao Du Yin 五味消毒饮	Five Ingredient Decoction to Eliminate Toxin	Five Ingredient Decoction to Eliminate Toxin
Wu Wei Zi Tang 五味子汤		Schizandra Decoction
Wu Zhi An Zhong Yin 五汁安中饮		Five Juices Drink to Calm the Middle
Wu Zhu Yu Tang 吴茱萸汤	Evodia Decoction	Evodia Combination
Wu Zi Yan Zong Wan 五子衍宗丸		Five Seed Ancestral (Qi) Amplifying Pill
Xian Fang Huo Ming Yin 仙方活命饮	Sublime Formula for Sustaining Life	Sublime Formula for Sustaining Life

Xiang Sha Liu Jun Zi Tang 香砂六君子汤	Six Gentlemen Decoction with Aucklandia and Amomum	Saussurea and Cardamon Combination
Xiang Sha Yang Wei Tang 香砂养胃汤	Nourish the Stomach Decoction with Aucklandia and Amomum	Nourish the Stomach Decoction with Aucklandia and Amomum
Xiang Su San 香苏散	Cyperus and Perilla Leaf Powder	Cyperus and Perilla Formula
Xiao Ban Xia Fu Ling Tang 小半夏茯苓汤		Minor Pinellia and Hoelen Combination
Xiao Chai Hu Tang 小柴胡汤	Minor Bupleurum Decoction	Minor Bupleurum Combination
Xiao Cheng Qi Tang 小承气汤	Minor Order the Qi Decoction	Minor Rhubarb Combination
Xiao Feng Zhi Yang Tang 消风止痒汤		Decoction to Eliminate Wind and Stop Itching
Xiao Huo Luo Dan 小活络丹	Minor Invigorate the Collaterals Special Pill	Minor Invigorate the Collaterals Special Pill
Xiao Ji Yin Zi 小蓟饮子	Cephalanoplos Decoction	Cephalanoplos Decoction
Xiao Jian Zhong Tang 小健中汤	Minor Construct the Middle Decoction	Minor Cinnamon and Peony Combination
Xiao Jiang Qi Tang 小降气汤		Minor Descending Qi Decoction
Xiao Luo Wan 消瘰丸	Reduce Scrophula Pill	Reduce Scrophula Pill
Xiao Qing Long Tang 小青龙汤	Minor Bluegreen Dragon Decoction	Minor Blue Dragon Combination
Xiao Xian Xiong Tang 小陷胸汤	Minor Sinking Into the Chest Decoction	Minor Sinking Into the Chest Decoction
Xiao Xu Ming Tang 小续命汤	Minor Prolong Life Decoction	Minor Prolong Life Decoction
Xiao Yao San 逍遥散	Rambling Powder	Bupleurum and Dang Gui Formula
Xiao Yu Tang 消瘀汤		Eliminate Blood Stasis Decoction
Xie Bai San 泻白散	Drain the White Powder	Morus and Lycium Formula
Xie Huang San 泻黄散	Drain the Yellow Powder	Drain the Yellow Powder
Xie Xin Tang 泻心汤	Drain the Epigastrium Decoction	Coptis and Rhubarb Combination
Xin Jia Xiang Ru Yin 新加香薷饮	Newly Augmented Elsholtzia Decoction	Newly Augmented Elsholtzia Decoction
Xin Yi Qing Fei Yin 辛夷清肺饮		Magnolia Flower Lung Clearing Decoction
Xin Yi San 辛夷散	Magnolia Flower Powder	Magnolia Flower Powder
Xing Jun San 行军散		Marching Powder
Xing Su San 杏苏散	Apricot Kernel and Perilla Leaf Powder	Apricot Kernel and Perilla Leaf Powder
Xing Wei Cheng Qi Tang 星蒌承气汤		Fading Star Order the Qi Decoction

PIN YIN	BENSKY AND GAMBLE	MACLEAN AND LYTTLETON
Xuan Fu Dai Zhe Tang 旋复代赭汤	Inula and Haematite Decoction	Inula and Haematite Decoction
Xuan Fu Hua Tang 旋复花汤		Inula Flower Decoction
Xuan Miao San 玄妙散		Wonderful Scrophularia Powder
Xue Fu Zhu Yu Tang 血府逐瘀汤	Drive Out Stasis in the Mansion of Blood Decoction	Achyranthes and Persica Combination
Yang He Tang 阳和汤	Yang Heartening Decoction	Yang Heartening Decoction
Yang Xin Tang 养心汤	Nourish the Heart Decoction	Nourish the Heart Decoction
Yang Yin Qing Re Tang 养阴清热汤		Decoction to Nourish Yin and Clear Heat
Yi Guan Jian 一贯煎	Linking Decoction	Linking Decoction
Yi Wei Tang 益胃汤	Benefit the Stomach Decoction	Benefit the Stomach Decoction
Yi Yi Fu Zi Bai Jiang San 意苡附子败酱散	Coicis, Prepared Aconite and Patrinia Powder	Coicis, Prepared Aconite and Patrinia Powder
Yi Zi Tang 乙字汤		Cimicifuga Combination
Yin Chen Hao Tang 茵陈蒿汤	Artemesia Yinchenhao Decoction	Capillaris Combination
Yin Chen Wu Ling San 茵陈五苓散	Artemesia Yinchenhao and Five-Ingredient Powder with Poria	Capillaris and Hoelen Five Formula
Yin Chen Zhu Fu Tang 茵陈术附汤	Artemesia Yinchenhao, Atractylodes and Prepared Aconite Decoction	Capillaris, Atractylodes and Aconite Combination
Yin Qiao Hong Jiang Jie Du Tang 银翘红酱解毒汤		Lonicera, Forsythia, Sargentodoxae and Patrinia Decoction to Eliminate Toxin
Yin Qiao San 银翘散	Honeysuckle and Forsythia Powder	Lonicera and Forsythia Formula
You Gui Wan 右归丸	Restore the (Right) Kidney Pill	Eucommia and Rehmannia Formula
Yu Nu Jian 玉女煎	Jade Woman Decoction	Jade Woman Decoction
Yu Ping Feng San 玉屏风散	Jade Windscreen Powder	Jade Screen Powder
Yu Shu Dan 玉枢丹		Jade Pivot Special Pill
Yu Zhen San 玉真散	True Jade Powder	True Jade Powder
Yue Bi Jia Zhu Tang 越婢加术汤	Maidservant from Yue Decoction plus Atractylodes	Atractylodes Combination
Yue Hua Wan 月华丸	Moonlight Pill	Moonlight Pill

Yue Ju Wan 越鞠丸	Escape Restraint Pill	Escape Restraint Pill
Zan Yu Dan 赞育丹	Special Pill to Aid Fertility	Special Pill to Aid Fertility
Zeng Ye Cheng Qi Tang 增液承气汤	Increase the Fluids and Order the Qi Decoction	Increase the Fluids and Order the Qi Decoction
Zeng Ye Tang 增液汤	Increase the Fluids Decoction	Increase the Fluids Decoction
Zhen Gan Xi Feng Tang 镇肝熄风汤	Sedate the Liver and Extinguish Wind Decoction	Sedate the Liver and Extinguish Wind Decoction
Zhen Ren Yang Zang Tang 真人养脏汤	True Man's Decoction to Nourish the Organs	True Man's Decoction to Nourish the Organs
Zhen Wu Tang 真武汤	True Warrior Decoction	True Warrior Decoction
Zheng Yang Li Lao Tang 拯阳理劳汤		Rescue Yang, Manage Exhaustion Decoction
Zheng Yin Li Lao Tang 拯阴理劳汤		Rescue Yin, Manage Exhaustion Decoction
Zhi Bai Ba Wei Wan 知柏八味丸	Anemarrhena, Phellodendron and Rehmannia Pill	Anemarrhena, Phellodendron and Rehmannia Formula
Zhi Bao Dan 至宝丹	Greatest Treasure Special Pill	Greatest Treasure Special Pill
Zhi Fei Jie He Ke Tan Xue Fang 治肺结核咳痰血方		Tuberculosis and Haemoptysis Formula
Zhi Gan Cao Tang 炙甘草汤	Honey Fried Licorice Decoction	Baked Licorice Combination
Zhi Lou Wan 痔漏丸		Fistula Pill
Zhi Shi Dao Zhi Wan 枳实导滞丸	Immature Bitter Orange Pill to Guide Out Stagnation	Immature Bitter Orange Pill to Guide Out Stagnation
Zhi Shi Li Zhong Wan 枳实理中丸	Immature Bitter Orange Pill to Regulate the Middle	Immature Bitter Orange Pill to Regulate the Middle
Zhi Sou San 止嗽散	Stop Coughing Powder	Stop Coughing Powder
Zhi Zhu Wan 枳术丸	Immature Bitter Orange and Atractylodes Macrocephala Pill	Immature Bitter Orange and Atractylodes Macrocephala Pill
Zhi Zi Dou Chi Tang 栀子豆豉汤	Gardenia and Prepared Soybean Decoction	Gardenia and Prepared Soybean Decoction
Zhong Man Fen Xiao Wan 中满分消丸	Separate and Reduce Fullness in the Middle Pill	Separate and Reduce Fullness in the Middle Pill

PIN YIN	BENSKY AND GAMBLE	MACLEAN AND LYTTLETON
Zhou Che Wan 舟车丸	Vessel and Vehicle Pill	Vessel and Vehicle Pill
Zhu Huang San 珠黄散		Mother of Pearl and Cow Gallstone Powder
Zhu Ju Wan 驻车丸		Stop the Chariot Pill
Zhu Ling Tang 猪苓汤	Polyporus Decoction	Polyporus Combination
Zhu Ru Tang 竹茹汤		Bamboo Shavings Decoction
Zhu Ye Huang Qi Tang 竹叶黄芪汤		Lophatherus and Astragalus Decoction
Zhu Ye Shi Gao Tang 竹叶石膏汤	Lophatherus and Gypsum Decoction	Lophatherus and Gypsum Decoction
Zhui Chong Wan 追虫丸		Pursue Parasites Pill
Zi Dang You 紫当油		Lithospermum and Angelica Oil
Zi Shen Tong Guan Wan 滋肾通关丸		Nourish Kidney, Open the Gate Pill
Zi Sheng Wan 资生丸		Aid Life Pill
Zi Wan Tang 紫菀汤		Aster Decoction
Zi Xue Dan 紫雪丹	Purple Snow Special Pill	Purple Snow Special Pill
Zi Yin Gan Lu Yin 滋阴甘露饮		Sweet Dew Decoction to Nourish Yin
Zuo Gui Wan 左归丸	Restore the Left (Kidney) Pill	Achyranthes and Rehmannia Formula
Zuo Gui Yin 左归饮	Restore the Left Decoction	Restore the Left Decoction
Zuo Jin Wan 左金丸	Left Metal Pill	Left Metal Pill

Index

Note: Page number followed by *f* refer to illustrations or flowcharts; page numbers followed by *t* refer to tables.

A

B

H

T

U

V

W

X

Z

BIBLIOGRAPHY

Chinese language sources

Ji Zheng Zhen Jiu 急症针灸
(Emergency Acupuncture) 1988
Zhang Ren, Peoples Medical Publishing Company, Beijing

Shi Yong Zhong Yi Nei Ke Xue 实用中医内科学
(Practical Traditional Chinese Internal Medicine) 1984
Huang Wen-Dong (Supervising editor), Shanghai Science and Technology Press, Shanghai

Shi Yong Zhong Yi Fu Ke Xue 实用中医妇科学
(Practical Traditional Chinese Gynaecology) 1985
Zhou Feng-Wu (ed.), Shandong Science and Technology Press, Shandong

Shi Yong Zhong Yi Wai Ke Xue 实用中医外科学
(Practical Traditional Chinese External Medicine) 1985
Gu Bo-Hua (Supervising editor), Shanghai Science and Technology Press, Shanghai

Shi Yong Zhong Yi Xue Ye Bing Xue 实用中医血液病学
(Practical Traditional Chinese Treatment of Blood Diseases) 1992
Wu Han-Xiang (Supervising editor), Shanghai Science and Technology Press, Shanghai

Shi Yong Zhong Yao Xue 实用中药学
(Practical Chinese Herbs) 1985
Zhou Feng-Wu (ed.), Shandong Science and Technology Press, Shandong

Shi Yong Fang Ji Xue 实用方剂学
(Practical Chinese Herbal Formulas) 1989
Zhou Feng-Wu (ed.), Shandong Science and Technology Press, Shandong

Shi Yong Zhong Yi Wai Ke Xue 实用中医外科学
(Practical Traditional Chinese External Medicine) 1985
Shang De-Jun (ed.), Shandong Science and Technology Press, Shandong

Shi Yong Zhong Yi Er Ke Xue 实用中医儿科学
(Practical Traditional Chinese Paediatrics) 1987
Jin Zu-Peng (ed.), Shandong Science and Technology Press, Shandong

Xiao Hua Ke Zhuan Bing 消化科专病
(Specific Gastroenterological Diseases) 2000
Luo Yun-Jian (ed.), Peoples Medical Publishing Company, Beijing

Zhen Jiu Zhi Liao Xue 针灸治疗学
(Acupuncture Therapeutics) 1985
Yang Zhang-Sen (ed.), Shanghai Science and Technology Press, Shanghai

Zhong Liu Ke Zhuan Bing 肿瘤科专病
(Specific Tumour Diseases) 2000
Liu Wei-Sheng (ed.), Peoples Medical Publishing Company, Beijing

Zhong Yi Nei Ke Ji Zheng Zheng Zhi 中医内科急症证治
(Proven TCM Treatments for Acute Internal Disorders) 1985
Huang Xing-Yuan (ed.), Peoples Medical Publishing Company, Beijing

Zhong Yi Nei Ke Lin Chuang Shou Ce 中医内科临床手册
(Clinical Handbook of Traditonal Chinese Internal Medicine) 1984
Dang You-Lian (ed.), Henan Science and Technology Press, Henan

Zhong Yi Er Bi Hou Ke Xue 中医耳鼻喉科学
(Traditional Chinese Otonasopharyngology) 1985
Wang De-Jian (ed.), Peoples Medical Publishing Company, Beijing

Zhong Yi Tan Bing Xue 中医痰病学
(Study of TCM Phlegm Diseases) 1984
Zhu Ceng-Bo, Hubei Science and Technology Press, Hubei

Zhong Yi Nei Ke Shou Ce 中医内科手册
(Handbook of TCM Internal Medicine) 1997
Chao En-Xiang (ed.), Fujian Science and Technology Press, Fujian

Zhong Yi Zhi Liao Yi Nan Za Bing Mi Yao 中医治疗疑难杂病秘要
(Treatment of Miscellaneous Difficult Diseases with Chinese Medicine) 1993 Zhang Jing-Ren (ed.), Wenhui Publishing

Zhong Guo Zhong Yi Mi Fang Da Quan 中国中医秘方大全
(A Compendium of Secret Chinese Medicine Formulas) 1991
Hu Xi-Ming (ed.), Wenhui Publishing

Zui Xin Fang Ji Shou Ce 最新方剂手册
(Handbook of the Latest Prescriptions) 1998
Fan Wei-Hong (ed.), Central Plains Publishing Company, Henan

English sources and references

Baldry PE (1993) *Acupuncture, Trigger Points and Musculoskeletal Pain*, Churchill Livingstone, Edinburgh

Bensky D and O'Connor (1985) *Acupuncture: A Comprehensive Text*, Eastland Press, Seattle, Washington

Bensky D and Gamble A (1993) *Chinese Herbal Medicine: Materia Medica*, Eastland Press, Seattle, Washington

Bensky D and Barolet R (1990) *Chinese Herbal Medicine: Formulas and Strategies*, Eastland Press, Seattle, Washington

Beers M and Berkow R, et al. (1999) *The Merck Manual* (17th Ed). Merck Research Laboratories, Whitehouse Station, New Jersey

Brown V (1984) The Differentiation and Treatment of Epigastric Pain by Acupuncture. The Journal of Chinese Medicine, 16:2-17

Clavey S (1995) *Fluid Physiology and Pathology in Traditional Chinese Medicine*, Churchill Livingstone, Melbourne

Deadman P, Al-Khafaji M and Baker K (1998) *A Manual of Acupuncture*, Journal of Chinese Medicine Publications, Hove, UK

Edwards CRW et al. (1995) *Davidson's Principles and Practice of Medicine* (17th Ed), Churchill Livingstone, Edinburgh

Ellis A and Wiseman N (1994) *Fundamentals of Chinese Medicine*, Paradigm Publications, Brookline, MA

Fruehauf H (1998) *Gu* syndrome. The Journal of Chinese Medicine, 57:10-17

Gascoigne S (1995) *The Manual of Conventional Medicine for Alternative Practitioners*, Jigme Press, Dorking, Surrey

Hsu HY (1980) *Commonly Used Chinese Herbal Formulas with Illustrations*, Oriental Healing Arts Institute, Los Angeles, California

Legge D (1997) *Close to the Bone*, Sydney College Press, Sydney

Leggett D (1999) *Recipes for Self Healing*, Meridian Press, Totnes, Devon

Leggett D (1998) *Helping Ourselves: A Guide to Traditional Chinese Food Energetics*, Meridian Press, Totnes, Devon

Lorenz P (1997) *Differential Diagnosis* (4th ed.) Social Science Press, Katoomba, NSW, Australia

Maciocia G (1989) *The Foundations of Chinese Medicine*, Churchill Livingstone, Edinburgh

Maciocia G (1994) *The Practice of Chinese Medicine*, Churchill Livingstone, Edinburgh

Maclean W (2000) *The Clinical Manual of Chinese Herbal Patent Medicines*, Pangolin Press, Sydney

Murtagh J (1996) *General Practice*, McGraw Hill Book Company, Sydney

Pitchford P (1993) *Healing with Whole Foods: Oriental Traditions and Modern Nutrition*. North Atlantic Books, Berkeley, California

Scott JP (1985) The Treatment of Diarrhoea and Constipation by Acupuncture. The Journal of Chinese Medicine, 19:2-11

Scott JP (1991) *Acupuncture in the Treatment of Children*, Eastland Press, Seatlle

Travell JG and Simons DG (1983) *Myofacial Pain and Dysfunction. The Trigger Point Manual*, Willians and Wilkins, Baltimore

Zhang Zhong-Jing (*c.* 210AD) Treatise on Febrile Diseases Caused By Cold with 500 Cases (Shang Han Lun). Translated by Luo Xi-Wen (1993) New World Press, Beijing, China

NOTES

NOTES

NOTES

NOTES